A Textbook of
DRUG DESIGN
and
DEVELOPMENT

A Textbook of DRUG DESIGN and DEVELOPMENT

SECOND EDITION

Edited by

Povl Krogsgaard-Larsen
Tommy Liljefors and Ulf Madsen
Royal Danish School of Pharmacy
Copenhagen Denmark

harwood academic publishers
Australia • Canada • China • France • Germany • India
Japan • Luxembourg • Malaysia • The Netherlands • Russia
Singapore • Switzerland • Thailand

Amsteldijk 166
1st Floor
1079 LH Amsterdam
The Netherlands

British Library Cataloguing in Publication Data

A textbook of drug design and development. – 2nd ed.
  1. Drugs – Design
  I. Krogsgaard-Larsen, Povl II. Liljefors, Tommy III. Madsen, Ulf
  615.1'9

ISBN 3-7186-5867-4

CONTENTS

CONTENTS

PREFACE

Studies of operational and regulatory cell mechanisms are in a state of rapid progress. The introduction of advanced biochemical, biophysical and physicochemical techniques in basic biological research has accelerated the disclosure of the complex mechanisms underlying cell function. Genetic technologies have revolutionized enzyme and receptor research and have made detailed mapping of receptor subtypes possible. Comparative studies of normal and diseased cells *in vivo* and *in vitro* have shed light on the nature of the biochemical and physiological malfunctions characterizing a number of diseases. These studies have disclosed potential targets for therapeutic attack in the relevant diseases.

Natural toxins and analogues of endogenous ligands have been used for the exploration of such sites and their susceptibility to pharmacological manipulation. Lack of specificity does, however, frequently limit the utility of such compounds. Using synthetic and enzymatic techniques it has been possible to convert non-specific toxins or ligands into compounds with highly specific actions on the cellular mechanisms under study. Such specific experimental tools represent the initial steps in the development of therapeutic agents.

Rational and systematic approaches along these lines have provided therapeutically useful drugs and are likely to lead to the development of novel classes of drugs against diseases, which, so far, have escaped effective treatment. In the present textbook all important aspects of modern drug design and development will be described and exemplified.

The first edition of this textbook, published in 1991, was co-edited by Professor Hans Bundgaard, who played an important role in the publication of the book and contributed a major chapter on design and application of prodrugs. From the early seventies and until his tragic and far too early death in 1992, Hans Bundgaard made an impressive series of original discoveries in this field of pharmaceutical sciences.

In light of the rapid, in some fields almost explosive, developments in industrial and academic drug research, we initiated the planning of the second edition of this textbook in 1994. The objective was to incorporate the major new developments in the field and to produce a new edition with even further emphasis on the educational level of the text. New topics in this second edition of the textbook include combinatorial approaches to lead discovery, computational pharmacophore mapping, recombinant receptors, design and development of peptidomimetics, ligands labelled with short-lived isotopes for imaging purposes, and examples of biostructure-based drug design.

Povl Krogsgaard-Larsen
Tommy Liljefors
Ulf Madsen

LIST OF CONTRIBUTORS

Chapter 1

Dr Michael Williams, Abbott Laboratories, 100 Abbott Park Road, Illinois 60064-3500, USA, Tel: +1 708 937 8186, Fax: +1 708 937 9195

Dr Eric M Gordon, Affymax Research Institute, 4001 Mirauda Avenue, Palo Alto, CA 94304-1218, USA

Chapter 2

Professor Uli Hacksell, Astra Draco AB, PO Box 34, S-221 00 Lund, Sweden, Tel: +46 46 33 6000, Fax: +46 46 33 6666

Chapter 3

Professor Tommy Liljefors, Royal Danish School of Pharmacy, Department of Medicinal Chemistry, 2 Universitetsparken, DK-2100 Copenhagen Ø, Denmark, Tel: +45 35 37 6777 ex. 505, Fax: +45 35 37 2209

Dr Ingrid Pettersson, Novo Nordisk A/S, Novo Nordisk Park, DK-2760 Måløv, Denmark, Tel: +45 44 43 4506, Fax: +45 44 43 4547

Chapter 4

Dr Thomas Högberg, Astra Draco AB, PO Box 34, S-221 00 Lund, Sweden, Tel: +46 46 33 6000, Fax: +46 46 33 6666

Dr Ulf Norinder, Astra Pain Control AB, S-15185 Södertälje, Sweden, Tel: +46 8 5532 5057, Fax: +46 8 5532 8877

Chapter 5

Dr Nanni Din, Department of Molecular Biology I, Bioscience, Novo Nordisk A/S, Novo Allé I (2C12), DK-2880 Bagsvaerd, Denmark, Tel: +45 44 42 6056, Fax: +45 44 98 0246

Dr Jens G L Petersen, Department of Protein Technology, Novo Nordisk A/S, Hagedornsvej 2, DK-2860 Gentofte, Denmark

Dr Henrik Dalbøge, Novo Nordisk A/S, Symbion, Fruebjergvej 3, DK-2100 København Ø, Denmark, Tel: +45 44 42 7815, Fax: +45 31 20 4213

Dr Søren Carlsen, Novo Nordisk A/S, Symbion, Fruebjergvej 3, DK-2100 København Ø, Denmark, Tel: +45 44 42 1220, Fax: +45 31 20 4213

Chapter 6

Professor Claus Braestrup, Pharmaceutical Division, Research Laboratories, Schering AG, Müllerstrasse 170-178, D-13342 Berlin, Germany, Tel: +49 30 468 1368, Fax: +49 30 4691 6740

Chapter 7

Dr Christer Halldin, Karolinska Institutet, Department of Clinical Neuroscience, Psychiatry Section, Karolinska Hospital, S-17176 Stockholm, Sweden, Tel: +46 87 29 2678, Fax: +46 8 34 6563

Dr Thomas Högberg, Astra Draco AB, PO Box 34, S-221 00 Lund, Sweden, Tel: +46 46 33 6000, Fax: +46 46 33 6666

LIST OF CONTRIBUTORS

Chapter 8
Professor David J Triggle, C 126 Cooke-Hochstetter Complex, School of Pharmacy, University at Buffalo, State University of New York, Box 601200, Buffalo, NY 14260-1200, USA, Tel: +1 716 645 2823, Fax: +1 716 645 3688

Chapter 9
Dr Ulf Madsen, Royal Danish School of Pharmacy, Department of Medicinal Chemistry, 2 Universitetsparken, DK-2100 Copenhagen Ø, Denmark, Tel: +45 35 37 6777 ex. 243, Fax: +45 35 37 2209

Chapter 10
Professor Povl Krogsgaard-Larsen, Royal Danish School of Pharmacy, Department of Medicinal Chemistry, 2 Universitetsparken, DK-2100 Copenhagen Ø, Denmark, Tel: +45 35 37 6777 ex. 247, Fax: +45 35 37 2209

Dr Bente Frølund, Royal Danish School of Pharmacy, Department of Medicinal Chemistry, 2 Universitetsparken, DK-2100 Copenhagen Ø, Denmark, Tel: +45 35 37 6777 ex. 495, Fax: +45 35 37 2209

Chapter 11
Dr Ian Ahnfelt-Rønne, Novo Nordisk A/S, Biopharmaceuticals Division – Research, Growth and Vascular Biology, Niels Steensens Vej 1, DK-2820 Gentofte, Denmark, Tel: +45 44 44 8888, Fax: +45 31 65 4574

Chapter 12
Dr Ole Jøns, Royal Danish School of Pharmacy, Department of Analytical and Pharmaceutical Chemistry, 2 Universitetsparken, DK-2100 Copenhagen Ø, Denmark, Tel: +45 35 37 6777 ex. 268, Fax: +45 35 37 5376

Dr Erik Sylvest Johansen, Royal Danish School of Pharmacy, Department of Analytical and Pharmaceutical Chemistry, 2 Universitetsparken, DK-2100 Copenhagen Ø, Denmark, Tel: +45 35 37 6777 ex. 267, Fax: +45 35 37 5376

Chapter 13
Dr Gitte Juel Friis, Royal Danish School of Pharmacy, Department of Analytical and Pharmaceutical Chemistry, 2 Universitetsparken, DK-2100 Copenhagen Ø, Denmark, Tel: +45 35 37 6777 ex. 466, Fax: +45 35 37 5376

Chapter 14
Professor Kristina Luthman, Department of Pharmacy, University of Tromsø, Forskningsparken, N-9037 Tromsø, Norway, Tel: +47 77 64 6605, Fax: +47 77 64 6151

Professor Uli Hacksell, Astra Draco AB, PO Box 34, S-221 00 Lund, Sweden, Tel: +46 46 33 6000, Fax: +46 46 33 6666

Chapter 15
Dr Fred Snyder, Oak Ridge Associated Universities, Medical Sciences Division, PO Box 117, Oak Ridge, TN 37831-0117, USA, Tel: +1 615 576 3110, Fax: +1 615 576 3194

Chapter 16
Dr P Herdewijn and Professor Erik De Clercq, Rega Institute, Katholieke Universiteit Leuven, Laboratory of Medicinal Chemistry, Minderbroedersstraat 10, B-3000 Leuven, Belgium, Tel: +32 16 33 7341, Fax: +32 16 33 7340

Chapter 17
Dr Ingrid Kjøller Larsen, Royal Danish School of Pharmacy, Department of Medicinal Chemistry, 2 Universitetsparken, DK-2100 Copenhagen Ø, Denmark, Tel: +45 35 37 6777 ex. 407, Fax: +45 35 37 2209

Chapter 18
Dr Joseph P Yevich, CNS Chemistry, Bristol-Myers Squibb, Pharmaceutical Research Institute, 5 Research Parkway, PO Box 5100, Wallingford, CT 06492-7660, USA, Tel: +1 203 284 6113, Fax: +1 203 284 7717

1. DRUG DISCOVERY: AN OVERVIEW

MICHAEL WILLIAMS and ERIC M. GORDON

CONTENTS

1.1 HISTORICAL PERSPECTIVE

1.1.1 Receptor concepts

A drug is generally envisaged as a chemical substance that can modify the response of a tissue to its environment. In a diseased or traumatized tissue where this response is modified in a manner detrimental to the long term survival of the organism, a drug is used to restore normal function. The conceptualization of a drug as a 'key' fitting into a 'lock' on the cell membrane arose from the seminal work of Langley and Ehrlich at the end of the 19th Century. Major advances in technology in both the chemical and biological arenas have yet to negate the 'lock and key' hypothesis, now a century old, as the seminal focus for compound design and drug targeting. For receptors, the recognition sites for hormones, neurotransmitters and neuromodulators, drugs may function as *agonists*, compounds that mimic the actions of the endogenous effector agent(s) or *antagonists*, compounds that block the actions of such agents.

Receptors exist as two main classes; G-protein coupled receptors (GPCRs) that are structurally represented by seven membrane spanning helices and are coupled to G-proteins, so described because of their functional dependence on the purine nucleotide, GTP, for activity; and ligand gated ion channels (LGICs) that are composed of several subunits, typically, but not always, a pentamer, that form an ion channel (see Chapter 6). α- and β-Adrenoceptors are classical GPCRs while $GABA_A$ and nicotinic receptors are LGICs. Two newer classes of receptor are represented by the thyroid hormone/steroid receptor superfamily, a group of drug recognition sites involved with the actions of certain steroids and retinoic acid on gene expression and the STATs (signal transducers and activators of transcription), drug recognition sites involved in transcriptional processes that include AP-1 and NFκB. In the case of enzymes, the catalytic units of cell activity, drugs may either function as inhibitors of the catalytic process, acting typically as false substrates, or as allosteric modulators which can modulate the catalytic process. Allosteric modulation of receptor function has also been demonstrated especially for LGICs (see Chapter 6).

Compounds that bind to the receptor (R) are known as ligands (L) and usually interact with the receptor according to the classical law of mass action in a reversible, competitive and saturable manner:

$$R + L \underset{k-1}{\overset{k+1}{\rightleftharpoons}} RL \overset{k+2}{\rightarrow} \text{Response} \tag{1.1}$$

The formation of the RL complex imparts on GPCRs the ability to alter cellular function via interaction with transmembrane signalling proteins that modulate the activity of a variety of systems within the cell that in turn alter the production of chemicals like cyclic AMP or phosphatidylinositol, or the intracellular levels of cations such as calcium. Such agents are known as second messengers. For LGICs, RL complex formation results in a change in ion flux. Receptor isolation and cloning studies have confirmed the long held hypothesis that the binding of a ligand to its receptor is an event distinct from that of coupling to the second messenger systems. RL complex formation thus results in either an alteration in the spatial relationship of the receptor to the transmembrane signaling proteins or, alternatively can cause a change in the steric conformation of the ligand thermodynamically favoring the transduction process.

For enzymes, the situation is somewhat similar to that for RL complex formation except that the enzyme – substrate – (ES) – complex results in the conversion of the substrate to a product:

$$E + S \underset{k-1}{\overset{k+1}{\rightleftharpoons}} ES \underset{k-2}{\overset{k+2}{\rightleftharpoons}} E + \text{Product} \tag{1.2}$$

Thus the substrate undergoes a catalytic conversion whereas with the RL interaction, the receptor and ligand remain unchanged at the end of the transduction process. For the ES complex, the reaction can also be driven backward in a feedback inhibitory mode in the presence of excess product. For an analogous situation with a receptor-mediated event, the extent of response can be diminished either by receptor downregulation, a decrease in receptor number, or uncoupling of the functional system.

For receptors, the ability of a compound to produce a functional response is a consequence of the intrinsic efficacy of the ligand. An agonist ligand that can elicit a full response in a defined biological system is defined as having an efficacy of 1.0 while an antagonist that is unable to produce any response but is able block the effects of agonist ligands is defined as having zero efficacy. In between full agonists and antagonists lie the partial agonists that are unable to produce a full response in a tissue system and have an efficacy ranging between zero and unity (Fig. 1.1). By definition such ligands are also partial antagonists. The factors that determine efficacy in a ligand remain unknown at this time.

1.1.2 Receptor technologies

The evaluation of new chemical entities (NCEs) for activity at either receptors or enzymes occurs at a number of hierarchical levels predicted on knowledge (and experience) in a given area of research. Until the 1970s, efforts were directed at largely empirical tissue or animal models that indirectly measured receptor function. Nonetheless, as evidenced by a continued stream of successful and often unexpected drug entities, this approach was a pragmatic one. Such compounds were often 'black box' in nature, producing effects that could result from a variety of receptor or enzyme related events. Major concerns existed in regard to delineating those factors responsible for the efficacy of a given compound from

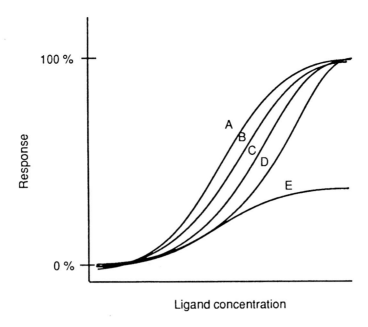

100 %

0 %

Response

Ligand concentration

Figure 1.1   Concentration response curves.

those eliciting unwanted side effects. The ratio between these two events, the therapeutic index, was consequently poorly understood and the search for active entities free from major side effects difficult to accomplish both conceptually and in practice. In the early 1970s, the technique of radioligand binding, developed as a research tool in the laboratories of Cuatrecasas and Roth at the NIH, Lefkowitz at Duke and Snyder at Johns Hopkins, provided a means to directly evaluate compounds for their ability to recognize a receptor or enzyme independent of efficacy. The principle of the radioligand binding assay is based on equation 1.1 where a selective radioactive ligand (L^*) is used to 'label' a given receptor or enzyme derived from mammalian tissues. In the absence of any other ligand, the RL^* complex will result in the binding of a given amount of radioactivity, tritium or iodine, that will by definition represent 100% of the 'recognition ability' of the receptor. In the presence of another ligand as shown in Figure 1.2, the total amount of radioactivity will be reduced on a proportional basis based on a competitive interaction where the receptor ligand complex can be represented as RL^*L. By convention, the activity of an unknown ligand is expressed in terms of its IC_{50} value, the ability to reduce specific binding of L^* by 50% expressed in molar units. The IC_{50} value can also be expressed as a K_i value using the Cheng-Prusoff equation where $K_i = IC_{50}/1 + c/Kd$; $c =$ the concentration of radioactive ligand and $Kd =$ the affinity constant of the ligand for the receptor. The K_i derivation thus has the advantage of correcting for variations in the concentration of radioligand used and the receptor affinity. As a result, the activity of a new compound across a series of binding assays can be appropriately compared.

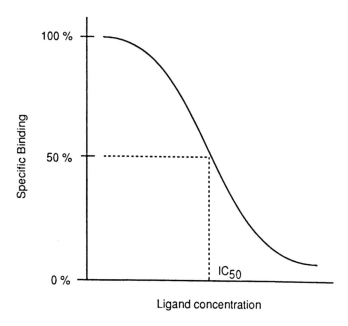

Figure 1.2 Schematic displacement curve.

For the medicinal chemist, the technique of radioligand binding and the many receptor reporter systems that it has given rise to have provided a rapid, cost effectively means to derive a structure-activity relationship (SAR) for a series of homologs at a given receptor or enzyme target thus providing a means to better design a compound to 'fit' the molecular site. The development of this screening technology and its adaptation to high throughput mode has contributed significantly to the development of the corresponding chemical technology, combinatorial chemistry (see Section 1.4.4).

Since only the recognition portion of the molecular target is under consideration, the intrinsic efficacy of the ligand is eliminated from the design equation resulting in an increased focus on the characteristics of a compound to recognize its molecular target. Binding assays are available for over 100 different classes of receptors and enzymes and have been used to identify new receptor classes and subtypes. It is thus possible to derive a binding profile for a given ligand that will measure its propensity to interact with a number of receptors or enzymes. If a given activity is thought to be responsible for a given side effect, the medicinal chemist is able to assess the disappearance of such activity through a concerted design effort while at the same time monitoring the activity thought to be important for therapeutic efficacy. Historically, and even in the era of receptor cloning and expression, the availability of selective antagonist ligands has been crucial to the delineation of receptor subtypes and their function in various tissue and animal models. Similarly, antagonist radioligands are more effective in labeling receptor populations *in vitro* due to their ability to recognize receptors in a variety of affinity states. While the efficacy of a compound can be determined in GPCR binding assays by assessing the effects of GTP on activity, agonists undergoing a decrease in affinity and antagonist binding remaining unchanged, this measure is not always reliable, true for every receptor or cost effective. A more reliable and informative measure is to use a classical functional assay to determine whether compounds are agonists or antagonists.

1.1.3 Functional assays

1.1.3.1 Classical approaches
The functional activity of a ligand can be determined by its ability to evoke a given response in a tissue preparation. A newly synthesized compound may thus be able to mimic the effects of a naturally occurring neurohumoral agent such as acetylcholine (ACh) or insulin by causing a muscle to contract or blood sugar to fall, respectively. In such instances, the degree to which the compound can elicit a response similar to that seen for the natural effector (Fig. 1.1) can determine whether it is a full or partial agonist. Conversely, a compound that blocks the actions of either ACh or insulin has antagonist activity. When using a tissue preparation to define such activity in a ligand, it is important to delineate between *pharmacological* and *functional* antagonism. Pharmacological antagonism describes the situation where a ligand can antagonize the effect of an agonist by blocking the actions of the latter directly at its molecular site of action. Such blockade may be competitive in nature with the antagonist interacting with the receptor in manner similar to that of the agonist. A non-competitive antagonist can influence the RL interaction process by binding to a site distinct from that of the natural ligand. Interaction with this site can either block access of the agonist to the receptor or allosterically alter the receptor or its interaction with transductional elements so that the ligand either cannot bind or is unable to elicit a functional response. Functional antagonism can manifest itself in a similar manner except that the antagonist ligand does not affect RL complex formation at the receptor with which the agonist interacts but acts at a distinct site one or several steps upstream. One example is a hypothetical system involving a $GABA_A$ receptor innervated by a dopaminergic pathway that itself is under the control of cholecystokinin (CCK) neurons. Pharmacologically, any response ascribed to $GABA_A$ receptor activation that is blocked by a compound could conceptually involve a $GABA_A$ antagonist. However, a dopamine receptor antagonist or a CCK-B (brain) receptor antagonist would produce a similar effect through an indirect route and thus represent a functional antagonist. A lack of appreciation of this concept may lead to a CCK-B antagonist being mistakenly characterized as a $GABA_A$ receptor antagonist representing a major drawback of *in vivo* compound evaluation in the absence of *in vitro* data. Accordingly, modern day drug discovery is generally hierarchical in nature, deriving the selectivity profile of a compound *in vitro* and subsequently using this information as the basis for the interpretation of tissue and *in vivo* studies.

1.1.3.2 Biochemical approaches
Functional activity may also be measured biochemically by assessing ligand-induced changes in receptor-linked second messenger systems or a gene reporter constructs. Using radiometric, radioimmunoassay or fluorescent dye readouts, receptor-mediated alterations in cyclic AMP formation, the arachidonic acid cascade, or calcium rise can easily be measured by a scintillation counter or microtiter plate reader. Reporter gene constructs using LGICs coupled to jellyfish green fluorescent protein (GFP) or GPCRs coupled to

melanophores or luciferase-dependent light formation provide similar readouts to rapidly assess the functional activity of a new ligand. There are however caveats to the reporter gene technology inasmuch as the transduction systems in expressed cell lines may not be representative of the situation where the receptor occurs naturally. Also, variations in the amount of receptor expressed can alter the readout giving false estimates of efficacy. Using such techniques, compounds can be evaluated for their ability to either mimic or block the actions of a reference agonist in a concentration-dependent manner. For enzymes, similar radiometric and spectrophotometric methods can be used to assess either the catalytic disappearance of substrate or appearance of product.

Once an NCE has been found to have functional activity, it is important that the *in vitro* selectivity be reassessed in appropriate systems. For instance, many different types of receptor mechanisms are known to alter cyclic AMP formation as can compounds that inhibit phosphodiesterase activity. Thus while a compound may be identified as selectively active at one receptor from its binding profile, there is always the possibility that it may alter second messenger production by more than one receptor-mediated mechanism in a functional system. The use of appropriate antagonists (or agonists in the case of an antagonist NCE) can help to clarify this situation.

1.1.4 Animal models

Functional activity in a given biochemical or tissue system for an NCE in terms of therapeutic potential is dependent on an assumption that the given mechanistic response under study has some role in the pathophysiology of the disease state being targeted. For instance while increased phosphatidyl-inositol (Pl) turnover is a measure of muscarinic cholinergic M_1 receptor activation, the hypothesis that M_1 receptor agonists can enhance cognitive function must be tested in appropriate animal models rather than assuming that the biochemical measure can be used *per se* to predict behavioral activity. Similarly while phosphodiesterase inhibitors can alter cardiac cyclic nucleotide metabolism, increasing contractile force, their ability to function as positive inotropic agents for the treatment of congestive heart failure must be assessed in an intact animal model. In addition to hypothesis validation, evaluation of compounds in animal models provides a measure of their bioavailability. An initial assumption that lack of activity *in vivo* is the result of the mechanism being uninvolved in the disease process targeted could be ascribed to the compound having insufficient bioavailabilty due to poor absorption, first pass metabolism or lack of access to the target.

1.2 MECHANISM-BASED DRUG DISCOVERY

Until the 1960s, many of the techniques used to discover new therapeutic entities were highly empirical. Anti-inflammatory agents were almost exclusively assessed for their ability to reduce the pain response associated with an injection of carageenin into the forepaw, antihypertensives by their ability to lower blood pressure in animal models and anticholinergics by their ability to increase pupil diameter. While such approaches had as an underlying theme, a receptor interaction, the localization and nature of the receptor were frequently unknown. Thus an effect elicited by serotonin could be measured at the tissue or whole animal level without reference to the type of receptor involved. Accordingly, side effects attributable to compound interactions with subtype b of receptor X, subtype a of which is responsible for its therapeutic action would be masked by a compound series that was equiactive at both a and b receptor subtypes. However, once a compound had been identified as having a relatively good therapeutic index, follow up studies can then be used to establish, in an iterative manner, the existence of receptor subtypes that in turn can be used to design second generation ligands that are typically more selective.

In general much, if not all, of modern drug discovery is based on the concept that receptor and enzyme subtypes exist and that these can be dissected using novel ligands to delineate between those whose modulation can produce a beneficial (e.g. therapeutic) effect and those responsible for the side effects.

The process of receptor (and enzyme) classification has historically been dependent on the discovery of novel ligands. For instance, the novel anti-anxiety agent, buspirone, was initially thought to produce its effects via a type of dopamine receptor. However, the discovery of the serotoninergic ligand, 8-OH-DPAT (8-hydroxy-2-(di-n-propylamino)tetralin) led to the identification of the $5HT_{1A}$ receptor subclass, and buspirone was found to be a partial agonist at this receptor. With the advent of recombinant DNA technologies, receptor identification and classification has become increasingly driven by cloning techniques such that receptor homologs are frequently identified before selective ligands are known. This has given rise to so-called 'orphan' receptors, typically members of the GPCR or thyroid hormone/retinoic acid superfamilies which show protein sequence homology to one or another of these receptor classes but which are different from identified receptors and for which the endogenous ligand is often unknown.

Based on the successful development by Black and co-workers of the syntopic antagonists, propranolol and cimetidine, for β-adrenergic and histamine H_2 receptors, respectively, and the angiotensin-converting enzyme (ACE) inhibitor, captopril by Cushman and Ondetti (see Chapter 11), drug development has become increasingly more mechanistic in focus. Following the identification of a molecular target, receptor or enzyme, the SARs of ligands or substrates, respectively, for these targets is examined in a highly interactive manner with close cooperation between medicinal chemist and biochemist. Black's studies on the H_2 receptor were based on using the neurotransmitter itself as a template for chemical synthetic effort, altering the molecule to an antagonist and concurrently providing definitive evidence for the existence of the gastric H_2 receptor (see Chapter 10).

1.3 TECHNOLOGICAL CHALLENGES

In identifying potential new drug targets and designing NCEs that interact with them, whether using the classical empirical approach or a mechanism-based one, the drug hunter is faced with a number of challenging problems. The iteration of the synthetic effort through *in vitro* and *in vivo* testing has no single, well defined path. As already indicated, affinity for a receptor, like the Km for an enzyme, is distinct from respectively, the intrinsic efficacy and catalytic Vmax for each type of molecular target. A compound with excellent *in vitro* activity and selectivity may be found *in vivo* to exhibit a totally unexpected side effect profile or, alternatively, no activity at all. The scientist has then to go back and either modify the hypothesis or the NCE. Many factors come into play at this point — the availability of a series of lead pharmacophores with differing properties and degrees of lipophilicity, the ability to examine lead structures in different functional models and awareness of potential species and tissue selective functional responses. Various permutations of these factors contribute to a lack of predictability in the discovery of NCEs. One means to circumvent such problems is to generate a profile for a compound in several systems and disease models and integrate the information obtained to make an educated judgment as to where to focus efforts. The ability to surmount problems in an objective manner is frequently as important as the discovery of the NCE. Interestingly, the most potent or most selective compound in a chemical series does not always make the optimal drug.

The use of human tissues (blood or samples from surgical procedures or cadavers) or cloned and expressed human receptors or enzymes to assess NCE activity represents an important facet of the compound evaluation process. In the area of inflammation, human blood cells are used to study complement, cytokine, leukotriene and prostacyclin receptor function. While intellectually rigorous, NCEs discovered in this manner have to eventually undergo evaluation in animal models relevant to the targeted disease state not only to validate the mechanistic hypothesis but also to provide information relevant to biological activity and bioavailability in the species used for toxicology. This situation is paradoxical in that an NCE designed to have activity and selectivity at the human target may behave very differently in lower species adding an additional layer of complexity to the characterization of a compound of interest.

1.4 TARGET SELECTION AND LEAD IDENTIFICATION

The process of drug discovery hinges on the ability to identify patentable NCEs that have the potential to treat a given disease state, the etiology of which may involve several discrete events (see Chapter 18). The choice of the target for a given disease approach may be based on: a therapeutic franchise for a given company; new scientific knowledge; unmet medical need; or a lead from high throughput screening. The availability of the necessary scientific and administrative skill bases in sufficient quantity to achieve a critical mass and management commitment are equally important and have been addressed by Weisbach and Moos. Management commitment and vision is of even greater importance when a company embarks on a strategic initiative to enter a new marketplace. Given that the greatest commercial successes are likely to occur in therapeutic areas where unmet medical need and risk are both high, the identification of new marketplaces using innovative approaches will be a major factor in ensuring success for the future.

1.4.1 Target selection

In therapeutic areas like hypertension, the science and the marketplace are of sufficient maturity to make drug discovery a highly predictable process. A compound that reduces blood pressure in the spontaneously hypertensive rat (SHR), unless it desensitizes the molecular target upon chronic administration or has a poor pharmacokinetic profile, will be active in humans. In other areas like Alzheimer's Disease (AD), rheumatoid arthritis (RA) and cancer, understanding of the disease process and consequently the mechanism of action of active drugs remains limited, making drug discovery and development both complex and unpredictable. In RA, many factors are thought to impact the chondyrocyte deterioration that represents one of the initial stages of the disease. Non-steroidal anti-inflammatory agents (NSAIDs) like aspirin, ibuprofen and diclofenac can treat the inflammation and pain associated with joint swelling but do not alter the disease process. Disease modifying antirheumatic drugs (DMARDs) like methotrexate and the steroids have a variable effect on disease attenuation with no single mode of action that represents a novel target with acceptable side effect liability. There is thus a growing need, concomitant with the growth in the aged population, for drugs that will effectively attenuate, reverse, or even prevent disease conditions such as RA.

In the past decade, many new blood derived inflammatory mediators have been identified including the cytokines. The possibility that these may be contributory factors in RA and related disease states is supported by their elevated levels in plasma samples from humans with RA. However, selection of one of these putative mediators as a drug target requires evaluation not only of NCEs, but also of the hypothesis that such factors are contributory to the disease etiology. Proteases e.g. stromolysin and mimics of endogenous protease inhibitors such as TIMP (tissue inhibitor of metalloproteinase) or STATs may also represent novel drug targets. In the context of new molecular targets, the drug discovery process depends on the identification of with selectivity and efficacy at the molecular level and their subsequent testing for proof of principle in the clinic. This process is expensive, iterative and unpredictable and thus represents a major component of the research and development (R & D) costs for a new drug especially when the hypothesis, only testable when the NCE is available, proves to be incorrect. Many such high risk research projects, because of the uncertainty component, are frequently terminated before the hypothesis is adequately tested making the whole endeavor the antithesis of a research based effort. Hypothesis testing, by definition, requires confirmatory or negatory data and when a decision is made to terminate a drug discovery project before such information is available, it is inevitable that the hypothesis, still unproven, will be revisited by others who will start the process again from scratch. Another example is that of AD where knowledge related to disease etiology is also at a very early stage making NCE evaluation, especially at the behavioral level in animals, exceedingly complex. As many as 80% of discovery projects, however well conceived, well planned and well funded fail to reach any level of commercial interest because of the nature of the 'cutting edge' research that the industry routinely conducts. As Maxwell has noted, some of the major by-products of industrial biomedical research are the NCEs that become research tools to elucidate biological mechanisms and disease etiology. Industry is thus part of an iterative cycle together with academia and government to define disease mechanisms and their potential treatment.

1.4.2 The flow chart

The flow chart (Fig. 1.3) is a vehicle frequently used to coordinate and prioritize the diverse scientific disciplines and resources present in a drug discovery project team. It provides the criteria for compound selection and characterization permitting sequential goal setting to achieve optimal synergies. The effectiveness of the project team is highly dependent on the quality of leadership and the individual membership. Williams and Stork have noted that 'good science' is but one part of the drug discovery equation, and there is a need to overcome constraints related to the different cultures of the various scientific

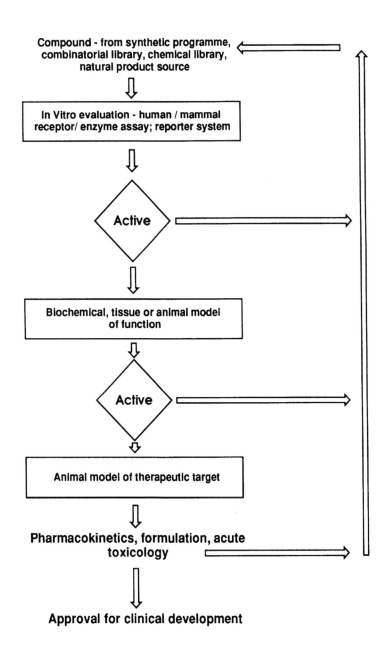

Figure 1.3 Generic Compound Flowchart.

disciplines to advance an NCE to the clinical testing stage. Ideally, a project is focused on the hierarchical evaluation of a compound moving from *in vitro* selectivity and target activity, to functional efficacy and selectivity, to activity in disease-predictive models. As the compound ascends through this process the criteria for its acceptance become increasingly stringent and there is often an iteration where an NCE is modified to improve bioavailability with a consequent change in efficacy. Balance is then achieved by treating the flow chart as a flexible mechanism to move from concept to execution rather than a "road map" set in concrete. Flow chart development, in terms of experimental procedures, criteria for activity, validation of reference compounds (if such entities exist), evaluation of measures of efficacy and selectivity can add considerably to the cost and time in initiating a project. This effort is again compounded by the absence of relevant animal models.

1.4.3 Compound sources

1.4.3.1 Synthetic effort
Chemical modification of a pharmacophore series to derive a structure activity relationship represents the major means to date by which NCEs are developed. The starting point for such an effort can be: the endogenous hormone or transmitter for the target enzyme or receptor; a 'lead' reported in the patent literature as possessing an interesting or unusual pharmacological profile; or a novel pharmacophore discovered by the targeted screening of a compound library or natural product sources. Many pharmaceutical companies have proprietary heterocycles that are a 'signature' of the company — for instance cyproheptadine at Merck and the benzodiazepines (BZs) at Roche. For many such structures, side-chain substitutions can confer many different pharmacological properties to a given heterocycle. This concept has been developed by Evans and colleagues at Merck to define the 1,4-BZ nucleus as a "privileged structure" that can recognize a large number of diverse peptide receptors.

In addition to the actual process of synthesizing targeted pharmacophores, modern synthetic approaches are highly dependent on the many skill bases in the area of structural biology to aid in understanding the necessary features in a molecule to both recognize the molecular target and initiate (or block) the transduction event. These technologies include computer-assisted molecular design (CAMD) based on space filling models of active compounds, isolation and point mutation of protein targets, X-ray crystallography and various means e.g. NMR, to model the ligand receptor interaction.

The traditional synthetic approach benefits from a highly focused effort that is iterative in real time. Newly synthesized compounds are thus immediately evaluated for activity and selectivity so that the information can be fed back into the synthetic planning process to aid in the design of subsequent compounds. The average cost of creating an NCE in a major pharmaceutical company in this manner is around $7500 per compound due to the "hand-crafted" nature of serial synthesis and testing of individual compounds. The development and utilization of high throughput, automated techniques has made possible the screening of hundreds of thousands of individual compounds each year at a selected drug target. This capability, combined with a global shift to reduce R & D costs by the pharmaceutical industry, the latter driven by health cost containment pressures, has expanded the need for continuous supplies of huge numbers of novel molecules. These may

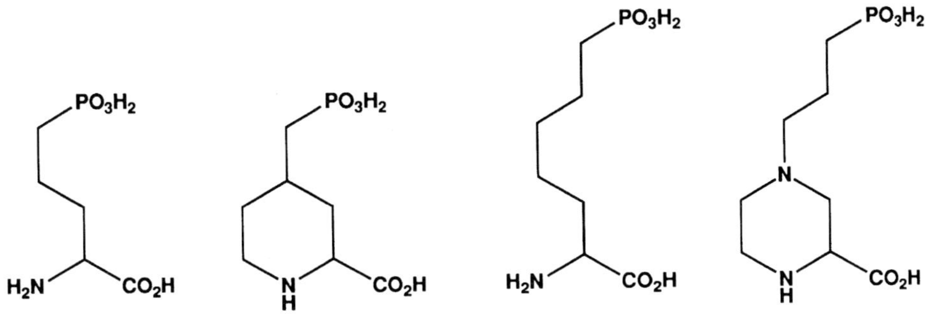

Figure 1.4 Structure of NMDA receptor antagonists.

be found in chemical libraries and natural product sources, or produced via combinatorial chemistry techniques.

1.4.3.2 High throughput screening

A novel lead pharmacophore is the single element that is crucial for the initiation and ultimate success of a drug discovery project. While it is still feasible to develop a compound from a competitor's structure based on information made available in human trials, the days in which fourth and fifth generation 'me-too' compounds can achieve commercial are a thing of the past. However, in taking a known compound as the starting point for a synthetic effort, several companies, unknown to one another can often arrive at the same proprietary structures within weeks or months. In the area of N-methyl-D aspartate (NMDA) receptor antagonists that have potential use in stroke, CGS 19755 (cis-4-phosphonomethyl-2-piperidinecarboxylic acid **1.2**; Fig. 1.4) was patented by Ciba-Geigy only weeks ahead of the Lilly group emphasizing the need for the timely and effective filing of patents. It also underlines the importance of identifying totally novel pharmacophores by serendipitously evaluating (or screening) other potential compound sources and sample collections.

By definition, screening is a random process even though the focus is on a defined molecular target, e.g. targeted screening. The a priori selection of compounds to be screened, as is frequently done in sifting through a compound library, can limit the usefulness of this highly serendipitous approach by limiting evaluation to those structures deemed to be of interest based on existing knowledge of the SAR of the receptor or enzyme. Ideally, screening should occur by total chance or by the use of chemically diverse structural libraries assembled from commercial sources.

Screening is less precise than the synthetic approach in that many thousands of compounds are evaluated at fixed concentrations to derive yes or no answers in terms of activity at a given target. The medicinal chemist is usually only involved peripherally in this effort until interesting leads are identified that require optimization.

1.4.3.3 Compound libraries

Pharmaceutical companies can complement their ongoing dedicated synthetic efforts by screening their compound libraries for activity using radioligand or target reporter screens for receptor and enzyme targets to identify novel pharmacophores to be used as templates for synthetic optimization. Chemical companies like Eastman Kodak have attempted to use this approach as a means to enter the pharmaceutical industry, in this particular instance in a very ineffectual manner as the recent sale of their Sterling-Winthrop subsidiary to Sanofi indicates. However, based on the legendary success of cimetidine (**1.10**) at Smith, Kline and French and ranitidine (**1.11**) at Glaxo, it only requires one major product to launch a company from the 'minor leagues' to a dominant position in the industry. Compound libraries in combination with novel screens represent a major source of potential new drugs.

The actual number of available compounds in a library is often overestimated because of decomposition and exhaustion of supplies. Compound supplies are limited to 100 mg or less (especially with reaction intermediates) and it is highly desirable that the maximum data be derived with the minimal amount of compound. As the tools of molecular biology are used to discover new molecular targets it can be anticipated that a new spectrum of potential drug targets will appear every 2–3 years or even more frequently such that sufficient compound will be needed to retest for activity as new assays are developed. Given that the majority of these entities (e.g. cytokines, trophic factors etc.) lack ligands other than those structurally modified from the natural ligand, these represent ideal targets for the ongoing retesting of compound libraries and natural product sources. Since many libraries reflect a large number of compounds with a limited number of dissimilar pharmacophores, diversity may often be absent.

Compound library resources can be maximized by weighing and solubilizing in 96-well microtiter plates. Portions of these can then be aliquoted using dilution stations to make 3–4 'copies' of the initial 'mother' plate. The copies can then be stored or distributed for testing throughout a research organization or to outside collaborators leaving the original plate as a resource for the retesting of compounds and reconfirmation of activity. In this manner, 3–4 mg of a compound can be used to assess activity in 20 or more assays. Such frugality assumes an even more important role when the current trend for synthesizing minimal amounts of an NCE is taken into account. Because radioligand binding assays are so efficient in providing data, many chemists are now making 10–20 mg samples of an NCE when 5 years ago the norm was 100–200 mg. Thus while older compound stores are being depleted, they are not being replaced by adequate supplies of newer compounds. One solution to this problem, resulting from changes in global geopolitics is the availability of chemical compound libraries from countries formerly part of the Soviet bloc. Another solution is that of combinatorial chemistry discussed below.

1.4.3.4 Natural product sources

While it has been estimated that as many as 60% of currently used medications owe their origins to microbial or plant sources, this well proven approach had for a period of time fallen into disfavor as a means to find new therapeutics. With the advent of radioligand binding and related *in vitro* assays, evaluation of samples from natural sources has become more resource efficient. In the late 1970s Hoffmann — La Roche's Institute for Marine Biology in Australia sought to exploit marine sources for new therapeutics. Among the compounds discovered were 1-methylisoguanosine (doridosine), an antihypertensive agent and a series of adenosine kinase (AK) and adenosine deaminase inhibitors. The strategic approach behind the Institute was however to take a marine organism and extract novel chemical structures and then test these for biological activity. This resulted in a very costly process, more so when the isolated material was found to be devoid of activity. The perceived poor return on investment from the Roche Institute resulted in a overly negative attitude to natural product screening due to the unfortunate focus on chemical structures to the exclusion of biological activity. Interestingly, one of the AK leads discovered, 5′-iodotubercidin, was used as the lead pharmacophore for Gensia's GP-1-515, an AK inhibitor entering clinical trials in 1995 for the potential treatment of septic shock.

Evaluation of natural product sources for interesting biological activity *before* attempts to isolate the active ingredient(s), while fraught with the possibility of losing active entities during the isolation process, is accepted as a far more sensible approach to natural product screening and one in keeping with the esthetics of pharmacognosy. The discovery of compounds such as the CCK-A receptor antagonist, asperlicin (**1.20**) and its derivative MK 329 (**1.21**) (see Fig. 1.13), the immunosupressants, cyclosporine and FK 506, the cholinesterase inhibitor, huperazine A and the cholesterol lowering acids have moved natural product evaluation from the realm of microbiology, antiinfectives and anticancer agents to a more general role in all therapeutic areas. This renewed interest has been further reinforced by the increased influence of Sino-Japanese holistic medicine as Mainland China has become more globally integrated. Since many "Kampoh"-type medicines have had a considerable human usage in defined disease states, these lend themselves to more focused approaches with defined therapeutic indications for their evaluation. Natural product sources include plants, microbial sources and marine flora and fauna. The National Cooperative Natural Products Discovery and Development Program has been established to provide an umbrella for industry-academia collaborations in the search for drugs from natural product sources.

1.4.3.5 Fermentation/microbial sources

The use of soil samples, fungi, symbiotic organisms and other microbial sources from around the world has a long and distinguished history in the anti-infective area. Commercial enterprises like Xenova and Mycosearch have their own proprietary collections of fungi while the Department of Energy's Savannah River Project has bacterial sources derived from the culturing of 'plugs' from subsurface drilling operations related to studies on the ecological consequences of nuclear waste storage. Similarly, many oil companies have plugs from deep sea drilling operations which have yet to be evaluated. Most major pharmaceutical companies have ongoing collection programs with their employees collecting soil and garbage samples during their travels.

1.4.3.6 Plant/herbal sources

The folklore of several continents has contributed significantly to medications currently in use. The poppy, belladonna, coffee, ginseng and Chinese cucumber plants are all rich and varied sources of substances active in man. Many other plants with a less well defined lineage have been documented for their therapeutic potential while others have yet to be adequately characterized. Evaluation of plant extracts in a comprehensive screen may yield many novel pharmacophores with drug potential like the recently discovered anticancer agent, taxol (see Chapter 18). Like the compound libraries however, the availability of natural product sources is finite since many are not being replenished. Of especial concern is the ongoing loss of ecological biodiversity as rain forests such as those in the Amazon are cleared. Merck has an ongoing arrangement with the government of Costa Rica to explore the rain forests of that country for novel pharmacophores while replenishing the natural resources.

1.4.3.7 Arachnid and amphibian sources

Secretions from spiders and frogs have provided some interesting new pharmacophores. The amine spider toxins, the agatoxins and conotoxins can affect glutamatergic neurotransmission and calcium channel function. A number of frogs secrete toxic substances through their skins presumably to deter predators. Epibatidine (**1.16**) (Fig. 1.12), discovered by Daly at the NIH is a novel and potent, yet unfortunately toxic, analgesic agent that produces its effects *via* neuronal nicotinic receptor activation. Interestingly, this compound is not found in frogs raised in captivity suggesting that the frog sequesters or produces epibatidine from some source in its natural habitat.

1.4.3.8 Marine sources

The oceans of the world represent another source of novel compounds. This was largely ignored before 1950 except in the case of therapeutics derived from seaweed in the Pacific Rim. The discovery of spongothymidine and the development of the antineoplastic agents, Ara-C and Ara-A, represented milestones in the development of marine sources as pharmaceuticals. Other anti-cancer agents discovered from marine sources include didemnin, bryostatin, dolasstatin and halichondrin B (see Chapter 17). Unlike surface derived natural product sources, the seabed is an inhospitable environment requiring the use of highly specialized equipment and personnel with attendant expense. Ocean Genetics, the Roche Institute (now owned by Suntory), the Australian Institute of Marine Science, Oceanix Biosciences/University of Maryland, Universities in Hawaii, Israel, New Zealand and California, and the Harbor Branch Oceanographic Institution represent major efforts in the collection of organisms from the world's oceans. The Japanese government has also initiated a consortium to finance purpose built ocean-going research laboratories and remotely operated seabed vehicles to enhance the collection of samples from marine sources.

1.4.3.9 Natural product isolation

As discussed the Roche example above, the approach to compound isolation is crucial in identification of the active principal. Fractionation of active extracts may lead to loss of the active principal. This may be caused by the latter entity only being present in small amounts, by the activity being due to a combination of discrete compounds or by the principal being unstable when isolated. This latter caveat can be addressed by ensuring that the biological testing is done proximal to the isolation chemistry laboratory as the fractions are prepared with an effective deconvolution strategy. Where the compound source is a fermentation extract, the organism may have undergone a change in metabolism during storage and is no longer able to produce the active principle(s). With plants and marine organisms, if the taxonomy of the initial sample and its location are not properly documented, it may be impossible to re-check activity on fresh samples.

	Number of Units	Number of Library Entities
Basis Set of 20 (e.g. Natural Amino Acids)	20^3 20^4 20^5	8, 000 160, 000 3.2 million
Basis Set of 100	100^3 100^4 100^5	1 Million 100 Million 10 Billion
Basis Set of 1000	1000^3 1000^4 1000^5	1 Billion 1 Trillion 1 Quadrillion

Figure 1.5   Basic building blocks.

1.4.4 Combinatorial approaches to chemical diversity

Combinatorial chemistry technologies allow the creation of "chemical libraries" as vast populations of molecules using a building block collection with the systematic assembly of these blocks in many combinations using chemical, biological, or biosynthetic procedures. The building block approach is used naturally for the creation of oligonucleotides, carbohydrates and peptides/proteins, through the combination of nucleosides, sugars and amino acids respectively. The universe of structural diversity accessible through assembly of even a small set of building block elements is potentially large, and the power inherent in the building block approach is crucial to the success of the combinatorial method in drug discovery. For example, exploitation of a basis set of 100 interchangeable building blocks with a molecular weight of approximately 150 each permits the theoretical synthesis of 100 million tetrameric or 10 billion pentameric low molecular weight chemical entities (Fig. 1.5).

1.4.4.1 Combinatorial approaches to peptide libraries

Synthetic combinatorial methods were first used to develop peptide libraries. The process was driven by the ready availability of a large and structurally diverse range of amino acid building blocks, a highly refined, generic coupling chemistry, and the fact that small peptides are of biological and pharmaceutical interest. The various technologies that have emerged for generating and screening peptide libraries may be fundamentally distinguished by the format in which the diversity is presented (tethered vs. soluble libraries;

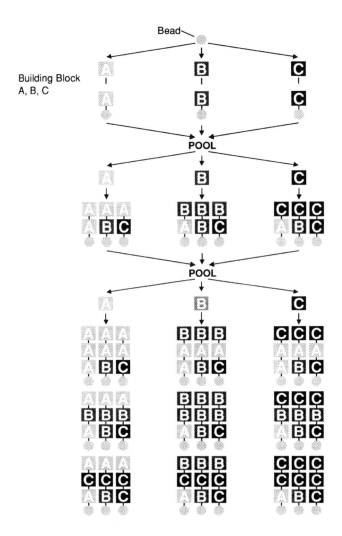

Figure 1.6   Preparation of a Combinatorial Library by the Split Bead Method.

physically segregated ligands vs. mixed pools). This in turn dictates the type of biological assay methods that may be utilized, influences the strategy followed in ligand structure elucidation and ultimately determines the size of libraries that can be practically screened. The common hallmark of these combinatorial techniques is that within each chemical coupling step, multiple compounds are generated simultaneously such that each synthesis cycle results in an exponential increase in library size.

An important yet simple mechanism for elaborating molecular diversity first reported by Furka and co-workers is known as *split-pool synthesis*. This procedure involves dividing the resin support (e.g beads) into n equal fractions, coupling a single monomer to each aliquot in a separate reaction and then thoroughly mixing all the resin particles together. Repeating this protocol for a total of x cycles can produce a stochastic collection of up to

n^x different peptides, as governed by the Poisson distribution. A schematic illustration of a split synthesis using three building blocks A, B and C to generate all 27 possible trimer combinations is shown in Figure 1.6. The "split synthesis" algorithm is readily adapted to generating equimolar mixtures of soluble peptides that may be screened in a variety of competition binding or functional bioassays.

In contrast, a different method of combinatorial synthesis in which the identity of a compound is given by its *location* on a synthesis substrate is termed a *spatially addressable synthesis*. Here, the combinatorial process is carried out by controlling the addition of a chemical reagent/building block to specific locations on a solid support. This technique as used at Affymax combines two well developed technologies: solid phase peptide synthesis chemistry and photolithography. The high coupling yields of Merrifield chemistry allow efficient peptide synthesis, and the spatial resolution of photolithography affords miniaturization. The merging of these two technologies is done through the use of photolabile amino protecting groups in the Merrifield synthetic procedure. Affymax researchers have developed this technology to perform library construction and analysis on "chips" containing thousands of compounds per chip.

1.4.4.2 Encoded combinatorial libraries

The generation and screening of very large combinatorial libraries assembled from an expanded set of molecular building blocks provide substantial challenges to current diversity technologies. For example, to screen an immobilized synthetic peptide library containing, for instance, 10^9 members constructed from a bead support as described above would require treating kilograms of resin with liters of soluble receptor, clearly an impractical undertaking. A decrease in the bead diameter might permit a library of this diversity to occupy a manageable volume, but the quantity of peptide associated with any selected particle would quickly fall below the threshold required for standard analysis.

In attempting to address some of these limitations, it was recognized that the products of a combinatorial synthesis on resin beads could be explicitly specified if it were possible to attach an identifier tag to the beads coincident with each monomer coupling step in the synthesis. Each tag would then convey which monomer was coupled in a particular step of the synthesis, and the overall structure of a ligand on any bead could be deduced by reading the set of tags on that bead (a type of molecular bar code). An encoded version of the combinatorial synthesis previously outlined in Figure1.6 is shown schematically in Figure 1.7.

Ideally, such tags should have a high information content, be amenable to very high sensitivity detection and decoding, and must be stable to reagents used in the ligand synthesis. A method using single stranded oligonucleotides to encode combinatorial peptide syntheses on 10 mm diameter polystyrene beads has recently been developed by Gallop and co-workers. Peptides and nucleotides are assembled in parallel, alternating syntheses so that each bead bears many copies of both a single peptide sequence and a unique oligonucleotide identifier tag. Each amino acid monomer used in the synthesis is assigned a distinct contiguous nucleotide sequence or "codon" and hence the structure of the peptide assembled on any bead is reflected in the oligonucleotide sequence of the corresponding tag. The oligonucleotides share common $5'$- and $3'$-PCR priming sites and thus the beads can serve as templates for the polymerase chain reaction (PCR), which is used to amplify the tag for sequencing/decoding.

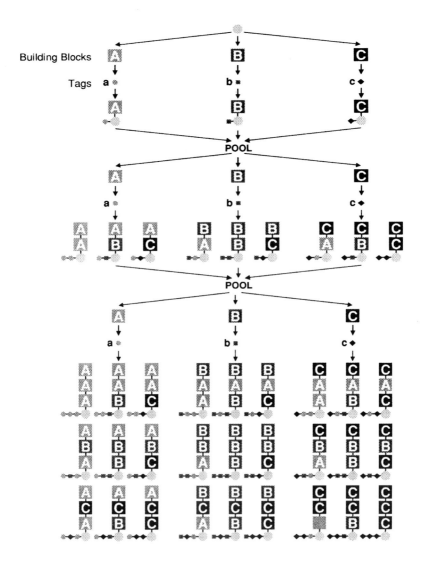

Figure 1.7   Schematic Assembly of an Encoded Synthetic Library.

Still and co-workers at Columbia University have reported an alternate approach to encoding combinatorial syntheses on resin beads wherein electron capture capillary gas chromatography (ECGC) is used in the analysis of the coding moieties. This scheme employs a series of chromatographically resolvable halocarbon derivatives as molecular tags which, when attached to reactive groups on the bead surface, can constitute a binary code that reflects the chemical history of any member of a library. In contrast to the oligonucleotide coding approach where the order of assembly of the chemical building blocks for any library member is preserved in the sequence of a single cognate tagging molecule, the binary strategy uses a uniquely defined mixture of tags to represent each building block at each particular step of the synthesis. Thus a set of N distinguishable tags can be used to encode the combinatorial synthesis of a library containing as many as 2^N different members. The chemically inert nature of the halocarbon tags is a particularly attractive feature of this coding approach, and facilitates the screening of non-sequenceable organic molecules prepared by multistep combinatorial synthesis.

1.4.4.3 Combinatorial organic synthesis (COS)

Generalization of peptide based combinatorial strategies has led to construction of collections of other natural polymers (e.g. oligonucleotides), and unnatural (synthetic) polymeric libraries. Medicinal chemistry is thus entering a new era in which vast numbers of small, non-polymeric molecules, of the types usually employed to make drugs, may be readily accessible by combinatorial approaches. Hence, the conventional paradigm of small molecule lead development, in which a compound undergoes many rounds of individualized, hand-crafted modification and biological testing en route to drug candidacy, will likely be dramatically accelerated by the application of combinatorial chemistry technologies to mass-produce and evaluate lead analogs.

A common feature of both peptide and COS paradigms is a reliance on solid phase synthesis methods to facilitate the assembly of combinatorial libraries. The work of Ellman at Berkeley on the solid phase synthesis of 1,4-BZs by inter-connection of three building blocks, each of different chemical families, to create a library of one of medicinal chemistry's most notable pharmacophores, represents one of the first examples of the application COS to non-polymeric organic compounds (Fig. 1.8). Many other examples of this style of synthesis have recently appeared in the literature and the refinement of solid phase COS will be an important research activity for the foreseeable future.

1.4.4.4 Assay and screening of combinatorial libraries

An essential element of the combinatorial discovery process is that *one must be able to extract the information made available by library screening*. Hence, the generation and screening of such immense numbers of compounds have demanded innovative tools for data handling and analysis. In broad terms, assay procedures can be grouped into three categories:

 (i) those that rely on affinity purification with an immobilized target receptor;
 (ii) those in which a soluble receptor binds to tethered ligands; and
(iii) those in which soluble compounds are tested for activity, either directly or in competition assays.

Each format presents different challenges with regard to the minimum affinity requirements for ligand detection, the demonstration of binding specificity, and the ability to discriminate among compounds in the library on the basis of their affinities for the target.

The different assay techniques are format specific and must clearly discriminate specific from non-specific binding. Since in a broad screening mode, one is almost always sampling a small percentage of the entire universe of diversity (10^{10} peptides are only 0.1% of the universe of 10 mers), it is crucial that appropriate assay techniques be competent to detect ligands with modest affinity. The identification of weak binders in any of the previously

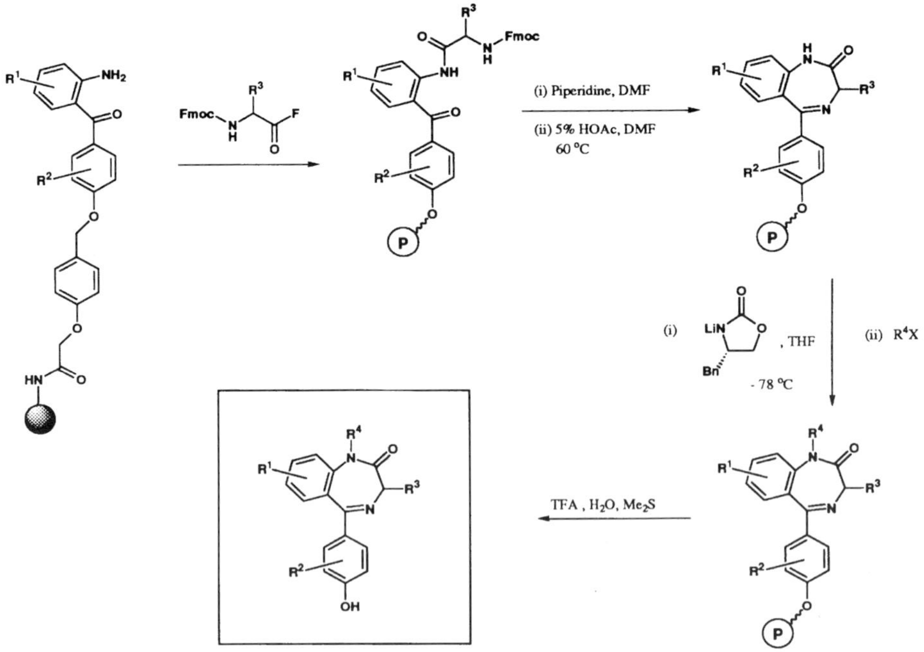

Figure 1.8   BZ Combinatorial.

mentioned approaches is very important, and leads directly to preparation of secondary libraries in which original "hits" become the centerpiece for more focused diversity creation. This is a consequential issue, since application of combinatorial technologies are best viewed as an iterative process and not a singular event. As the emphasis in a project shifts from lead discovery to analog evaluation, assays must then be capable of affinity discrimination between closely related library members.

1.4.4.5 Combinatorial libraries — future innovations

As the field of combinatorial chemistry attracts increasing attention from the pharmaceutical establishment, it seems likely that the contents of chemical libraries will continue to evolve to look more and more like the type of compounds which have previously lead to drugs. In spite of the complexity that early parts of the process may pose to the combinatorial chemist, a hidden advantage that combinatorially-derived molecules offer is that any "hit" will be readily synthesizable — by definition. This should be contrasted with a natural product driven approach to drug discovery and development, where often the structural complexity of the lead compound may hamper the rapid preparation of analog molecules and the acquisition of SAR. To be sure, it is anticipated that combinatorial chemistry will not replace any of the traditional methods of lead finding and development, but will certainly be a useful adjunct to them.

Though combinatorial technologies may soon prove their worth in the drug discovery process by delivering new leads quickly and cheaply, in order to completely fulfill the promise of "making drugs" an important question will be whether some of the common major obstacles to drug development (e.g. cell penetration, bioavailability, pharmacokinetics, metabolism) can be productively addressed through the application of combinatorial approaches (i.e. *combinatorial drug development*).

Combinatorial technologies diverge sharply from historical precedent through a change in emphasis from the consideration of individual molecules to thinking in terms of populations of molecules. *The notion of intentionally biasing a chemical library is thus a form of drug design*, not applied to individuals but rather to groups or populations of molecules. The drug design of populations versus individuals is analogous to fishing with a net rather than just a hook. As more knowledge of workable strategies for combinatorial synthesis are understood, it is expected that structural and computational input, and other rational design information will be integrated into a broad combinatorial medicinal chemistry approach.

1.4.5 Lead optimization

1.4.5.1 Selectivity and activity
Once an active compound, originating from either the medicinal chemistry laboratory or isolated from the screening of natural product sources, has been shown to have activity, it then becomes a lead structure. At this point, the focus is to enhance, activity, selectivity and bioavailability for the molecular target. This can be done using experience from other series, substituting bioisosteric groups that enhance activity, by modeling the receptor ligands or enzyme substrates using either Drieding models or CAMD approaches. In addition, once an active conformation suggests itself to the chemist, a substructure search can be undertaken using a Molecular Access System (MACCS) based data base to select related compounds from either a company's compound library or the Aldrich, Bader or Maybridge catalogs. Ideally, using the format of the flow chart, an iterative process can thus be undertaken to derive the most active compound. CAMD approaches can provide a significant level of sophistication to the drug design process. However, many assumptions are made regarding the minimal energy conformation and water content of a molecule and the compounds designed, based on the optimal three dimensional modeling of a homologue series, are very often inactive in the biological test system. This does not however discount the usefulness of the technique but rather emphasizes the nature of the learning curve and the limited data bases currently available. Information regarding the crystalline structure of the ligand, can provide an additional template to model the recognition site while point mutations in the known structure of the molecular target, where available, can be used to ascertain the importance of individual amino acids to the recognition of ligands. Additional information can be derived from dimensional NMR of the receptor — ligand or enzyme-substrate complex.

As one example of the approaches used to impart selectivity and affinity into a molecule, Hutchison and co-workers at CIBA-Geigy in developing the selective, high affinity adenosine A_{2a} receptor agonist, CGS 21680C (2-[p-(2-carboxyethyl)phenethylamino]-5'-N-ethylcarboxamidoadenosine) (**1.8**) used prior art that showed that 5'-N-ethylcarboxamido-adenosine (NECA; **1.5**; Fig. 1.9.) was the most potent adenosine A_2 receptor agonist known. This compound was however, non-selective having activity at A_1, A_{2a} and A_{2b} receptors. A 2-substituted adenosine analog, CV 1808 (2-phenylaminoadenosine, **1.6**; Fig. 1.9), a compound with coronary vasodilatory activity, developed by Takeda, while 10-fold less

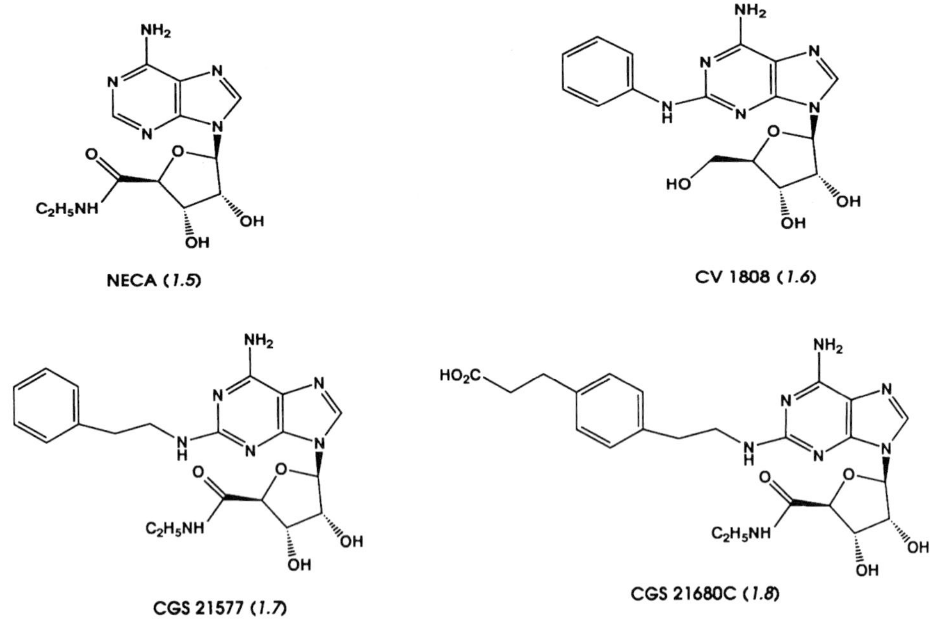

Figure 1.9   Adenosine.

active than NECA showed 5-8-fold selectivity for the A_{2a} receptor. Anecdotally, selective modification of the 2-substituent of the adenine ring was considered to have little effect on receptor selectivity while significantly reducing binding activity. Nonetheless, Hutchison and co-workers increased the size and length of the carbon side chain at the 2-position of NECA. The first compound synthesized, 2-phenethylamino-NECA, CGS 21577 (**1.7**; Fig. 1.9) retained the A_{2a} receptor activity of NECA with a dramatic reduction in A_1 activity. In contrast to NECA, which was non-selective, CGS 21577 was 59-fold selective for the A_{2a} receptor. Subsequent addition of a carboxyethyl group to the 2-position side chain ostensibly to reduce blood-brain barrier access, resulted in CGS 21680C which again retained the A_{2a} activity of NECA but underwent a further reduction in A_1 receptor activity such that the compound was 140-fold selective for the A_{2a} receptor. This compound was the first selective ligand for the adenosine A_{2a} receptor. It is noteworthy that it was made without recourse to computer modeling.

1.4.5.2 Efficacy and bioavailability
The concept of functional efficacy remains an enigma from the molecular design standpoint. Despite considerable data, it is not known what mechanisms contribute to the process that translates binding of a ligand to a functional response. Based on classical enzyme theory it had been generally considered that ligand binding induced a change in the receptor to facilitate its interaction with the transmembrane G-proteins to elicit activation of an enzyme or ion channel second messenger system. Indeed, in the early days of receptor binding,

based on the Monod/Koshland models of allosteric enzymes it had even been suggested that agonist and antagonist ligands differed in their ability to induce an 'active' form of the receptor. While the 'receptor change' concept remains a working hypothesis, studies with cholinergic receptors, both muscarinic and nicotinic, have suggested that the binding of ligand to the receptor can induce an conformational change in the ligand to assume the correct spatial orientation to facilitate a functional response. Thus the ligand conformation for recognition can differ from that required for transduction, implying a sequential process.

Compound bioavailability is a phenomenon that is not adequately addressed by current approaches to the molecular design process. Frequently, highly potent and selective NCEs lack *in vivo* activity. This may be ascribed to metabolic factors or species differences. However, the inability of a compound to reach its site of action due to lack of absorption from the gut, first pass metabolism in the liver or lack of penetration of the blood-brain barrier can make its potential as a drug candidate limited unless alternative dosage forms can overcome these obstacles. The factors affecting bioavailability are slowly being understood but, to date, there are no hard and fast rules that can be applied across a chemical series with any degree of reasonable predictability. The soft drug approach of Bodor, where an esterified form of a drug is able to cross the blood-brain barrier where it is then transformed and cleaved by esterases within the brain reducing its ability to recross the blood-brain barrier is a chemical approach to this problem (see Chapter 13). Another is that of vectored delivery using antibodies or other ligand dependent carrier systems. Selective ligand binding to the tissue of interest can then theoretically act to facilitate the concentration of the active principal at the site of action.

1.4.6 The bioisosteric approach

Bioisosteric replacement is the substitution of atoms or groups of atoms in the parent molecule to produce compounds with broadly similar biological properties to the parent with an attendant structural diversity. This approach has been used in a wide range of pharmacophores (see Chapter 10) and a program, RANGEX, has been developed to select bioisosteres for a given analog from a series of substitutent constants. Classical isosteres include groups of atoms in which the peripheral layers of electrons are considered identical and include the elements of each group of the periodic table and annular equivalents. Non-classical isosteres represent atoms or groups of atoms that do not necessarily overlap but have steric, electronic or other properties similar to the parent. Examples of some common and broadly applicable bioisosteres are shown in Table 1.1. Since no two atoms or atom groups are identical, substitutions often result in alterations of the size, shape (bond angles, hybridization), electronic distribution, pKa, water and lipid solubility, hydrogen bonding capabilities, chemical reactivity and susceptibility to enzymatic modification of the parent compound. NCEs can thus be developed that have improved or altered selectivity, potency, stability, pharmacokinetic and metabolic profiles, novel antagonist activity, decreased toxicity and enhanced duration of action. A given replacement will generally modify some, but not all, of these parameters in a molecule or series, the changes and magnitude being dependent on the particular role that the moiety plays in the molecule. It also should be emphasized that a favorable bioisostere in one compound series will not necessarily be acceptable in another. Discovery of novel bioisosteric replacements for a known class of drug can provide structurally unique and patentable agents, permitting rapid entry into a therapeutic market. An example of this approach are the H_2-receptor antagonists, cimetidine (**1.10**) and ranitidine (**1.11**). One of the initial H_2-blockers, metiamide (**1.9**; Fig. 1.10) caused granulocytopenia. This side effect was overcome by researchers at Smith, Kline and French *via* the isosteric replacement of the thiourea with a cyanoguanidine to give cimetidine (**1.10**). In turn, the nitrogen heterocycle in **1.10** was replaced by Glaxo chemists with dimethylaminomethylfuran and the cyanoguanidine with a nitromethyleneguanidine group to give ranitidine (**1.11**). Two further examples of the bioisostere approach involve cholinergic agonists. Researchers at Merck, using a finding by chemists at Ferrosan that replacement of the ester function in BZs by an oxadiazole increased efficacy, modified the muscarinic agonist, arecoline (**1.12**; Fig. 1.11) to give the stable analog, **1.13**. This was modified to the quinuclidine, **1.14** and eventually to L-670,207 (**1.15**) one of the most potent known ligands for the M_1 receptor. The nicotinic cholinergic receptor agonist, ABT 418 (**1.18**; Fig. 1.12.) from Abbott is an isoxazole bioisostere of (S)-(−)-nicotine (**1.17**) having the same efficacy as (S)-(−)-nicotine in terms of cognition enhancement with a significant reduction in cardiovascular and dependence liability side effects.

Table 1.1   Bioisosteric relpacements.

Classical

Monovalent	$-F$, $-OH$, $-NH_2$, $-CH_3$, $-SH$, $-t-C_4H_9$, $-i-C_3H_7$
Brivalent	$-O-$, $-S-$, $-SE-$, $-CH_2-$, $-NH-$, COOR, COSR, $COCH_2R$
Trivalent	$-N=$, $-P=$, $-CH=$, As=
Annual equivalent	$-CH=CH-$, $=CH-$, $-S-$, $=N-$, $-O-$, $-S-$, $-CH_2-$, $-NH-$

Non-classical

Hydroxyl	OH, CH_2OH, NHCOR, $NHSO_2R$, $NHCONH_2$, NHCN
Carbonyl	CO, $C=C(CN)_2$, SO_2NRR', $CONRR'$, =CHCN
Carboxyl	CO_2H, SO_2NHR, SO_3H, $PO(OH)NH_2$, CONHOH

	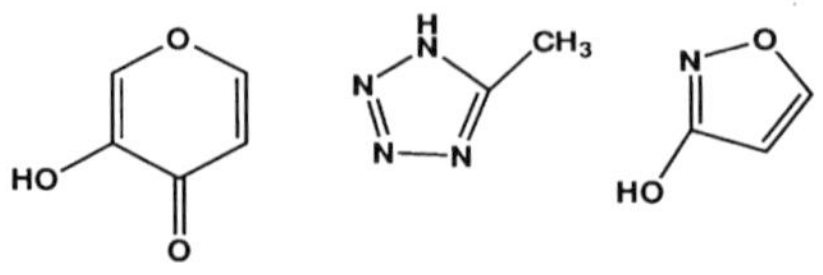
Halogen	Cl, CF_3, CN, $N(CN)_2$, $C(CN)_3$

Pyridine	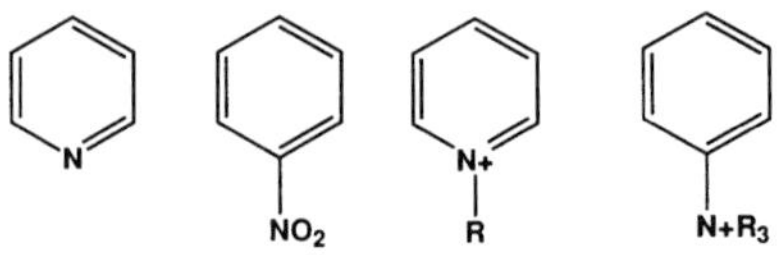

Spacer groups	$-(CH_2)_3-$ 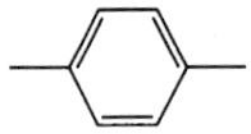

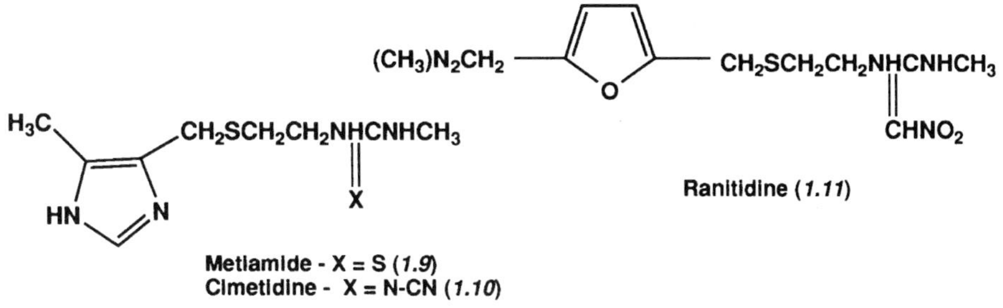

$(CH_3)N_2CH_2$ —

$CH_2SCH_2CH_2NHCNHCH_3$

$CHNO_2$

Ranitidine (1.11)

H_3C

$CH_2SCH_2CH_2NHCNHCH_3$

X

HN   N

Metiamide - X = S (1.9)
Cimetidine - X = N-CN (1.10)

Figure 1.10   Histamine.

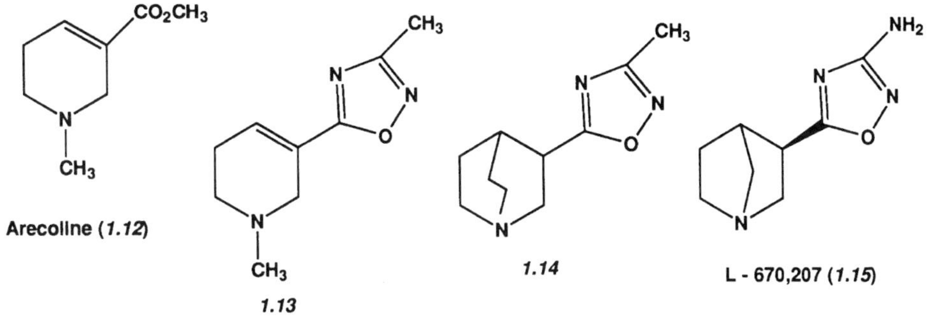

CO_2CH_3

CH_3

CH_3

NH_2

N   N

N   N

N   N

O

O

O

CH_3

N

CH_3

Arecoline (1.12)

N

CH_3

1.13

N

1.14

N

L - 670,207 (1.15)

Figure 1.11   Muscarinic.

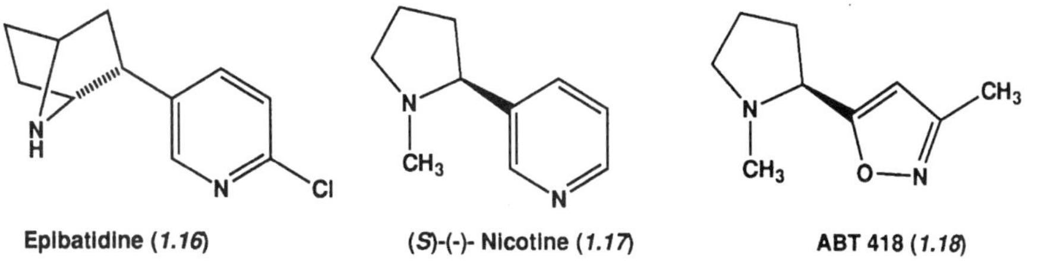

N
H

N   Cl

Epibatidine (1.16)

N

CH_3

N

(S)-(-)- Nicotine (1.17)

N

CH_3

CH_3

O—N

ABT 418 (1.18)

Figure 1.12   Nicotinic ligands.

1.4.7 Peptides and biologics as drug candidates

Many of the newer receptors identified in the past decade have peptides as their endogenous ligands. Such targets are generally considered to be more subtle in terms of their effects on biological function due to their indirect effects and neuromodulatory rather than neurotransmitter roles. Accordingly, neuropeptide receptors have received much attention as potential drug targets. Hormonal receptors e.g. insulin have proved amenable to replacement therapy, in this particular instance, insulin itself, either derived from porcine pancreas or genetically engineered as in Lilly/Hybridtech's Humulin^{TM}. Since hormones are by definition vascular entities, such replacement therapy has been highly successful.

In intact nervous tissue, either peripheral or central, the ability to deliver peptides to their proposed site of action has proved to be a formidable task. Oral bioavailability, first pass metabolism and in the case of the brain, penetration of the blood brain barrier are, sequentially, major obstacles in compound development.

The generic example of a peptide neuromodulator has been that of the opiate peptides, the enkephalins. Their discovery in the mid 1970s sent several major drug companies scurrying to modify these relatively simple pentapeptides to increase stability, bioavailability, receptor selectivity and affinity in order to produce novel analgesic agents that would be free of the respiratory depression, dependence liability and dysphoria associated with the the use of morphine and its congeners. Some 20 years later, after the expenditure of many millions of dollars, morphine remains the major analgesic in current usage. The recent cloning of the opiate receptor family that has provided important information on how ligands bind to the receptors may be anticipated to renew interest in this area.

The lack of significant success in the opiate area should be contrasted with progress in the area of CCK receptor antagonists at Merck. Using as a starting point a radioligand binding assay, Chang and colleagues screened many fermentation broths to discover the non-peptidic CCK-A receptor antagonist, asperlicin (**1.20**; Fig. 1.13). This was used as a lead pharmacophore to develop MK 329 (**1.21**; Fig. 1.13), a novel benzodiazepine with high affinity and selectivity for the CCK-A receptor.

Significant progress has been made in the area of non-peptide antagonists using the screening approach for neurokinin (NK) and neurotensin receptors (Fig. 1.14). SR 48692 (**1.22**) is a non-peptide neurotensin antagonist while a number of non-peptides including CP 99994 (**1.23**), WIN 51708 (**1.24**), RP 67580 (**1.25**) and SR 48968 (**1.26**) are antagonists at various peptide receptors.

At one time, it was estimated that 80% of the pharmacopea in the year 2010 would be biologic in nature, including various biological response modifiers (BRMs), lymphokines, cytokines, catalytic antibodies, antisense oligonucleotides, trophic factors, hormones and paracrine modulators. As such entities have made their way into clinical trials it has become apparent that problems with efficacy and side effect liability are not unique to conventional small molecule approaches. The initial trials of recombinant mouse NGF in Alzheimer's Disease were a disaster due to latent virus induction while clinical trials for CNTF (ciliary neurotrophic factor) in the treatment for ALS (amyotrophic lateral sclerosis) were discontinued due to unacceptable side effect liabilities. In the area of septic shock, the monoclonal antibodies ebacumab (Centor), edobacomnab (E5; Xoma/ Pfizer) and T-88 (Chiron), the IL-1 antagonist anakinra (IL1ra; Synergen) and the bradykinin antagonist, CP-0127 (Cortech) failed to demonstrate any benefit in terms of mortality outcomes in

Asp-Tyr(SO₃H)-Met-Gly-Trp-Met-Asp-Phe-NH₂

CCK-8 (*1.19*)

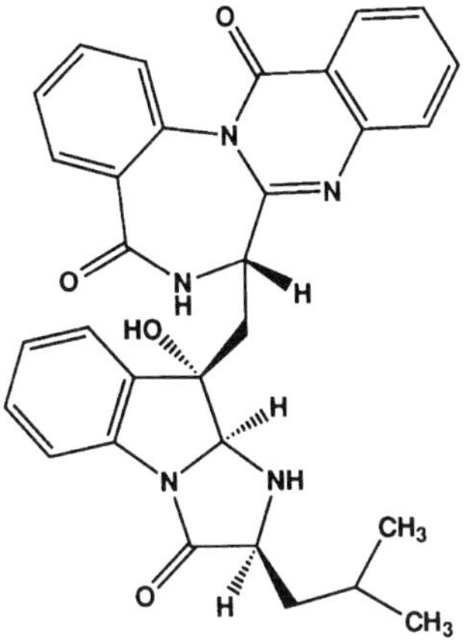

Asperlicin (*1.20*)

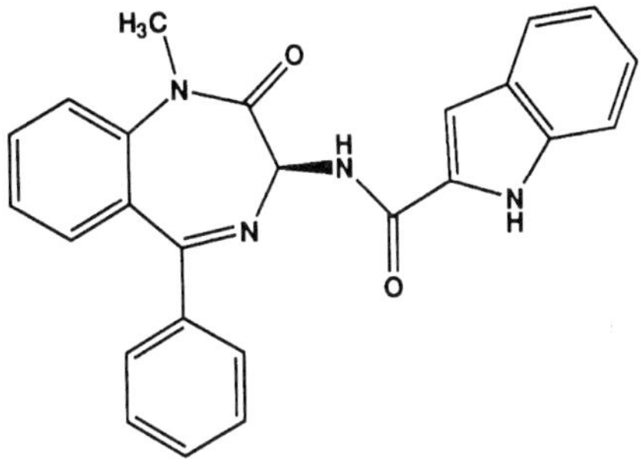

MK 329 (*1.21*)

Figure 1.13 CCK antagonists.

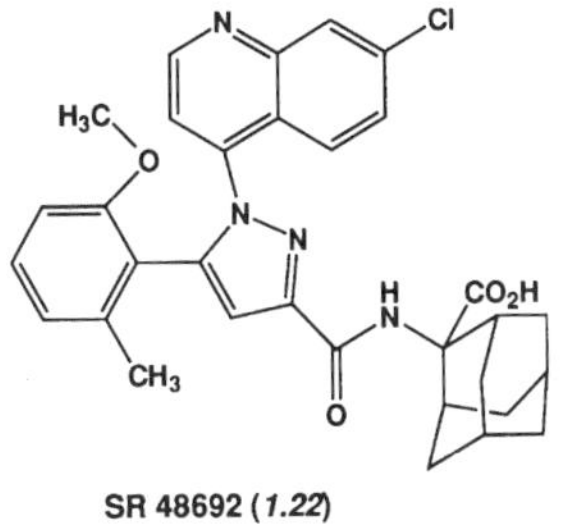

SR 48692 (*1.22*)

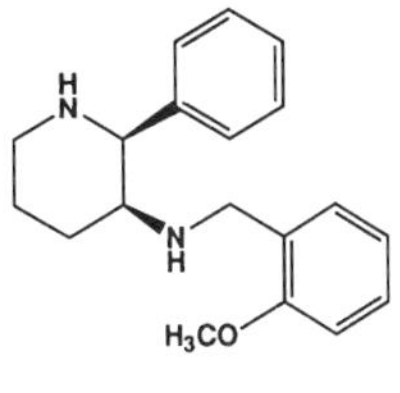

CP 99994 (*1.23*)

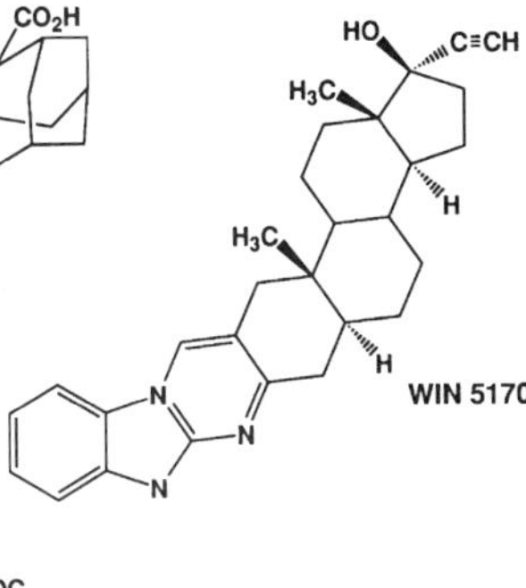

WIN 51708 (*1.24*)

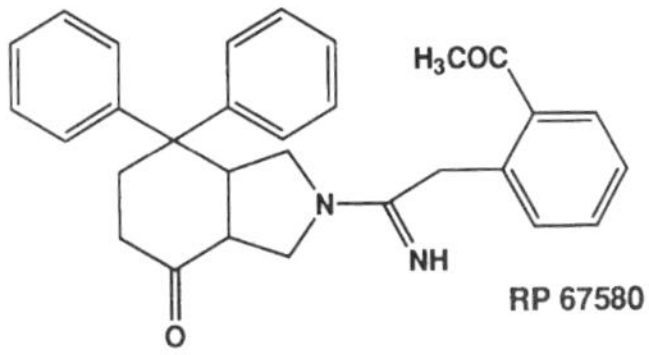

RP 67580 (*1.25*)

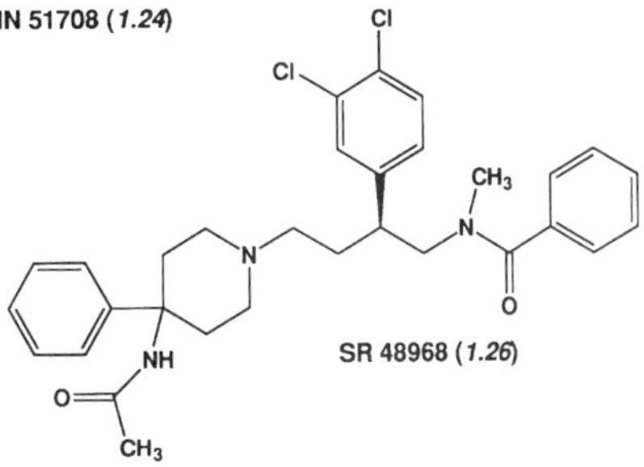

SR 48968 (*1.26*)

Figure 1.14 Non-peptide peptide antagonists.

clinical trials. All five biologics have been withdrawn from human trials with varying financial impact on the companies involved.

The net result of these recent clinical developments is a reappraisal of the usefulness of biologics as the 'wave of the future' in therapeutics. It is no longer a given that such agents, because of their natural occurrence, would have relatively fewer side effects than conventional small molecules.

1.5 COMPOUND DEVELOPMENT

1.5.1 Absorption, distribution, metabolism and excretion (ADME)

In assessing the *in vivo* activity of an NCE, it is important that some correlation be demonstrated between drug efficacy and the presence of either the parent compound or its metabolites in plasma. For this reason pharmacokinetic and pharmacodynamic studies, otherwise referred to as ADME studies represent an important part of the new drug application package (IND), and while never having been unimportant are now receiving considerably more attention as the cost of drug trials continues to escalate. Once cold (as opposed to radioisotope) HPLC methodology is developed for a lead compound and its metabolite(s), ADME studies can provide a quantifiable measure of drug availability. This can then be correlated with biological data and the temporal relationship between efficacy and drug levels and metabolites formed and their elimination established. Once a reasonable relationship has been established, taking into account different drug vehicles, doses, routes of administration and dosing regimens, ADME studies can be use to both design and monitor clinical trials for an NCE thus eliminating much in the way of trial and error in using biological efficacy as the only readout (see Chapter 18).

1.5.2 Toxicological evaluation

Once a compound has evolved to lead status its safety has to be evaluated in available *in vitro* and animal models. A compound is initially evaluated *in vitro* in cell culture to assess effects on bacterial and mammalian cell replication to assess toxicity. The Ames test, a measure of mutagenicity in bacteria, can be used to assess the effects of an NCE on gene function and is one of the first toxicological test procedures carried out on a new compound series.

Following *in vitro* testing, the compound series is evaluated in a rising dose study, usually 7–14 days to find out at what dose signs of toxicity can be observed. Initial *in vivo* testing is for 14 or 90 days. While both time periods are classified as subchronic, the former provides sufficient safety data to do a single dose Phase I study and the latter, a full fledged clinical evaluation, the amount of planning and tissue assessment required for an *in vivo* toxicological evaluation can take up to 9 months for a 14 day study and from 2–3 years for a 90 day study. Toxicological evaluation is extremely labor and cost intensive. Following primary evaluation, an NCE in clinical trials will also be evaluated over an 18–24 month period for reproductive effects, teratogenicity and immunological and behavioral toxicity both in adult mammals and their offspring. Carcinogenicity studies can take in excess of three years for completion.

An often overlooked part of the toxicological evaluation process is the quantity of material required. In most instances, biological evaluation of efficacy and selectivity at the preclinical level can be completed with 5–10 g of the NCE. For toxicological evaluation, quantities from 250 g–1 kg are routinely required. The synthesis of bulk drug usually requires an optimization of the synthetic route to increase yield and reduce cost of compound produced. A fifteen step synthesis at the pre-toxicological stage that cannot be cost-effectively reduced to a more cost effective 4 or 5 steps in process chemistry at the 'kilo-lab' stage is often a major factor in deciding whether to continue development of a compound as a drug candidate. From a price perspective, the more efficacious the compound, the less is required to achieve a therapeutic effect and consequently the less active ingredient is required in the final formulation. Synthesis and purity of bulk drug, often called 'Batch 0', are regulated in many countries by government regulations generically called "Good Manufacturing Practices" or GMP after the U.S. Food and Drug Administration (FDA) regulations. A company is required to file a 'new process' registration for the scale-up synthesis of the compound. Three separate lots of the compound are then synthesized according to this protocol which are then used to assess the physical properties of the compound over extended time periods. If process chemistry is brought into the synthetic process at an early enough stage, economies can be effected by having the time to develop new synthetic routes and even modified structures that have acceptable efficacy and are more cost effective to manufacture.

Attempts to reduce animal usage by emphasizing *in vitro* test procedures are the focus of a major effort in the pharmaceutical industry both to increase the turnaround time to generate useful data and reduce costs. Like bioavailability, the structure activity relationship for toxicity is not well understood.

1.5.3 Clinical evaluation

Clinical development is divided into four distinct phases (frequently abbreviated to PL) preceded by the filing of a Notice of Claimed Investigational Exemption for a New Drug — the IND in the US, the Clinical Trial Certificate (CTC) outside the U.S. to the FDA (Food and Drug Administration) in the US, EMEA (European Medications Evaluation Agency) in the EU or their equivalents in Japan. This document runs to many thousands of pages collating the preclinical safety and efficacy studies performed on an NCE. The four phases of clinical trials are:

Phase I: Clinical pharmacology and toxicity — these studies are concerned with safety and are typically performed on healthy volunteers. Rising dose studies are done with the compound of interest to determine an acceptable single drug dosage *via* the route of administration deemed to be of interest — the dose derived being that which can be given without eliciting serious side effects. Drug metabolism and bioavailability studies are also carried out at this time and may include multiple dosing regimens in preparation for the Phase II trials. Depending on the targeted disease, patients may also be included in the Phase I trials to more accurately reflect the targeted population, e.g. geriatric patients.

Phase II: Initial clinical investigation for treatment effect — these studies continue evaluation of the safety of a new compound and begin to monitor efficacy in the selected patient population. Phase II is colloquially divided into a and b stages, the former a limited trial to ascertain some degree of efficacy followed by Phase IIb, a more broad range (and expensive) trial involving a larger number of patients. During Phase II trials, biochemical indices of drug efficacy are routinely sought as more objective endpoints of drug action. Clinical trials are usually conducted on a "double-blind" basis rather than "open". In double blind studies, neither the patient nor those involved in providing health care have knowledge of whether a placebo, a vehicle formulation identical to that used for the active principle of the NCE without the NCE, or the drug is being given. This can rule out psychological aspects of drug treatment especially when evaluating CNS drugs. In those instances where there is no known treatment for a disease, it is ethical, as laid down in the revised (1975) Declaration of Helsinki, in order to prove efficacy, that the control group remains untreated. It has been documented that oral placebo drug therapy can be effective in a large number of instances. Open studies are usually carried out without a code and in some instances without an adequate control group. The phrase 'breaking the code' refers to the identification of which treatment a patient has received. A phase II "signal" — the first indication of efficacy in the targeted population, is a major milestone in the clinical development of an NCE.

Regulatory agencies frequently require, in addition to a placebo arm, a comparative or positive control arm with a known drug (if available) to validate both the trial and to demonstrate that the NCE has comparable or superior efficacy and an equivalent or superior safety profile. If the positive control arm, say fluoxetine for an antidepressant, ibuprofen for an antiinflammatory and ciprofloxin for an antibiotic fails to show efficacy then the trial can be considered a failure.

Phase III: Full-scale evaluation of treatment — the multicenter comparison of the new compound in a large patient population with known treatments and comparison with placebo. The dosage used in this stage is critical as Phase III data are those upon which regulatory decisions are made and which support the marketing of the compound. The number of patients involved in the portion of compound development can be several hundred to two to three thousand. Once sufficient data have been accumulated from a Phase III trial (which can take from 2–8 years), a company may then file a New Drug Application (NDA) to the FDA in the U.S. to request approval to market the NCE as a drug. The NDA is 5000–100,000 pages in length containing efficacy data as a basis for the claimed indications as well as safety information and a summary of the risks and benefits for the agent. In the European Union, the Product License Application (PLA) is the equivalent of the NDA.

Phase IV: Postmarketing surveillance — this portion of the clinical trial occurs after the drug is approved and undertakes the monitoring of adverse effects and additional long term, large-scale studies of drug efficacy. In addition, Phase IV trials can be used to monitor both additional uses for a new drug for a subsequent NDA as well as gathering information to assess the cost — benefit ratios for the introduction of a new treatment modality. Such information can be used to convince health care payers that the use of a new drug offers significant benefit over existing therapy (surgery or other drugs) to the extent that there are savings in either initial or long terms as reflected in time for patient recovery and quality of life.

Many pharmaceutical companies have established clinical research units at major research hospitals across the world to facilitate the monitoring of compound development. In addition, several companies are accelerating compound evaluation in man by the use of Exploratory Clinical Research Units, small Phase I units that are geared to take novel, mechanism based compounds that have undergone toxicology to FDA standards into limited human evaluations to assess efficacy and proof of principle. Such units are especially important when a compound is developed preclinically on the basis of a novel mechanism of action which requires hypothesis testing in humans without the expense of full clinical evaluation (for further details, see Chapter 18).

ACKNOWLEDGEMENT

MW would like to recognize the contribution of Alex M. Nadzan to the previous version of this chapter in the First Edition which was used as the basis for this update.

FURTHER READING

Annual Reports In Medicinal Chemistry. An indispensable yearly review publication on current topics in medicinal chemistry published by the American Chemical Society.

Black, J.W. (1989) Drugs from emasculated hormones: the principle of syntopic antagonism. *Science*, **245**, 486. The Nobel laureate's acceptance speech for his major contributions to science and health care in the discovery and development of propranolol and cimetidine.

Bunin, B.A. and Ellman, J.A. (1992) A general and expedient method for the solid-phase synthesis of 1,4-benzodiazepine derivatives. *J. Am. Chem. Soc.*, **114**, 10997.

Cutler, N.R. *et al.* (1994) *Alzheimer's Disease. Optimizing Drug Development Strategies.* Wiley, Chichester, U.K. While this book focuses on one disease, Chapter 9 "Finding the dose: the bridging study" provides an excellent overview to problems encountered in moving from Phase I studies in healthy volunteers to Phase II studies in the patient population.

Dooley, C.T. *et al.*, (1994) An all D-amino acid opiod peptide with central analgesic activity from a combinatorial library. *Science*, **266**, 2019. A paper that describes the combinatorial synthesis of 52 million or so hexamers one of which, AC-rfwink-NH^2 is a high affinity ligand (Ki = 16–41 nM) for μ opiate receptors and has *in vivo* central analgesic activity.

Evans, B.E. *et al.* (1987) *J. Med. Chem.*, **30**, 1229.

Flam, F. (1994) Chemical prospectors scour the seas for promising drugs. *Science*, **266**, 1324.

Furka, A. *et al.* (1991) General method for rapid synthesis of multicomponent peptide mixtures. *Int. J. Peptide Protein Res.*, **37**, 487.

Gallop, M. *et al.* (1994) Applications of combinatorial technologies I. Background and peptide combinatorial libraries. *J. Med. Chem.*, **37**, 1233. An excellent, in-depth overview of combinatorial chemistry.

Gordon, E.M. *et al.* (1994) Applications of combinatorial technologies II. Combinatorial organic synthesis, library screening strategies and future directions. *J. Med. Chem.*, **37**, 1385. Part 2 of the most current update on combinatorial chemistry.

Greer, J. *et al.* (1994) Application of the three-dimensional structures of protein target molecules in structure-based drug design. *J. Med. Chem.*, **37**, 1035. An account of three success stories in structure based drug design.

Hirschmann, R. (1991) Medicinal Chemistry in the Golden Age of Biology: Lessons from Steroid and Peptide Research. *Angew. Chem.*, **30**, 1278.

Jack, D. (1989) The challenge of drug discovery. *Drug Design Deliv.*, **4**, 167. The architect of Glaxo's rise to one of the top five drug companies in the world describes his approach to drug discovery.

Jacobs, J.W. and Fodor, S.P.A. (1994) Combinatorial Chemistry: Applications of Light Directed Chemical Synthesis. *Trends Biotechnol.*, **12**, 19–26.

Joyce, C. (1994) *Earthly Goods. Medicine Hunting in the Rain Forest.* Little, Brown, Boston. A current account on natural products as drug sources.

Kenakin, T. (1993) *Pharmacologic Analysis of Drug-Receptor Interaction. 2nd Edn.* Raven, New York. The second edition of a seminal text on basic pharmacology. An essential part of the drug discoverer's library.

Needels, M.N. *et al.* (1993) Generation and screening of an oligonucleotide-encoded synthetic peptide library. *Proc. Natl. Acad. Sci., USA*, **90**, 10700.

Ohlmeyer, M.H.J. *et al.* (1994) Complex synthetic chemical libraries indexed with molecular tags. *Proc. Natl. Acad. Sci. USA*, **90**, 10922.

Patchett, A.A. (1993) Excursions in Drug Discovery. *J. Med. Chem.*, **36**, 2051.

Ramsden, C.A. (1990) Quantitative drug design. *Comp. Med. Chem.*, Vol 4. Pergamon, Oxford.

Roussel, P.A., Saad, K.N. and Erickson, T.J. (1991) *Third Generation R & D. Managing the link to Corporate Strategy.* Harvard Business School Press, Boston, MA. An impressive book from the A.D. Little group on how innovative high tech research should be conducted. Well written, easy to follow and applicable to the pharmaceutical industry.

Sebestyen, F. *et al.* (1993) Chemical synthesis of peptide libraries. *Bioorg. Med. Chem. Lett.*, **3**, 413.

Spilker, B. (1991) *Guide to Clinical Trials.* Raven, New York. The most comprehensive and user friendly guide to clinical trials.

Spilker, B. (1994) *Multinational Drug Companies. Issues in Drug Discovery and Development.* Raven, New York. The second edition of a highly personalized account of all facets of drug discovery by the pharmaceutical industry's most prolific writer. Essential.

Sweetnam, P.M. *et al.* (1993) The role of receptor binding in drug discovery. *J. Natural Products*, **56**, 441. Excellent overview of the screening process.

Weisbach, J. and Moos, W.H. (1995) Diagnosing the decline in major pharmaceutical research laboratories: a prescription for drug companies. *Drug. Dev. Res.*, **34**, 243. An outstanding and provocative consideration of the role of venture capital funded 'biotech' companies in the pharmaceutical industry of the 21st century. A tour de force

Werth, B. (1994) *The Billion Dollar Molecule.* Simon and Schuster, New York. One of *Business Week's* top books for 1994, a wonderful, insightful account of the evolution of Vertex Pharmaceuticals.

Williams, M. (1993). Strategies for drug discovery, *NIDA Res. Monograph*, **134**, 1. An overview of the tactics for drug discovery including organizational structures.

Williams, M. and Stork, D. (1994) Setting up the R & D team. *AMA Management Handbook*, Ed. J.J. Hampton, AMACOM, New York, 7–25.

Williams, M., Deecher, D.C. and Sullivan, J.P. (1994) Drug receptors, In *Burger's Medicinal Chemistry and Drug Discovery, 5th Edition.* Part I. Ed. M.E. Wolff, Wiley, New York, 349.

Williams, M. *et al.* (1993) Biotechnology in the drug discovery process: strategic and management issues. *Med. Res. Rev.*, **13**, 399. The impact of biotechnology on how drug-related research is conducted and the need for its integration into the mainstream process.

Zukermann, R.N. *et al.* (1994) Discovery of nanomolar ligands for 7-transmembrane G-protein coupled receptors from a diverse (N-substituted) glycine peptoid library. *J. Med. Chem.*, **37**, 2678. A research paper on Chiron's success in a combinatorial library strategy that led to the identification of a 7 nM alpha-adrenergic lead.

2. STRUCTURAL AND PHYSICOCHEMICAL FACTORS IN DRUG ACTION

ULI HACKSELL

CONTENTS

2.1 IMPORTANT PROPERTIES OF DRUGS

The ability of a drug to elicit its effect is related to its concentration at the site of action and its ability to interact with (block or stimulate) the biological target. Thus, in order to properly describe the action of a drug we have to consider properties and events which are fundamentally different. The concentration of the drug at the site of action is discussed in terms of pharmacokinetics whereas its pharmacodynamic properties are relevant to the specific interaction with the biological target. Even if a drug elicits a pronounced effect in an isolated tissue, it may be inactive when administered *in vivo*. On the other hand, a drug may be inactive *in vitro* but active *in vivo* provided that it is bioactivated. A number of events preceding the interaction with the biological target have to be considered in addition to those responsible for the action of primary interest. These involve adsorption, distribution, metabolism and elimination (Fig. 2.1). In order to assess the importance of each of these factors on drug action we have to take into account structural and physicochemical properties of the drug.

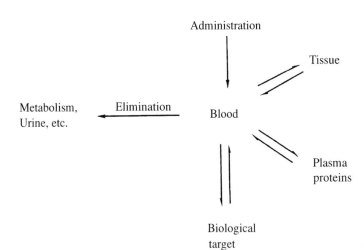

Figure 2.1   Simplified representation of the fate of a drug in the human organism.

2.2 PHYSICOCHEMICAL ASPECTS

2.2.1 Lipophilicity

Lipophilicity (hydrophobicity) is a molecular property which is related to the ability of a compound to partition between water and a nonpolar solvent. Traditionally, log P, the logarithm of the partition coefficient between water and 1-octanol, has been used to define lipophilicity (eq. 2.1).

$$\log P = \log[(\text{drug})_{1-\text{octanol}}/(\text{drug})_{\text{water}}] \tag{2.1}$$

The lipophilicity of a particular substituent may be obtained by equation 2.2 in which x may be any substituent. Like the Hammet constants, π values are additive. Some π values are given in Table 2.1 and many more are available in the literature. Therefore, it is frequently possible to accurately predict lipophilicities for compounds in a series provided that the lipophilicity for one compound in the series has been determined experimentally.

$$\pi_x = \log P_x - \log P_H \tag{2.2}$$

The lipophilicity of a drug considerably affects a number of pharmacokinetic parameters since it normally has to pass various biological membranes by passive diffusion. A more lipophilic drug is adsorbed better after peroral administration than a less lipophilic analog. Similarly, lipophilic drugs more readily pass the blood-brain barrier and are thus better distributed to the brain. However, it appears to be a parabolic relationship between distribution over biological cell membranes and lipophilicity. This is not surprising since biological membranes have properties which are very different from n-octanol.

Table 2.1 Lipophilicity (π-values) of some selected aromatic substituents[a].

Substituent	π-value
$-C_6(CH_3)_3$	1.98
$-C_6H_5$	1.96
$-I$	1.12
$-Br$	0.86
$-Cl$	0.71
$-SCH_3$	0.61
$-CH_3$	0.56
$-F$	0.14
$-H$	0.00
$-COOCH_3$	-0.01
$-OCH_3$	-0.02
$-NO_2$	-0.28
$-COCH_3$	-0.55
$-CONH_2$	-1.49

[a]Values are taken from C. Hansch, and A.Leo: Substituent constants for correlation analysis in chemistry and biology. Wiley, New York, 1979.

An optimal lipophilicity for penetration through the blood-brain barrier appears to exist at about log $P = 2$. Muscarinic antagonists such as mepensolate (2.1) have a quaternary

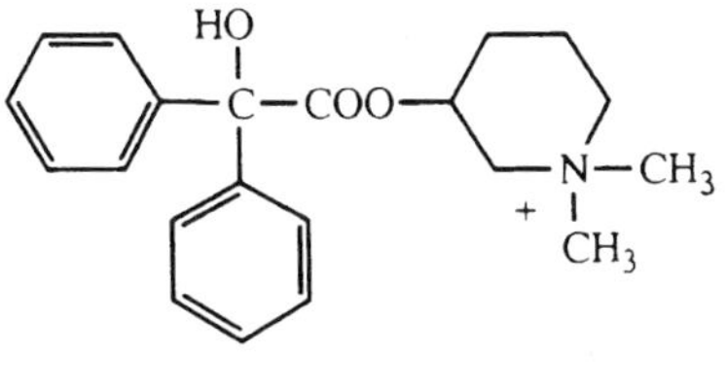

Mepensolate

(2.1)

ammonium group and are permanent cations. Such drugs will be very polar regardless of the pH of the environment. Consequently, quaternary cholinergic muscarinic antagonists are absorbed poorly from the gastrointestinal area and into the brain. The fact that permanent cations are absorbed at all may be related to the formation of lipophilic ion-pairs. Some hydrophilic drugs may utilize specific uptake mechanisms for absorption. One example is provided by L-DOPA (2.2) which readily enters the brain although it is more polar than the neurotransmitter dopamine (DA, 2.3) which is poorly transported over the blood brain barrier. It should also be noted that the site of absorbtion of acids or bases after peroral administration is partly related to their pKa-values since the pH in the GI tract varies from about 1 in the stomach to about 5 in the duodenum and then steadily increases. Thus, the adsorption of a basic drug from the stomach will be negligible (compare Table 2.2).

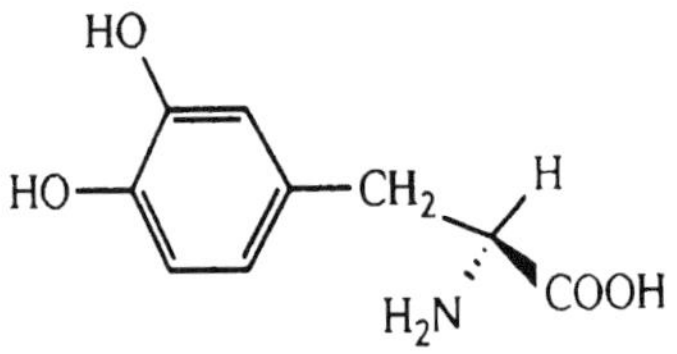

L-DOPA (2.2)

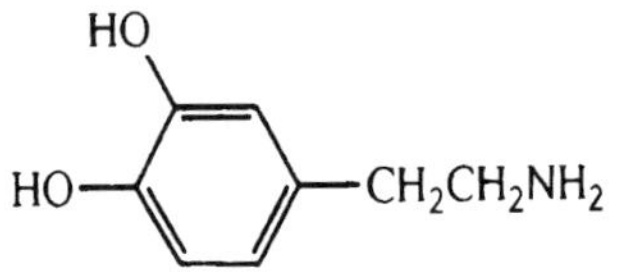

DA (2.3)

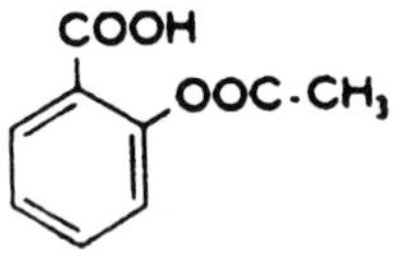

(2.4)

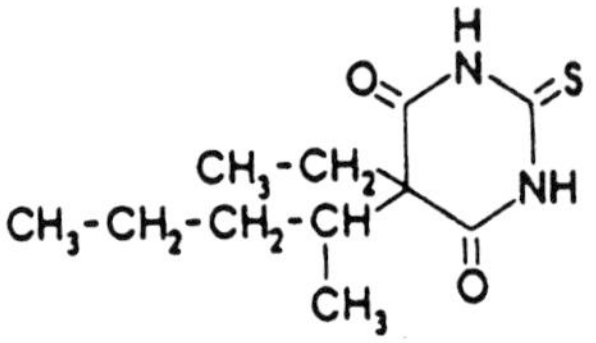

(2.5)

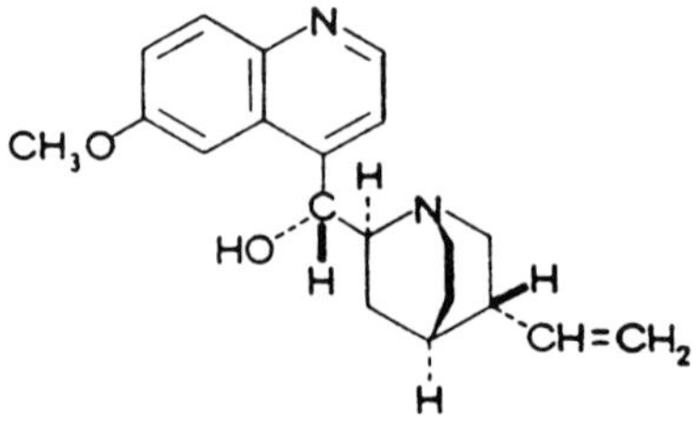

(2.6)

2.2.2 Important intermolecular forces

Most drugs exhibit an effect as the result of a specific interaction with a receptor or an enzyme and even rather small structural changes in the drug lead to a change in the biological response. Therefore, such drugs are called "structurally specific." There are, however, drugs which are "structurally nonspecific," that is, small structural changes do not

Table 2.2   Percent compound absorbed during 1 h from rat stomach at different pH-values[a]

Compound	pKa	% absorption	
		pH = 1	pH = 8.0–8.3
Acidic compounds			
Acetylsalicylic acid (2.4)	3.5	61	13
Thiopental (2.5)	7.6	46	34
Basic compounds			
Aniline	4.6	6	56
Quinine (2.6)	8.4	0	18

[a]Data taken from L.S. Shanker, *J. Pharm. Exp. Ther.*, 1957, **120**, 528.

lead to changes in the biological effect. The classical example is provided by anesthetics that are administered by inhalation. According to Ferguson's rule the activity of such drugs is related to the ratio of the partial vapor pressure of the substance in air and the vapor pressure of the substance. Typically, structurally nonspecific drugs are active only in high concentrations whereas structurally specific drugs may produce a biological response at very low concentrations. One reason is that structurally specific drugs may utilize some of the very efficient amplification processes, such as the production of second messengers as the result of receptor activation, which are used by cells. Structurally specific drugs interact with specific targets, normally biomacromolecules such as receptor proteins or enzymes in order to exert an effect. This interaction may be best described as the formation of a bimolecular complex. The drug-receptor complex may be stabilized by various forces (for simplicity, in the present chapter the receptor concept will be used in a sense that accommodates most types of drug targets).

The covalent bond.   The formation of a covalent bond between the target and the drug is the strongest possible interaction. Intermolecular covalent ("irreversible") bond formation is of interest mainly in chemotherapy. In order for drugs to react covalently their reactivity has to be increased and, thus, the desired selectivity may be lost. A highly electrophilic drug will not discriminate between nucleophiles at the desired site of action and other endogenous nucleophiles, the latter being in large majority. In addition, covalent bonds are much less reversible than other intermolecular bonds and reversibility of drug action is desirable since, for example it may be necessary to interrupt drug therapy rapidly if severe side effects occur.

Alkylating receptor ligands have been used frequently as tools in basic drug research. If the selectivity is high enough they may be used in combination with photoaffinity labeling techniques to characterize the ligand binding site of receptors or to inactivate a fraction of receptors.

Potent and selective receptor ligands may be modified into useful biochemical tools by introduction of isotopic labels and functionalities which can be converted into highly reactive functional groups under photolytical conditions. The basic idea is that a reactive species should be generated and trapped near or at the binding site of the receptor by photolysis. The isotopic labels will then help in identifying receptor proteins irreversibly bound to the ligand. Provided that the desired selectivity is obtained, this strategy appears very promising. One such example is provided by compound (**2.7**) which is converted into a carbene (**2.8**) under photolysis. Another alternative for photoaffinity labeling is provided by the arylazide derivative **2.9** which may be converted into a reactive nitrene (**2.10**) by photolysis (Scheme 2.1). Both (**2.7**) and (**2.9**) are derivatives of 8-OH DPAT (**2.11**) which is a highly potent and selective ligand for a subtype of serotonin receptors denoted 5-HT$_{1A}$. Selective manipulation of such receptors may be of interest in the treatment of anxiety and depression.

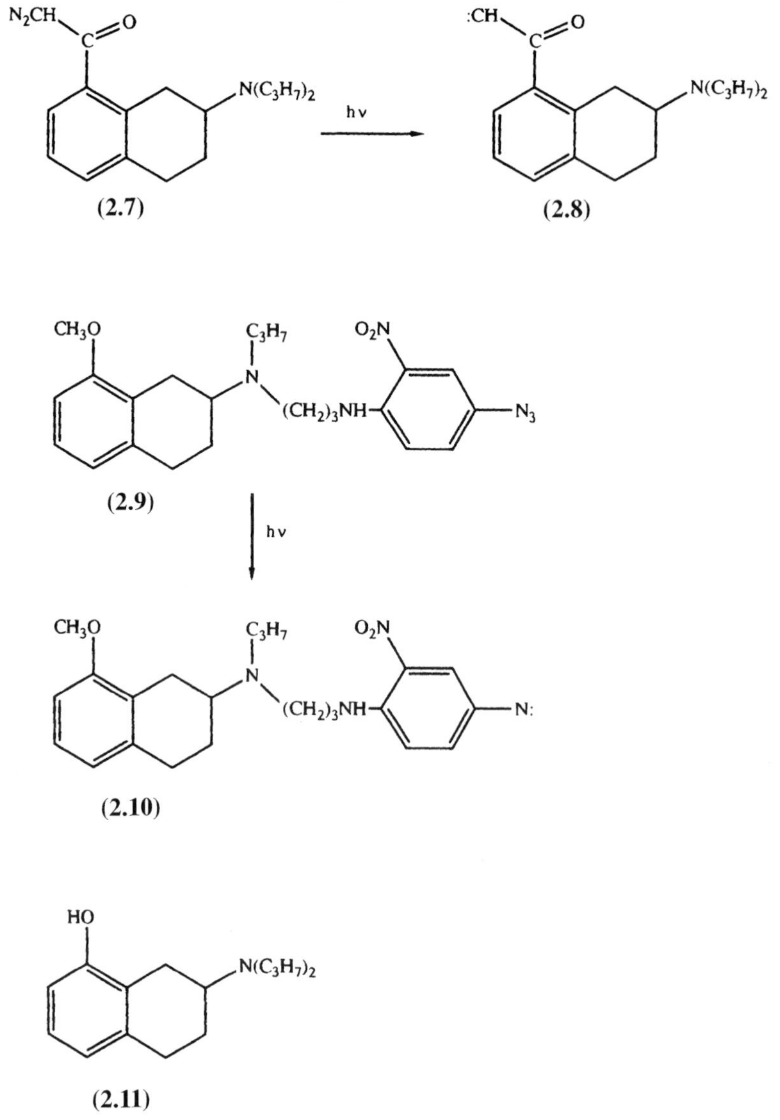

Scheme 2.1

Receptor agonist with equal affinities may differ in their ability to elicit a response from a receptor, i.e., they may have different potencies. Various parameters such as intrinsic activity (α), efficacy (e) and intrinsic efficacy (E) have been used to rationalize these differences. By definition, an antagonist does not have intrinsic activity, efficacy of intrinsic efficacy. These terms may be derived (equations 2.3–2.5) from the maximal response (E) of a particular agonist when compared to the maximal response of a full agonist (E_{max}) by taking into account the number of occupied receptors, DR, and total number of receptors, R_T:

$$\frac{E}{E_{max}} = \frac{\alpha[DR]}{[R_T]} \tag{2.3}$$

$$\frac{E}{E_{max}} = f\left(\frac{e[DR]}{[R_T]}\right) \tag{2.4}$$

$$\frac{E}{E_{max}} = f(\varepsilon[DR]) \tag{2.5}$$

Alkylating ligands may be used in pharmacological experiments in which so called spare receptors are inactivated. This may enable accurate determinations of efficacies, e.g., propylbenzilylcholine mustard (**2.12**) may be used to selectively inactivate a desired number

(2.12)

of muscarinic receptors. The mustard itself is of fairly low reactivity in its protonated form, however, upon deprotonation, it rapidly cyclizes to a much more reactive aziridinium ion (see also Chapter 6). By use of this ligand to inactivate spare receptors it has been possible to compare relative efficacies of muscarinic agonists which may be of interest as therapeutic agents in the treatment of senile dementia (Table 2.3). It is apparent that a much better understanding of the receptor interaction is obtained using this approach than in experiments in which only direct measures of potencies are obtained since the relative potencies of the enantiomers differ from their relative efficacies.

Non-covalent interactions. Although alkylating agents are of significant interest in both therapy and basic research, the majority of all drugs do not form covalent bonds with their receptors. Instead, a combination of rather weak intermolecular attractions such as electrostatic forces, dispersion forces, hydrogen bonds and the hydrophobic effect make major contributions to the formation of complexes between receptors and drugs (see Table 2.4 for a summary of intermolecular forces and related energies). In a more fundamental sense, the energy between molecules (atoms) may be described in terms of five components:

(i) The *electrostatic attraction* may be due to an ion-ion, an ion-dipole or a dipole-dipole interaction. The distance dependence increases in that order, that is, whereas the energy for an ion-ion interaction decreases with $1/r$ (r is the distance between interacting nuclei), the energy for a dipole-dipole interaction decreases with $1/r^3$.

(ii) The *polarization energy* is related to a charge redistribution (polarization) which may occur when two molecules approach each other. It may be of the ion-induced dipole or dipole-induced dipole type.

(iii) The *charge-transfer energy* is due to a small flow of electrons between interacting molecules. Thus, π-deficient aromatic rings may form weak complexes with π-rich counterparts.

(iv) The *exchange repulsion energy* is a repulsive term which results from the fundamental principle that electrons with the same spin should be separated in space. This term diminishes exponentially with the distance between atoms.

(v) The *dispersion energy* contributes to the attraction between polarizable molecules (atoms) even if permanent dipoles are absent. It is the only energy component which accounts for the formation of dimers of the rare gases. The strength of the dispersion interaction increases with the ease of polarizability of the interacting nuclei. Thus, the dispersion stabilization of Xe-Xe is stronger than that of Ne-Ne. The dispersion component of the complex energy is often referred to as London or van der Waals attraction.

In biological systems, electrostatic bonds, hydrogen bonds, van der Waals bonds, effects related to electron-transfer and the hydrophobic effect are of major importance. In solvents with low dielectric constants, the electrostatic forces between ions are by far the strongest of the noncovalent intermolecular forces. In water, these forces become less important because of solvation. It is hard to appreciate the strength of the electrostatic interaction in drug

Table 2.3   Relative efficacies and potencies of the muscarinic oxotremorine and BM-5 in the ileum.

Compd	Structure	Relative efficacy	Relative potency
Oxotremorine		1.00	1.00
(R)-BM-5		0.095	0.25
(S)-BM-5		0.11	0.015

Table 2.4   Approximate energies of intermolecular interactions[a].

Interaction	energy (KJ/mol)
Reinforced ionic bond	40
Ionic bond	20
Hydrogen bond	4–30
Ion-dipole interaction	4–30
Dipole-dipole interaction	4–30
van der Waals interaction	2–4

[a] Adapted from W.O.F. Foye: Principles of Medicinal Chemistry, Lea and Febiger, Philadelphia, 1981.

receptor complexes since the water content of the environment is unknown. Nevertheless, the electrostatic interaction appears to be the primary/dominating interaction between drugs and receptors. The strength of this interaction decreases rapidly with the distance between interacting nuclei.

Most neurotransmitter receptor proteins seem to contain acidic amino acid residues which may anchor positively charged endogenous neurotransmitters or exogenous drugs. In this context, it may be noted that most drugs that act on these receptors contain a basic nitrogen which will be protonated at physiological pH. The electrostatic interaction may be amplified by the participation of a hydrogen bond — thereby forming a reinforced ionic bond.

van der Waals (dispersion) forces are weak and decrease rapidly with the distance between interacting nuclei ($E = 1/r^6$). They are present in interactions between most types of molecules and arise from fluctuations in the electron distribution, which occur even in non-polar molecules, and which generate temporary electrical fields. Although a van der Waals bond is relatively weak, the summation of all the van der Waals bonds between two molecules in a complex may result in a very important energy contribution.

The hydrogen bond is fairly weak but is of paramount importance in biological systems. Hydrogen bonds probably contain contributions from all the five energy components described above but the major contribution usually comes from the electrostatic component. It may be described as a weak association between an electronegative atom (the hydrogen bond acceptor) and a hydrogen covalently linked to another electronegative atom (the hydrogen bond donor). A reinforced hydrogen bond involves an ion-ion interaction in addition to the hydrogen bond; an example is the interaction between a carboxylate ion and a protonated amine. The energy content of a hydrogen bond varies with the solvent but in water it is normally between 4–20 kJ/mol. The energy varies with the distance and angle between the interacting nuclei. It appears that the hydrogen bond in $C = O \cdots H-N$ becomes stronger when it is formed in the plane of the carbonyl group and along one of the lone pair sp^2-orbitals. This indicates that orbital overlap is important. The most spectacular example of hydrogen bonds is found in DNA which contains numerous hydrogen bonds between the various base pairs that stabilize its particular three-dimensional arrangement (Fig. 2.2).

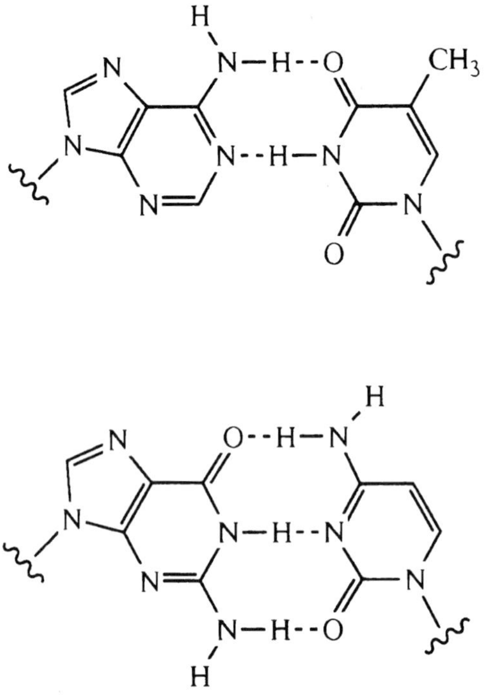

Figure 2.2 Hydrogen bonds that stabilize adenine-tymine (top) and guanine-cytosine (bottom) interaction in DNA.

The hydrophobic effect plays an important role in drug-receptor interactions. It is sometimes
called a hydrophobic bond which is misleading since the effect is due to an increased entropy
for the drug receptor complex and its environment. The hydrophobic effect is related to the
structure of water. Water alone is a dynamic system formed by water molecules connected
by hydrogen bonds which are constantly formed and broken (it has, however, a rather low
entropy even at 37 °C). When non-polar compounds are dissolved in water, the entropy
decreases since the water molecules at the surface of the solute form a highly ordered
hydrogen bonded network. The larger the surface of the solute, the lower the entropy and
the higher becomes the energy of the system. In order for the net-entropy of the system
to increase, non-polar solutes tend to aggregate to decrease the total surface area. Thus,
the hydrophobic effect is due to entropic changes in a system. However, intermolecular
interactions are also affected by another entropic change, a decreased structural mobility
of each of the two molecules interacting with each other. Thus, whereas chemical reactions
may often be properly modeled on the basis of entalphy changes, many intermolecular
processes may depend more on entropy. In fact, many biological processes may be entropy-
controlled.

Table 2.5   Selected biological stereoselectivities.

drug	observation
Disopyramide	The (S)-enantiomer is 4–5 times more potent as an anti-arrhythmic drug whereas the (R)-enantiomer is more potent in producing inotropic effects.
Indomethacin	Only the (S)-enantiomer is an anti-inflammatory agent.
α-Methyl dopa	Only the (S)-enantiomer produces hypotension and only this enantiomer inhibits the aromatic amino acid decarboxylase
Nicotine	The (R)-enantiomer is substrate for N-methyl whereas the (S)-enantiomer is a competitive inhibitor.
Penicillamine	The L-enantiomer is highly toxic
Propranolol	The (S)-enantiomer is hundred fold more potent than the antipode in blocking inotropic and chronotropic effects due to β_1 and β_2-stimulation.
Tranylcypromins	The (1S, 2R)-enantiomer is a more powerful blocker of MAO whereas the (1R, 2S)-enantiomer is more potent in blocking monoaminergic uptake mechanisms.
Warfarin	The (R)-enantiomer is metabolized mainly by reduction of the carbonyl moiety and by C6- or C8-hydroxylation. The (S)-enantiomer is predominantly metabolized by C7-hydroxylation.

2.3 STERIC AND CONFORMATIONAL ASPECTS

A drug must possess a certain structural complementarity to the receptor in order to bind with high affinity. This implies that conformational and stereochemical factors may play an important role in drug action. In fact, this has been demonstrated repeatedly. As early as 1858, Pasteur observed that (+)-tartaric acid inhibited the growth of the mold *Penicillium glaucum*. In contrast, the (−)-enantiomer appeared to be inactive in this respect. In 1908, Muller showed that (−)-adrenalin is the more potent hypertensive enantiomer in dogs. More recently, numerous examples of pharmacological stereoselectivity have emerged in the literature, some examples are given in Table 2.5. It should be noted that stereoselectivity is not confined to the drug-receptor interaction. Stereoisomers may, e.g. undergo stereoselective metabolism or uptake. In fact, only rarely, if at all, do enantiomers have identical biological properties. Thus, over the past thirty years it has become increasingly apparent that stereoselectivity has to be considered in drug development. In the fifties and sixties, it happened that mixtures of diastereomers were registered as drugs. Today, this would not be considered as acceptable. However, racemates are still being developed into drugs and of 521 chiral synthetic drugs marketed worldwide today, only 61 are marketed as single enantiomers. When it comes to drugs from natural sources and semisynthetic drugs, the picture is different: of 517 chiral drugs, only 8 are marketed as racemates. From a regulatory point of view, it has become increasingly apparent that the use of a pure enantiomer of a drug may offer therapeutic advantages as compared to the racemate. Therefore, it will be much more difficult to register racemates as drugs in the future.

There are many reasons for the large number of racemic drugs, most of them of economic and practical nature. It used to be difficult to synthesize enantiomers. Today, however, synthetic chemists may produce enantiomerically pure compounds by a variety of methods (Schemes 2.2 and 2.3). These may, e.g., involve asymmetric synthesis, synthesis from the chiral pool, enzymatic synthesis, and the classical resolution of diastereomeric salts

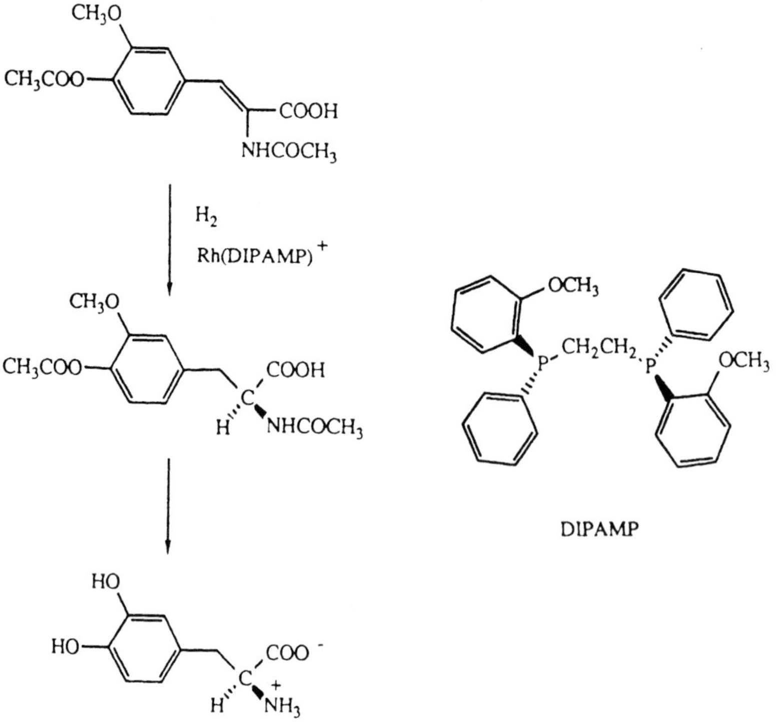

Scheme 2.2   Asymmetric hydrogenation applied to the synthesis of L-DOPA.

by fractional crystallization (see also Chapter 1). In addition, chromatography on chiral columns may be used to separate enantiomers even in large scale. It used to be very difficult to analyze enantiomers but progress in this area has been as impressive as in synthetic chemistry. Thus, numerous methods for analyzing enantiomers chromatograph- ically have emerged during the last decade. Unfortunately, the fact that it is impossible to unambiguously establish pharmacokinetic and pharmacodynamic properties of a chiral drug by studying the racemate has not been universally understood. Still, many scientists work with racemates without grasping the limitations and, therefore, overinterpreting the results.

To explain biological stereoselectivity, models involving three attachment points between drugs and receptors have been frequently used. According to such models (Fig. 2.3) the more potent enantiomer can develop three (intermolecular) bonds to the receptor surface whereas the less potent enantiomer only is able to form two bonds. This is a consequence of the idea that the drug has to adopt one particular orientation in relation to the receptor site. If we consider less abstract models it becomes apparent that the less potent enantiomer is

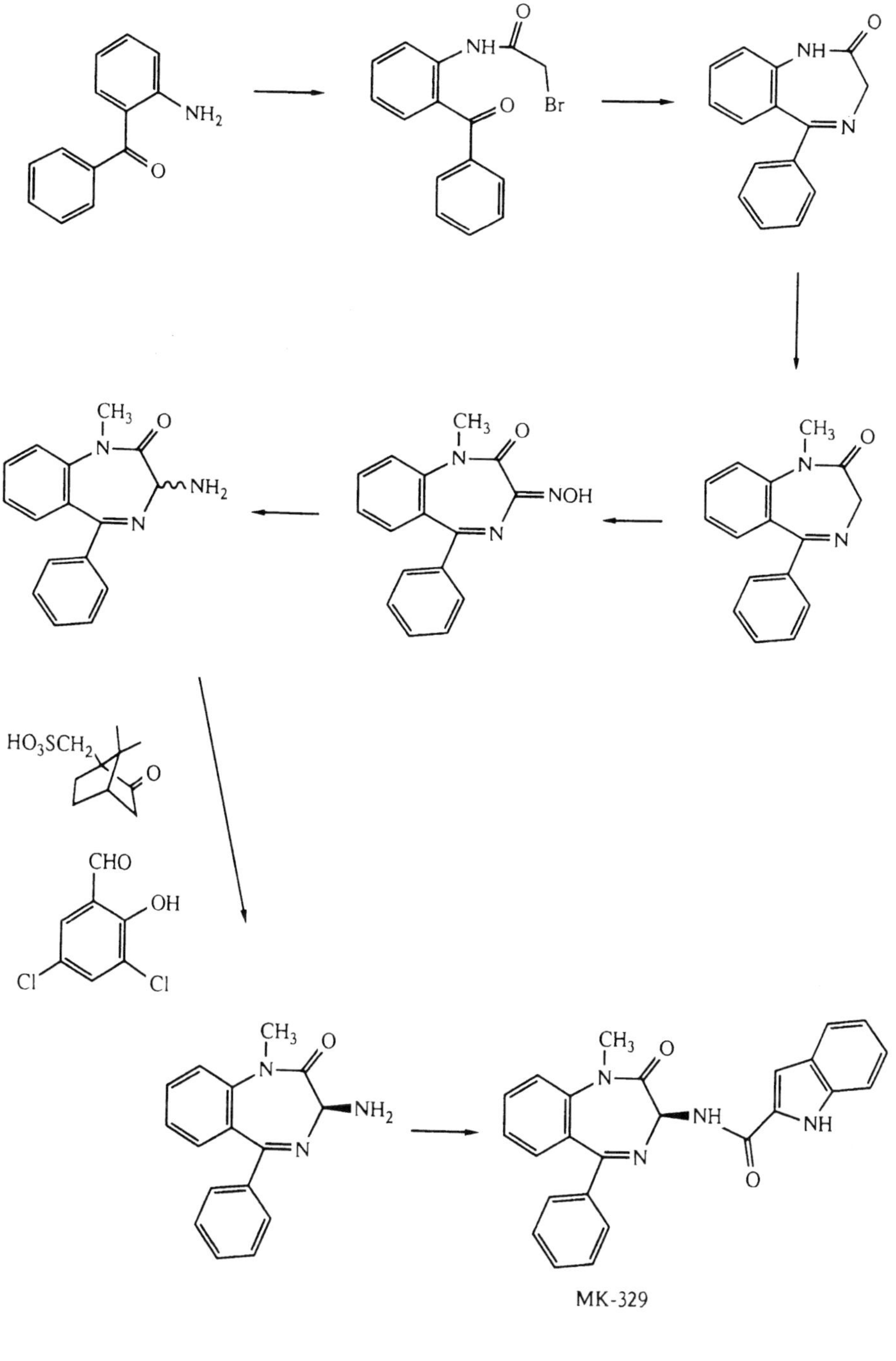

Scheme 2.3   Synthesis of the potent cholecystokinin A (CCK A) receptor antagonist MK-329. The key step is the crystallization-induced transformation of the racemic primary amino derivative into the desired (S)-enantiomer.

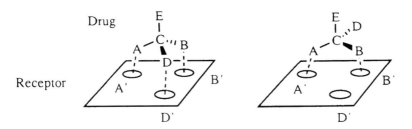

Figure 2.3   Traditional simplified model used to rationalize drug stereoselectivity. Only one of the enantiomers
   (left) has the spatial arrangement that allows for development of three intermolecular bonds to the receptor.

also able to develop three intermolecular bonds to the receptor provided that it approaches
the receptor site in a different manner. Thus, the picture is much more complicated than
generally believed. In addition, a three point attachment is not at all necessary to explain
stereoselectivity. Three interaction points, repulsive or attractive, are sufficient. Thus, one
attachment point and two obstacles may be equally effective to model a stereoselective
interaction. However, when docking e.g. a substrate with the active site of an enzyme
it becomes apparent that numerous contacts between the receptor and the ligand are
possible. An additional factor to consider is that a mutual structural rearrangement of both
enzyme/receptor and substrate/ligand may occur during complex formation. Thus, not only
stereochemistry but also conformational mobility has to be considered when evaluating
possible modes of binding of drugs. It may very well be that the bioactive conformations
of two enantiomers are different and, in addition, the receptor sites may be different due to
a conformational adaptation of the receptor site to the enantiomer.

2.4 METHODS TO STUDY MOLECULAR STRUCTURES

To study the structure of a drug, various physical and theoretical methods may be used.
Determinations of absolute configurations are most frequently done by use of X-ray
crystallography or by chemical correlation. In studies of enzyme-substrate interactions,
X-ray crystallography has become a very powerful tool since it allows investigation of
not only the enzyme but also of the enzyme-bound conformation of a drug. In addition,
the information obtained from such studies may be used in modeling and design. If the
preferred solution conformation of a compound is known, circular dichroism may be used
to deduce the configuration.

During the last decade, NMR-spectroscopy has undergone a tremendous development.
Powerful instruments are available at reasonable prices and numerous new pulse sequences
which provide exciting possibilities are constantly being developed. Today, 2D-NMR
spectroscopy on instruments with high resolution (above 200 MHz) and various heteronu-
clear NMR-applications may be considered as routine. Determinations of conformational
preferences rely heavily on NMR-experiments. Geometries of preferred conformations are
deduced based primarily on vicinal coupling constants and nuclear Overhauser effects

(NOEs). The magnitude of a vicinal coupling is related to the dihedral angle between the interacting nuclei. Therefore, these coupling constants may provide valuable geometrical information. It should be noted that not only vicinal proton-proton couplings provide information on dihedral angles. Also couplings between other nuclei, e.g. between a carbon and a vicinal hydrogen may provide geometrical angular information. NOE data, which are related to distances between nuclei, offer additional information. In particular, NOE data are useful in such cases where vicinal couplings are absent and in studies of macromolecules. However, NMR data are weighted averages of various co-existing conformers present at equilibrium. Since several conformations frequently may be present in solution this limitation may be difficult to overcome, in particular when dealing with large molecules such as polypeptides.

The conformational mobility of a compound may also be studied theoretically by molecular mechanics or quantum mechanical calculations (see Chapter 3).

2.5 DOPAMINE AND SEROTONIN-RECEPTOR AGONISTS AND ANTAGONISTS

The effects of various structural parameters on the DA and serotonin (5-HT, **2.13**) receptor stimulating ability of interesting DA- and 5-HT-analogs will be used to illustrate the importance of structural factors on drug action.

5-HT

(2.13)

The details of the function and regulation of the dopaminergic systems in the brain are not well understood but the following is generally accepted: There are two major subtypes of DA receptors — D_1 and D_2 like receptors — which interact with each other in an apparently synergistic fashion. The D_2-receptors belong to what is commonly referred to as the G-protein coupled receptor-superfamily. Other members in this class involve five muscarinic receptor subtypes, several serotonergic receptors, including the 5-HT_{1A}-, the 5-HT_{1C}- and the 5-HT_2-receptors, the beta adrenergic receptors and many peptidergic receptors. All receptor proteins in this superfamily are believed to have a particular structural feature in common — they appear to possess seven lipophilic regions which pass back and forth through the cell membrane (see also Chapters 9 and 10).

D_2 receptors are present on presynaptic nerve terminals and are also located postsynapti-cally. Stimulation of the presynaptic nerve terminals results in an inhibition of the enzyme tyrosine hydroxylase which is responsible for the conversion of tyrosine (**2.14**) into DOPA (Fig. 2.4). In addition, a presynaptic stimulation is believed to decrease the release of DA. Thus, the presynaptic receptors are part of a feedback system which is used to counteract

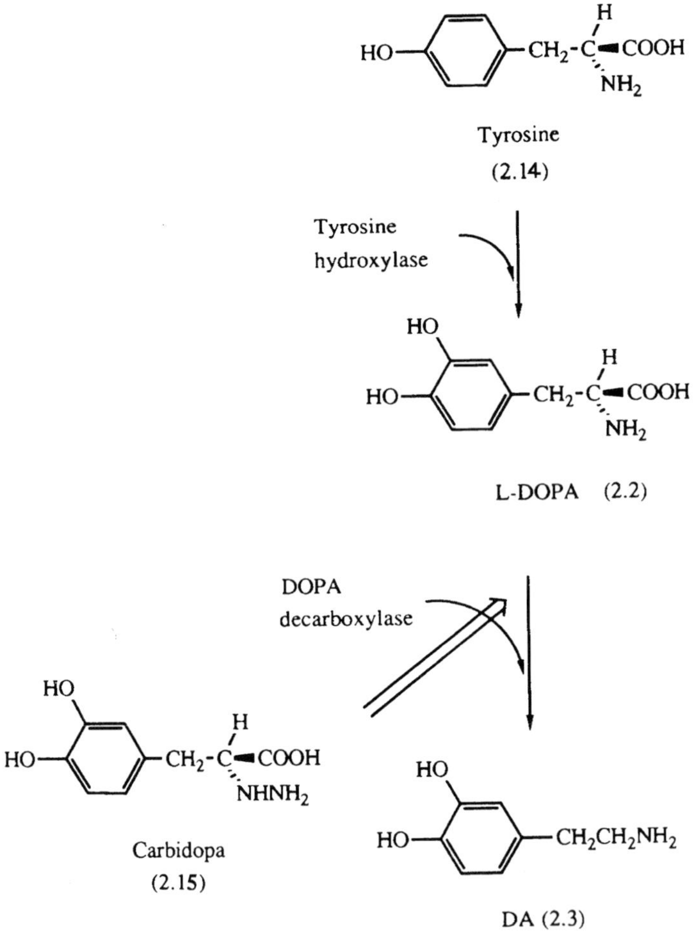

Figure 2.4   Biosynthesis of dopamine (DA). The enzyme responsible for decarboxylation of L-DOPA is inhibited by carbidopa (**2.15**).

excessive concentrations of DA in the synaptic cleft. In addition to this system, also other feedback systems may be utilized by the dopaminergic neuron.

Stimulation of the presynaptic D_2-receptors inhibits DA synthesis and release. Thus, selective stimulation of presynaptic D_2-receptors should produce a response equivalent to that observed after a postsynaptic D_2-receptor blockade. By analogy, inhibition of the presynaptic receptors would be functionally equivalent to stimulation of postsynaptic D_2-receptors. Thus, a DA-receptor agonist with high selectivity for presynaptic over postsynaptic D_2-receptors may offer an alternative to use postsynaptic antagonists in the treatment of psychosis.

DA is not suitable as a centrally active drug due to a variety of reasons, e.g. its catechol function is easily oxidized, it is very poorly distributed into the brain and it is readily

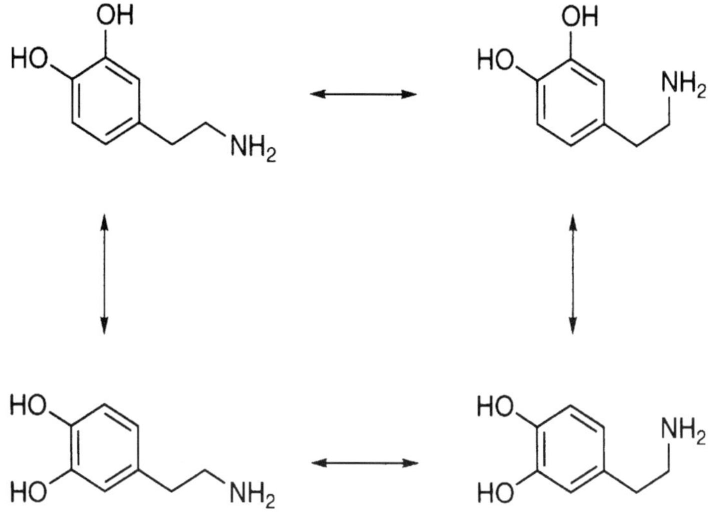

Figure 2.5 Four interconvertible conformations of the flexible neurotransmitter dopamine.

degraded by e.g. MAO and various other enzymes. In addition, it is not selective for a particular subtype of DA receptors. The problem with the poor bioavailability has been solved in an elegant fashion by administration of the biosynthetic precursor L-DOPA together with a DOPA decarboxylase inhibitor, for example carbidopa (**2.15**, Fig. 2.4) which is unable to pass the blood-brain barrier. DOPA, on the other hand, which is less lipophilic than DA, is transported into the brain by an active transport system. By this "trick", peripheral side effects due to excessive DA levels in the periphery are minimized. L-DOPA therapy has proven rather useful in Parkinson's disease in which the symptoms arise because of a degeneration of dopaminergic neurons and a resulting imbalance between dopaminergic and cholinergic output in the brain.

DA is a flexible molecule (Fig. 2.5) but a number of investigators have tried to establish the "active" conformation of DA using the assumption that it should be equivalent to the minimum-energy conformation in a particular aggregation state. The following observations have been made: In the solid state, DA hydrochloride adopts an anti conformation with the ethylamine chain extended and almost perpendicular to the plane of the benzene ring. In aqueous solution, however, there are about equal amounts of the anti and gauche conformers and the latter has a folded ethylamine chain. It has also been demonstrated using calculational chemistry that various other conformations of DA are possible. Thus, it is impossible to draw conclusions on the receptor bound conformation of a flexible compound since this conformation does not necessarily correspond to the global minimum-energy conformation. In fact, fairly large energy penalties may be allowed even for potent compounds since the stabilizing interactions in a receptor-ligand complex may become quite large. Therefore, more information may be gained from studies of series of conformationally restricted analogs.

3-PPP (2.16)

3-PPP (**2.16**) was synthesized as a conformationally restricted DA-analog. It contains a stereogenic centre and, thus, two enantiomers exist of 3-PPP. In most test systems, racemic 3-PPP behaves as a highly selective agonist for presynaptic DA receptors. Thus, it inhibits DA synthesis in reserpine-pretreated rats (in which the monoamine stores are depleted) without being able to counteract the reserpine-induced akinesia (immobility). Post- and presynaptic DA-receptor agonists, such as (*R*)-apomorphine (**2.17**, Scheme 2.5), produce the same inhibition of DA-synthesis but also counteract the reserpine-induced akinesia. The latter effect is supposed to be due to postsynaptic stimulation. Thus, (±)-3-PPP behaves as a DA-receptor agonist with a selective action on presynaptic receptors and it became a prototype for a new type of dopaminergic agents with potential use in central disturbances related to dopaminergic overactivity (such as schizophrenia). However, when the pure enantiomers were investigated pharmacologically, it turned out that the apparent selectivity of the racemate was due to counteracting effects of the enantiomers on the postsynaptic DA D_2-receptors: (*R*)-3-PPP behaved as a typical DA-receptor agonist both on pre- and postsynaptic DA-receptors. In contrast, in most test systems, the (*S*)-enantiomer acts as an antagonist on postsynaptic receptors and as an agonist on presynaptic receptors. In fact, this strange profile of (*S*)-3-PPP is typical for a weak partial agonist. That is, the efficacy of (*S*)-3-PPP is too weak to induce an effect on the postsynaptic DA D_2-receptors which are less sensitive for agonist stimulation than presynaptic receptors. It has been suggested

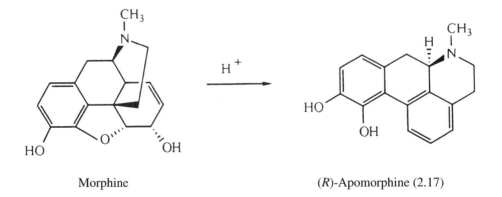

Morphine   (*R*)-Apomorphine (2.17)

Scheme 2.4   (*R*)-Apomorphine is readily prepared from natural morphine by an acid-catalyzed rearrangement.

that less stable conformers of both (*R*)- and (*S*)-3-PPP would interact with DA-receptors and that their different efficacies would be due to different abilities to interact with a "propyl group binding site" at the receptor. It is noteworthy, that other examples of interesting stereoselectivities may be found among the dopaminergic 2-aminotetralins.

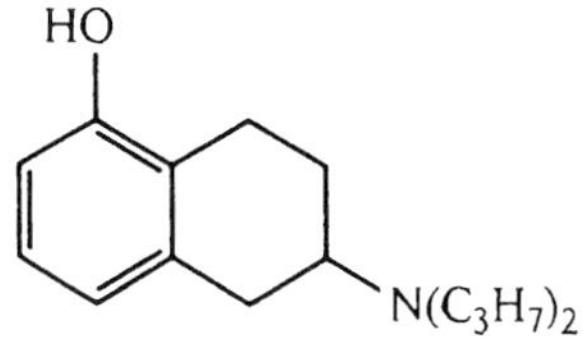

HO

5-OH DPAT

N(C$_3$H$_7$)$_2$

(2.18)

5-OH DPAT (**2.18**) is a DA-receptor agonist of much higher potency than 3-PPP and with a higher selectivity for D$_2$- over D$_1$-receptors than (*R*)-apomorphine. Like 3-PPP, 5-OH DPAT is a conformationally restricted DA-analog with one stereogenic centre (at C2). The agonist potency of 5-OH DPAT resides in the (*S*)-enantiomer. In contrast, (*R*)-5-OH DPAT is a DA D$_2$-receptor antagonist, but more than 100-fold less potent as a DA-receptor ligand than (*S*)-5-OH DPAT. Therefore, the profile of racemic 5-OH DPAT is indistinguishable from that of the (*S*)-enantiomer. When the hydroxyl group is moved from C5 to the other aromatic positions, interesting effects are observed (Table 2.6). 6-OH DPAT (**2.19**) loses most of the dopaminergic potency whereas 7-OH DPAT (**2.20**) is a potent DA-receptor ligand. 8-OH DPAT (**2.11**) is not a DA-receptor agonist but a potent and selective serotonergic 5-HT$_{1A}$-receptor agonist.

Table 2.6   Pharmacological profiles of some phenolic 2-dipropylaminotetralins.

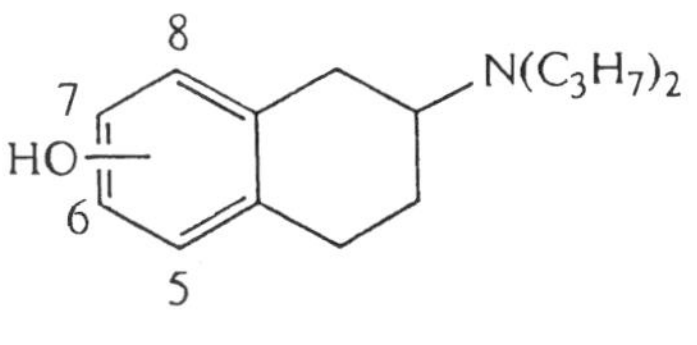

OH-position	abs. config	pharmacological profile
5	(*S*)	potent DA D$_2$-receptor agonist
5	(*R*)	weakly potent DA D$_2$-receptor antagonist
6	(±)	weakly potent dopaminergic agonist
7	(*S*)	inactive (?)
7	(*R*)	potent DA D$_2$-receptor agonist
8	(*S*)	potent 5-HT$_{1A}$-receptor agonist
8	(*R*)	potent 5-HT$_{1A}$-receptor agonist

HO — [structure]

6-OH DPAT
(2.19)

N(C₃H₇)₂ → $N(C_3H_7)_2$

7-OH DPAT
(2.20)

HO — [structure] — $N(C_3H_7)_2$

HO — [structure] — $N—C_3H_7$

(2.21)

To be able to discuss conformational factors of importance for the biological activity it is necessary to compare conformers to a pharmacophore model (Chapter 3). Such models are most readily obtained by structural comparisons of fairly rigid structures. In the DA-area, several such compounds are available. It is possible to derive a DA D_2-pharmacophore from the potent and fairly rigid agonists (R)-apomorphine and octahydrobenzo[f]quinoline derivative **2.21** by computer-aided comparisons of all possible conformations of the two compounds. Based on structure-activity studies it has been deduced that DA-receptor agonists related to 5-OH DPAT interact with the receptor basically through a reinforced ionic bond from the protonated nitrogen, hydrogen bonding from the phenolic hydroxyl (or an isosteric hydrogen donating functionality such as an indole N-H) and an electrostatic interaction which includes the aromatic ring. As stated above, the primary interaction between amine-containing neurotransmitter analogs is believed to be a reinforced ionic interaction. The conformations that produce the best fit of these pharmacophore elements should contain the pharmacophore groups in a bioactive conformation. It turns out that the best fit of the pharmacophore points/groups of (R)-apomorphine and **2.21** is obtained with their minimum-energy conformations and the fit defines a dopaminergic pharmacophore in three dimensions (Fig. 2.6). Thus, the energetically favored half chair conformation with a pseudoequatorial dipropylammonium group of (S)-5-OH DPAT should correspond to a pharmacophore conformation. 7-OH DPAT possesses almost the same agonist potency as 5-OH DPAT but its stereoselectivity is reversed. Thus, (R)-7-OH DPAT is responsible for the dopaminergic activity of the racemate. In order to obtain the same relative orientation of the three pharmacophore elements, it has been suggested that the 5- and 7-hydroxylated regioisomers should adopt the relative orientations shown in Figure 2.7. This is a reasonable model since the two potent analogs will adopt the same orientation of their N^+–H moieties.

The dopaminergic phenolic 2-aminotetralins are fairly flexible molecules and offer an opportunity to demonstrate the importance of conformational factors in drug action.

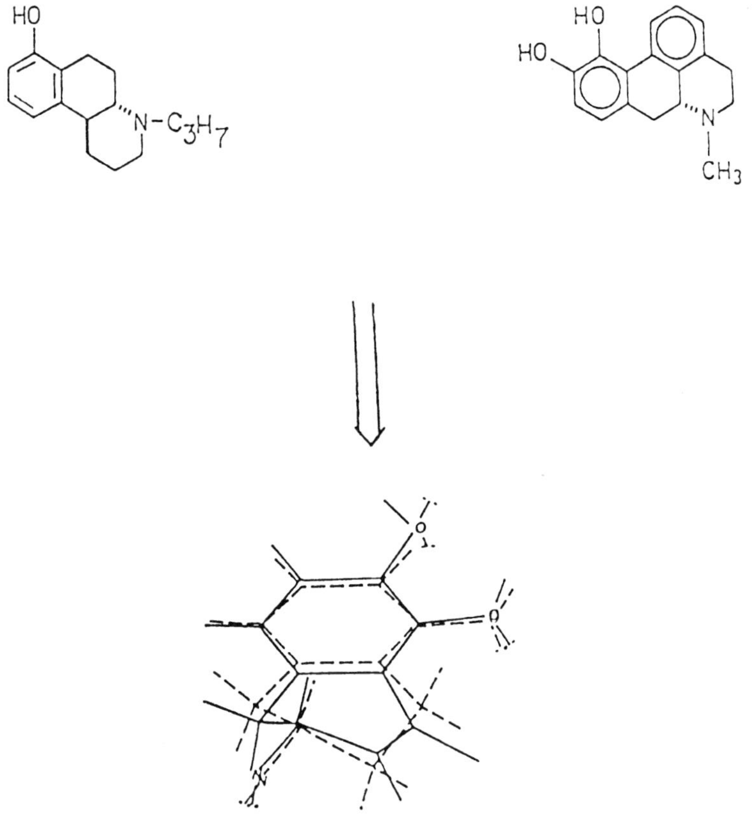

Figure 2.6   Generation of a dopaminergic pharmacophore conformation (bottom) for 2-aminotetralins by the best possible superposition of two conformationally restricted DA D_2-receptor agonists, 2.18 and (R)-apomorphine.

The series of compounds in Table 2.7 consists of a number of derivatives of 5-OH DPAT in which methyl substituents have been inserted. With one notable exception, the C3-methylated *cis*-derivative **2.24** (the synthesis is described in Scheme 2.5), the methyl derivatives are less or much less potent than 5-OH DPAT, itself. The lower potency of most of the compounds may be rationalized in conformational terms. Thus the weakly potent *trans*-C1-methyl derivative **2.23** does not readily adopt a conformation which fits to the DA D_2-pharmacophore discussed above. In fact, this compound differs from the other by readily adopting conformations with a pseudoaxial dipropylammonium substituent. The *trans*-C3-methyl derivative **2.25**, which is also weakly potent, preferentially adopts conformations with a pseudoequatorial C2-substituent but only unwillingly dipropylammonium substituents with the optimal N^+–H orientation. Although the *cis*-C1-methyl derivative **2.22** readily adopts pharmacophore conformations, it is only of moderate potency as a DA-receptor agonist. Since the loss in activity as compared to 5-OH DPAT is not due to conformational factors, it may be attributed to the steric bulk of the methyl group

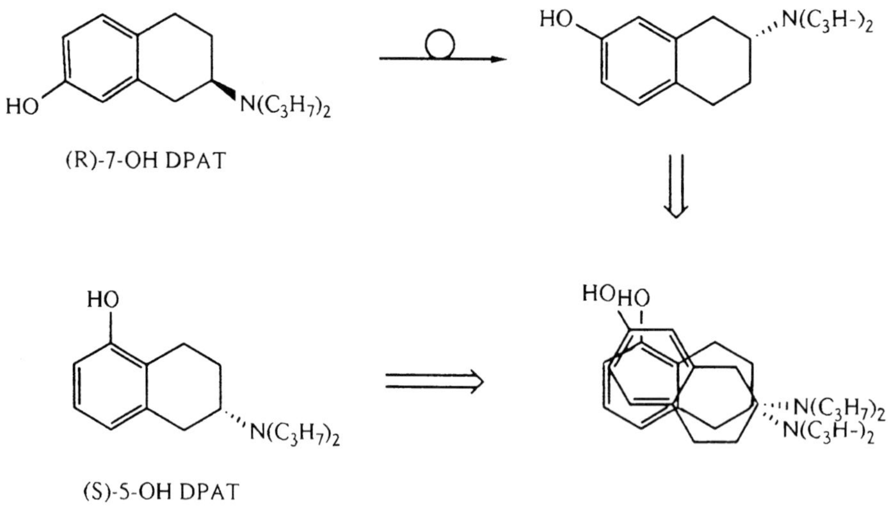

(R)-7-OH DPAT

(S)-5-OH DPAT

Figure 2.7 The opposite stereoselectivities of the dopamine receptor agonists 5- and 7-OH DPAT may be rationalized by a "flip" of 7-OH DPAT.

which may prevent an optimal receptor interaction. The C2-methyl derivative **2.26**, which shows a complex pharmacological profile involving serotonergic components, is not a DA-receptor agonist. This particular derivative prefers to adopt conformations with the dipropylammonium substituent in a pseudoaxial position. However, it has not been possible to unambiguously establish whether the inactivity is due to conformational factors or to the steric bulk of the C2-methyl substituent.

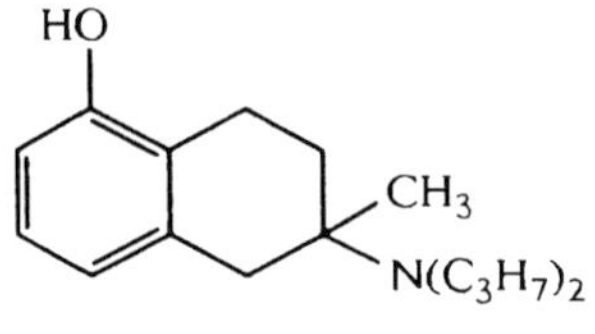

(2.26)

In contrast to 5-OH DPAT which is a highly stereoselective dopaminergic agent, 8-OH DPAT (**2.11**) is a potent serotonergic 5-HT$_{1A}$-receptor agonist with low stereoselectivity, the potency and affinity of the (R)-enantiomer being only about two times larger than that of the antipode. This low stereoselectivity indicates that the receptor interaction between the 5-HT$_{1A}$-receptor and 8-OH DPAT is different from that of 5-OH DPAT and the DA D$_2$-receptor. Indeed, SAR data indicate that the hydroxyl group in 5-OH DPAT serves as a hydrogen bond donor whereas the hydroxyl group in 8-OH DPAT does not. In fact, the presence of a C8-substituent does not appear to be necessary for potent serotonergic

Table 2.7 Dopaminergic potencies and relative steric energies of the pharmacophore conformation of some 2-aminotetralins

Compound		Dopaminergic agonist potency	Relative steric energy of the pharmacophore conformation (kcal/mol)
(S) 5-OH-DPAT (**2.18**)		very potent	0.5
(1R, 2S)-UH-242 (**2.22**)		potent	0
(1S, 2S)-AJ-116 (**2.23**)		weakly potent	2.4
(2R, 3S)-AJ-166 (**2.24**)		very potent	0
(2R, 3R)-AJ-164 (**2.25**)		weakly potent	>2.5

activity. Therefore, one only has to consider two primary interaction points (pharmacophore elements) in preliminary models of 5-HT$_{1A}$-receptor agonists — one protonated nitrogen and an aromatic ring.

Introduction of methyl groups in the nonaromatic ring of 8-OH DPAT (**2.11**) leads to a considerable increase in stereoselectivity. The most impressive stereoselectivity is shown by the *cis*-C1-methyl substituted derivative **2.27** in which the affinity of the (1S, 2R)-enantiomer is more than 1000 times greater than that of the distomer (the less potent enantiomer). In contrast, when a *cis*-C1-methyl group is introduced in the dopaminergic 5-OH DPAT, producing **2.22**, the enantiomeric affinity ratio changes from about 100 to about 1. *Cis*- and

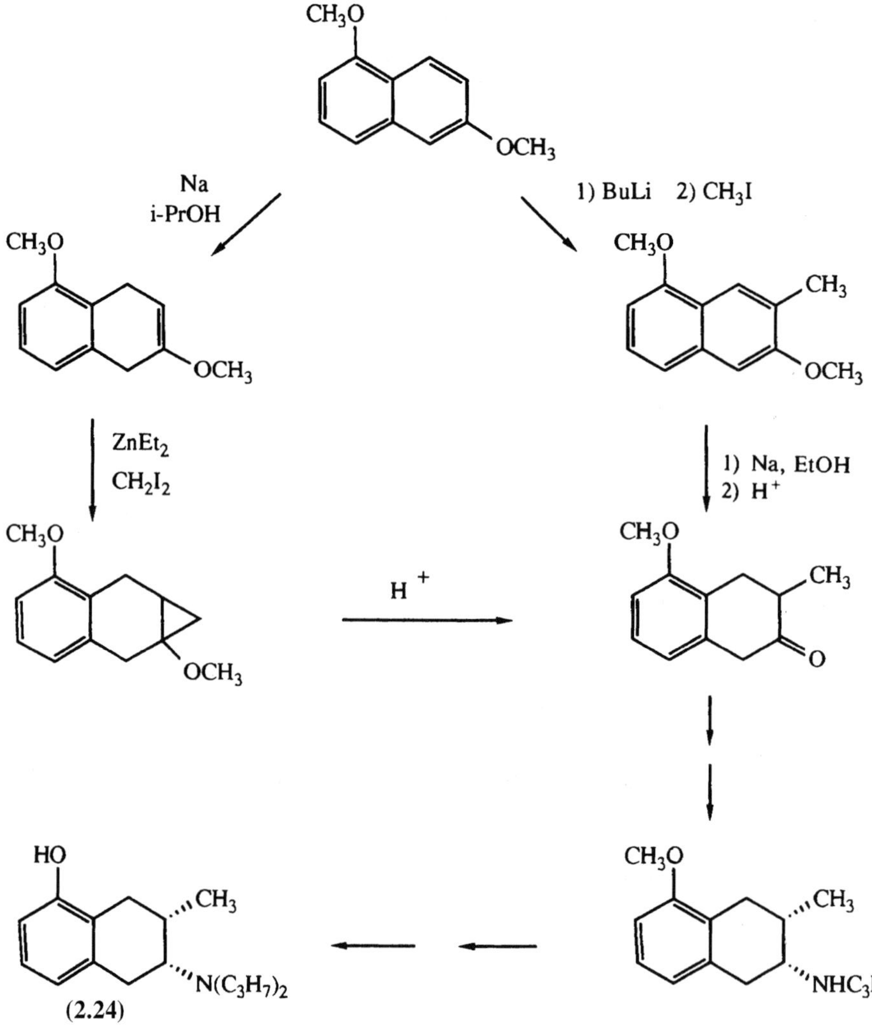

Scheme 2.5

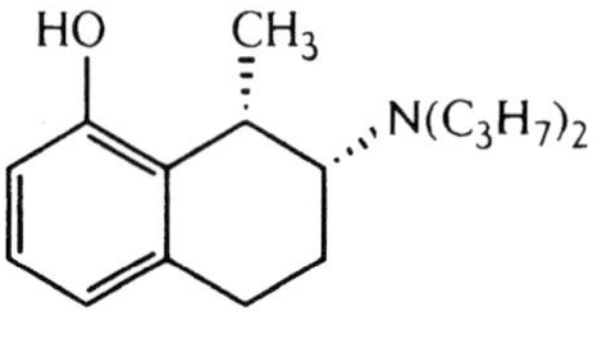

(1S, 2R)-ALK-3 (2.27)

(2.28)

trans-C3-methyl substitution in 8-OH DPAT also enhance stereoselectivity considerably but decrease potency and affinity.

A spectacular case of stereoselectivity has been observed in a fluorinated 8-OH DPAT analog. Racemic **2.28** was devoid of serotonergic activity when tested *in vivo*. However, when the enantiomers were investigated it became apparent that (*R*)-**2.28** was a typical 5-HT$_{1A}$-receptor agonist that produced all effects expected from an agonist of this type whereas the (*S*)-enantiomer behaved as an antagonist. Thus, the inactivity of the racemate was due to counteracting effects of the enantiomers. This example clearly points to the neccessity of studying pure enantiomers since data obtained with racemates may be misleading.

REFERENCES

Andrews, P. (1986) Functional groups, drug-receptor interactions and drug design. *Trends Pharmacol. Sci.*, 148–151.

Ariens, E.J., Soudijn, W. and Timmerman, P.B.M.W.M. (1983) *Stereochemistry and biological activity of drugs*, Blackwell, Oxford.

Brown, C. (1990) *Chirality in drug design and synthesis.* Academic Press, London.

Dean, P.M. (1987) *Molecular foundations of drug-receptor interactions.* Cambridge University Press, Cambridge.

Karlen, A., Helander, A., Kenne, L. and Hacksell, U. (1989) Topography and conformational preferences of 6,7,8,9-tetrahydro-1-hydroxy-N,N-dipropyl-5H-benzocyclohepten-6-ylamine. A rationale for the dopaminergic inactivity. *J. Med. Chem.*, **32**, 765.

Karlen, A., Helander, A., Johansson, A.M., Kenne, L., Sundell, S. and Hacksell, U. (1993) Conformational analysis of 2-aminotetralins: Molecular mechanics calculations, X-ray crystallography and nuclear magnetic resonance spectroscopy. *J. Chem. Res. (S)*, 448.

Malmberg, Å., Nordvall, G., Johansson, A.M., Mohell, N. and Hacksell, U. (1994) Molecular basis for the binding of 2-aminotetralins to human dopamine D$_{2A}$ and D$_3$ receptors. *Mol. Pharmacol.*, **46**, 299.

Wainer, I.W. and Drayer, D.E. (1988) *Drug stereochemistry: analytical methods and pharmacology.* Marcel Dekker, New York.

Yalkowsky, S.H., Sinkula, A.A. and Valvani, S.C. (1980) *Physical chemical properties of drugs.* Marcel Dekker, New York.

3. COMPUTER-AIDED DEVELOPMENT OF THREE-DIMENSIONAL PHARMACOPHORE MODELS

TOMMY LILJEFORS and INGRID PETTERSSON

CONTENTS

3.1 DIRECT AND INDIRECT COMPUTER-AIDED LIGAND DESIGN

The development of a new drug is a very expensive process which often takes a decade or more to complete. More than ten thousand compounds may be synthesized and tested in a drug development project before a new drug can reach the market (see Chapters 1 and 18).

The explosive development of computer technology and of methodology to calculate molecular properties have increasingly made it possible to use computer techniques to aid the drug development process with the aim of making it more rational. The so-called *rational drug design* methods employ computational chemistry in an attempt to develop new ligands which are able to bind to the target enzyme or receptor. The use of computer techniques in this context is often called *computer-aided drug design*, but since the development of a drug involves a large number of steps in addition to the development of a high-affinity ligand (bioavailability, toxicity and metabolism must also be taken into account as discussed in Chapter 1), a more appropriate name is *computer-aided ligand design*.

If the three-dimensional (3D) structure of the target enzyme or receptor is available from X-ray crystallography, preferentially with a co-crystallized ligand so that the binding site and binding mode of the ligand is known, it is feasible to study the biomacromolecule-ligand complex in a direct way by interactive computer graphics techniques and computational chemistry. In this way a detailed knowledge of the interactions between the ligand and the enzyme/receptor may be obtained. New candidate ligands may be "docked" into the binding site in order to study if the new structure can interact with the receptor in an optimal way. This procedure is known as *structure-based ligand design* or *receptor fitting* (Fig. 3.1). An example of the use of this type of ligand design in the development of new high-affinity ligands for dihydrofolate reductase (DHFR) is discussed in Chapter 17.

It may seem straightforward to develop new ligands for known enzyme or receptor structures, but there are many difficult problems involved. For instance, conformational changes of the ligand and/or the biomacromolecule may be necessary for an optimal binding. In addition, conformational energies, multiple binding modes and differential solvation effects must be taken into account. However, much progress in this field have been made in recent years and several successful examples of the use of structure-based ligand design in a drug development process have been reported. A particularly useful strategy is the iterative use of computer-aided receptor fitting, synthesis and testing of the designed ligand followed by X-ray crystallographic determination of the ligand-enzyme complex.

Structure-based ligand design requires that the 3D-structure of the biomacromolecule is known. Many target receptors of high interest in connection with drug development, for instance receptors for neurotransmitters, are membrane-bound and all attempts to crystallize and determine the structure of these receptors by X-ray crystallography have

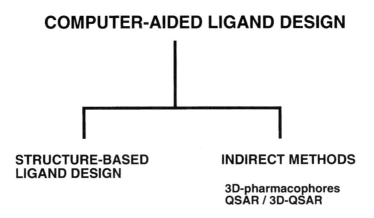

Figure 3.1   Direct and indirect methods in computer-aided ligand design.

so far been unsuccessful. In the absence of an experimentally determined 3D-structure for the receptor, rational ligand design may be performed by the use of an *indirect strategy* based on the analysis and comparison of molecular properties and receptor binding data for known receptor ligands (Fig. 3.1). In the present chapter, the development and use of 3D-pharmacophores will be discussed. The QSAR and 3D-QSAR methods are discussed in Chapter 4.

The underlying hypothesis of the indirect methods is a shape and electronic complementarity between the receptor and the ligand. In 3D-pharmacophore studies, the concept of *pharmacophore* is employed in an attempt to deduce the spatial relationships between those parts of the ligand which are essential for its binding to the receptor — the *3D-pharmacophore*. On the basis of this, a comparison of the molecular volumes of active and inactive compounds may additionally yield information about the dimensions of the binding cavity. High-affinity ligands are characterized by being capable of assuming a conformation which presents those parts of the ligand which are crucial for the affinity in such a way that they are complementary to the 3D-arrangement of the corresponding receptor binding sites. An additional requirement for high affinity is that the ligand in its receptor-bound conformation must not compete with the receptor for space.

A successful development of a 3D-pharmacophore model, including information about the dimensions of the receptor binding cavity, may be employed to design new ligands which fit the model. In contrast to the traditional Quantitative Structure-Activity Relationship (QSAR) methods (Chapter 4), this approach is useful not only for the optimization of a lead structure but also for design of novel lead structures for a target receptor.

It should be noted that 3D-pharmacophore models do not yield quantitative predictions of receptor affinities. The use of such models is restricted to the *classification* of candidate ligands as active or inactive (high or low affinity). Such a classification may be used in the selection of new molecules to be synthesized in a drug development project. However, 3D-pharmacophore models are the basis of the 3D-QSAR methodology (see Chapter 4) by which quantitative predictions may be made.

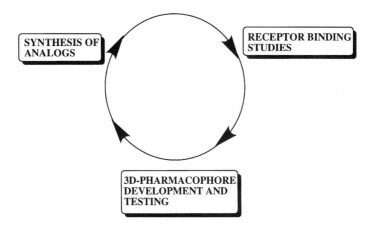

Figure 3.2 An iterative and multi-disciplinary approach is required for the development and use of a 3D-pharmacophore model.

The development of a 3D-pharmacophore model and its use for ligand design is necessarily an iterative and multi-disciplinary process (Fig. 3.2). The initial model, based on known ligands, is used to design new compounds to test the model and the outcome of receptor binding studies of the new compounds is used to refine (or discard) the model.

3.2 THE PHARMACOPHORE CONCEPT AND ITS USE

Pharmacophore and pharmacophore elements are central concepts in medicinal chemistry. The idea behind these concepts comes from the common observation that variations of some parts of the molecular structure of a compound drastically influence the activity at a target receptor, whereas variations of other parts only cause minor activity changes. (In the following the term receptor is used in a general sense for the biomacromolecular component and no distinction of enzymes and receptors are made).

A *pharmacophore element* is traditionally defined as an atom or a group of atoms (a functional group) common for active compounds with respect to a receptor and crucial for the activity of the compounds. However the concept of pharmacophore element may be fruitfully extended to include representations of interactions with receptor sites as discussed in Section 3.2.3. The *pharmacophore* is the collection of pharmacophore elements and the concept of *3D-pharmacophore* may be used when the relative spatial positions of the pharmacophore elements are included in the analysis. Thus, a 3D-pharmacophore consists of a specific 3D-arrangement of pharmacophore elements. The pharmacophore concept has been used for a long time in medicinal chemistry in a topological sense (2D), however the use of computer techniques has enormously facilitated the topographical (3D) use of the concept.

3.2.1 Steps in 3D-pharmacophore identification

It is useful for the following discussion to separate the 3D-pharmacophore identification process into a number of discrete steps.

Step 1. A set of high affinity ligands for the target receptor is collected and pharmacophore elements are selected. The molecules in the set should have as diverse structural frameworks as possible. Pharmacophore elements and their representation are discussed in Sections 3.2.2 and 3.2.3. The number of pharmacophore elements should be the same for all molecules in the set and it is a great advantage if the pharmacophore elements are identical for all compounds in the set. However, pharmacophore elements which are bioisosteres may be fruitfully used. In order to facilitate the next step in the process, the selected compounds should have as few torsional degrees of freedom as possible. The receptor binding data for the selected compounds, preferentially obtained by a radioligand binding assay, should be of high quality and preferably from the same laboratory.

Step 2. A conformational analysis is performed for each compound in the set in order to identify low-energy conformations for each active molecule. Conformational analysis is discussed in Section 3.3.2.

Step 3. Molecular superimposition techniques are used to identify low-energy conformations of each high-affinity molecule in the set, conformations for which the selected pharmacophore elements superimpose (see Section 3.4). The aim of this step is to find a common 3D-pharmacophore for all high-affinity compounds. If none is found, the selected pharmacophore elements should be reconsidered. If more than one common 3D-pharmacophore is found, there is probably too low diversity in the set of compounds and more compounds need to be added to the set.

The use of molecular superimpositions assumes that all compounds bind in a single binding mode. However, there may be sets of compounds for which this is not true and a common 3D-pharmacophore cannot be obtained. In such cases, the set may be divided into subsets corresponding to molecules with the same binding mode (see Section 3.2.4).

Step 4. When a common 3D-pharmacophore for all high-affinity compounds have been identified, inactive or low-affinity compounds which fit the 3D-pharmacophore may be used to explore the dimensions of the receptor cavity and to identify the receptor-excluded and receptor-essential volumes. This is discussed in Section 3.5.

3.2.2 Selection of pharmacophore elements

The selection of pharmacophore elements is generally based on experimental observations about parts (atoms, functional groups) of a set of active molecules which are common for these molecules and essential for the activity. Pharmacophore elements used in the development of 3D-pharmacophore models are most often atoms or functional groups (or derived from atoms or functional groups) which may interact with receptor binding sites *via* hydrogen bonds, electrostatic forces or van der Waals forces (for a discussion of such interactions see Chapter 2). Thus, heteroatoms such as oxygens and nitrogens and polar functional groups such as carboxylic acids, amides and hydroxy groups are commonly used as pharmacophore elements. Drug molecules frequently include aromatic ring systems.

Since such ring systems may strongly interact with, for instance, aromatic side-chains of the receptor they are very often selected as pharmacophore elements.

Many potent dopamine D-2 receptor agonists are derived from the structure of dopamine itself (**3.1**). Thus, their structures often include an *ortho*-dihydroxy phenyl (catechol) moiety and a nitrogen atom as exemplified by (**3.2**). However, only the *meta*-hydroxy group is necessary for activity as shown by the active compound (**3.3**). Furthermore, it has been demonstrated that the catechol/phenol moiety may be bioisosterically replaced by, for instance, an indole ring (**3.4**) or a pyrazole ring (**3.5**). Considering these experimental observations, suitable pharmacophore elements for dopamine D-2 receptor agonists may include the nitrogen atom corresponding to the one in (**3.1**), the aromatic ring and the *meta*-hydroxy group or its bioisosteric equivalent. A closer analysis of the structures suggests that it may be desirable to include the hydrogen bond donating and/or accepting properties of the hydroxy group in the pharmacophore. Similarly, explicit inclusion of the direction of the nitrogen atom-lone pair, or in the protonated case the N-H bond vectors, may extend the usefulness of the pharmacophore. Such extended pharmacophore elements are discussed in Section 3.2.2.

Although the pharmacophore concept originally was formulated in terms of atoms and functional groups, multi-atom functional groups as such are in general not useful in computer-aided 3D-pharmacophore identification. The reason for this is that most molecular superimposition techniques require the pharmacophore elements to be represented as points. If all atoms of a multi-atom functional group are used as pharmacophore elements, the statistical weight of such a group distorts the comparison of molecules by molecular least-squares superimposition techniques. Instead, geometrically well defined points representing the entire functional group may be used. Alternatively, as discussed in the next section, the functional group may be represented by its interactions with the receptor.

3.2.3 Representation of pharmacophore elements as ligand points or site points

If we consider a hydroxy group as a pharmacophore element, the important properties of this functional group in connection with its binding to the receptor are its hydrogen bond donating and accepting properties. The hydroxy group pharmacophore element may be represented in various ways as shown in Figure 3.3.

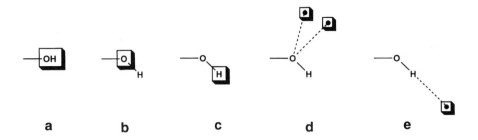

a   b   c   d   e

Figure 3.3   Various representations of a hydroxy group as a pharmacophore element.

The representation in Figure 3.3a does not specify any particular properties of the hydroxy group and a pharmacophore built on the selection of such a pharmacophore element merely requires that a hydroxy group is located at a particular location in 3D-space in all active compounds.

In Figure 3.3b,c the hydrogen bond accepting and donating properties, respectively, are indirectly specified. The use of the oxygen or the hydrogen atom as a pharmacophore element (a *ligand point*) implies that the corresponding atoms should superimpose in space in all active compounds. However, this does not take into account that a hydroxy group of a set of ligands may bind equally well to the receptor, even if the atoms of the functional group in different ligands have different locations in space. For instance, as illustrated in Figure 3.4, the hydroxy group may bond hydrogen equally well to a carbonyl group of a receptor binding site without requiring that the hydroxy hydrogen atom or oxygen atom in all active compounds are superimposable.

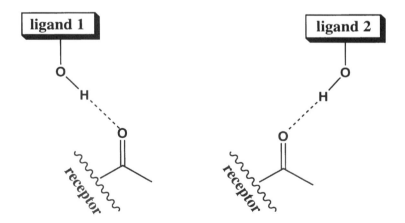

Figure 3.4   A hydroxy group may interact equally well with a carbonyl group in a ligand-receptor interaction without the requirement that the atoms of the hydroxy group in different ligands superimpose.

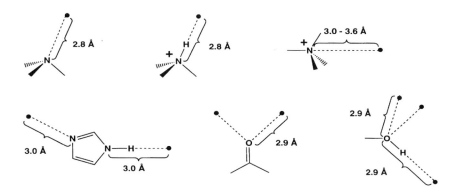

Figure 3.5   Site points for some oxygen and nitrogen containing functional groups.

The extension of the pharmacophore concept to include *site points* as shown in Figure 3.3d,e is a great advance in 3D-pharmacophore development. The connection between a site point and a ligand functional group represents an interaction with a receptor site and the site point itself represents the interacting amino acid residue. Suitable site points for some nitrogen and oxygen containing functional groups are shown in Figure 3.5.

The site points in Figure 3.5 for primary, secondary and tertiary amines and for ammonium groups and the imidazole group simulate hydrogen bonding interactions with a receptor site. The site points are placed in the direction of the N-lone pair or N-H bond. Depending on the structures and the structural diversity of the set of molecules to be analyzed, various combinations of site points and ligand points may be used. The use of the site point *and* the nitrogen atom as pharmacophore elements implies that not only the amino group as such is important, but that a specific direction of the interaction between the amine and the receptor is crucial for the activity. If *only* the site point is used and not the nitrogen atom, the implication is that the interaction with the receptor site represented by the site point may take place from different directions. The site point for an ammonium group may be used to simulate an electrostatic interaction with an anionic or aromatic side-chain in the receptor binding cavity.

An aromatic system such as a phenyl group is often represented by a ligand point positioned at the center of the aromatic ring (Fig. 3.6). Specification of all carbon atoms in the ring will give such a ring an unrealistically large weight in a molecular least-squares superimposition (see Section 3.4). In some applications it is useful to employ site points for an aromatic system located on the normal passing through the centroid of the aromatic system, above and below the ring plane (Fig. 3.6). Such points may represent electrostatic and van der Waals interactions between the aromatic group and amino acid residues in the receptor binding site.

3.2.4 Beyond single site points

It is sometimes found in 3D-pharmacophore identification studies that the originally selected set of ligands must be split into two (or more) classes. This indicates that the selected ligands

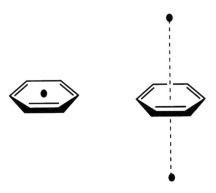

Figure 3.6   Ligand point and site points commonly used to represent a phenyl ring or other aromatic systems.

may have different binding modes. A possible reason for the necessity to separate the set of ligands into different classes may be that they interact with different atoms of a multi-atom amino acid residue.

Neurotransmitters as norepinephrine, dopamine and serotonin and agonists and antagonists for the receptors of these neurotransmitters are primary, secondary or tertiary amines (or ammonium ions). Site-directed mutagenesis studies indicate that these compounds bind to an aspartic acid/aspartate residue. The protonation state of the interaction is not known, but in the ion pair as well as in the neutral case different binding options are available as shown in Figure 3.7. An ammonium group may bind to a carboxylate anion from different directions, resulting in different ligand binding modes. However, it may be possible that ligands have similar binding modes, but that an ammonium group interacts with different oxygen atoms of a carboxylate anion or an amino group with an OH group in different positions obtained by a conformational (or tautomeric) change of the carboxylic acid. These interactions can only to a crude approximation be modeled by a single site-point. For instance, the binding of an ammonium ion to a carboxylate anion could equally well occur with the ammonium group in the two different spatial positions shown in Figure 3.8. The two ligands may bind equally well to the carboxylate anion without requiring that the site-points in the direction of the N-H bonds superimpose.

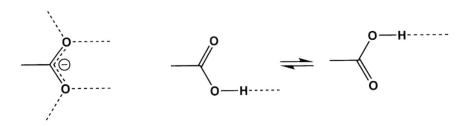

Figure 3.7   Possible directions of interaction between a carboxylate anion and an ammonium group (left) and between a carboxylic acid and an amino group (right).

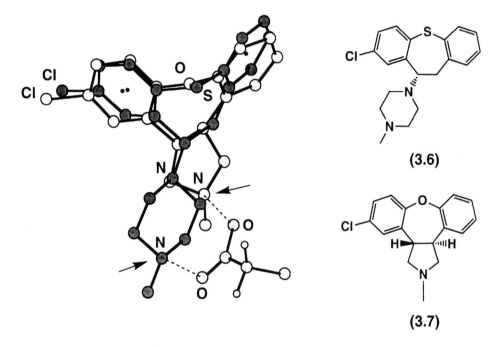

Figure 3.8   The ammonium group of two ligands with similar binding modes but interacting with different oxygens of a carboxylate anion.

Figure 3.9   Superimposition of compounds (**3.6**) and (**3.7**) (hydrogen atoms are omitted for clarity) based on fitting of the two tricyclic ring systems. The relevant nitrogen atoms (indicated with arrows) in the two compounds are then located in such positions that may interact with different oxygen atoms of a carboxylate anion.

Compounds (**3.6**) and (**3.7**) (Fig. 3.9) have high affinities for the dopamine D-2 receptor. In compound (**3.6**) the distal nitrogen is known to be the relevant one for binding to the receptor, presumably to an aspartate residue. If the tricyclic systems are superimposed, the nitrogens will be far apart as seen in the superimposition in Figure 3.9. The use of a single site point model for the carboxylate anion will not significantly improve the situation. However, the relative positions of the nitrogens are such that they may optimally interact with different oxygen atoms of a carboxylate anion of an aspartate residue. Thus, dopamine D-2 receptor antagonists of the two classes represented by (**3.6**) and (**3.7**) may be included in the same 3D-pharmacophore model, provided that a pharmacophore element representation of the carboxylate anion beyond single site points is employed.

3.3 THE RECEPTOR-BOUND OR "ACTIVE" CONFORMATION

3.3.1 Thermodynamic considerations

The great majority of drug molecules are flexible, which means that they through rotations about bonds and/or inversions about atomic centers may adopt a large number of conformations, giving the molecule a correspondingly large number of different 3D-shapes. In the context of the pharmacophore concept, this means that a ligand in general may exhibit a large number of possible spatial relationships between its pharmacophore elements. The pharmacophore hypothesis implies that one of these shapes is optimally complementary to the receptor binding sites and that the ligand, when bound to the receptor, is characterized by a specific molecular conformation.

The single most important (and certainly most difficult) problem in 3D-pharmacophore identification is to identify the *receptor-bound (bioactive) conformation*. If this can be accomplished, the spatial relationships of the pharmacophore elements in this conformation defines the 3D-pharmacophore and new candidate ligands may be tested to investigate if they fit this 3D-pharmacophore. Inactive molecules which fit the 3D-pharmacophore are of special interest since they may contain extra molecular volume which can be used for mapping of the dimensions of the receptor cavity (see Section 3.5).

The probability of finding the molecule in a particular conformation is related to its conformational free energy. This is defined as the difference in free energy between the actual conformation and the lowest energy conformation of the molecule. It is important to note that the bioactive conformation is not necessarily the lowest energy conformation of the molecule in solution, in the crystal or in the gas phase. It may not even correspond to an energy minimum structure in any of these phases. Thus, experimental data on structures and conformational equilibria alone are of limited use in attempts to identify the bioactive conformation. A computational approach is required and the entire conformational space must be investigated.

Unless the ligand-receptor interaction is characterized by extensive hydrogen bonding or a large number of other strong interactions, it is highly probable that the ligand binds in a conformation which corresponds to a low energy conformation for the molecule *in vacuo* (see Section 3.3.3). This is supported by observed conformations of ligands in crystal structures of ligand-enzyme complexes.

The ligand-receptor interaction is characterized by the equilibrium (3.1), as illustrated in Figure 3.10.

$$\text{ligand} + \text{receptor} \overset{K}{\rightleftharpoons} \text{ligand} - \text{receptor complex} \tag{3.1}$$

The free energy difference ΔG is given by equation (3.2) where K is the equilibrium constant, R the gas constant (8.314 J K^{-1} mol^{-1}), T the absolute temperature in Kelvin, and K_d the dissociation constant.

$$\Delta G = -RT \ln K, \quad K_d = 1/K \tag{3.2}$$

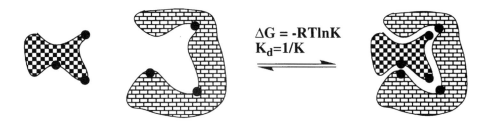

Figure 3.10   The equilibrium between the ligand and the receptor and the ligand-receptor complex.

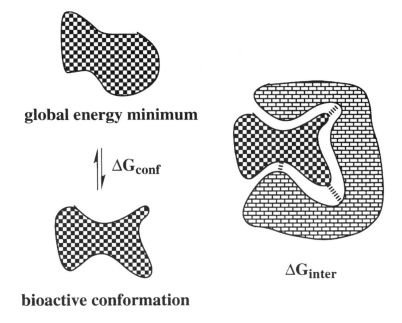

Figure 3.11   Contributions to the free energy of binding assuming that the ligand has two accessible conformations and that the active conformation is the higher energy one.

It is convenient for the discussion of receptor binding to define a free energy of binding, ΔG_{bind} (equation (3.3)). A stronger binding gives a more positive ΔG_{bind}.

$$\Delta G_{\text{bind}} = -\Delta G \qquad (3.3)$$

If we for the moment neglect energy contributions from solvation of the ligand, the receptor and the ligand-receptor complex, the overall free energy of binding may be separated into two components as shown in equation (3.4) and Figure 3.11 (solvation effects are discussed in Section 3.6).

$$\Delta G_{\text{bind}} = \Delta G_{\text{inter}} - \Delta G_{\text{conf}} \qquad (3.4)$$

ΔG_{conf} is the free energy required for the ligand to assume the bioactive conformation. ΔG_{inter} corresponds to the intermolecular interaction of this conformation with the receptor. In terms of the pharmacophore concept, ΔG_{inter} is due to binding interactions between the pharmacophore elements and the complementary binding sites. ΔG_{conf} is related to the Bolzmann probability of the active conformation (P_{conf}) by equation (3.5).

$$\Delta G_{\text{conf}} = -RT \ln P_{\text{conf}} \qquad (3.5)$$

P_{conf} may be approximately calculated using equation (3.6) where E_{conf} is the calculated energy of the bioactive conformation, and E_i are conformational energies of all accessible conformations.

$$P_{\text{conf}} \approx \frac{e^{-E_{\text{conf}}/RT}}{\sum_i e^{-E_i/RT}} \qquad (3.6)$$

If we compare the affinities of two flexible compounds with the same pharmacophore elements, and if we assume that ΔG_{inter} for the two compounds is very similar, i.e. $\Delta\Delta G_{\text{inter}} \approx 0$, the difference in affinity, $\Delta\Delta G_{\text{bind}}$, is $\approx \Delta\Delta G_{\text{conf}}$. Thus, for closely similar molecules, differences in conformational free energies may determine relative affinities.

If ΔG_{conf} is not equal to zero, i.e. the receptor-bound conformation is not the lowest energy conformation of the free molecule, there is always a decrease in the affinity due to this "conformational effect". The factor of decrease (K_{conf}) may be calculated from equation (3.7) ($T = 310$ K).

$$\Delta G_{\text{conf}} = RT \ln K_{\text{conf}} = 5.9 \log K_{\text{conf}} \qquad (3.7)$$

Thus, if the active conformation has a conformational energy of 5.9 kJ mol^{-1} the decrease in the affinity (corresponding to an increase of the dissociation constant) is a factor of 10 due to this "conformational effect". For each additional 5.9 kJ mol^{-1} of conformational free energy, the affinity decreases by a further factor of 10.

Equation (3.8) gives the corresponding relationship between differences in conformational energies of two ligands and their relative affinities due to the conformational effect.

$$\Delta\Delta G_{\text{conf}} = \Delta G_{\text{conf}}(B) - \Delta G_{\text{conf}}(A) = 5.9 \log \frac{K_{\text{conf}}(B)}{K_{\text{conf}}(A)} \qquad (3.8)$$

The relationships between differences in conformational energies and relative receptor affinities in the general case should not be used alone for purposes of quantitative predictions. However, these relations may be fruitfully used as tools in the development of a 3D-pharmacophore model and also for the rough estimation of relative affinities of structurally closely related compounds which fit the model. High affinity ligands should in general have low conformational energies, and high conformational energies should correspond to low affinity ligands. Relative affinities between structurally similar molecules, which fit a pharmacophore model, should be related to their differences in conformational free energies according to equation (3.8).

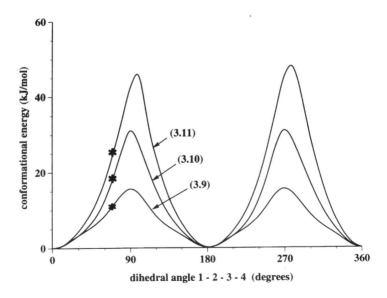

Compound (**3.8**) is a potent dopamine D-2 receptor agonist. The receptor-bound conformations of the related compounds (**3.9**)–(**3.11**) have been deduced by using (**3.8**) as a template and the conformational energies of the bioactive conformations (*in vacuo*) have been calculated by molecular mechanics (see Section 3.3.2.1). These conformations are labeled with asterisks in Figure 3.12. The affinities as well as the agonist activities of (**3.9**)–(**3.11**) are significantly lower than that of (**3.8**). Furthermore, the affinities and the agonist activities of (**3.9**)–(**3.11**) are in the order (**3.9**) > (**3.10**) > (**3.11**). These data are nicely accounted for by the calculated conformational energies of the bioactive conformations of (**3.9**)–(**3.11**) as shown in Figure 3.12. Note that the deduced bioactive conformations of (**3.9**)–(**3.11**) are not energy minimum conformations, i.e. they do not correspond to stable conformations *in vacuo*.

Figure 3.12   Calculated potential energy curves for rotation about the central bond in (**3.9**)–(**3.11**). The asterisks denote the deduced bioactive conformations of the compounds.

3.3.2 Conformational analysis

There are two groups of methods which may be used for the calculation of conformational properties of molecules (*i*) quantum chemical methods and (*ii*) molecular mechanics or force field methods. In the quantum chemical methods the Schrödinger equation is solved, treating the molecule as a collection of positive nuclei and negative electrons moving under the influence of Coulombic potentials. A hierarchy of quantum chemical methods at different levels of approximation are being used in computational chemistry.

In the quantum chemical *ab initio* methods, all electrons are included in the calculations, whereas in the *semi-empirical methods* only the outer (valence) electrons are explicitly included in the calculations and many terms are not calculated but fitted to experimental data. Explicit calculations of electron distribution in the field of the nuclei limit quantum chemical calculations, especially of the *ab initio* type, to small molecular systems. Although several of these methods are being used in connection with problems in medicinal chemistry, the methods necessary to yield reliable results are, at the present time, in general much too time-consuming to be of practical use for the extensive search of conformational space, which is needed in connection with 3D-pharmacophore identification. These methods will thus not be considered here.

The other group of computational methods, molecular mechanics or force field methods, are well suited for extensive calculations on conformational properties of molecules of interest in medicinal chemistry and may also be used for calculations on biomacromolecules.

3.3.2.1 Molecular mechanics (force field) calculations

Molecular mechanics is a method for the calculation of molecular structures, conformational energies and other molecular properties using concepts from classical mechanics. A molecule is considered as a collection of atoms held together by classical forces. These forces are described by potential energy functions of structural features like bond lengths, bond angles, torsional (dihedral) angles, etc.

The energy (E) of the the molecule is calculated as a sum of terms as in equation (3.9).

$$E = E_{stretching} + E_{bending} + E_{torsion} + E_{van der Waals} + E_{electrostatic}$$
$$+ E_{hydrogen bond} + \text{cross terms} \tag{3.9}$$

The first four terms in the sum are the energies due to deviations of bond lengths, bond angles, torsional angles and non-bonded distances, respectively, from their reference or "ideal" values. $E_{electrostatic}$ gives the electrostatic attraction or repulsion between bond dipoles or partial atomic charges. Although a large part of the hydrogen bonding is included in the electrostatic energy component, many molecular mechanics methods include an additional hydrogen bonding term ($E_{hydrogen bond}$) to fine-tune the energies and geometries of a hydrogen bond interaction. More advanced force fields include cross terms such as stretch-bend, bend-bend, torsion-stretch etc. These terms are of importance for the accurate calculation of geometric properties of small rings (stretch-bend term) or for the calculation of vibrational frequencies (bend-bend term).

The energies are calculated using analytical potential energy functions similar to those used in classical mechanics. The functional forms of the potential energy functions for the

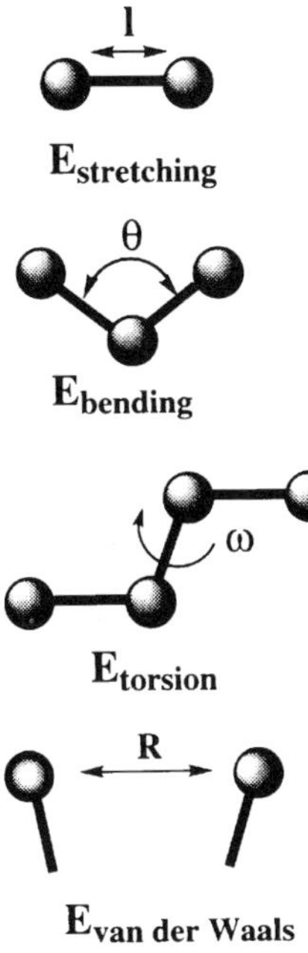

$$E_{\text{stretching}} \qquad \frac{k_s}{2}(l-l_o)^2 + \frac{k_{3s}}{2}(l-l_o)^3 + \frac{k_{4s}}{2}(l-l_o)^4$$

$$E_{\text{bending}} \qquad \frac{k_b}{2}(\theta-\theta_o)^2 + \frac{k_{3b}}{2}(\theta-\theta_o)^3 + \frac{k_{4b}}{2}(\theta-\theta_o)^4 + \frac{k_{5b}}{2}(\theta-\theta_o)^5 + \frac{k_{6b}}{2}(\theta-\theta_o)^6$$

$$E_{\text{torsion}} \qquad \frac{V_1}{2}(1+\cos\omega) + \frac{V_2}{2}(1-\cos2\omega) + \frac{V_3}{2}(1+\cos3\omega)$$

$$E_{\text{van der Waals}} \qquad \sqrt{\varepsilon_i\varepsilon_j}\,(a\,e^{(-bP)} - c\,P^6)\;;\qquad P = \frac{r_i + r_k}{R}$$

Figure 3.13   Some potential energy functions included in the MM3 force field.

first four terms in equation (3.9) are shown in Figure 3.13. The potential functions shown are those included in the MM3 force field.

The quadratic terms in the functions for stretching and angle bending in Figure 3.13 simply correspond to Hookes' law and the higher order terms are corrections for anharmonicity. In the van der Waals function the first term corresponds to non-bonded repulsion, whereas the second term describes non-bonded attraction (London dispersion forces).

The subscripted letters in Figure 3.13 are force-field parameters which are parameterized for each atom or atom combination by the use of experimental data (or possibly high-quality quantum chemical *ab initio* results). The set of energy functions and the corresponding parameters are called a *force field*.

The molecular mechanics method calculates the energy as a function of the nuclear coordinates and energy minimization is an integral part of the method. A trial molecular geometry is constructed, most often by using computer graphics techniques, and the atoms are iteratively moved (without breaking bonds) using an energy minimization technique until the net forces on all atoms vanish and the total energy of the molecule reaches a minimum. The 3D-structure of the molecule corresponding to this energy minimum is one of the stable conformations of the molecule but *not necessarily* the most stable one (Fig. 3.14). Since the energy minimization methods cannot move the molecule across energy barriers, the minimization of a trial molecule continues until the first *local energy minimum* is found. Other local energy minima including the lowest energy one (the *global energy minimum*)

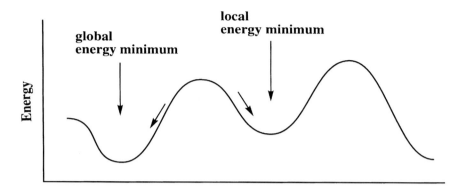

Figure 3.14   Energy minimization proceeds downhill to the nearest energy minimum.

may be found by repeating the calculation with another start geometry or more efficiently by the use of a conformational search method (see Section 3.3.2.2).

By itself, E in equation (3.9) has no direct physical meaning. However, the difference in E (ΔE) between two conformations corresponds closely to the enthalpy difference (ΔH). Very often, entropy differences between conformations are small and then $\Delta H \approx \Delta G$. In some molecular mechanics methods it is possible to calculate entropies from vibrational frequencies and thus explicitly the free energy difference between two conformers ($\Delta G = \Delta H - T\Delta S$).

In general, the calculated results from a molecular mechanics calculation refer to the isolated molecule (*in vacuo*). Thus effects of the environment are generally not included. In order to simulate a polar environment, an often used (but crude) approximation is to employ a dielectric constant higher than that for gas phase (1.0) in the calculations of the electrostatic energy contributions. However, other more accurate methods have recently been developed by which solvent effects may be included in the calculation.

The best molecular mechanics force fields currently available may calculate bond lengths, bond angles, dihedral angles, and energies to within 0.005 Å, 1 degree, 5 degrees, and 2 kJ mol^{-1}, respectively, provided that the necessary force field parameters have been accurately determined.

3.3.2.2 *Conformational search methods*

As described above in Section 3.3.2.1, the energy minimization procedure moves the molecule from the initial (trial) geometry to the *closest* local energy minimum. For molecules with just one or two degrees of torsional freedom, various trial conformations may be generated manually and energy minimized, but for molecules with three or more rotatable bonds, computer implemented search methods are in general necessary. Many methods for conformational search have been devised but only the major ones, systematic search in torsional space and the random search methods, will be described here. If well implemented, both methods are of similar efficiency and may be feasible for up to 10–15 rotatable bonds with current computer resources.

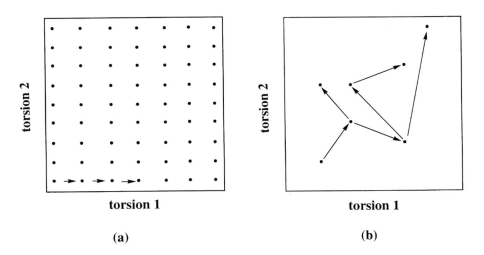

Figure 3.15 The generation of trial conformations in (a) systematic search in torsional space. (b) random torsional search.

The systematic conformational search methodology is in principle simple and straight-forward. New structures are generated using all combinations of torsional angle values at a preset resolution (angle increment) which gives a uniform grid search in torsional space (Fig. 3.15a).

In the one-dimensional (one rotatable bond) or two-dimensional (two rotatable bonds) cases, so-called *torsional driving* is feasible. Each torsional angle is incremented by a user defined value and the dihedral value is then kept fixed while the molecule is energy-minimized with respect to all other degrees of freedom. The result of a calculation using torsional driving is a potential energy curve or a potential energy (conformational) map which displays not only energy minima but also energy barriers and pathways for conformational interconversions. This type of calculations is very time consuming and is therefore seldom used for problems involving more than two rotatable bonds. Examples of potential energy curves calculated by the torsional driving method are shown in Figure 3.12 above and in Section 3.7.3 below.

For three and more rotatable bonds, conformational search methods in general focus on finding (low) energy minima. The main problem involved in such calculations is the large number of conformations which must be handled. This number can be calculated from equation (3.10) where n is the number of rotatable bonds and m is the angle increment in degrees.

$$\text{number of conformations} = (360/m)^n \qquad (3.10)$$

Thus, for six rotatable bond, as in (**3.12**), the number of conformations to consider is 46 656 for an angle increment of 60 degrees and 2 985 984 for an increment of 30 degrees.

(3.12)

The number of conformations increases very fast with increasing number of rotatable bonds and with decreasing angle increment (the combinatorial explosion) and it is not feasible to energy minimize all of these trial conformations. The efficiency of a particular systematic conformational search method depends on how efficient the method can reduce the number of conformations to be energy minimized. Most methods check for close non-bonded contacts in each generated conformation. The rational for this is that if two or more atoms are too close to each other in the trial structure, energy minimization will probably lead to a high energy conformation and the trial structure can be discarded in a search for low energy conformations. Various other methods have been developed in order to keep the number of conformations to be energy-minimized as low as possible.

In random conformational search methods, random numbers are used to determine how many and which torsional angles to be incremented and by how much (torsional space) or how much and in which directions the x, y and z-coordinates of each atom are to be translated. The trial conformation generated in this way is then energy minimized and the resulting conformation is compared with those already stored. If it is a new conformation it is added to the storage. The procedure is repeated a large number of times and the completeness of the search may be estimated by how many times each stored conformation have been found. An advantage of this methodology is that it can be halted at any time and restarted and the results from repeated runs may be combined.

The development of new methods for searching conformational space is currently a very active area of research.

3.3.3 Conformational energy cut-off

A much debated problem in connection with conformational search and 3D-pharmacophore identification is which energy cut-off to use in a search for possible candidates for the receptor-bound conformation of a ligand. That is, how high conformational energy can the receptor-bound conformation of a high-affinity ligand have?

The relationship between conformational energy (ΔG_{conf}) and affinity derived in Section 3.3.1 shows that each conformational energy increase of 5.9 kJ mol^{-1} decreases the affinity (i.e., increases the K_d value) by a factor of 10. Considering a single ligand-receptor complex, the conformational energy penalty that can be tolerated depends on how strong the intermolecular interactions (ΔG_{inter}) between the ligand and the receptor are. If unusually extensive and strong hydrogen bonding or strong electrostatic interactions are present, a substantial conformational energy penalty may be overcome and the ligand may still have a high affinity for the receptor. (Favourable free energy of solvation may also contribute to this, see Section 3.6). Thus, in an absolute sense it is difficult to specify a general cut-off, but in the absence of particularly strong ligand-receptor interactions, our experience is that a conformational free energy of up to 10–12 kJ mol^{-1} may be tolerated. It should be noted that if a receptor-bound conformation for a flexible ligand has a high conformational energy it should, in principle, be possible to design a structurally related but conformationally constrained analogue with a lower conformational energy and consequently with a significantly higher affinity.

Conformational energies are most straightforwardly used in a comparison of two similar high affinity ligands with identical (or bioisosteric) pharmacophore elements. For a valid 3D-pharmacophore such compounds should have similar conformational energies. Thus, if two structurally related high affinity compounds have substantially different conformational energies (>10–12 kJ mol^{-1}) the 3D-pharmacophore should be reconsidered.

3.4 MOLECULAR SUPERIMPOSITION

3.4.1 Least-squares superimposition and template forcing

A 3D-pharmacophore model is characterized by a particular 3D-arrangement of pharmacophore elements. Active (high affinity) ligands are able to assume a low energy conformation in which the pharmacophore elements are positioned at closely similar relative positions in space as those of the 3D-pharmacophore model. In order to investigate similarities and differences in the spatial relationships of pharmacophore elements between different conformations of the same molecule, between conformations of different molecules or between conformations of a molecule and a 3D-pharmacophore model, molecular superimposition techniques are being used.

Such superimposition techniques assume that the ligands studied have a common binding mode and that the receptor binding site is relatively fixed. If receptor binding data and molecular structures suggest that the ligands may have different binding modes, the compounds may be separated into different classes, as discussed above, and analyzed separately. Later it may be possible to merge the separate classes and models into a single model, but this may not always be the case. For instance, early attempts to develop 3D-pharmacophore models for dopamine receptor ligands included agonists as well as antagonists in the same model. This met with considerable difficulties and predictions made from such models were not successful. The development of separate 3D-pharmacophore models for dopamine receptor agonists and antagonists have been much more successful.

The most commonly used molecular superimposition method is the *least-squares superimposition* of pharmacophore elements represented as ligand points or site points. The root mean square deviation (rms) between selected points in the test molecule and the corresponding points in the reference molecule is minimized by displacing and rotating the test molecule as a rigid body. The rms value of the resulting least-squares fit is given by equation (3.11).

$$\text{rms} = \sqrt{\frac{\sum_{i=1}^{N} R_i^2}{N}} \qquad (3.11)$$

R_i in equation (3.11) is the distance between the ith pair of ligand or site points and N is the number of such pairs. The rms value is zero (Å) for a perfect fit and increases as the fit is decreased.

The minimum energy conformations obtained from a conformational search and then used in a molecular least-squares superimposition study may not be the optimal ones. The receptor-bound conformation is not necessarily a local energy minimum and deviations of torsional angles from the values for a stable conformation of the molecule *in vacuo* may be necessary for an optimal binding to the receptor. Molecular superimposition algorithms often include possibilities to perform *flexible fitting* by systematic variations of the torsional angles of user defined rotatable bonds until an optimal fit between fitting points (pharmacophore elements) are found.

An alternative to the least-squares superimposition method is to connect the fitting points to be superimposed by an isotropic spring, which by the use of an energy minimization procedure forces the test molecule to be fitted to the reference molecule ("template forcing").

3.4.2 The use of molecular superimposition techniques

When a 3D-pharmacophore model has been developed, an important use of molecular superimposition techniques is to investigate if inactive (low affinity) compounds fit the model. If such a compound does not fit the model in any conformation, the obvious rationalization of its low affinity is its inability to present the pharmacophore elements in a correct way. If the compound fits the model but in a high energy conformation, the equally straightforward rationalization of its lack of affinity is that the energy penalty for binding to the receptor is too high. However, if the inactive compound fits the model in a low energy conformation there are three possibilities to rationalize its inactivity: (*i*) the compound is too voluminous in some direction(s) causing steric repulsive interactions with the receptor (see Section 3.5), (*ii*) the compound has a very unfavourable free energy of solvation (see Section 3.6), or (*iii*) the electronic properties of the ligand are not complementary to the receptor binding site (see Section 3.4.3). If none of the cases (*i*), (*ii*) and (*iii*) is probable, the 3D-pharmacophore model is seriously in doubt and should be reconsidered. Thus, molecular superimposition studies may corroborate or discard a 3D-pharmacophore model. Testing of the 3D-pharmacophore model with all available high and low affinity ligands should be done before the design of new molecules based on the model is attempted. The ultimate use of a 3D-pharmacophore model is of course in the design of new ligands. Molecular superimposition techniques are then indispensable tools for testing if newly designed ligands fit the model in low energy conformations. Molecular superimpositions and their use are exemplified in Section 3.7.

3.4.3 Future directions — property and field fitting

New molecular superimposition techniques have recently been developed in which molecular properties and fields are being fitted instead of ligand points and site points. The most interesting of these methods are based on the fact that in addition to shape complementarity, electronic complementarity is important for molecular recognition. That is, positively and negatively charged parts of the molecular surface should interact with oppositely charged parts in the receptor binding cavity. Thus, methods have been devised to identify a common

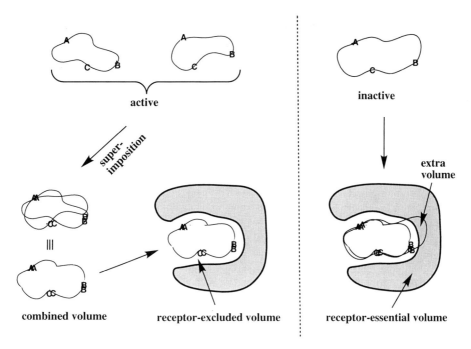

Figure 3.16   The *combined volume* gives an estimate of the lower-bound of receptor volume available for ligand binding (*receptor-excluded volume*). Inactive compounds may have an *extra volume* which overlaps the *receptor-essential volume* and thus causes steric repulsive interactions between the ligand and the receptor.

charge pattern or even better a common pattern of electrostatic potentials on or just outside the molecular surface of low energy conformations of a set of high-affinity ligands. (The electrostatic potential is the potential energy between a unitary positive charge placed at a position in space and the molecular charge distribution).

3.5 RECEPTOR-EXCLUDED AND RECEPTOR-ESSENTIAL VOLUMES

The volume of a molecule may be computed and graphically displayed in terms of the sum of atomic van der Waals radii. For a superimposed set of high affinity ligands for the target receptor, the *combined volume* may be calculated as the union of the volumes for all the molecules in the set (Fig. 3.16). This volume should be readily accomodated by the receptor and the combined volume gives an estimate of the lower bound of the receptor volume available for binding of ligands (the *receptor-excluded volume*). The volume occupied by the receptor is called the *receptor-essential volume* and is not available for ligand binding (Fig. 3.16). The analysis of molecular volumes on the basis of a 3D-pharmacophore model may give valuable information about the dimensions of the receptor cavity. An inactive or low affinity compound which fits the 3D-pharmacophore model in a low energy conformation may have a van der Waals volume larger than the combined volume of the high

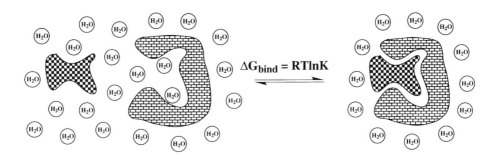

Figure 3.17   The ligand receptor interaction in an aqueous environment. The ligand must be desolvated before it can enter the binding cavity of the receptor.

affinity set of molecules (*extra volume*). For a valid 3D-pharmacophore model, the extra volume of the inactive compound indicates positions in space, where the ligand volume is in conflict with the receptor-essential volume (Fig. 3.16). This information is extremely valuable in connection with design of new ligands based on a 3D-pharmacophore model as it provides knowledge about positions in space where ligand fragments should not be present.

3.6 SOLVATION EFFECTS

The free energy of ligand-receptor binding does not only depend on the intermolecular interactions between ligand and receptor and the possible conformational effects discussed in Section 3.3.1. Solvation in aqueous solution of the molecular species involved must also be taken into account. Before it can enter the binding cavity of the receptor, the ligand must be desolvated and a better solvated ligand requires more free energy for the desolvation process. Consider the equilibrium characterizing the receptor binding in water solution shown in Figure 3.17. For a more water soluble ligand the equilibrium in Figure 3.17 is shifted to the left, the equilibrium constant K is smaller and thus, the free energy of binding (the affinity) is smaller.

The illustration in Figure 3.17 represents the case of water soluble enzymes. For membrane-bound receptors, part of the biomacromolecule has a membrane bilayer environment and for some highly lipophilic ligands, partitioning into the lipid bilayer and binding to the receptor via the bilayer may occur. In this case the overall equilibrium constant is a composite of an intramembrane equilibrium constant and the partition coefficient and this affects the interpretation of the equilibrium constant. In the following it is assumed that the ligand enters the binding cavity directly from the aqueous phase.

If we make the reasonable assumption that the ligand-receptor complexes for two ligands are equally well solvated, an approximate relationship between the difference in free energy of binding for the molecules *in vacuo* ($\Delta\Delta G_{bind}$(vacuo)) and the difference in free energy of binding in water $\Delta\Delta G_{bind}$ (aq) is given by equation (3.12).

$$\Delta\Delta G_{bind}\ (aq) = \Delta\Delta G_{bind}(vacuo) + \Delta\Delta G_{solv} \tag{3.12}$$

$\Delta\Delta G_{bind}$(vacuo) represents differences in intermolecular interactions with the receptor as well as possible differences in conformational energies of the bioactive conformations of the two ligands (see Section 3.3.1). $\Delta\Delta G_{solv}$ is the difference in free energies of solvation in water (a better solvated ligand has a more negative ΔG_{solv}). Thus, even if the two ligands interact equally well with the receptor ($\Delta\Delta G_{vacuo} = 0$), the affinities for the receptor, as measured by $\Delta\Delta G_{bind}$ (aq), could be significantly different due to differences in ΔG_{solv}. Similarily, if one ligand interacts less well with the receptor, this could be compensated for by a smaller free energy of desolvation, that is, a more positive free energy of solvation in water.

(3.13)   **(3.14)**

As an example of this, compound (**3.13**) binds to the zinc-requiring endopeptidase thermolysin. X-ray crystallography of the ligand-enzyme complex shows that the NH group, indicated by an arrow, hydrogen bonds to a carbonyl oxygen of the enzyme binding site. However, compound (**3.14**) binds equally well to the enzyme in spite of the fact that the CH$_2$ group in (**3.14**), replacing the NH group in (**3.13**), cannot hydrogen bond to the enzyme. Computer simulations of the equilibrium in Figure 3.17 show that (**3.14**) interacts less well with the enzyme by 10 kJ mol^{-1}, but has a more positive free energy of solvation in water by 11 kJ mol^{-1}. The net effect is that (**3.13**) and (**3.14**) have essentially the same affinities for the enzyme.

In the development of 3D-pharmacophore models, the possibility of differential solvent effects must be taken into account. This may be done by only including compounds with similar free energies of solvation in the set on which the model is built. Otherwise such effects must be qualitatively estimated or explicitly calculated. Various methods for the calculation of free energies of hydration have recently been developed and the further development of such methods is currently a very active area of research.

3.7 EXAMPLES OF 3D-PHARMACOPHORES AND THEIR USE

3.7.1 A 3D-pharmacophore for muscarinic acetylcholine receptor agonists

In early attempts to identify the 3D-pharmacophore for agonists at the muscarinic acetylcholine receptor, solid state conformations were used in order to find common patterns

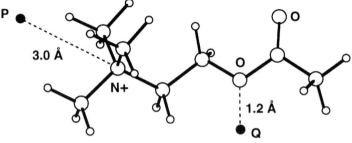

acetylcholine

Figure 3.18   Site points used in the development of a muscarinic 3D-pharmacophore and the deduced bioactive conformation of acetylcholine.

of torsional angles. This approach did not meet with much success, which demonstrates the very limited use of X-ray structures in 3D-pharmacophore identification.

In a more unbiased approach, a 3D-pharmacophore for the recognition of agonists containing the N-C-C-O-C-C backbone by the muscarinic acetylcholine receptor has been developed on the basis of site-points and conformational analysis of a series of muscarinic agonists. The 3D-pharmacophore and the deduced bioactive conformation of acetylcholine is shown in Figure 3.18. Point P represents a specifically oriented interaction between the cationic head group and an anionic receptor site. This point lies on the three-fold axis of the trimethylammonium group. Point Q represents an electrostatic or hydrogen bonding interaction with the receptor. It is assumed that the distance PQ is essentially constant for high-affinity agonists.

Instead of using the N-C-C-O and C-C-O-C dihedral angles in the search for receptor-bound conformations, the P-N-O-Q "interaction" dihedral angle was employed. For all agonists in the series, conformations calculated to be within 13–17 kJ mol^{-1} of the lowest energy conformation and displaying a common PQ distance (6.6–6.8 Å) were selected for further analysis. In this analysis it was found that the P-N-O-Q dihedral angle must be in the range of 110–117 degrees for active compounds. Acetylcholine itself satisfies these requirements in a conformation with C-C-O-C and N-C-C-O dihedral angles of 189 and 132 degrees, respectively. These angles are significantly different from the corresponding angles in X-ray structures of acetylcholine. The bromide salt displays dihedral angles of 79 and 77 degrees and the chloride salt has angles of 193 and 85 degrees, respectively.

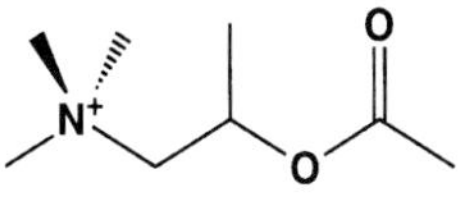

(3.15) 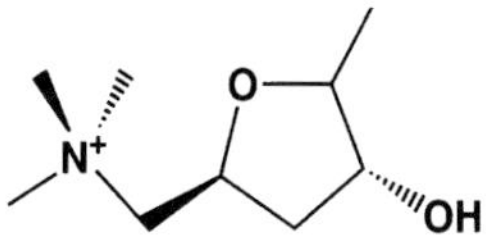 (3.16) 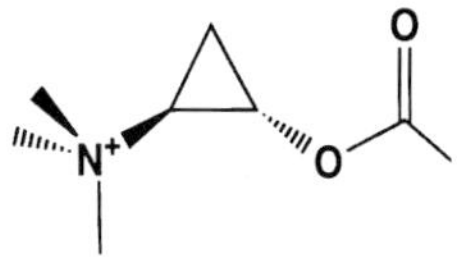 (3.17)

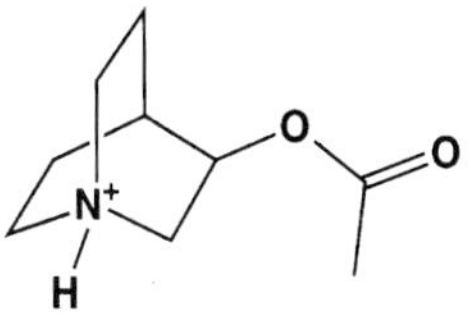

(3.18) 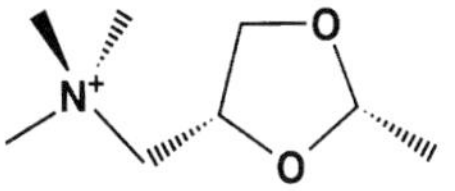 (3.19)

The 3D-pharmacophore model in Figure 3.18 is capable of rationalizing the stereoselec-tivities of the agonists β-methylacetylcholine (**3.15**), muscarine (**3.16**), *trans*-acetoxycyclo-propyltrimethylammonium (**3.17**), 3-acetoxyquinuclidine (**3.18**), and *cis*-2-methyl-4-trimethylammoniummethyl-1,3-dioxolan (**3.19**). The inactive (or less active) stereoisomers are found to require conformational energies significantly higher than 17 kJ mol^{-1} to fit the 3D-pharmacophore.

3.7.2 Apomorphine congeners — conformational energies *vs.* agonist activities

An often used strategy in the structural elaboration of a lead compound is a simplification of the lead structure by ring-cleavage and/or deletion of rings. Compounds (**3.21**)–(**3.30**) are examples of such compounds, derived from the structure of the potent dopamine D-2 receptor agonist apomorphine (**3.20**).

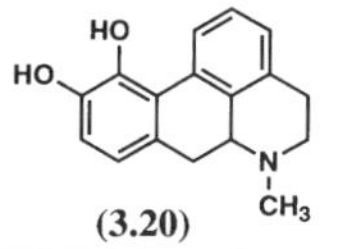

(3.20) 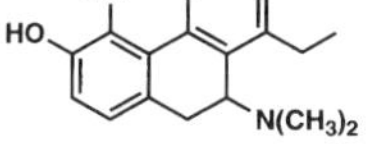 (3.21) 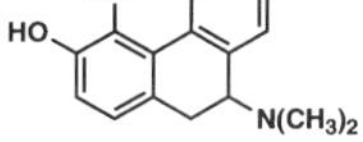 (3.22) 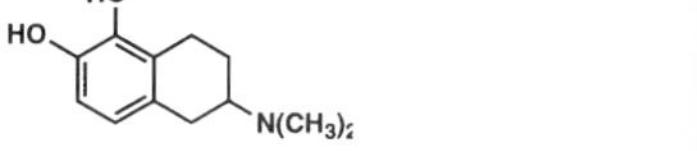 (3.23)

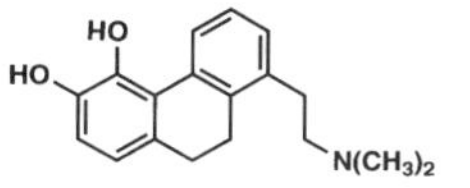

(3.24) 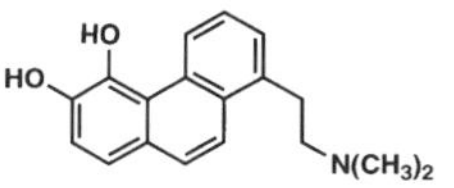 (3.25) 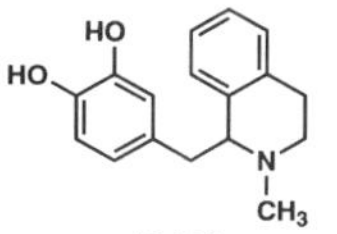 (3.26) 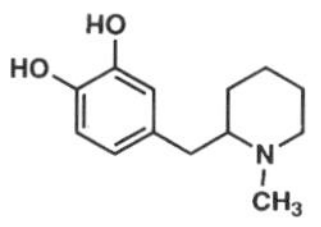 (3.27)

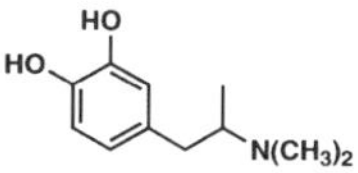

(3.28) 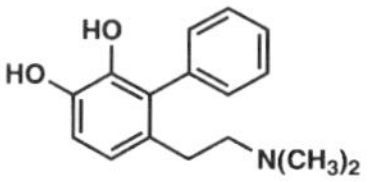 (3.29) 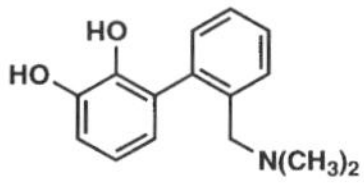 (3.30)

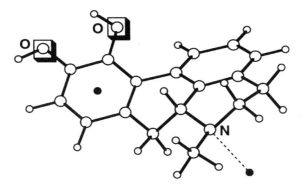

Figure 3.19 A 3D-pharmacophore model for dopamine D-2 agonists of the catechol type. The oxygen atoms, the center of the catechol ring and a site point 2.8 Å from the nitrogen atom in the direction of the nitrogen lone electron pair are employed as pharmacophore elements.

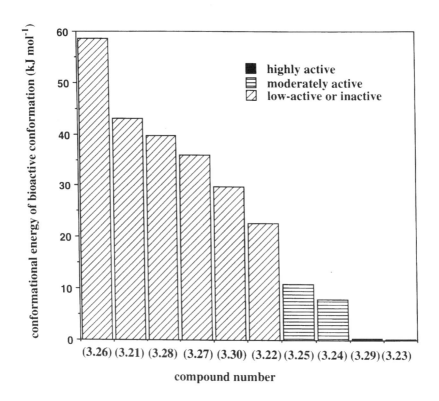

Figure 3.20 Calculated conformational energies of the deduced active conformations of compounds (**3.21**)–(**3.30**) *vs.* their dopamine receptor agonist activities.

Figure 3.19 displays a 3D-pharmacophore for dopamine D-2 receptor agonists of the catechol type, based on three ligand points and a site point. Topologically (2D), compounds (**3.21**)–(**3.30**) all may display the same relative positions of the pharma-cophore elements as (**3.20**). However, when (**3.21**)–(**3.30**) are subjected to conformational analysis by molecular mechanics, it is found that most of the compounds require high conformational energies to fit the 3D-pharmacophore defined in Figure 3.19. Figure 3.20 displays the relationship between calculated conformational energies for the bioactive conformations of (**3.21**)–(**3.30**) and their agonist activities. The highly active com-pounds (**3.23**) and (**3.29**) have conformational energies of less than 2 kJ mol^{-1}, whereas the moderately active compounds (**3.24**) and (**3.25**) display conformational energies of 8 and 11 kJ mol^{-1} respectively. All low active or inactive compounds have conforma-tional energies in excess of 20 kJ mol^{-1}. This clearly demonstrates that conformational energies must be taken into account in the design of new ligands from a template structure.

3.7.3 A 3D-pharmacophore model for dopamine D-2 receptor antagonists

(1R, 3S)-Tefludazine (**3.31**) and (S)-octoclothepin (S)-(**3.32**) are high-affinity dopamine D-2 receptor antagonists (Fig. 3.21). On the basis of these compounds a 3D-pharmacophore for D-2 receptor antagonists has been developed. The pharmacophore elements chosen are the centers of the aromatic rings, the nitrogen atoms encircled in Figure 3.21, and a site point in each molecule, 2.8 Å from the nitrogen atom in the direction of the nitrogen lone electron pair (Fig. 3.21).

Based on exhaustive conformational analysis of the two compounds by molecular mechanics and molecular least-squares superimposition studies, the superimposition shown in Figure 3.22 was obtained (rms = 0.23 Å). A closer inspection of this superimposition reveals that a simultaneous rotation in (**3.31**) and (S)-(**3.32**) about the C-N bond connecting the piperazine ring to the tricyclic ring system, preserves the excellent superimposition of the pharmacophore elements. However, such a simultaneous rotation generates an infinite number of possible 3D-pharmacophore candidates. It will be demonstrated below that calculated conformational energies may be used to select among these candidates.

Figure 3.23 displays calculated potential energy curves for the reorientation of the piperazine rings in (**3.31**) and (S)-(**3.32**). The two curves are slightly displaced so that the pair of dihedral angles giving an optimal fit of the pharmacophore elements are placed directly above each other. Thus, the superimposition shown in Figure 3.22 corresponds to dihedral angles of 290 degrees for (S)-(**3.32**) and 300 degrees for (**3.31**).

The potential energy curve for (**3.31**) displays several low-energy regions corresponding to possible receptor-bound conformations. However, the potential energy curve for (S)-(**3.32**) displays only a few such regions — only a small region with dihedral angles in the range of 260–315 degrees, lies below 12 kJ mol^{-1}. Since the corresponding region in the potential energy curve of (**3.31**) (270–325 degrees) has conformational energies well below 10 kJ mol^{-1}, the receptor-bound conformations for (**3.31**) and (S)-(**3.32**) are most probably to be found for dihedral angles in these regions. The conformations for (**3.31**) and (S)-(**3.32**) displayed in the superimposition in Figure 3.22 correspond to the lowest-energy conformations in these regions.

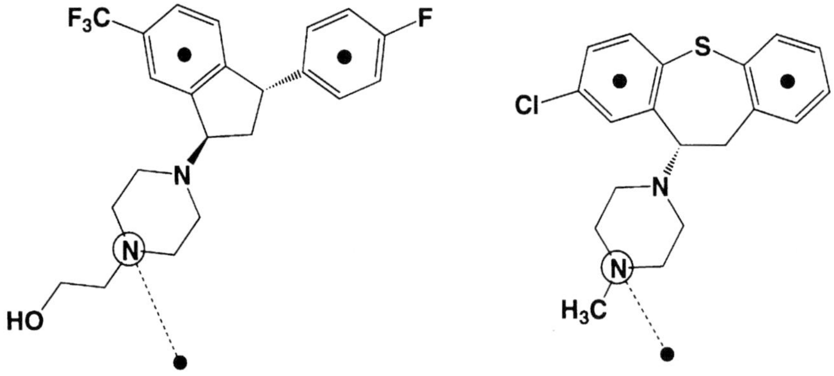

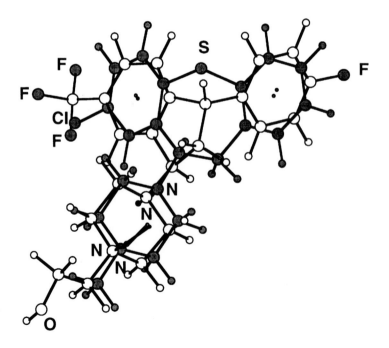

(3.31)   (S)-(3.32)

Figure 3.21   Pharmacophore elements used in the development of a 3D-pharmacophore model for dopamine D-2 receptor antagonists.

Figure 3.22   A least-squares molecular superimposition of compounds (3.31) and (S)-(3.32). Note that the trifluoromethyl group in (3.31) and the chloro substituent in (S)-(3.32) (the "neuroleptic substituents") are very similarily positioned in space.

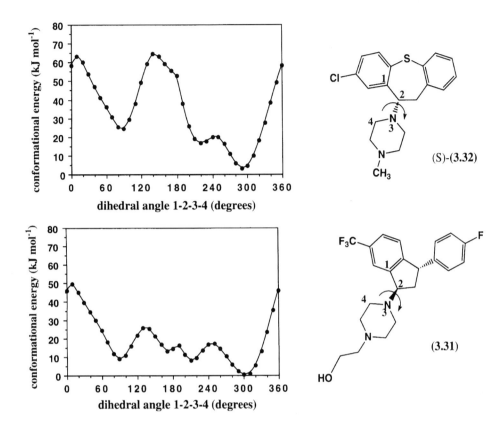

Figure 3.23   Potential energy curves calculated using molecular mechanics for the rotation about the C2-N3 bond in (**3.31**) and (S)-(**3.32**). Note that the global energy conformation for (S)-(**3.32**), (corresponding to a conformational energy of 0.0 kJ mol^{-1}) is not included in the potential energy curve. The global energy conformation has another conformation of the tricyclic ring system.

The enantiomers of (**3.32**) may be used to test the proposed receptor-bound conformation for (S)-(**3.32**). The conformational properties of (S)- and (R)-(**3.32**) are such that it is possible to find a conformation for (R)-(**3.32**) which extremely well superimposes with the proposed receptor-bound conformation of (S)-(**3.32**). This superimposition is shown in Figure 3.24. Note that in the superimposition, the two enantiomers have different conformations of their tricyclic ring systems.

The very high degree of similarity displayed by the two enantiomers in their proposed bioactive conformations implies that energy contributions to ΔG_{bind} due to intermolecular interactions with receptor sites (ΔG_{inter}) should be essentially the same for the enantiomers. ΔG_{bind} should consequently be determined by the difference in conformational energies of the conformations shown in Figure 3.24, as discussed in Section 3.3. The experimental ΔG_{bind} for (R)-(**3.32**) determined by radioligand receptor binding is 4.2 kJ mol^{-1} higher than that for (S)-(**3.32**). The conformational energy difference calculated by molecular

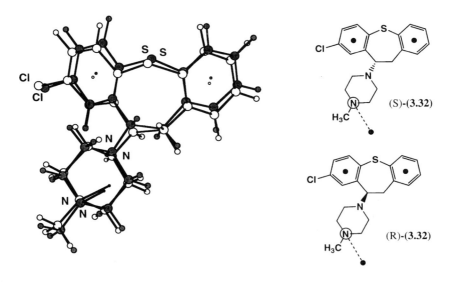

Figure 3.24 A molecular least-squares superimposition (rms = 0.28 Å) of (S)-(**3.32**) (grey atoms) and (R)-(**3.32**). The pharmacophore elements used in the superimposition are included in the structural formulas.

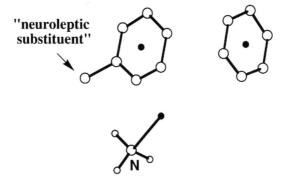

Figure 3.25 A representation of the basic 3D-pharmacophore model for dopamine D-2 receptor antagonists. The position of the "neuroleptic substituent" which generally increases the affinity of the molecule for the dopamine D-2 receptor is included in the model.

mechanics is 5.8 kJ mol^{-1}. Since energy contributions to ΔG_{bind} due to desolvation, hydrophobicity, loss of entropy etc. are identical for enantiomers, the calculated number may be directly compared with the experimental ΔG_{bind}. The good agreement between calculated and experimental results corroborates the proposed receptor-bound conformation for (S)-(**3.32**) (and thus for (**3.31**)). This analysis demonstrates that enantiomers having such conformational properties that pharmacophore elements are able to superimpose may be

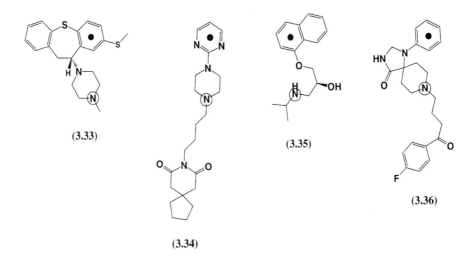

Figure 3.26   5-HT$_{1A}$ receptor antagonists used for the development of a 3D-pharmacophore. The compounds are oriented as in the superimposition discussed in the text.

valuable tools in 3D-pharmacophore identification. However, the enantiomeric purity must be very high in order to make it possible to determine a meaningful $\Delta\Delta G_{bind}$ by receptor binding studies.

A representation in terms of disconnected fragments of the 3D-pharmacophore derived from the superimposition in Figure 3.22 is shown in Figure 3.25.

3.7.4 Design of selective serotonin 5-HT$_{1A}$ receptor antagonists using 3D-pharmacophores

(*R*)-Methiothepin (**3.33**), buspirone (**3.34**), (*S*)-propranolol (**3.35**) and spiperone (**3.36**) are serotonin 5-HT$_{1A}$ receptor antagonists. However, their selectivities with respect to, for instance, 5-HT$_{1B}$ and 5HT$_{2A}$ receptors are low.

These compounds have been used to develop a 3D-pharmacophore for 5-HT$_{1A}$ antagonism with the aim of developing new antagonists with increased affinity and selectivity. Several different sets of pharmacophore elements were tried and the best set was found to be (*i*) the nitrogen atom encircled in Figure 3.26 (*ii*) a 2 Å long vector, orthogonal to the plane of the labeled aromatic ring and through the centroid shown in Figure 3.26.

Conformational analysis (with the replacement of the substituents of the encircled nitrogens in (**3.33**)–(**3.36**) by a methyl group) was performed for each compound using a conformational search procedure and conformations which display closely similar relative 3D-locations of the pharmacophore elements were identified. In the deduced bioactive conformations of each of (**3.33**)–(**3.36**), the mean distance between the center of the aromatic ring and the nitrogen atom was found to be 5.6 Å and the nitrogen atom was located on the average 1.6 Å above the aromatic ring plane (Fig. 3.27).

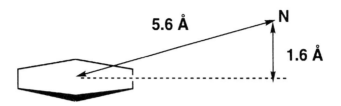

Figure 3.27   A basic 3D-pharmacophore for 5-HT$_{1A}$ receptor antagonists.

The superimpositions and the model in Figure 3.27 was used to design several new ligands. One of these novel ligands is the benzodioxan (**3.37**). Radioligand receptor binding studies on (**3.37**) showed that this compound indeed has a very high affinity for the 5-HT$_{1A}$ receptor.

(**3.37**)   (**3.38**)

Furthermore, it was found to be very selective with respect to the 5-HT$_{1B}$, the 5HT$_{2A}$, and the dopamine D-2 receptors, and also to have low affinity for the α_2-adrenoceptor. However, it still displayed significant affinity for the α_1-adrenoceptor. Comparison of the receptor-excluded volume (see Section 3.5) of the 5-HT$_{1A}$ receptor, computed using the superimposition of compounds (**3.33**)–(**3.36**), and that of the α_1-adrenoceptor suggested that compound (**3.38**) should have a decreased affinity for the α_1-adrenoceptor compared to (**3.37**) without affecting the affinity for the 5-HT$_{1A}$ receptor. This prediction was shown to be correct by radioligand receptor binding studies.

This study exemplifies the use of a rational computer-aided design of a high-affinity and highly selective ligand based on 3D-pharmacophore models.

REFERENCES AND FURTHER READING

References for the examples in Section 3.7:

Schulman, J.M., Sabio, M.L. and Disch, R.L. (1983) Recognition of cholinergic agonists by the muscarinic receptor. 1. Acetylcholine and other agonists with the NCCOCC backbone. *J. Med. Chem.*, **26**, 817–823.

Pettersson, I. and Liljefors, T. (1987) Structure-activity relationships for apomorphine congeners. Conformational energies *vs.* biological activities. *J. Computer-Aided Mol. Design*, **1**, 143–152.

Liljefors, T. and Bøgesø, K.P. (1988) Conformational analysis and structural comparisons of 1R, 3S-(+)-, 1S, 3R-(−)-tefludazine, S-(+)-octoclothepin and (+)-dexclamol in relation to dopamine receptor antagonism and amine-uptake inhibition. *J. Med. Chem.*, **31**, 306–312.

Bøgesø, K.P., Liljefors, T., Arnt, J., Hyttel, J. and Pedersen, H. (1991) Octoclothepin enantiomers. A reinvestigation of their biochemical and pharmacological activity in relation to a new model for dopamine D-2 receptor antagonists. *J. Med. Chem.*, **34**, 2023.

Hibert, M.F., Gittos, M.W., Middlemiss, D.N., Mir, A.K. and Fozard, J.R. (1988) Graphics computer-aided receptor mapping as a predictive tool for drug design. Development of potent, selective, and stereospecific ligands for the 5-HT$_{1A}$ receptor. *J. Med. Chem.*, **31**, 1087–1093.

Suggested further reading:

Burkert, U. and Allinger, N.L. (1982) *Molecular Mechanics, ACS Monograph 177*, Washington D.C.: American Chemical Society.

Cramer, C.J. and Truhlar, D.G. (1992) AM1-SM2 and PM3-SM3 Parameterized SCF Solvation Models for Free Energies in Aqueous Solution. *J. Computer-Aided Mol. Design*, **6**, 629–666.

Golender, V.E. and Vorpagel, E.R. (1993) Computer-Assisted Pharmacophore Identification. In *3D QSAR in Drug Design. Theory, Methods and Applications*, edited by H. Kubinyi, pp. 137–149. Leiden: Escom Science Publishers.

Leach, A.R. (1991) A Survey of Methods for Searching the Conformational Space of Small and Medium-Sized Molecules. In *Reviews in Computational Chemistry, Vol. 2*, edited by K.B. Lipkowitz and D.B. Boyd, pp. 1–55, New York: VCH Publishers.

Marshall, G.R. (1993) Binding Site Modeling of Unknown Receptors. In *3D QSAR in Drug Design. Theory, Methods and Applications*, edited by H. Kubinyi, pp. 80–116. Leiden: Escom Science Publishers.

Merz Jr., K.M. and Kollman, P.A. (1989) Free Energy Perturbation Simulations of the Inhibition of Thermolysin. Prediction of the Free Energy of Binding of a New Inhibitor. *J. Med. Chem.*, **111**, 5649–5658.

Ripka, W.C. and Blaney J.M. (1991) Computer Graphics and Molecular Modeling in the Analysis of Synthetic Targets. In *Topics In Stereochemisty, Vol. 20*, edited by E.L. Eliel and S.H. Wilen, pp. 1–85. New York: J. Wiley & Sons.

Siebel, G.L. and Kollman, P.A. (1990) Molecular Mechanics and the Modeling of Drug Structures. In *Comprehensive Medicinal Chemistry, Vol. 4*, edited by C. Hansch, P.G. Sammes, J.B. Taylor and C.A. Ramsden, pp. 125–138. Oxford: Pergamon Press.

Still, W.C., Tempczyk, A., Hawley, R.C. and Hendrickson, T. (1990) Semianalytical Treatment of Solvation for Molecular Mechanics and Dynamics. *J. Amer. Chem. Soc.*, **112**, 6127–6129.

Wermuth, C.-G. and Langer, T. (1993) Pharmacophore Identification. In *3D QSAR in Drug Design. Theory, Methods and Applications*, edited by H. Kubinyi, pp. 117–136. Leiden: Escom Science Publishers.

4. QUANTITATIVE STRUCTURE-ACTIVITY RELATIONSHIPS AND EXPERIMENTAL DESIGN

THOMAS HÖGBERG and ULF NORINDER

CONTENTS

4.1 INTRODUCTION

Pharmacophoric mapping is of great value in generating new chemical lead structures, especially when a limited number of compounds are available or when different chemical classes are used (see Chapter 3). A steric fit, reflected by the 3-D geometry of a structure in its active conformation is a necessary but not sufficient cause of activity, since electronic and hydrophobic forces between ligand and receptor are required for the response. An inherent limitation with pharmacophoric modeling techniques like the active analogue approach is their inability to quantitatively describe the effect, i.e. one can usually only distinguish active from inactive compounds. In the process of optimizing a lead structure it is necessary to utilize the information from quantitative activity data and from other structural properties in a more efficient way in order to predict more active congeners. Furthermore, quantitative structure-activity relationships (QSAR) can provide a great deal of information regarding the nature of ligand-target protein interactions. In series of homologous derivatives, various quantitative structure-activity analyses utilizing linear free energy relationships, multiple linear regression, and pattern recognition techniques have been applied. Furthermore, recent progress has been made in combining molecular modeling and statistical models, which allows for handling of non-congeneric series.

4.2 HANSCH ANALYSIS

4.2.1 Hydrophobic correlations

The biological activity can be regarded as a function of the physicochemical and structural properties of the ligand. Already at the turn of the century, Meyer and Overton observed independently of each other that the anesthetic potency of simple organic molecules increases linearly with their oil/water partition coefficients (P). Four decades later Ferguson connected the narcotic activity and partition coefficients with thermodynamic principles. He stated that under equilibrium conditions, narcotic activity was correlated to the relative saturation of membranes by the gaseous narcotic substance. However, Hansch reasoned that too lipophilic molecules will partition into the first line of lipid membranes and be retained there. Likewise, too hydrophilic molecules will not readily partition from the first aqueous compartment into the lipid of a membrane. Accordingly Hansch and coworkers observed in the 1960s that the biological activity for several sets of congeners conformed with a parabolic dependence on lipophilicity ($\log P$) according to equation (4.1). Thus, an optimal $\log P$ value would correspond to the maximum probability of a compound to reach a receptor protein on a random walk between various lipophilic and hydrophilic compartments. The optimal lipophilic value, $\log P_o = a/2b$, is obtained from the derivative $d(\log 1/C)/d \log P$ being equal to zero. The biological activity is usually expressed as the logarithm of the inverse concentration or dose [$\log(1/C)$ or pC] which produces some standard response, e.g. $\log(1/IC_{50})$ or $\log(1/ED_{50})$.

$$\text{biological activity } (\log 1/C) = a \log P - b(\log P)^2 + c \tag{4.1}$$

Phenomena involved in the transport of the ligand to its site of action and the hydrophobic interactions with the receptor are mainly determined by equation (4.1). For several classes of CNS active substances it has been found that the activity and thus the penetration over the blood-brain barrier (BBB) is optimal for $\log P_o$ (octanol) values in the range of 1.5–2.7, with a mean value of 2.1 (see also Section 4.5.5 for a more recent view).

Kubinyi has developed an alternative model to describe biphasic relationships with a bilinear equation (4.2) which is especially useful when the positive and negative slopes are different, or in cases where one slope may be zero. This equation fits many sets of experimental data better than the quadratic equation (4.1). However, it is more cumbersome to use, since the calculation involves an iterative determination of the β-value in equation (4.2).

$$\log(1/C) = a \log P - b \log(\beta P + 1) + c \tag{4.2}$$

The observation of different negative and positive slopes in biphasic QSARs has also been argued to be due to receptor binding rather than transport phenomena. Thus, a linear dependence on $\log P$ can be expected up to a point where the hydrophobic region of the receptor is covered and thereafter the activity decreases due to steric hindrance during the interaction of ligand and receptor. In several cases, the whole lipophilicity range may not have been investigated and, thus, only a linear dependence is revealed.

4.2.2 Multifactorial correlations

In order to take other types of molecular interactions into account, Hansch and Fujita included descriptors for steric, electronic and hydrophobic (= lipophilic) properties in the QSAR equation (4.3), which is based on the fact that the variables can be related to free energies in a linear free energy relationship (LFER).

$$\log(1/C) = a(\text{hydrophobic parameter}) + b(\text{electronic parameter})$$

$$+ c(\text{steric parameter}) + d(\text{other descriptor}) + e \tag{4.3}$$

where a, b, c, d and e are the regression coefficients determined by least squares regression analysis, often referred to as a Hansch analysis. Different physicochemical parameters have been used to describe the global properties of the molecule or the contribution from individual substituents. The most commonly used substituent parameters are shown in Table 4.1. These independent variables (parameters and descriptors) can be collinear, i.e. the same information is carried by the parameters, which will lead to false correlations. By including indicator variables one can for example describe the presence or absence of a certain substituent or other structural characteristics (cf. Section 4.3.1). In the ideal case,

Table 4.1   Physicochemical parameters used in QSAR.

Parameter	Symbol
Hydrophobic parameters	
Partition coefficient	$\log P$, CLOGP, PrologP
Substituent constant	π
Hydrophobic fragmental constant	f, f'
Distribution coefficient	$\log D$
Apparent partition coefficient (fixed pH)	$\log P'$, $\log P_{app}$
Capacity factor in HPLC	$\log k$, $\log k_w$
Solubility parameter	δ
Electronic descriptors	
Hammett constants	$\sigma, \sigma^-, \sigma^+$
Taft's inductive (polar) constants	σ^*, σ_I
Swain and Lupton field parameter	$\mathfrak{I}$
Swain and Lupton resonance parameter	$\mathfrak{R}$
Ionization constant	pKa, ΔpKa
Chemical shifts (^{13}C and ^{1}H)	δ
Theoretical parameters	
Atomic net charge	q^σ, q^π
Superdelocalizability	S^N, S^E, S^R
Energy of highest occupied molecular orbital	E_{HOMO}
Energy of lowest unoccupied molecular orbital	E_{LUMO}
Electrostatic potentials	V (r)
Steric descriptors	
Taft's steric parameter	E_S, E^c
Molar volume	MV
Molecular weight	MW
Van der Waals radius	r
Van der Waals volume	V_W
Molar refractivity	MR
Parachor	P_r
STERIMOL parameters	$L, B_1, B_5(B_2, B_3, B_4)$

the biological data and physicochemical parameters should be spread evenly and over a large range as will be discussed in the following Section 4.8.

The number of compounds (n) in the correlation must be considerably larger than the number of parameters (k) used, i.e. four to six compounds (data points) per variable for medium sized data sets in order to avoid chance correlations. In the PLS method described in Section 4.6 this is not a limitation even if redundant variables should be avoided. The correlation coefficient r, the relative measure of the quality of fit, should be around 0.9 for *in vitro* data, i.e. the explained variance r^2 should be over 80%, for acceptable regression equations. The standard deviation s, the absolute measure of the quality of fit, should not exceed the standard deviation in the biological data set too much. The regression coefficients (a, b, c, d, etc.) should make sense from a physicochemical standpoint (cf. ρ-values in physical organic chemistry) and be justified by confidence intervals at the 95% level (not shown in the following equations). The F-value, i.e. the ratio between explained and unexplained variance for the available degrees of freedom ($n - k - 1$), should be larger than the 95% significance limits.

Importantly, the physicochemical descriptors contain information that will give direct insight about properties essential for the transport to the site of action and for the interaction with the target protein required for the biological activity. Thus, one should select and statistically justify independent (low intercorrelation coefficients) variables, which describe different structural properties. In the analysis, one should aim for the simplest model to describe the data (principle of parsimony).

4.3 FREE-WILSON ANALYSIS

4.3.1 Additivity models

Free and Wilson reasoned that the biological activity for a set of congeners can be described by the additive properties of the activity contributions from substituents or structural elements present in a parent structure. Thus, the presence and absence of structural element is indicated by the values 1 and 0, respectively. The addition of an indicator variable to the Hansch equation (4.3) can be thought of as a combination of the Fujita-Ban modification of the Free-Wilson analysis and Hansch analysis, where the (other descriptor) term includes the indicator variables describing certain structural features, e.g. substructures, chiral centers and special substituents. The formulation of the Fujita-Ban modification of the Free-Wilson methodology, which is the technique used today and often referred to as 'Free-Wilson analysis', is presented in equation (4.4)

$$\log (1/C_i) = \sum a_j X_{ij} + \mu \tag{4.4}$$

where a_j is the group contribution of the structural feature X in position j in molecule i and μ is the theoretical biological activity value of a reference compound. The descriptor X_{ij} has a value of 1 if the feature is present in position j in molecule i and 0 in the absence of that feature.

Kubinyi has applied Free-Wilson analysis to a set of α-bromophenethylamines (**4.1**) investigated as adrenergic blockers (Table 4.2). The compounds, which antagonize the effects of epinephrine in the rat, have been used as a pilot example in many calculations (cf. equations (4.22) and (4.23)). A relationship according to equation (4.5) explains 94% of the variance in the data set and the relative contributions of the halogen and methyl substituents in the *meta* and *para* positions are easily seen.

$$\log (1/\text{ED}_{50}) = -0.301[m\text{--F}] + 0.27[m\text{--Cl}] + 0.434[m\text{--Br}] + 0.579[m\text{--I}]$$

$$+ 0.454[m\text{--Me}] + 0.340[p\text{--F}] + 0.768[p\text{--Cl}] + 1.020[p\text{--Br}]$$

$$+ 1.429[p\text{--I}] + 1.256[p\text{--Me}] + 7.821$$

$$n = 22, r^2 = 0.94, s = 0.194, F = 17.0 \tag{4.5}$$

The application of Free-Wilson analysis to chiral compounds is represented by an example involving norepinephrine-uptake inhibition in isolated rat heart ($1/\text{IC}_{50}$) by optically active phenethylamines (**4.2**). The structural description and results are given in Table 4.3 and by equation (4.6), respectively.

(4.1)   (4.2)

Table 4.2   Free-Wilson structural description of the α-bromophenethylamines (**4.1**).

#	meta	para	meta-					para-				
	(X)	(Y)	F	Cl	Br	I	Me	F	Cl	Br	I	Me
1	H	H										
2	H	F						1				
3	H	Cl							1			
4	H	Br								1		
5	H	I									1	
6	H	Me										1
7	F	H	1									
8	Cl	H		1								
9	Br	H			1							
10	I	H				1						
11	Me	H					1					
12	Cl	F		1				1				
13	Br	F			1			1				
14	Me	F					1	1				
15	Cl	Cl		1					1			
16	Br	Cl			1				1			
17	Me	Cl					1		1			
18	Cl	Br		1						1		
19	Br	Br			1					1		
20	Me	Br					1			1		
21	Me	Me					1					1
22	Br	Me			1							1

The parent compound in this study was the unsubstituted phenethylamine, which means that all hydrogen columns are removed from the structural matrix (Table 4.3). A 50:50 mixture is assumed for the substituents (Table 4.3) in racemates, which transfers to an assigned value of 0.5 in the corresponding columns.

$$\log\left(1/\mathrm{IC}_{50}\right) = 0.355[\mathrm{OH}(X)] - 0.879[\mathrm{OMe}(X)] + 0.417[\mathrm{OH}(Y)]$$

$$- 1.410[\mathrm{OMe}(Y)] - 0.379[\mathrm{OH}(R_1)] - 0.785[\mathrm{OH}(R_2)]$$

$$- 0.288[\mathrm{Me}(R_3)] + 0.763[\mathrm{Me}(R_4)] - 0.467[\mathrm{Me}(R_5)] + 1.975$$

$$n = 30, r^2 = 0.93, s = 0.276, F = 28.8 \tag{4.6}$$

Table 4.3   Structural description of sympathomimetic amines (**4.2**).

#	chirality	X OH	X OMe	Y OH	Y OMe	R_1 OH	R_2 OH	R_3 Me	R_4 Me	R_5 Me
1	–			1		1				
2		1		1						
3	+/–	1		1				0.5	0.5	
4	+								1	
5	+/–	1						0.5	0.5	
6	–	1		1		1			1	
7	–	1		1		1				
8	+/–	1		1		0.5	0.5	0.5	0.5	
9		1								
10	+/–							0.5	0.5	
11				1						
12	+								1	1
13	+/–	1		1		0.5	0.5			
14		1		1						1
15	–	1		1		1				1
16								1	1	1
17										
18	+/–	1				0.5	0.5			
19	+	1		1			1			
20	+/–	1		1		0.5	0.5			1
21	+/–					0.5	0.5	0.5	0.5	
22	–					1			1	1
23	–							1		
24	+/–					0.5	0.5			
25	–			1		1				1
26			1							
27	+/–	1				0.5	0.5			1
28	+/–	1			1	0.5	0.5			1
29	+/–	1			1	0.5	0.5			
30			1		1					

A drawback with the Free-Wilson analysis is that the structural description in many cases give rise to a large number of parameters, which may represent a statistical problem if multiple linear regression (MLR) techniques are used. This situation can, however, be circumvented by instead using pattern recognition methods such as PLS (see Section 4.6 for a description of the method) for delineating the relationship between structures and biological activities. Norinder has investigated the PLS application to Free-Wilson analysis for some N-alkylmorphine-6-one opioids. The 41 opioids were described by 74 variables and the PLS analysis resulted in the following statistics: $n = 41$, $r^2 = 0.81$, cross-validated $r^2 = 0.64$, $s = 0.267$, $F = 51.66$, which represents an improvement compared with an earlier investigation by Hernandez-Gallegos and Lehmann F using MLR.

4.3.2 Pros and cons

The Free-Wilson methodology is simple to apply and can provide valuable information regarding the importance of different structural features in an easy manner without the need for more elaborate variables, which may be hard to come by for certain types of substituents and/or substructures. However, the Free-Wilson technique has some severe limitations:

1. The method is strictly interpolative from a structural point of view, i.e. only structural features described in the derived model by the set of investigated compounds can be used. The method can not, as opposed to techniques based upon a physicochemical description of the structures, be used for extrapolative purposes to find new structural elements that are predicted to be of potential interest. Usually this means that only a relatively small number of new analogues can be predicted from Free-Wilson models.

2. Also, as mentioned before in this section, a relatively large number of variables are usually required in a model to describe a rather limited number of structural features.

3. Especially troublesome are the instances when a structural feature only occurs once in the data set studied, a so called single-point determination, because the corresponding structural contribution will then contain the entire experimental error of the dependent property, e.g. biological activity.

4. The Free-Wilson description of a structure, although useful for deriving meaningful QSAR models, are also questionable from a similarity/dissimilarity point of view. All structural features and/or substituents are considered to be equally dissimilar. For example, the change from a methyl group to an ethyl group can hardly be represented as being of the same physicochemical magnitude as that from a methyl group to a sulfonamide moiety. Furthermore, even though the indicator variables will display which particular group and/or structural feature that is the most favorable in a certain position, these descriptors will neither reveal the physicochemical reasons why a certain structural element is preferred, nor give any indication as to in what way that element could be modified chemically to give rise to compounds with new and improved biological properties.

4.4 PHYSICOCHEMICAL PROPERTIES

4.4.1 Electronic descriptors

The first and still most widely used electronic substituent parameter σ was developed by Hammett 1935 on the basis of ionization constants for benzoic acid derivatives. The Hammett equation (4.7) is expressed as

$$\rho\sigma = \log K_X - \log K_H \tag{4.7}$$

where K_H and K_X are the ionization constants for benzoic acid and a *para* or *meta* substituted derivative, respectively, and $\rho = 1$ for measurements in water at 25 °C. Positive σ values represent electron withdrawing properties ($X = CN, NO_2, CF_3$) and negative σ values electron donating properties ($X = NH_2, CH_3$).

A number of related Hammett parameters applicable for special circumstances, e.g. $\sigma_p^-, \sigma_p^+, \sigma_m$ and σ_p, can provide mechanistic insight on the nature of the interaction if a considerably better correlation is obtained with a particular constant (cf. equations (4.23) and (4.24) below).

The inductive field (polar) component of the electronic substituent effect could be separated from the resonance part. Swain and Lupton described the Hammett σ constant as a linear combination of a resonance effect $\mathfrak{R}$ and a field effect $\mathfrak{I}$. These parameters are not position-dependent, which makes them useful and easy to handle in QSAR (cf. equation (4.26)). The Hammett constant σ is related to the $\mathfrak{I}$ and $\mathfrak{R}$ values as expressed in equation (4.8)

$$\sigma = f\mathfrak{I} + r\mathfrak{R} \tag{4.8}$$

where f and r are weighting factors.

4.4.2 Hydrophobic parameters

Analogous to the derivation of the Hammett constant, the substituent constant π for hydrophobic effect can be described by equation (4.9),

$$\pi = \log P_X - \log P_H \tag{4.9}$$

where P_X is the partition coefficient of a substituted derivative and P_H that of the parent compound. The distribution is measured between an organic solvent and water and the partition coefficient P is the ratio of the same solute in the two immiscible solvents. Octanol is the accepted standard system used and it has been justified as a suitable model for lipid constituents in biomembranes by the slightly amphiphilic nature introduced by the hydroxyl group in the long alkyl chain. The hydrogen bond donating and accepting properties facilitate the interaction with several types of solutes and octanol also dissolves an appreciable amount of water during equilibrium conditions. The partitioning to other solvent systems can be calculated by the Collander equation (4.10). This linear relationship between log P obtained in different systems make it reasonable to apply one arbitrary standard system (octanol) even if limitations have been pointed out.

$$\log P_1 = a \log P_2 + c \tag{4.10}$$

A positive π corresponds to a lipophilic character and negative π to a hydrophilic character relative to hydrogen. In the case of ionizable solutes, log P for the nonionized species can be determined from the distribution coefficient D, which is dependent on pH, by inclusion of the ionization constant(s) in the calculation (e.g. equations (4.11) and (4.12)). Partition through membranes is usually regarded to be associated with the nonionized molecules.

$$\log D_{\text{acid}} = \log P - \log[1 + 10^{(\text{pH} - \text{pKa})}] \tag{4.11}$$

$$\log D_{\text{base}} = \log P - \log[1 + 10^{(\text{pKa} - \text{pH})}] \tag{4.12}$$

However, the determination of partition coefficients by the classical shake flask technique is connected with several practical problems, e.g. disturbances from minor impurities, effects of ions in aqueous buffers, difficulties to analyze solutes in both phases especially for compounds with extreme log P values, necessity to work with very low concentrations of solute to diminish aggregation, and establishment of equilibrium conditions. These problems to determine log P values can largely be overcome by use of HPLC-derived hydrophobicity data. The HPLC methodology can also be applied to small and impure amounts of material and gives accurate data by frequent use of calibration standards. Furthermore, no quantitative methods for the determination of the solutes are required. The chromatographically derived values are not unique, but they can be converted into the familiar octanol/water partition coefficients. This makes HPLC the method of choice for experimental determination of log P values.

The slope a in equation (4.1) has been found to have values in the range from about 0.2 to 1.4. It has been argued that a-values of about unity implies complete desolvation and binding deep into a lipophilic pocket (cf. equations (4.17), (4.18), (4.21), (4.23) and (4.31)), whereas a-values of about 0.5 reflects only partial desolvation and binding along the surface of a protein (cf. equations (4.16) and (4.19)). However, this view is under debate, since binding to a highly structured membrane reduces the freedom of an alkyl chain, which will diminish the slope a and the π values.

The additive properties of the π values make it possible to estimate log P of a new compound, either completely from tables or by combination of experimental values and tabulated data. For example, the log P value for xylene can be estimated with a high degree of accuracy from the log P values of benzene and toluene by the following simple calculation.

$$\pi_{Me} = \log P_{Ph-Me} - \log P_{Ph-H} = 2.69 - 2.13 = 0.56$$

$$\log P_{xylene} = \log P_{Ph-Me} + \pi_{Me} = 2.69 + 0.56 = 3.25 \qquad \text{(Experimental 3.20)}$$

However, in several cases, especially for aliphatic compounds, large differences between observed log P values and partition coefficients calculated from π values are found. To overcome these limitations, Rekker introduced the concept of fragmental constants f, which are related to the π values according to equation (4.13). The fragmental constants, which were statistically derived from over thousand log P determinations, measure the absolute lipophilicity contribution of a given structural fragment i, which occurs a_i number of times in a structure. Interaction factors F were also introduced in order to correct for intramolecular electronic, steric or hydrogen bond interactions between fragments according to equation (4.14).

$$f_X = f_H + \pi_X \qquad (4.13)$$

$$\log P = \sum a_i f_X + \sum F_i \qquad (4.14)$$

The fragmental constant system has been modified by Leo and Hansch based on a small number of accurately determined log P values instead of the statistical approach used by Rekker. Based on this concept a computer program CLOGP was developed by Chou and Jurs, which allows for more facile calculations of log P values.

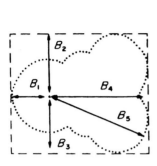 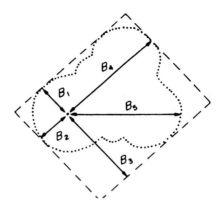

Figure 4.1   Definition of STERIMOL parameters for the methoxy group. L (orthogonal to paper) is the length of the substituent along its axis of attachment and the width parameters B are all orthogonal to L. B_1 is the minimum and B_5 is the maximum width. Two different possibilities to select B_1 result in different definitions of the perpendicular B_2, B_3 and B_4. The new B_5 parameter has no directional relationship to B_1. Reproduced with permission from Pergamon Press and Corwin Hansch.

4.4.3 Steric descriptors

The description of steric bulk of a substituent is difficult to assess, since the conformation may vary among the ligands in the test series as well as for the target protein. However, several parameters have been successfully applied. The steric effect has been described by Taft's steric parameter E_S, derived from acidic hydrolysis of esters (X-CH_2COOR). E_S is more negative for larger groups [t-Bu, CCl_3] and more positive for smaller groups (H, F, OH).

In order to better account for the shape of the substituents, Verloop has developed a set of parameters using the STERIMOL program based on CPK-models. The length parameter L and the four width parameters B_1, B_2, B_3, and B_4 which describe the dimensions of the group along fixed axes, were originally used. The STERIMOL length parameter L and the minimum distance parameter B_1 have been retained and a new maximum width parameter B_5 has been introduced (cf. equation (4.18)). By using ratios of L/B_1 and B_5/B_1 one might get information on any directionality of importance for the receptor interaction. The definitions of STERIMOL parameters are shown in Figure 4.1.

Alternatively, the van der Waals radii and the molar volume $MV = MW/d$ have been used. The molar refractivity (MR) is related to the molar volume by the Lorentz-Lorenz equation (4.15).

$$MR = [(n^2 - 1)/(n^2 + 2)](MW/d) \qquad (4.15)$$

where n is the refraction index, d is the density and MW is the molecular weight. Fragment values have been calculated since MR is an additive property of the molecule. A larger MR value for a substituent corresponds to a larger steric bulk and a greater tendency to interact via dispersion forces. A compilation of commonly used parameters for aromatic substituents is shown in Table 4.4.

Table 4.4 Commonly used aromatic substituent parameters and principal properties (PP) calculated from the complete set of parameters by principal component analysis (Section 4.6).

Subst.	σ_m	σ_p	$\mathfrak{I}$	$\mathfrak{R}$	π	MR	L	B_1	B_5	PP_1	PP_2	PP_3
H	0.00	0.00	0.00	0.00	0.00	1.03	2.06	1.00	1.00	1.35	−3.00	−0.39
F	0.34	0.06	0.43	−0.34	0.14	0.92	2.65	1.35	1.35	2.38	−1.95	0.45
Cl	0.37	0.23	0.41	−0.15	0.71	6.03	3.52	1.80	1.80	2.22	−0.15	−0.57
Br	0.39	0.23	0.44	−0.17	0.86	8.88	3.82	1.95	1.95	2.08	0.38	−0.74
I	0.35	0.18	0.40	−0.19	1.12	13.94	4.23	2.15	2.15	1.49	1.00	−1.21
NO$_2$	0.71	0.78	0.67	0.16	−0.28	7.36	3.44	1.70	2.44	4.12	1.12	0.87
CH$_3$	−0.07	−0.17	−0.04	−0.13	0.56	5.65	2.87	1.52	2.04	0.25	−1.84	−1.36
CCH	0.21	0.23	0.19	0.05	0.40	9.55	4.66	1.60	1.60	1.30	−0.01	−0.60
CHCH$_2$	0.05	−0.02	0.07	−0.08	0.82	10.99	4.29	1.60	3.09	−0.09	−0.18	−0.65
C$_2$H$_5$	−0.07	−0.15	−0.05	−0.10	1.02	10.30	4.11	1.52	3.17	−0.71	−0.65	−0.90
C$_3$H$_5$	−0.07	−0.21	−0.03	−0.19	1.14	13.53	4.14	1.55	3.24	−1.02	−0.56	−0.83
C$_3$H$_7$	−0.07	−0.13	−0.06	−0.08	1.55	14.96	4.92	1.52	3.49	−1.35	0.15	−0.78
CH(CH$_3$)$_2$	−0.07	−0.15	−0.05	−0.10	1.53	14.98	4.11	1.90	3.17	−0.87	0.16	−1.89
C$_4$H$_9$	−0.08	−0.16	−0.06	−0.11	2.13	19.59	6.17	1.52	4.54	−2.43	1.22	−0.32
CH$_2$CH(CH$_3$)$_2$	−0.10	−0.20	−0.07	−0.13	1.98	19.62	4.92	1.52	4.45	−2.16	0.61	−0.55
C(CH$_3$)$_3$	−0.10	−0.20	−0.07	−0.13	1.98	19.62	4.11	2.60	3.17	−1.03	1.20	−3.70
C$_5$H$_{11}$	−0.08	−0.15	−0.06	−0.09	2.67	24.25	7.17	1.52	5.23	−3.22	2.21	−0.03
C$_6$H$_5$	0.06	−0.01	0.08	−0.08	1.96	25.36	6.28	1.71	3.11	−1.51	1.73	−0.64
C$_6$H$_{11}$	−0.15	−0.22	−0.13	−0.10	2.51	26.69	6.17	1.91	3.49	−2.68	1.67	−1.83
CF$_3$	0.43	0.54	0.38	0.19	0.88	5.02	3.30	1.99	2.61	2.83	1.00	−1.10
CN	0.56	0.66	0.51	0.19	−0.57	6.33	4.23	1.60	1.60	3.59	0.57	0.52
CHO	0.35	0.42	0.31	0.13	−0.65	6.88	3.53	1.60	2.36	2.51	−0.13	0.05
CH$_2$OH	0.00	0.00	0.00	0.00	−1.03	7.19	3.97	1.52	2.70	0.62	−1.22	−0.44
COCH$_3$	0.38	0.50	0.32	0.20	−0.55	11.18	4.06	1.60	3.13	2.13	0.73	0.42
COC$_6$H$_5$	0.34	0.43	0.30	0.16	1.05	30.33	5.81	1.60	5.98	−0.71	3.40	1.37
CONH$_2$	0.28	0.36	0.24	0.14	−1.49	9.81	4.06	1.50	3.07	1.90	−0.12	0.63
COOH	0.37	0.45	0.33	0.15	−0.32	6.93	3.91	1.60	2.66	2.36	0.28	0.17
COOCH$_3$	0.37	0.45	0.33	0.15	−0.01	12.87	4.73	1.64	3.36	1.60	1.21	0.42
COOC$_2$H$_5$	0.37	0.45	0.33	0.15	0.51	17.47	5.95	1.64	4.41	0.62	2.33	0.88
NH$_2$	−0.16	−0.66	0.02	−0.68	−1.23	5.42	2.78	1.35	1.97	−0.36	−3.85	−0.12
NHCH$_3$	−0.30	−0.84	−0.11	−0.74	−0.47	10.33	3.53	1.35	3.08	−2.03	−3.29	−0.18
N(CH$_3$)$_2$	−0.15	−0.83	0.10	−0.92	0.18	15.55	3.53	1.35	3.08	−1.97	−2.76	0.46
NHC$_4$H$_9$	−0.34	−0.51	−0.28	−0.25	1.45	24.26	6.88	1.35	4.87	−4.18	0.46	−0.11
N(C$_2$H$_5$)$_2$	−0.23	−0.90	0.01	−0.91	1.18	24.85	4.83	1.35	4.39	−3.76	−1.37	0.66
NHC$_6$H$_5$	−0.12	−0.40	−0.02	−0.38	1.37	30.04	4.53	1.35	5.95	−3.30	0.53	0.82
NHCOCH$_3$	0.21	0.00	0.28	−0.26	−0.97	14.93	5.09	1.35	3.61	0.23	−0.27	1.54
NHCONH$_2$	−0.03	−0.24	0.04	−0.28	−1.30	13.72	5.06	1.35	3.61	−0.74	−1.11	0.84
OH	0.12	−0.37	0.29	−0.64	−0.67	2.85	2.74	1.35	1.93	0.96	−3.02	0.54
OCF$_3$	0.38	0.35	0.38	0.00	1.04	7.86	4.57	1.35	3.61	1.25	0.71	1.04
OCH$_3$	0.12	−0.27	0.26	−0.51	−0.02	7.87	3.98	1.35	3.07	0.06	−1.57	0.85
OC$_2$H$_5$	0.10	−0.24	0.22	−0.44	0.38	12.47	4.80	1.35	3.36	−0.57	−0.78	0.88
OCH(CH$_3$)$_2$	0.10	−0.25	0.22	−0.45	1.05	17.06	6.05	1.35	4.42	−1.62	0.37	1.31
OC$_4$H$_9$	0.10	−0.32	0.25	−0.55	1.55	21.66	6.86	1.35	4.79	−2.40	0.97	1.62
OCH(CH$_3$)$_2$	0.10	−0.45	0.30	−0.72	0.36	17.06	4.80	1.35	4.10	−1.33	−0.85	1.53
OC$_6$H$_5$	0.25	−0.03	0.34	−0.35	2.08	27.68	4.51	1.35	5.89	−1.64	1.63	1.74
SH	0.25	0.15	0.28	−0.11	0.39	9.22	3.47	1.70	2.33	1.47	−0.31	−0.48
SCF$_3$	0.40	0.50	0.35	0.18	1.44	13.81	4.89	1.70	3.94	1.16	2.11	0.17
SCH$_3$	0.15	0.00	0.20	−0.18	0.61	13.82	4.30	1.70	3.26	0.17	0.15	−0.28
SO$_2$NH$_2$	0.46	0.57	0.41	0.19	−1.82	12.28	4.02	2.04	3.05	3.04	1.08	−0.04

4.4.4 Biological relevance

Recently, the relevance of several statistical correlations on enzyme inhibitors have been supported by computer modeling in cases where the solid state structure of the enzymes have been determined (cf. equation (4.1)). For example, binding with substituents in certain positions correlated with hydrophobicity (π) whereas in other positions with molar refractivity (*MR*). The significance of the π terms in the correlation equations could be rationalized by van der Waals contacts with hydrophobic regions (see Chapter 2), where desolvation is the major driving force. On the other hand, correlations of substituents with *MR* appeared in polar regions of the protein where binding mainly involves dispersion forces. This means that it is possible not only to retrospectively correlate the data and predict more active congeners but also to gain mechanistic information on the nature of the interactions between the ligand/substrate and the receptor/enzyme.

4.5 APPLICATIONS OF HANSCH EQUATIONS

4.5.1 Hydrophobic and steric factors

A wide range of biological activities have been correlated with linear free energy-related parameters and a selection of examples will be given to show some of the information that can be obtained. For simple *in vitro* systems, e.g. enzyme inhibition data, simpler and more accurate relationships may be derived than for more complex biological systems which involve a combination of transport, distribution and receptor-interaction phenomena.

Protein binding is a non-specific interaction to hydrophobic areas of serum proteins and a linear relationship between $\log K$ (binding constant) and $\log P$ has indeed been found. Equation (4.16) shows the relationship for binding of sulfonylurea derivatives to bovine serum albumin (BSA) and the small (0.33) regression coefficient indicates binding of an only partly desolvated compound.

$$\log K = 0.33 \log P + 0.24 \, \mathrm{pK}_a + 1.48$$

$$n = 15, r^2 = 0.90, s = 0.090 \tag{4.16}$$

In concordance with the Meyer-Overton findings, the narcotic effect on tadpoles of a set of structurally diverse compounds was simply explained by the lipophilicity according to equation (4.17), which supports a non-specific interaction. In this case the regression coefficient is close to unity, which is in line with a complete accumulation of the molecules in a lipophilic bioenvironment similar to that in octanol.

$$\log (1/C) = 0.94 \log P + 0.87$$

$$n = 51, r^2 = 0.94 \tag{4.17}$$

(4.3)   (4.4)

The muscarinic effect of a series of *meta*-substituted benzyltrimethylammonium deriva-tives (**4.3**) expressed as pD_2 determined on isolated rat jejunum could be modeled by equation (4.18), which indicates binding of the *meta*-substituent X into a lipophilic pocket (large regression coefficient for the hydrophobic parameter π) of limited size (negative coefficient for the STERIMOL parameter B_5).

$$pD_2 = 1.30\,\pi - 0.41 B_5 + 5.68$$

$$n = 10,\, r^2 = 0.90,\, s = 0.186 \tag{4.18}$$

The displacement of the benzodiazepine [^{3}H]flunitrazepam from bovine brain mem-branes of a series of quinolinones (**4.4**) was significantly correlated to steric and hydrophobic parameters, however for different positions, according to equation (4.19). The positive coefficient of Taft's steric constant for the *ortho*-positions might indicate a required coplanar arrangement of the phenyl ring during the receptor binding, which is abolished by too much bulk in these positions. However, lipophilic (and large) groups are favorable in other positions and the intermediate size of the π coefficient reflects a partial desolvation during the hydrophobic interaction of the *meta*-substituents.

$$\log\,(1/IC_{50}) = 0.481\,E_S(2,6) + 0.606\,\pi(3,5) + 4.81$$

$$n = 20,\, r^2 = 0.76,\, s = 0.278,\, F = 24.8 \tag{4.19}$$

4.5.2 Influence of electronic and other factors

The *in vivo* activity of a series of 17 tricyclic antipsychotics (**4.5**) related to octoclothepin ($X = Cl$) have been correlated with the electronic and steric parameters of the X substituent according to equation (4.20).

$$\log\,(1/ED_{50}) = 0.698\,\sigma_p + 0.347\,E_S + 0.0458\,MV - 0.00059\,MV^2 + 0.297$$

$$n = 17,\, r^2 = 0.93,\, s = 0.128,\, F = 40.4 \tag{4.20}$$

(4.5)   (4.6)

An electron-withdrawing X group will enhance the activity as shown by the positive value of the coefficient for σ_p. The parabolic dependence on MV indicate that a too large X group could be detrimental for the activity by steric interference but smaller substituents interact favorably with the dopamine receptor, which is believed to mediate the antipsychotic activity. The latter aspect is also supported by the positive coefficient of E_S. In this case the lipophilic parameters π and π^2 were not significantly involved.

The influence of the aromatic substituent X in a series of 12 mono-substituted potential antipsychotic salicylamides (4.6) on their ability to displace [³H]spiperone from the dopamine D_2 receptors *in vitro* has been investigated (Fig. 4.2). The parabolic dependence on lipophilicity is clear from equation (4.21), which indicates that a limited size of the substituent X can be tolerated by the dopamine D_2 receptor since transportation effects should be negligible in this type of assay.

$$\log\left(1/IC_{50}\right) = 1.28\,\pi - 0.518\,\pi^2 - 0.692\,\sigma_m + 1.495$$

$$n = 12,\, r^2 = 0.94,\, s = 0.399,\, F = 19.9 \qquad (4.21)$$

The same set of antiadrenergic α-bromophenethylamines (4.1) that was investigated by the Free-Wilson analysis shown in equation (4.5) (Section 4.3.1) has been analyzed by use of the Hansch approach according to equation (4.22). A strong dependence was found on lipophilicity and the Hammett σ constant, but an even better correlation was obtained with σ^+, when the data later was reanalyzed by Unger and Hansch (equation (4.23)). The σ^+ constants are derived from the ionization of t-cumyl chlorides in aqueous acetone and used to reflect a direct resonance stabilization of electron-deficient centers ($\sigma_m^+ = \sigma_m$ and $\sigma_p^+ \neq \sigma_p$).

$$\log\left(1/ED_{50}\right) = 1.22\,\pi - 1.59\,\sigma + 7.89$$

$$n = 22,\, r^2 = 0.84,\, s = 0.238 \qquad (4.22)$$

$$\log\left(1/ED_{50}\right) = 1.15\,\pi - 1.47\,\sigma^+ + 7.82$$

$$n = 22,\, r^2 = 0.89,\, s = 0.197 \qquad (4.23)$$

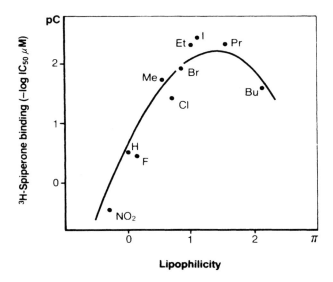

Figure 4.2 Relationship between the inhibition of [³H]spiperone binding and lipophilicity (π) of the 3-substituent (X) of 6-methoxysalicylamides (**4.6**). Reproduced with permission of the American Chemical Society.

The highly negative regression coefficients (ρ value) in both equations and the better correlation with σ^+ compared to σ is in accordance with a proposed reaction mechanism for these derivatives, which has been postulated to involve a benzylic carbonium ion intermediate, as shown in Scheme 4.1. The compounds (**4.1**) are unstable at physiological pH and reacts presumably with a nucleophilic center at the α-receptor site to inhibit the pressor action of epinephrine.

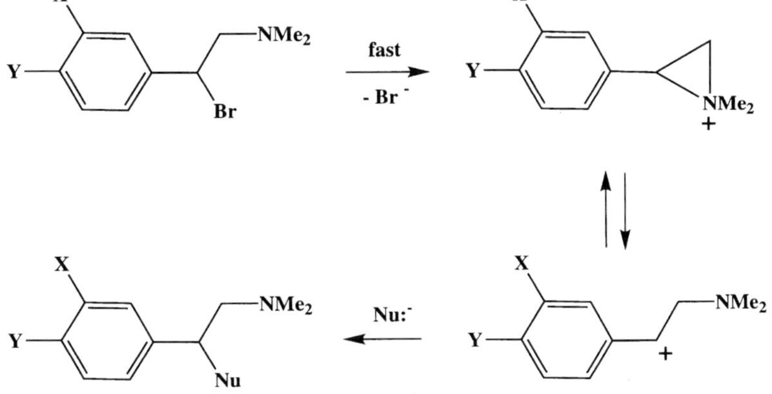

Scheme 4.1

(4.7)   (4.8)

The fungicidal activity against *Cladosporium cucumerinum* of a series of arylethynsulfones (**4.7**) could be explained by electronic, lipophilic and steric descriptors in equation (4.24). A favorable correlation was obtained with σ^-, which is based on ionization of substituted phenols in water and used for correlation of reactions having an electron-rich reaction center in conjugation with electron withdrawing substituents. The correlation with this electronic substituent with a positive coefficient (ρ value) argues for a nucleophilic attack on the triple bond to be of importance for the biological action.

$$pC = 1.10\ \sigma^- + 0.84\ \pi - 0.07\ \pi^2 + 2.10\ E_S + 4.17$$

$$n = 25, r^2 = 0.89, s = 0.248 \tag{4.24}$$

4.5.3 Ionization constants

The acidity of the phenolic group in the antipsychotic 6-methoxysalicylamides (**4.8**) has been considered to be of importance for the biological activity. To better understand the effects of the substituents on the acidity a number of models with steric and electronic descriptors were investigated. The most significant regression equation (4.25) was obtained with a σ parameter for the *ortho* substituent X and the modified Taft parameter E^c for the *para* substituent Y. The regression coefficient of σ_o is in accordance with the well-known stabilization of anionic forms by electron withdrawing *ortho* substituents. The steric effect induced by the *para* substituent can be rationalized by the influence on the conformation of the methoxy substituent. A more perpendicular orientation of the methoxy group inflicted by a more bulky Y substituent could lead to a weakening of the OH–O=C hydrogen bond, an effect which increases the acidity of the phenol.

$$pK_{a1} = -1.66\ \sigma_o - 1.36\ E^c_p + 7.98$$

$$n = 9, r^2 = 0.92, s = 0.37 \tag{4.25}$$

4.5.4 Predictions from equations

A series of substituted benzamides (**4.9**) of the clebopride ($4 = NH_2$, $5 = Cl$, $6 = H$) type containing both phenols ($n = 12$) and non-phenols ($n = 10$) with substituents in the 3-, 4-, and 5-positions were treated in a Hansch analysis. The indicator variable I_{OH} is set to unity for phenols and zero for non-phenols (cf. example on PLS analysis of benzamides with pyrrolidine side chains in Section 4.6). The affinity for the [^{3}H]spiperone binding site

(OH)   O
5
4
3   CH$_3$

(4.9)

OH   O
Br
H$_3$C—O   CH$_3$

(4.10)

could be modeled by a small number of variables describing electronic properties, e.g. Swain and Lupton resonance parameters for the substituent in the 4-position ($\Re_4$) and the sum for the 3- and 5-substituents ($\Re_{(3+5)}$) as shown in equation (4.26).

$$\log\left(1/IC_{50}\right) = -1.75\,\Re_4 - 3.69\,\Re_{(3+5)} + 0.80\,I_{OH} + 0.04$$

$$n = 22,\, r^2 = 0.82,\, s = 0.321,\, F = 27.1 \tag{4.26}$$

The equation (4.26) could be used to predict that compound (**4.10**) should have an IC$_{50}$ value of 0.45 nM, i.e. 10-fold more active than the previous most potent member of the series. Synthesis and testing of this compound showed that the activity (IC$_{50}$ = 0.36 nM) conformed with the predicted value to a degree we had not dare to expect. Figure 4.3 shows the new potent benzamide (**4.10**) included in the regression equation (4.27). Notably, the regression coefficients are virtually unchanged compared to equation (4.26), which is in accordance with the good prediction.

It should be emphasized, however, that extrapolation outside the data set most often leads to large differences between predicted and found values, since the original model does not necessarily take the descriptors properly into account. In this case we had included all the substituents used in the original test set, but the combinations of substituents were different in the predicted compound.

4.5.5 Blood-brain barrier penetration

As mentioned in Section 4.2.1, the optimal log P for penetration of the blood-brain barrier (BBB) is around 2.1 for a wide range of compounds. In a study aiming for centrally acting histamine H$_2$ antagonists, the physicochemical properties of importance for the brain penetration was investigated in detail by Young and coworkers. A better correlation was found between the logarithms of the equilibrium brain/blood concentration ratios in the rat and the partition parameter $\Delta \log P$ (equation (4.28)) than for log P in octanol (equation (4.29)).

$$\log\left(C_{\text{brain}}/C_{\text{blood}}\right) = -0.604\,\Delta \log P + 1.23$$

$$n = 6,\, r^2 = 0.96,\, s = 0.249,\, F = 98.0 \tag{4.28}$$

$$\log\left(C_{\text{brain}}/C_{\text{blood}}\right) = 0.150 \log P_{\text{oct}} - 0.96$$

$$n = 6,\, r^2 = 0.026,\, s = 1.241 \tag{4.29}$$

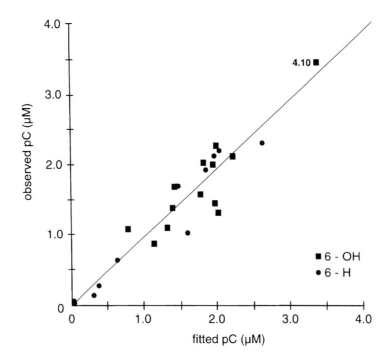

Figure 4.3   Found pC (log $1/IC_{50}$; μM) values for [^{3}H]spiperone binding shown as a function of data calculated according to the equation (4.27):

$$\log (1/IC_{50}) = -1.76\,\Re_4 - 3.75\,\Re_{(3+5)} + 0.81 I_{OH} + 0.02$$

$$n = 23,\ r^2 = 0.87,\ s = 0.313,\ F = 41.8 \tag{4.27}$$

Seiler introduced the $\Delta \log P$ parameter, as the difference between the octanol/water and cyclohexane/water log P values, which is related to the overall hydrogen-bonding capacity of a compound by equation (4.30).

$$\Delta \log P = \log P_{oct} - \log P_{cyh} = \sum I_H - 0.16$$

$$n = 195,\ r^2 = 0.94,\ s = 0.333,\ F = 107 \tag{4.30}$$

where I_H is the hydrogen-bonding ability for a given substituent. The larger the I_H value the more prone a substituent is to donate or accept a hydrogen bond, e.g. 2.60 for Ar–OH, 1.18 for Ar–NH$_2$, 0.45 for –NO$_2$, 0.31 for C=O, and 0.11 for ether –O–. Thus, the BBB penetration can be increased by lowering the overall hydrogen-bonding ability of a compound by, for example, encouraging intramolecular hydrogen bonding, shielding with nonpolar groups and by making less polar prodrugs. The principles could be utilized in the design of potent histamine H$_2$ antagonists, which readily cross the BBB, such as zolantidine (**4.11**) with a $\Delta \log P$ of 1.69 and a log P_{oct} of 5.41.

(4.11)   (4.12)

4.5.6 Relations to molecular modeling

In a classical paper from the Hansch and Langridge groups (1982) the QSAR models for
papain hydrolysis of phenyl hippurates (**4.12**) were compared with X-ray crystallography-
based molecular modeling. Papain is a cystein protease which hydrolyzes a number of esters,
amides and peptides. A QSAR with the equation (4.31) was derived for a set of substituted
phenyl hippurates.

$$\log 1/K_m = 0.57\, \sigma + 1.03\, \pi_3' + 0.61\, MR_4 + 3.80$$

$$n = 25, r^2 = 0.82, s = 0.208 \tag{4.31}$$

where σ refers to substituents in any positions, MR_4 (scaled with 0.1 to be comparable
with the other parameters) for the *para* substituents and π_3' indicates that only π for the
most hydrophobic group in the *meta* position is considered significant. The latter parameter
makes mechanistic sense, since substituents that are hydrophobic ($\pi > 0$) partition into the
enzyme, whereas those with negative values cause a rotation around the phenyl ring to place
the less hydrophilic hydrogen onto the enzyme while the X-substituent is oriented into the
aqueous phase. The term MR_4 cannot be replaced with π, which indicates that the *para*
substituent does not contact a lipophilic surface. On the other hand, the most lipophilic *meta*
substituent is making a hydrophobic interaction with complete desolvation as indicated by
the correlation coefficient (1.03).

The solid state structure has been determined for an enzyme-inhibitor complex (benzyl-
oxycarbonyl-L-phenylalanyl-L-alanylmethylene-papain, ZPA-papain), which allows for a
proper orientation of the phenyl hippurates in the active site. The derived model was used
to validate the QSAR equation (4.31) and indeed all terms could be shown to accommodate
the modeling data. Thus, the 4-substituents collide with a highly polar amide moiety in
Gln-142 and remain exposed to solvent. The hydrophobic *meta*-substituent is completely
buried (desolvated) within a shallow hydrophobic pocket, whereas the other *meta*-position
is oriented into the solvent as shown in Figure 4.4.

4.6 PATTERN RECOGNITION

4.6.1 PCR and PLS methods

In some cases where a structure-activity model is to be derived there are more variables,
i.e. characteristics of the structures under investigation, than there are compounds.

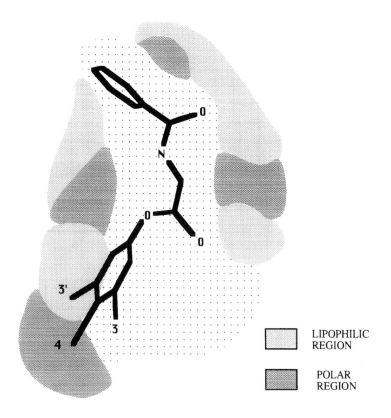

LIPOPHILIC
REGION

POLAR
REGION

Figure 4.4   A cartoon of the phenyl hippurates (**4.12**) oriented in the active site of papain. The different shadings indicating hydrophobic and polar regions have been adopted by Magnus Jendbro according to the original modeling work by Hansch, Langridge and coworkers.

In such instances traditional methods such as multiple linear regression (MLR; see previous Section 4.2) can not be used since there are more unknown variables than available equations (one equation for each compound in the test set). This situation is especially true for the 3D-QSAR models (see Section 4.7) where the number of variables typically exceeds the number of compounds by a factor of a 100. Pattern recognition methods, such as PLS (Partial least squares projections to latent structures) and PCR (Principal component regression), can be used to analyze these kinds of problems. Both these methods contract (reduce) the original description of each molecule into a few descriptive dimensions, so-called principal components (PCs). Thus, these methods reexpress the original matrix of data (X) for the compounds under investigation as mean vector (X_m) plus the product of a score matrix T times a row matrix P' (Fig. 4.5). The scores, where each investigated compound has a computed set of score values, give the best summary of X and can be seen as the underlying factors of the studied system. Furthermore, the scores are, using the method described above, linear combinations of the original variables (equation (4.32)).

$$t_1 = C_1 V_1 + C_2 V_2 + C_3 V_3 + \ldots + C_n V_n \tag{4.32}$$

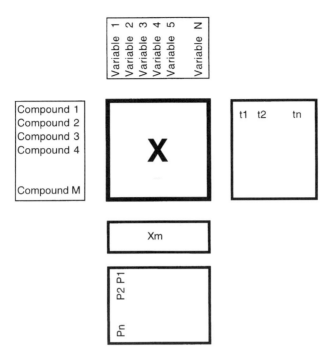

Figure 4.5   Schematic representation of the deconvolution of the structural descriptor matrix X into a score vector T $(t_1, t_2, \dots, t_n)$ and a loading vector $P'(P_1, P_2, \dots, P_n)$.

where C_n are the weighting constants (loadings), V_n the original variables and t_1 is the first score value for a molecule (see Fig. 4.5).

How are the principal components then calculated? Starting from the description of the investigated compounds (the mean centered data matrix X) the first PC is computed with the objective to explain as much information as possible in matrix X. This gives rise to the first score vector t_1 and the first row vector P'_1. The information contained in the first PC is then subtracted from the matrix X by subtracting the $t_1 P'_1$ matrix from X. A second PC with the same objective as that of the first PC, i.e. to explain as much information as possible in the new, updated matrix X is then calculated and so on for additional PCs. This means that each PC is orthogonal (independent) to all other PCs and that the first PC (PC_1) contains the largest part of explained variance (information content) in the data. Subsequent PCs contain decreasingly smaller amounts of explained variance. It is desirable to first center the data matrix by subtracting the mean value from each column. Otherwise, the first PC will contain no interesting structural information but will instead represent a vector from origo to the point represented by the mean values.

How many components should then be calculated (extracted), i.e. used to describe the properties of the investigated compounds? Certainly one should only extract relevant information and stop when the amount of noise becomes too large in a calculated component. The term "extracted" is mostly used in the literature instead of "calculated", when dealing with PCs. A cross-validation (CV) procedure described by Wold is used to determine the stoppage point. In CV a portion of the data is left out, a PC is extracted and a model is created with the remaining data. The left out data are then predicted by the model. As long as the prediction of the left out data becomes better, the extracted component is judged to be significant and is kept in the model. When the prediction of the left out data does not improve any more, the extraction of components is stopped and the resulting model is based on the previously extracted significant components.

There is a fundamental difference between PLS and PCR in deriving the PCs. PCR is composed of two steps. In the first step a principal component analysis (PCA) is applied to the description of the structures (the X matrix; see Fig. 4.5) and a relevant number of PCs are extracted. These PCs are then, in a second step, correlated against the biological activity using MLR. In PLS a correlation between the chemical descriptors (variables) and biological activity (or other properties) is obtained where PLS uses the available biological information (biological activity) during the extraction of PCs. Thus, PLS tries to derive PCs that explain as much as possible of the biological information while PCR in the first step, the PCA, tries to explain as much as possible of the structural description of the molecules and then, in the second step, uses the derived PCs to derive a good model with respect to the measured activities. This means that the PCs from PLS and PCR differ from each other. Since PLS is targeted at explaining the activities this also means that PLS usually produces somewhat better QSARs compared with PCR. Some of the advantages of using PLS/PCR compared with multiple regression techniques are the following:

i. The number of compounds in the analysis can be significantly smaller than the number of variables used.
ii. There are no collinearities between final variables since PLS/PCR is PC based, which means that addition of relevant variables will improve the relationship.
iii. The original data set of chemical descriptor may contain "missing data", i.e. a number of variables have not been assigned a value for some reason and are missing. PLS/PCR tolerates a certain number of such data depending on the distribution in the data matrix X.

All evidence suggest that PLS gives at least as good relationships (predictions) as other regression techniques and sometimes much better.

4.6.2 Application of PLS

PLS has been used by Norinder and Högberg to study the QSAR between the *in vitro* affinity to [^{3}H]spiperone binding sites of mono- and disubstituted benzamides (**4.13**) with a large number of physicochemical descriptors for size, lipophilicity and electronic characteristics. Each of the 3- and 5-substituents were described by the original physicochemical parameters (σ_m, σ_p, $\Im$, $\Re$, π, MR, L, B_1 and B_5 in Table 4.1) and the corresponding squared values. Since only two choices exist for position 2 (R_2 = H, OH) a so called indicator variable (I_2) was also used. This variable can assume two values; $I_2 = 0$ for R_2 = H and $I_2 = 1$ for R_2 = OH. A similar indicator variable (I_S) was also used to represent the stereochemistry of the side chain (I_S; $R = -1$, $S = 1$, racemate = 0). In total 38 variables were used to describe each compound.

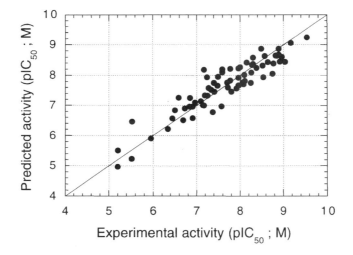

(**4.13**)

The PLS analysis resulted in 4 PCs which explained 86% of the variance (information) in binding affinity (see Fig. 4.6). The analysis pointed out the major importance of size, lipophilicity and electronic properties of the 3-substituent as well as a (S)-configuration of the side chain.

4.7 3D-QSAR METHODOLOGIES

4.7.1 Methods and strategy

Structure-activity relationships of traditional type, e.g. Hansch analysis or pattern recognition methods as discussed above, usually do not take the three dimensional structures of the investigated compounds into account in an explicit manner. Instead they use substituent parameters and indicator variables to describe the structural variations.

Figure 4.6   Plot of predicted versus experimental [^{3}H]spiperone displacing activity (pIC$_{50}$; M) of substituted salicylamides (**4.13**). The QSAR was made with the PLS method as described in Section 4.6.

Today it is well recognized that, at the molecular level, the interactions that produce an observed biological effect are usually non-covalent and that such steric and electrostatic interactions can account for many of the observed molecular properties. Recently, an extension to the traditional QSAR approaches have been developed which explicitly uses the three dimensional geometry of the structures during the development of a QSAR model. These new technologies are commonly referred to as 3D-QSAR methodologies. The presently most used technique, Comparative Molecular Field Analysis (CoMFA), was developed by Cramer and coworkers.

The following steps have to be considered when trying to develop a 3D-QSAR model:

1. Identification of active conformation(s)
2. Alignment rule
3. 3D grid construction
4. Calculation of field values
5. Selection of training set compounds
6. PLS analysis
7. Interpretation of results (contour maps)
8. Predictions of new compounds

One of the most fundamental problems when trying to develop a good and predictive 3D-QSAR model is the identification of the bioactive conformation(s) (cf. the detailed discussion in Chapter 3) of the investigated compounds and how to align them (steps 1 and 2). This becomes especially critical when one is dealing with a set of structurally diverse compounds. There are several available methods, such as APEX-3D, Catalyst, DISCO and SUPER, by which atoms or molecular properties are superimposed onto a reference compound or a set of reference compounds. However, for flexible molecules there is usually not one unique "best" way of identifying bioactive conformations and superimposing the geometries. In the end the researcher must decide which superimpositioning scheme to use for the 3D-QSAR model. If a predictive model was developed then this may serve as an indication that the choice of alignment scheme was a reasonable one.

Once the choice of molecular alignments and conformations is made then a 3D grid box is spanned around the molecules under investigation. The box is filled with grid points (see Fig. 4.7) with an internal distance of usually between 1–2 Å (step 3).

A probe atom with, in the case used here as an example (see below), the van der Waals properties of a sp^3 carbon and a charge of +1 is placed at each grid point and two forces (interactions) related to non-bonded and charge interactions are calculated for each molecule (step 4). Thus, all the computed values become a "fingerprint" for each molecule. All values are stored in a large data matrix (see Fig. 4.5) where each row is related to a compound. Each of the two sets of calculated forces (non-bonded and electrostatic, respectively) are usually referred to as a field. Thus, in this example we have a non-bonded field and an electrostatic field. To delineate the relationship between biological activity and structural description, where the number of variables greatly exceeds the number of compounds, the method of partial least squares (PLS) is used (step 6). Again, cross-validation is used to judge the predictivity and statistical quality of the derived 3D-QSAR model by leaving a portion of the compounds out from the data set and building a model with the remaining compounds (see Section 4.6 for more details on cross-validation). The results of a 3D-QSAR model is usually depicted as 3D contour maps. Each grid point in the box spanned around

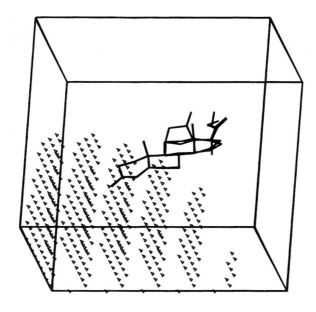

Figure 4.7   The 3D box, with partially depicted grid points, used in the 3D-QSAR example in Section 4.7. Only steroids 1 and 11 are shown with hydrogens omitted for clarity.

the molecules is associated with, in this case, two coefficients from the PLS analysis. One coefficient is related to the non-bonded field and the other coefficient is related to the electrostatic field. Each of the two sets of coefficients are displayed as iso-contour maps (step 7). In most cases it is not a trivial task to choose the appropriate iso-contour level in order to create a meaningful picture. The interpretation of contour maps will be discussed in Section 4.7.2.

4.7.2 Application to steroids

Here the 3D-QSAR methodology will be exemplified by a data set of 30 steroids with affinities for human corticosteroid-binding globulins (CBG). This example is often used as a benchmark in 3D-QSAR investigations. Since all the compounds possess a common substructure, the steroid skeleton, the numbered atoms containing an asterisk in Figure 4.8 were used to superimpose compounds 2–30 onto compound 1 (see Fig. 4.9).

Compounds 1–21 were used as training set (step 5) and the remaining steroids (22–30) were used as test set for which the affinities should be predicted by the derived 3D-QSAR model (step 8). A 3D grid with an internal separation of 1.5 Å between grid points was constructed based on the training set. Two fields (non-bonded and electrostatic) were computed. Each steroid was defined by 4704 variables. A so called leave-one-out cross-validation scheme was used to determine the number of relevant PLS components. In a leave-one-out procedure one compound is held out and the remaining compounds are used

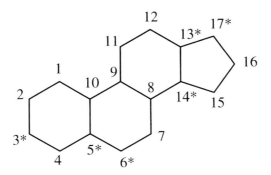

Figure 4.8　Steroid skeleton with atomic numbering system. Atoms indicated with an asterisk were used to superimpose steroids 2–30 in Figure 4.9 onto steroid 1.

to develop a model. The activity of the held-out compound is then predicted by the model. Then all but the second molecule are used to generate a model that predicted the activity of the second molecule and so on. This procedure resulted in 2 significant PLS components. The Q^2 value was 0.791 for the training set and Q^2 is defined in equation (4.33).

$$Q^2 = 1.0 - \left\{ \sum (\text{Pred}_i - \text{Exp}_i)^2 / \sum (\text{Exp}_i - \text{Exp}_m)^2 \right\} \qquad (4.33)$$

where Pred_i and Exp_i are the predicted and experimental activity for the held-out compound i, respectively. Exp_m is the mean value of the experimental activities of all compounds and the summation in equation (4.33) runs over all compounds.

The R^2 value, where R^2 is defined analogous to Q^2, for the test set compounds 22–30 was 0.560 which is a value indicating that the model has fair predictivity. The resulting PLS coefficients related to the grid points were transformed so that the coefficient with the highest absolute value, i.e disregarding the sign, was set to 100 or −100 depending on the sign of the coefficient and the rest of the coefficients were scaled accordingly. The contours for the electrostatic interactions are displayed here as an iso-contour map at −30 (Fig. 4.10).

How can these iso-contour maps (Fig. 4.10) be interpreted and used for the development of new compounds? Let us examine the resulting negative electrostatic contour map from the 3D-QSAR model based on steroids 1–21. The negative region is mainly concentrated around (outside) the 3 position of the steroids. This location coincides very well with the keto moiety present in a large number of the steroids in the training set. Thus changing the electrostatic nature of this oxygen atom into something more positive or, to some extent, the direction of the atom, as in steroids 2, 3, 5, 9, 16, 17 and 18, will result in compounds with lower affinity. The non-bonded iso-contour maps (not displayed in this example) can be interpreted in a similar manner. Thus areas of positive non-bonded regions indicate that it is favorable to have a substituent or substructure present close to these domains, while the opposite is true for the areas close to negative non-bonded iso-contours.

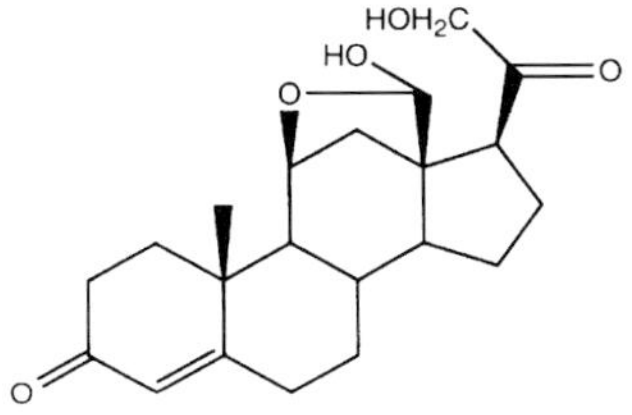

1

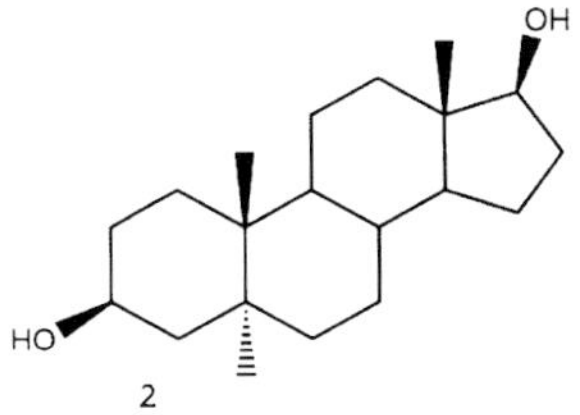

2

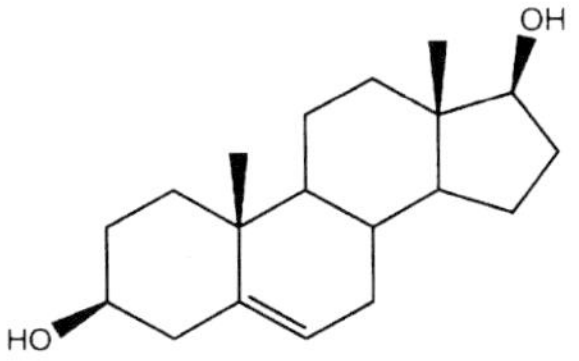

3

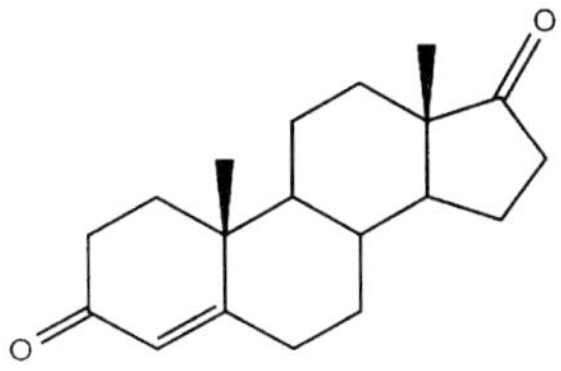

4

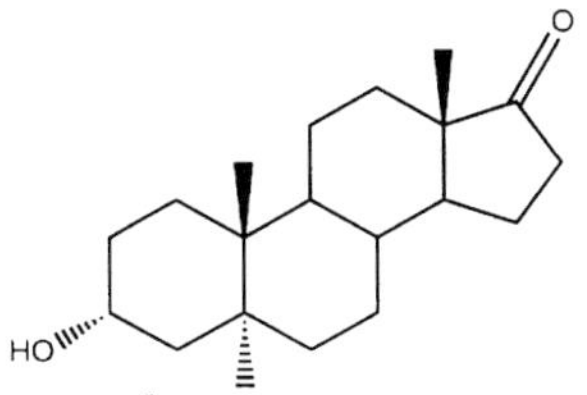

5

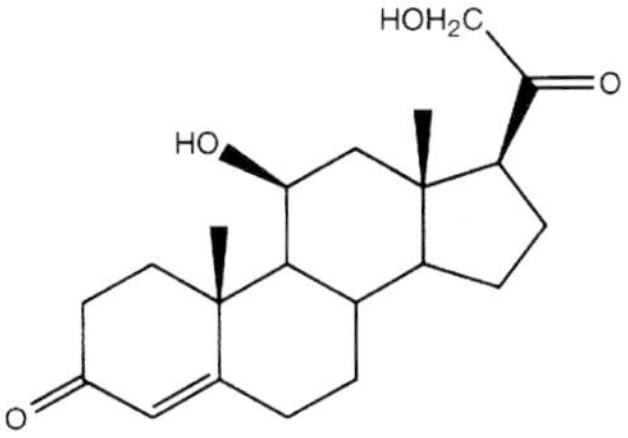

6

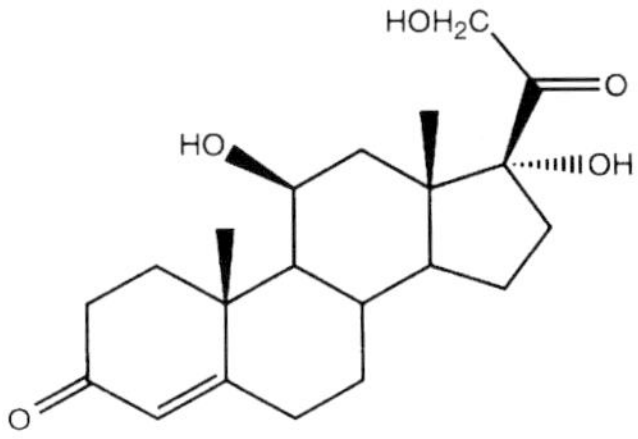

7

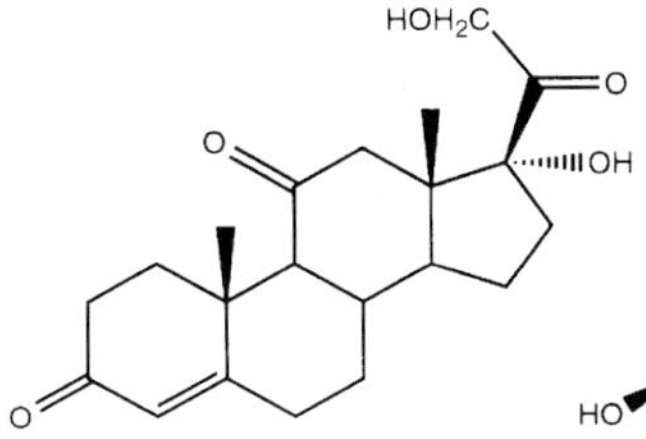

8

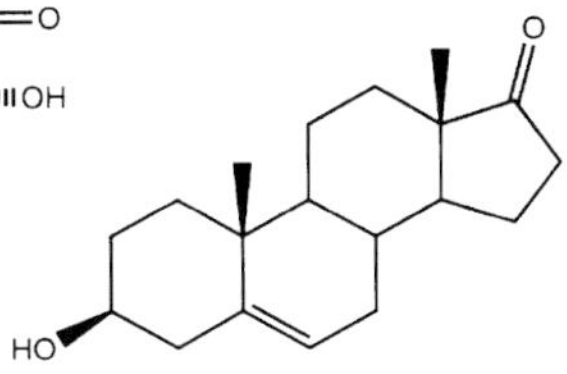

9

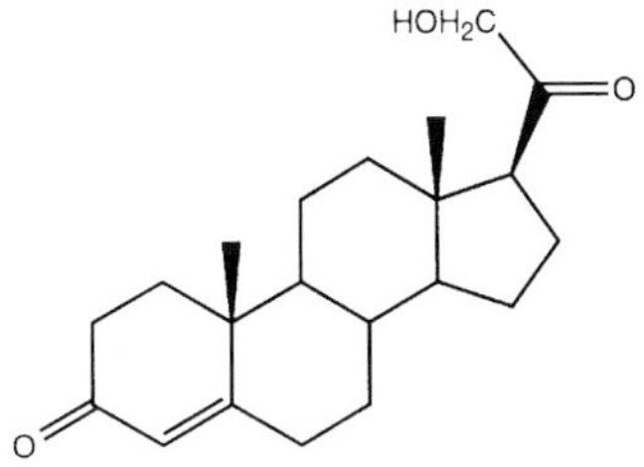

10

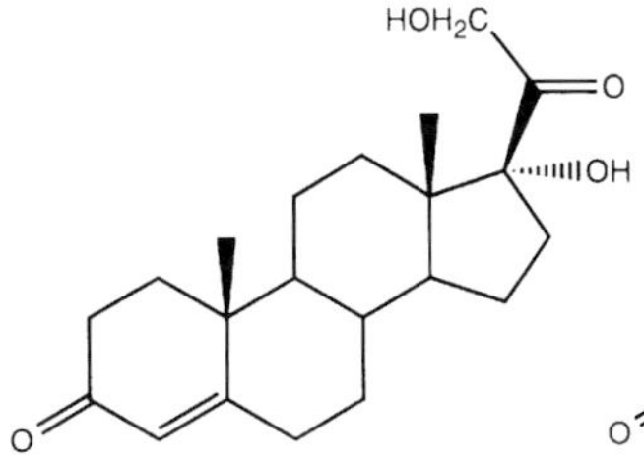

11

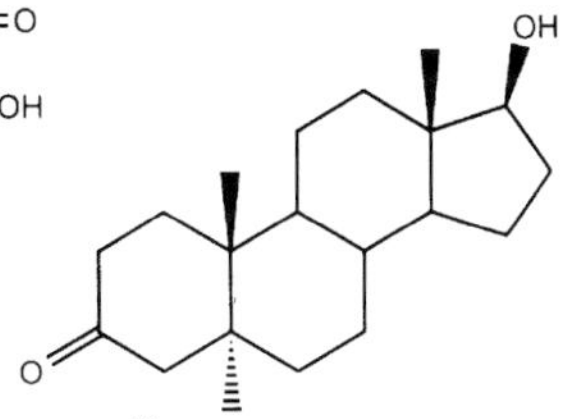

12

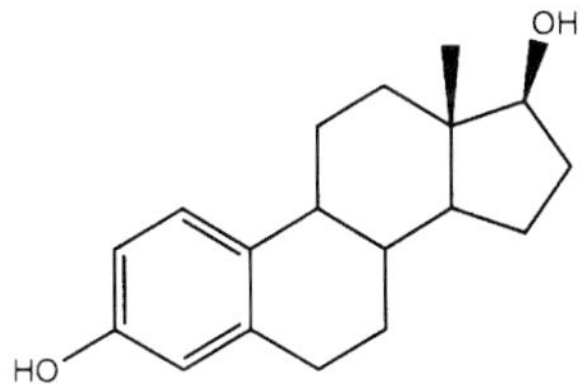

13

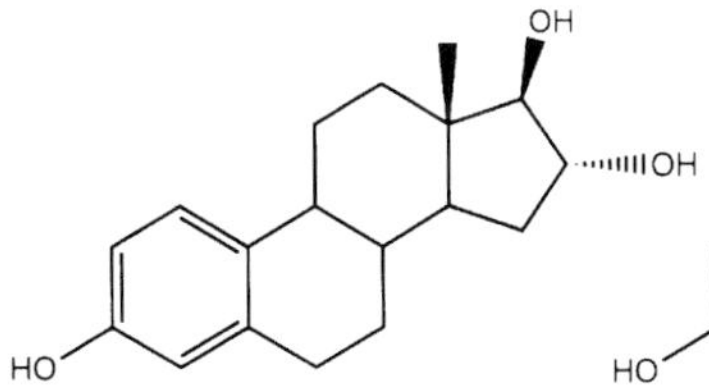

14

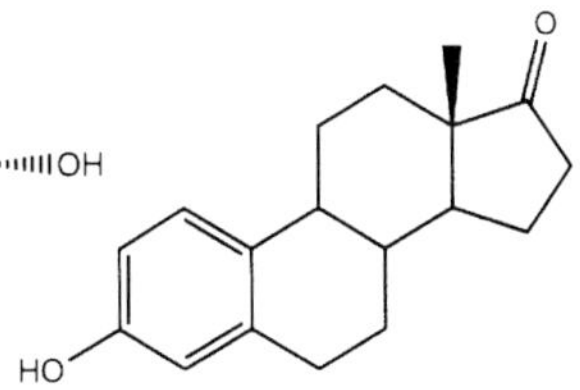

15

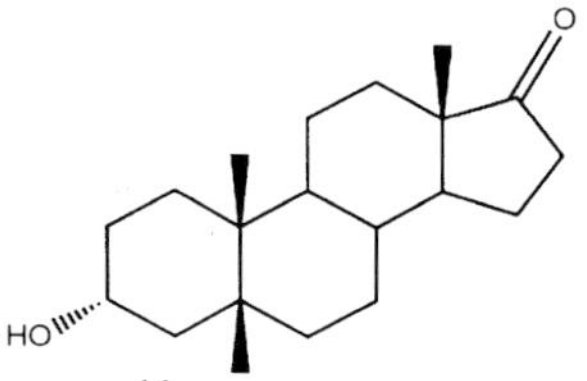

16

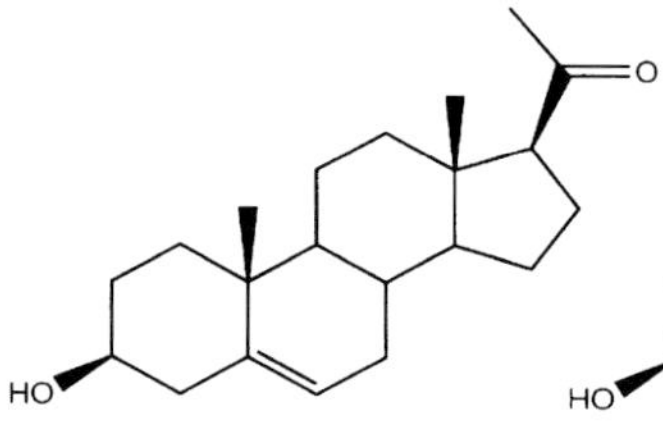

17

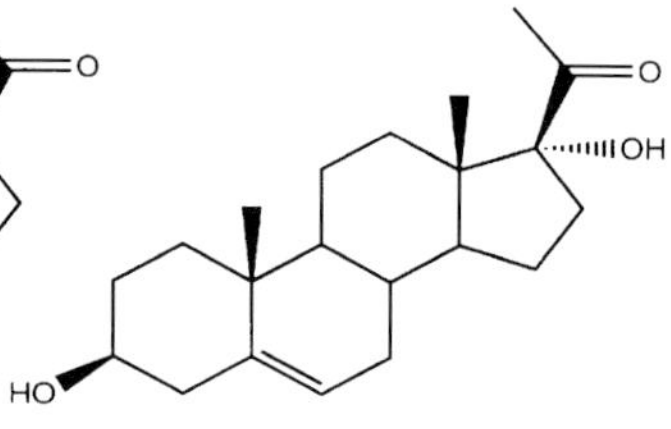

18

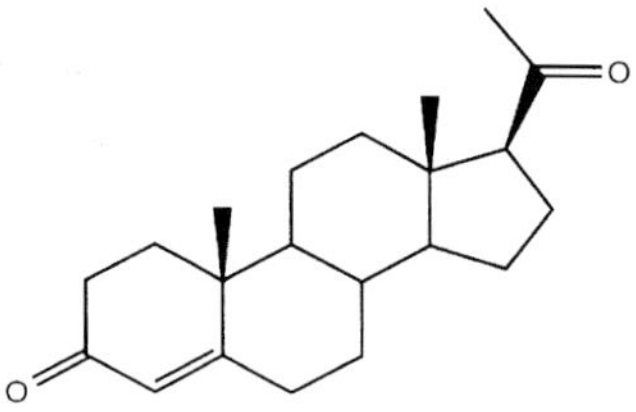

19

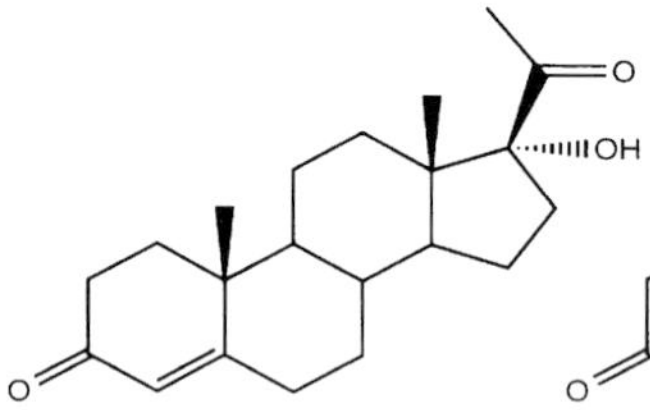

20

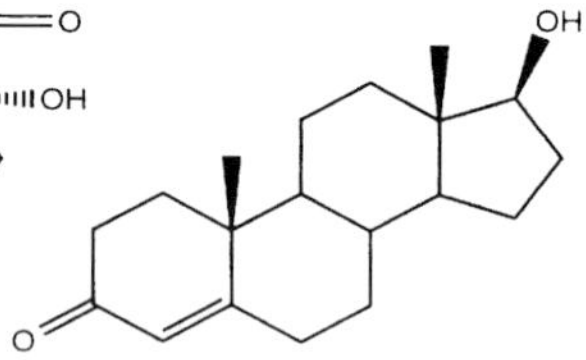

21

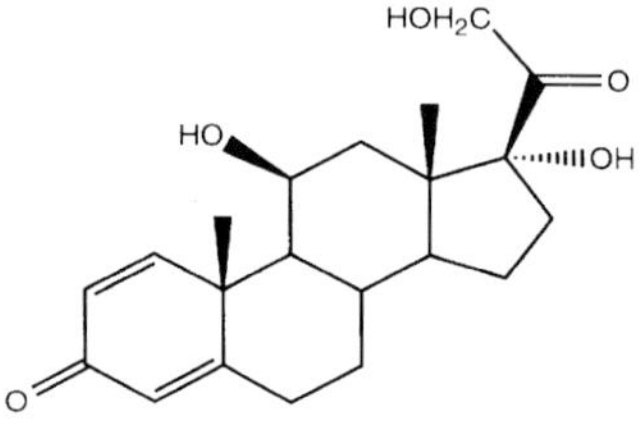

22

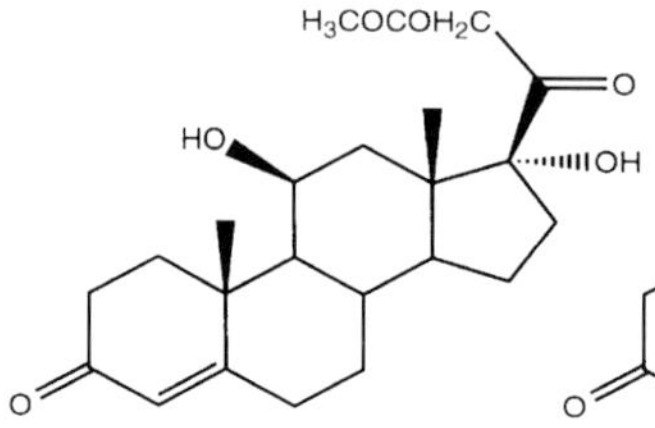

23

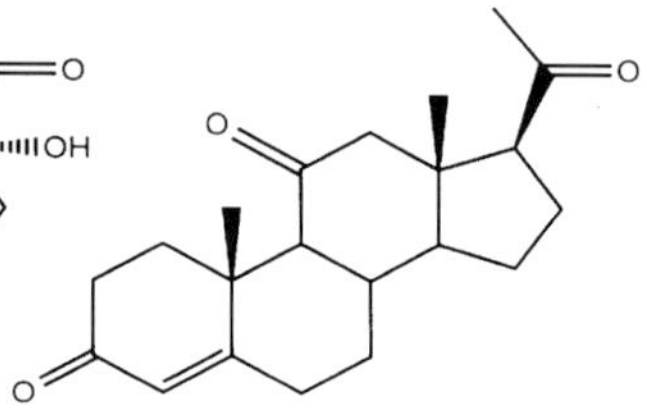

24

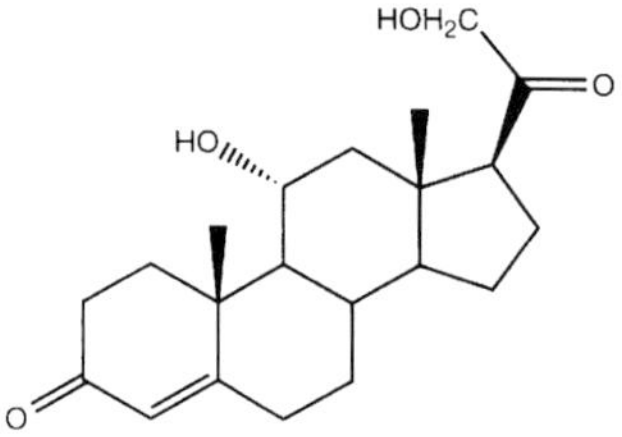

25

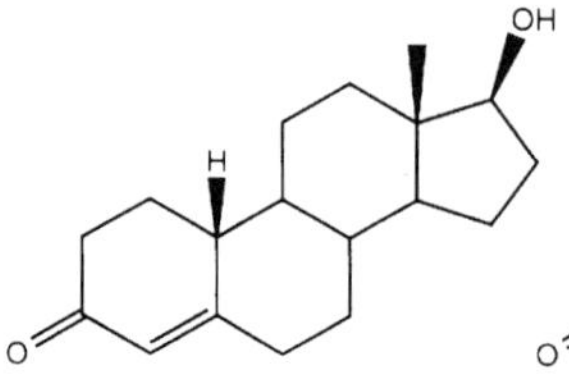

26

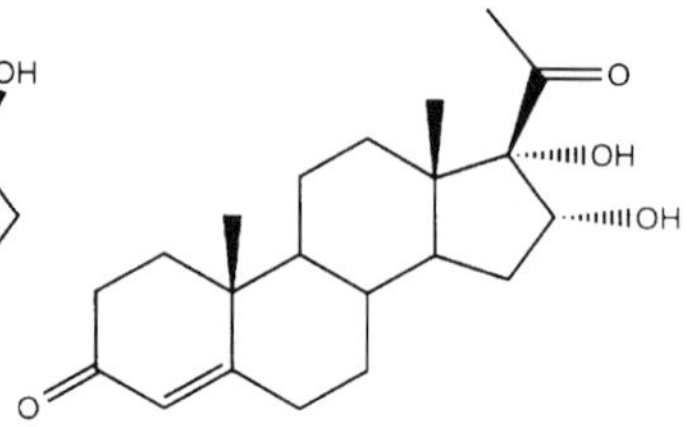

27

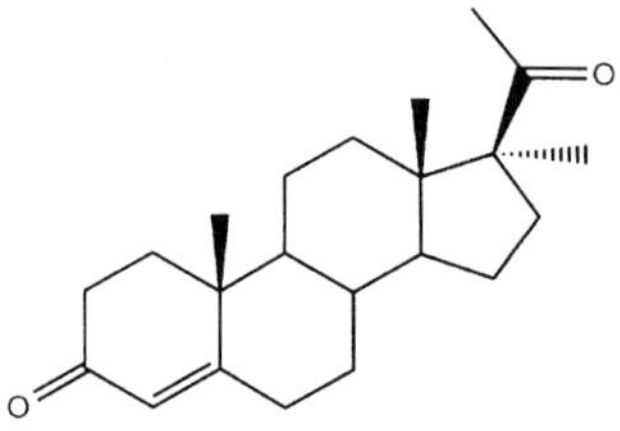

28

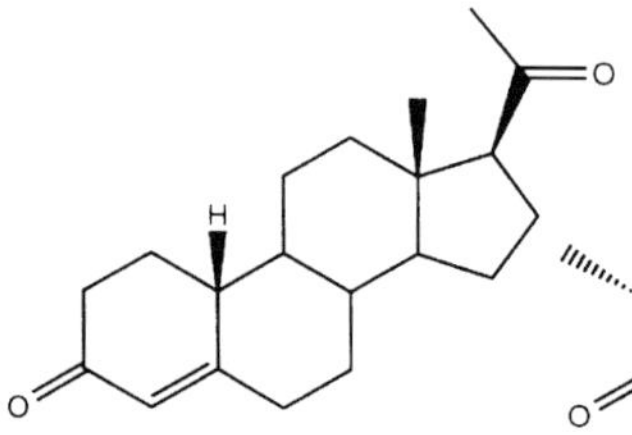

29

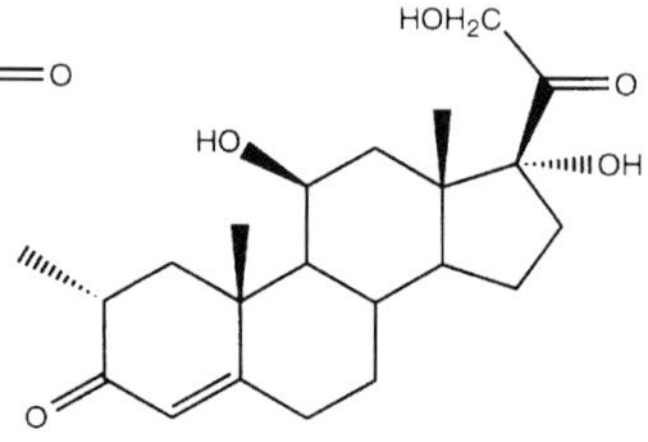

30

Figure 4.9 Structures of the steroids 1–30 used in the 3D-QSAR analysis in Section 4.7.

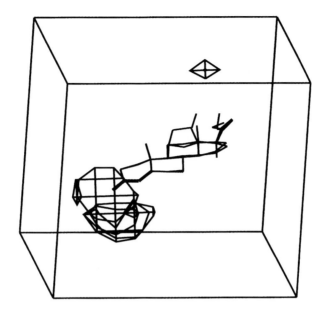

Figure 4.10   Electrostatic contour map resulting from the 3D-QSAR analysis of steroids 1–21. The contours are depicted at a level of –30. Only steroids 1 and 11 are shown with hydrogens omitted for clarity.

4.7.3 Pros and cons

One advantage with 3D-QSAR studies is that the same protocol, i.e. steps 1–8 mentioned in Section 4.7.1, can be used for every new problem of interest. Also, the method can handle data sets to be investigated that contain structurally different compounds and predict new compounds of potential interest containing slightly different scaffolds than originally present among the training set compounds.

A limitation of the technique is that the models are only predictive in 3D space which have been covered by substructures of sufficient variation. Thus, if in a certain position only a methyl-, ethyl-, and a propyl group have been present in the investigated structures the 3D-QSAR model cannot make a reasonable prediction for the longer alkyl side chains such as butyl, pentyl and so on. A QSAR model based on some physicochemical description, such as the 3D dimensions of the side chain, can at least make a prediction for the latter group of substituents even though it represents an extrapolation. Also, if certain parts of 3D space have only been covered by structural features of one compound then the 3D-QSAR model, using many variables in those 3D domains to represent the substructure, is nothing but an elaborate 3D version of the Free-Wilson description based upon only one or a few variables.

One interesting aspect of the contour maps of the derived 3D-QSAR models is their relationship to important drug-receptor interactions. Let us consider a case where the 3D structure of the active site in a receptor is known. The compounds investigated in the study have been aligned by docking them into the active site. Each drug-receptor complex has then been brought into a common reference system by superimposing the receptor protein in each case onto each other. The compounds in their aligned orientations have then been taken out from the complex and used to derive a 3D-QSAR model. When the contour maps, which have the investigated compounds as reference, are overlaid on the drug-receptor complexes the spacial positioning of the most important parts of the contour maps may, in favorable cases, be located onto certain amino acid residues of the receptor protein. This, in turn, may provide a more qualitative description of exactly how important various drug-receptor interactions seem to be. The different impact (importance) in the 3D-QSAR model associated with these contours may then be used to upgrade and/or downgrade the interactions of certain amino acid residues in the docking process. Hopefully, this will then in the end lead to a more refined docking scheme which, in turn, results in a better and more predictive 3D-QSAR model. Thus, protein chemistry and biology, biotechnology, molecular modeling, conformational analysis, computational chemistry (to derive charges and other descriptors) and QSAR form a closely interlinked interdisciplinary entity in drug development.

4.8 EXPERIMENTAL DESIGN

4.8.1 Factorial design and principal properties

In order to be able to create a useful QSAR with good predictability one wants the compounds included in the model (usually called the training set) to cover a large number of substituent and/or structural variation. However, at the same time it is desirable to keep the number of compounds to be synthesized and tested at a minimum. To obtain as much information as possible with a minimum of observations, one needs a protocol (experimental or statistical design) where the structures are varied in a carefully selected manner. Such protocols are found in the field of experimental design. There are several different types of protocols available but most often are factorial design schemes used due, in part, to the ease of evaluating these set-ups.

In a factorial design each variable is assigned to a certain number of levels. A two level factorial design, which is most frequently used in chemistry, with four variables (a, b, c, d) involves sixteen experiments (2^4). Each variable is designated a high level (+) and a low level (–) and the protocol is given in Table 4.5. The outcome of the sixteen experiments may then be evaluated by some least squares method (like PLS).

Chemical substituents, however, are characterized by a large number of physicochemical properties. To perform a complete two level factorial or fractional factorial (reduced scheme) design using the original variables would involve too many compounds and be practically impossible. One method to circumvent this problem involves utilization of so called "principal properties" (PPs), which are principal component derived variables (scores) from the original physicochemical parameters. However, since the PPs are not continuous due to a limited number of substituents it is not possible to construct a factorial design with exactly defined high and low levels. Instead the substituents are classified according to the size and sign of their PPs. Table 4.4 shows the first three PPs of a number of aromatic substituents.

Table 4.5   Experimental design protocol for a two level factorial design.

#	a	b	c	d
1	+	+	+	+
2	−	+	+	+
3	+	−	+	+
4	−	−	+	+
5	+	+	−	+
6	−	+	−	+
7	+	−	−	+
8	−	−	−	+
9	+	+	+	−
10	−	+	+	−
11	+	−	+	−
12	−	−	+	−
13	+	+	−	−
14	−	+	−	−
15	+	−	−	−
16	−	−	−	−

Practically, however, PPs are usually derived separately for each study since the objective is to span the chemical property space of the available substituents for the investigated compounds as effectively as possible. This will then, in turn, help to select compounds having a large variation in the mentioned physicochemical property space. However, since different sets of substituents are used for different investigations and the purpose of each PCA is to explain as much information as possible with each PC the numerical values of the PPs may differ considerably between different PCAs (see Tables 4.4 and 4.6). Again, one must look upon these values (PPs) as guidance when selecting substituents having a large difference and variation in physicochemical properties and pay less attention to the exact numerical values. The QSAR equations that are subsequently derived from the selected compounds, the training set, are based on the original physicochemical variables. However, an alternative approach is to use the PPs directly as variables in the QSAR model. In this case all substituents must have the same framework. Thus, one must include all the substituents to be used both for the training set compounds as well as for those compounds that are to be predicted from the derived QSAR model in the PCA when one calculates the PPs, since the exact numerical values will be used in this case to derive the QSAR equation.

4.8.2 Applications of factorial design

An example of using PPs as design variables for some substituted benzamides (**4.13**) (the same compounds as used in Section 4.6) is given below. The number of different available 3- and 5-substituents were few (F, CN, NO_2, Cl, H, OH, NH_2, Me, OMe, I, Br, Et, n-Pr, n-Bu) in this retrospective study and the PPs derived for this subset are shown in Table 4.6.

The fractional factorial design protocol and the choice of substituents are listed in Table 4.7. The sixteen selected compounds were then used to construct a model by which the activities of the remaining 54 benzamides were predicted using PLS.

Table 4.6   Design levels for the R_3- and R_5-substituents used in retrospective study of some benzamides (**4.13**).

Substituent	PP_1	PP_2	FDL^a
F	2.17	0.16	+ +
CN	0.79	2.51	
NO_2	0.56	2.94	
Cl	0.35	1.34	
H	2.46	−0.65	+ −
OH	2.11	−1.46	
NH_2	1.92	−2.56	
Me	0.52	−0.62	
OMe	0.09	−1.29	
I	−1.34	1.65	− +
Br	−0.28	1.57	
Et	−1.30	−0.72	− −
n-Pr	−2.56	−0.69	
n-Bu	−4.38	−0.93	

^{a}FDL = factorial design levels.

Table 4.7   Experimental design protocol and selected substituents for the benzamides (**4.13**)^a

#	R_3 a	b	R_5 c	d	R_2 abcd	R_3	R_5	R_2
1	+	+	+	+	+	Cl	Cl	OH
2	−	+	+	+	−	Br	OH	H
3	+	−	+	+	(−)	OMe	Cl	OH
4	−	−	+	+	+	Pr	Cl	OH
5	+	+	−	+	(−)	NO_2	Br	OH
6	−	+	−	+	(+)	Br	Br	H
7	+	−	−	+	+	Me	Br	OH
8	−	−	−	+	−	Et	Br	H
9	+	+	+	−	−	Br	OMe	H
10	−	+	+	−	(+)	I	OMe	H
11	+	−	+	−	(+)	Me	OMe	H
12	−	−	+	−	(−)	Pr	Me	OH
13	+	+	−	−	+	Cl	Pr	OH
14	−	+	−	−	(−)	Br	Et	OH'
15	+	−	−	−	(−)	H	Et	OH
16	−	−	−	−	+	Et	Et	OH

^{a}Parenthesis indicate a deviation from the protocol in selecting the substituent.

Three significant components were extracted. They explained 89% of the variance in binding affinity. The model explained 61% of the variance of the biological data for the test set of 54 benzamides (**4.13**). Figure 4.11 shows a plot a calculated vs. experimental activities. The substituents R_3 and R_5 were described by a total of 38 variables, i.e. the parameters $\sigma_m, \sigma_p, \Im, \Re, \pi, MR, L, B_1$ and B_5 (cf. Table 4.1), the corresponding squared values and indicator values for R_2 and stereochemistry (*), in the same way as in the PLS analysis in Section 4.6. As can be seen in Figure 4.11, the small training set predicts the

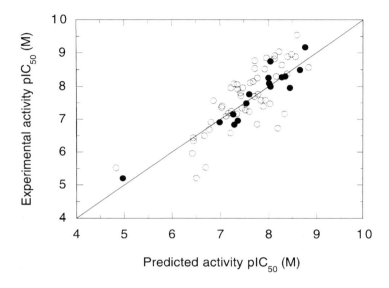

Figure 4.11   Plot of predicted versus experimental [^{3}H]spiperone displacing activity (pIC$_{50}$; M) of substituted salicylamides (**4.13**). The QSAR was made with the PLS method as described in Section 4.6. Solid and open circles represent the training set and test set compounds, respectively.

activity quite well and covers a large activity span which is quite frequently the consequence of the experimental design procedure. The model also predicts the remaining 54 benzamides in the test set reasonably well.

The second example is related to a set of β-adrenergic blockers analyzed by Norinder. The 101 compounds available are of the phenoxypropanolamine type (**4.14**) with a reasonable structural variation. Again a two level PP fractional factorial design was applied and eight compounds were selected according to the design protocol (Table 4.10). Substituents R_1 and X were treated with indicator variables since only two choices existed in each case {$R_1 = t$-Bu (+1), i-Pr (-1); X = direct attached (-1), NH (+1)}. Substituents R and R_2 were characterized by the following physicochemical variables: $R = MR, f, L, B_1, B_5$; $R_2 = \Im, \Re, \pi, MR, L, B_1, B_5$. See Tables 4.8 and 4.9 for the calculated PPs of R- and R_2-substituents, respectively, using PCA on the original physicochemical parameters.

(**4.14**)

Table 4.8   Calculated   score   vectors   for R-substituents   in phenoxypropanolamine derivatives (**4.14**).

Substituent	PC_1	PC_2	FDL^a
H	−4.06	−1.00	− −
$(CH_2)_2OCH_3$	−0.42	−0.73	
CH_2CHCH_2	−0.33	−0.36	
$(CH_2)_2CH_3$	−0.30	−0.23	
CH_3	−2.60	0.18	− +
CH_2CH_3	−1.24	−0.13	
$CH(CH_2)_2$	−0.95	−0.04	
$CH(CH_3)_2$	−0.52	0.98	
$(CH_2)_3CH_3$	1.02	−0.53	+ −
$CH_2C_6H_5$	1.83	−0.46	
$(CH_2)_4CH_3$	2.15	−0.72	
$(CH_2)_5CH_3$	3.31	−0.93	
$CH_2CH(CH_3)_2$	0.45	2.99	+ +
C_6H_5	0.80	0.18	
$CH(CH_2)_4$	0.86	0.81	

^{a}Designated factorial design levels.

Table 4.9   Calculated   score   vectors   for R_2-substituents   in phenoxypropanolamine derivatives (**4.14**).

Substituent	PC_1	PC_2	FDL^a
CH_2CHCH_2	−3.10	−0.92	− −
$(CH_2)_2CH_3$	−3.04	−0.76	
CH_2CH_3	−1.62	−1.09	
OCH_2CH_3	−1.20	−0.52	
SCH_3	−1.43	0.44	− +
I	−0.92	2.21	
$COCH_3$	0.00	1.28	
OCH_3	0.19	−0.79	+ −
CH_3	0.42	−1.52	
OH	2.46	−1.28	
H	2.58	−2.48	
Br	0.27	1.75	+ +
Cl	0.91	1.20	
NO_2	1.65	2.75	

^{a}Designated factorial design levels.

The PLS analysis resulted in three significant components which explained 92% of the variance of the biological data in the training set (the eight compounds in Table 4.11). The model explained 67% of the variance of the biological data of the remaining 93 compounds. The model predicts compounds A–D (Table 4.11) to be interesting new structures with high activity.

Table 4.10   Fractional factorial design protocol and choice of training set compounds of phenoxypropanolamine derivatives (**4.14**).

| | R | | $R_1{}^a$ | R_2 | | X^b | | |
#	a	b	c	abc	ab	bc	R	R_2
1	+	+	+	+	+	(+)	$CH(CH_2)_4$	Cl
2	–	+	+	–	–	+	CH_2CH_3	CH_2CHCH_2
3	+	–	+	–	–	–	$(CH_2)_5CH_3$	CH_2CHCH_2
4	–	–	+	+	(+)	(–)	H	H
5	+	+	–	(–)	+	–	C_6H_5	Cl
6	–	+	–	+	–	–	$(CH_2)_2CH_3$	OCH_3
7	+	–	–	+	–	+	$(CH_2)_3CH_3$	CH_3
8	–	–	–	(–)	(+)	+	CH_2CHCH_2	CH_3

Parenthesis indicate a choice for the training set of a substituent which deviates from the protocol.
[a] R_1 has only two choices: (+) = $C(CH_3)_3$, (–) = $CH(CH_3)_2$.
[b] X has only two choices: (+) = $-NH-$, (–) = amide group directly attached to phenyl ring.

Table 4.11   Predicted activities for compounds A–D of phenoxypropanolamine derivatives (**4.14**).

Compound	R	R_1	R_2	X	Pred. Act.
A	$(CH_2)_3CH_3$	$C(CH_3)_3$	I	NH	7.54
B	$(CH_2)_3CH_3$	$C(CH_3)_3$	Br	NH	7.42
C	$(CH_2)_3CH_3$	$C(CH_3)_3$	$(CH_2)_2CH_3$	NH	7.43
D	$(CH_2)_3CH_3$	$C(CH_3)_3$	Cl	NH	7.34

If one uses all of the 101 available compounds to derive a model the same four compounds (A–D) are predicted by this model to possess high activity. Thus, not much new information was added to the model by incorporating an additional 93 compounds, which is also indicated by the fact that the PLS regression coefficients were virtually the same for both models. This further proves the power of using experimental design to cover the available structural variation by a small number of compounds in a good manner.

Thus, using the predictive power of these models one can design compounds with the desired potency in a very efficient way, which is advantageous in the drug development phase. This also shows the usefulness of statistical design whereby structural variation is performed in an organized manner. These methods provide a broad basis for constructing a QSAR with good predictability which makes it possible to keep the number of compounds to be synthesized and tested at a minimum.

FURTHER READING

Ramsden, C.A., Ed. (1990) Quantitative Drug Design. In *Comprehensive Medicinal Chemistry*, Vol. 4, edited by C. Hansch, P.G. Sammes and J.B. Taylor. Oxford: Pergamon Press. This book provides a full and critical account of all aspects of QSAR by experts in the field.
Kubinyi, H. (1993) QSAR: Hansch Analysis and Related Approaches. In *Methods and Principles in Medicinal Chemistry*, edited by R. Mannhold, P. Krogsgaard-Larsen and H. Timmermann. Weinheim: VCH. This book provides an excellent overview of the different techniques in the field.

Hansch, C. and Leo, A.J. (1979) *Substituent Constants for Correlation Analysis in Chemistry and Biology.* New York: Wiley.

van de Waterbeemd, H. and Testa, B. (1987) The Parametrization of Lipophilicity and Other Structural Properties in Drug Design. In *Advances in Drug Research*, Vol. 16, edited by B. Testa, pp. 85–225. London: Academic Press.

Dean, P.M. (1987) *Molecular foundations of drug-receptor interaction.* Cambridge: Cambridge University Press.

Perun, T.J. and Propst, C.L. (1989) *Computer-Aided Drug Design. Methods and Applications.* New York: Marcel Dekker.

Fauchère, J.L., Ed. (1989) *QSAR: Quantitative Structure-Activity Relationships in Drug Design.* New York: Alan R. Liss.

Wermuth, C.G., Ed. (1993) *Trends in QSAR and Molecular Modeling 92.* Leiden: ESCOM Science Publishers.

Kubinyi, H., Ed. (1993) *3D QSAR in Drug Design. Theory, Methods and Applications.* Leiden: ESCOM Science Publishers.

Box, G.E.P., Hunter, W.G. and Hunter, J.S. (1978) *Statistics for Experimenters.* New York: Wiley.

Wold, S. and Dunn III, W.J. (1983) Multivariate Quantitative Structure-Activity Relationships (QSAR). Conditions for Their Applicability. *J. Chem. Inf. Comp. Sci.*, **23**, 6–13.

Wold, S. (1979) Cross-Validatory Estimation of the Number of Components in Factor and Principal Components Models. *Technometrics*, **20**, 379–405.

Gupta, S.P. (1989) QSAR Studies on Drugs Acting at the Central Nervous System. *Chem. Rev.*, **89**, 1765–1800.

de Paulis, T., Hall, H., Kumar, Y., Rämsby, S., Ögren, S.O. and Högberg, T. (1990) Potential antipsychotic agents. 6. Synthesis and antidopaminergic properties of substituted N-(1-benzyl-4-piperidinyl)salicylamides and related compounds. QSAR based design of more active members. *Eur. J. Med. Chem.*, **25**, 507–517.

Norinder, U. and Högberg, T. (1991) QSAR on Substituted Salicylamides Using PLS with Implementation of 3D MEP Descriptors. *Quant. Struct.-Act. Relat.*, **10**, 1–5.

Norinder, U. and Högberg, T. (1992) A quantitative structure-activity relationship for some dopamine D_2 antagonists of benzamide type. *Acta Pharm. Nord.*, **4**, 73–78.

Tsai, R.-S., Carrupt, P.-A., Testa, B., Gaillard, P., El Tayar, N. and Högberg, T. (1993) Effects ot Solvation on the Ionization and Conformation of Raclopride and Other Anti-dopaminergic 6-Methoxysalicylamides: Insight into the Pharmacophore. *J. Med. Chem.*, **36**, 196–204.

Young, R.C., Mitchell, R.C., Brown, T.H., Ganellin, C.R., Griffiths, R., Jones, M., Rana, K.K., Saunders, D., Smith, I.R., Sore, N.E. and Wilks, T.J. (1988) Development of a New Physicochemical Model for Brain Penetration and Its Application to the Design of Centrally Acting H_2 Receptor Histamines Antagonists. *J. Med. Chem.*, **31**, 656–671.

Nelson Smith, R., Hansch, C., Kim, K.H., Omiya, B., Fukumura, G., Dias Selassie, C., Jow, P.Y.C., Blaney, J.M. and Langridge, R. (1982) The Use of Crystallography, Graphics, and Quantitative Structure-Activity Relationships in the Analysis of the Papain Hydrolysis of X-Phenyl Hippurates. *Arch. Biochem. Biophys.*, **215**, 319–328.

Cramer, R.D., Patterson, D.E. and Bunce, J.D. (1988) Comparative Molecular Field Analysis (CoMFA). I. Effect of Shape on Binding of Steroids to Carrier Proteins. *J. Am. Chem. Soc.*, **110**, 5959–5967.

Norinder, U. (1993) Multivariate Free-Wilson Analysis of Some N-Alkylmorphinan-6-one Opioids Using PLS. *Quant. Struct.-Act. Relat.*, **12**, 119–123.

Norinder, U. (1991) An Experimental Design Based Quantitative Structure-Activity Relationship Study On β-Adrenergic Blocking Agents Using PLS. *Drug. Des. Discov.*, **8**, 127–136.

5. GENE TECHNOLOGY IN PHARMACEUTICAL RESEARCH AND PRODUCTION

NANNI DIN, JENS G.L. PETERSEN, HENRIK DALBØGE and SØREN CARLSEN

CONTENTS

5.1 INTRODUCTION

Gene technology is one of several terms used to describe the methods which have evolved as a result of research on the structure and function of genes. Other terms used to describe these methods are "recombinant DNA (rDNA) technology", "genetic engineering" and "gene splicing". As the names imply, this technology involves taking genetic material from one source and recombining it with genetic material from another.

Genetic engineering can be used to introduce a gene coding for a desired protein into a biological environment where this protein can be produced in large quantities. This possibility has been one of the main reasons for the immediate interest of the pharmaceutical industry in adopting genetic engineering methods. Using these methods, manufacturers can in principle produce unlimited quantities of biologically active proteins and peptides, as has already been convincingly demonstrated in many cases. The first approved human therapeutics produced by the aid of gene technology appeared in 1982. This landmark drug was insulin, a peptide hormone used to treat diabetes. At present (end of 1994), around a dozen different peptides or proteins produced by gene technology methods have been approved as human therapeutics, and more are about to follow. In contrast to insulin, which has been produced by extraction from the pancreases of pig or ox for many years, some of the other approved gene technology products have never been in regular use as drugs before, because they were impossible to produce in sufficient quantities. This possibility of producing substances that have hitherto been so elusive as to make their use as pharmaceuticals completely remote, is one of the real promises of the new technology.

Another advantage of gene technology is that with this technique modifications can easily be introduced in proteins at desired positions. The modifications may be a few changes in the amino acid sequence, made by introducing specific mutations in the gene encoding the protein. Such changes might lead to desirable altered physico-chemical characteristics, e.g. new solubility properties or a different physiological half life of an active polypeptide. However, more profound changes are also possible.

Gene technology has also proven an invaluable tool in pharmaceutical research and development. Thus, the technique is already extensively used to provide materials for the development of non-peptide drugs. Further, the new understanding of cellular and physiological processes that are gained by the aid of gene technology is of paramount importance in devising new avenues for disease intervention.

5.2 GENERAL METHODS IN GENE TECHNOLOGY

5.2.1 Basic DNA cloning tools

At the beginning of the 1970s, many new methods of significant importance for the recombinant DNA technology were developed. Since then the methods have been improved and new have emerged, but the principles are still based on the same tools: enzymes, DNA vectors and host cells (Fig. 5.1).

A key factor in the breakthrough of the 1970s was the discovery of two types of enzymes, the restriction enzymes and the DNA ligases. Restriction enzymes are endonucleases that recognize and cleave DNA at specific sequences, typically 4–8 base pairs long. As a result specific DNA fragments are generated, some of which may contain a single complete gene.

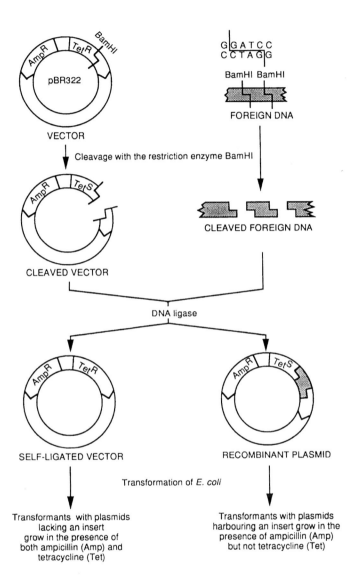

Figure 5.1 **Cloning of foreign DNA using the *E. coli* vector pBR322**. The plasmid pBR322 carries genes which confer resistance to the antibiotics ampicillin (Amp^R) and tetracycline (Tet^R). It contains a unique site for restriction endonuclease BamHI located in the tetracycline resistance gene. When a DNA fragment is inserted into the BamHI site, the resistance gene is destroyed giving sensitivity to tetracycline (Tet^S). In order to clone DNA fragments into this site, vector and foreign DNA are cleaved with BamHI, mixed and joined by the aid of the enzyme DNA ligase. The mixture of ligated DNA molecules is transformed into *E. coli*. Cells which have received a plasmid will grow in the presence of ampicillin. Transformant colonies harbouring a recombinant plasmid are identified by their sensitivity to tetracycline.

Restriction endonucleases can be isolated from a variety of microorganisms, and a large range of enzymes, each with a specific recognition site, is now commercially available. As an example, the restriction enzyme BamHI (endonuclease $\underline{I}$ isolated from $\underline{Bacillus}$ $\underline{amyloliquefaciens}$ $\underline{H}$) cleaves at the sequence GGATCC. DNA ligases have no specific sequence requirement but are capable of joining DNA molecules together. These features of the restriction enzymes and DNA ligases make it possible to perform *in vitro* cleavage and rejoining ("splicing") of DNA fragments.

In order to clone a DNA molecule it must be introduced into a host cell in a form which allows it to be replicated. Replication requires the presence of specific sequences which are not found universally in DNA, but can be provided by so-called vector DNA. Therefore, to generate clonable DNA, a restriction fragment is joined to a vector which can mediate replication in a suitable host cell. A very important host-vector system is the bacterium *Escherichia coli* and its naturally occurring small (2–10,000 base pairs) circular "minichromosomes" called plasmids.Some of these plasmids have been modified so that they are particularly useful for cloning purposes. An important feature of the vector is the presence of a gene coding for a selectable marker, such as resistance to an antibiotic. When recombinant plasmids are introduced into *E. coli* (in a process called transformation), the resistance gene will allow the cells to grow in the presence of the antibiotic, whereas cells without the plasmid will be eliminated. A recombinant plasmid is able to multiply until each cell contains several copies (often in the range from 20 to 200), and as the doubling time for *E. coli* under optimal conditions is 20–30 minutes, it is possible to multiply one single copy of the recombinant plasmid to more than 10^{10} molecules within 12 hours. Thus, this host-vector system allows the production of high amounts of identical plasmid molecules, thereby making further manipulation of a particular gene possible.

5.2.2 Cloning of cDNA

Cloning and expression of human genes, which are of special interest within pharmaceutical contexts, present special challenges. This is due to the fact that most human genes contain internal regions that do not code for any part of the corresponding protein. These regions, named introns or intervening sequences, are often much larger than the coding regions, also called exons (Fig. 5.2). Thus, human genes can be more than 200,000 base pairs long, which makes it difficult to generate a restriction fragment containing an intact gene. Another problem is that large DNA fragments are difficult to maintain stably in bacterial vectors. Further, *E. coli* is unable to express intron-containing genes correctly due to lack of the necessary processing functions.

Fortunately a method has been devised that allows cloning of a DNA fragment containing only the coding regions of a human gene. This method takes advantage of the fact that eukaryotic transcription and processing machineries generate mature mRNA molecules in which the intron regions have been removed. By an enzymatic *in vitro* reaction using a viral enzyme called reverse transcriptase it is possible to make a DNA copy of the mRNA. This DNA copy (called cDNA for copy DNA or complementary DNA) contains an uninterrupted coding region which can be cloned and expressed in *E. coli* (Fig. 5.3).

To generate cDNA coding for a protein of interest, mRNA is isolated from specific tissues or organs known to synthesize this protein. The isolated mRNA is a population of molecules representing all the genes expressed in the tissue. Hence, only a small proportion

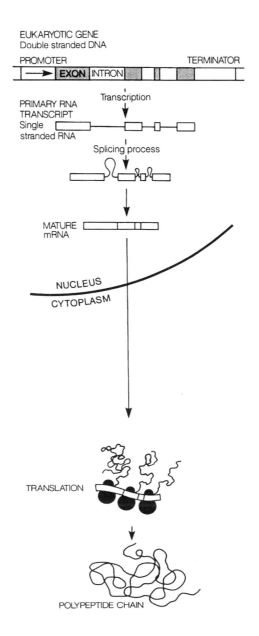

Figure 5.2 **Structure and expression of a eukaryotic gene**. Most eukaryotic genes are composed of coding regions (exons) interspersed with non-coding regions (introns). Expression starts with transcription which is initiated at the so-called promoter and terminated at the terminator. The resulting primary transcript is converted to the mature mRNA without introns by special RNA splicing enzymes located in the nucleus of the cell. The mature mRNA is subsequently exported to the cytoplasm of the cell and translated into a polypeptide chain.

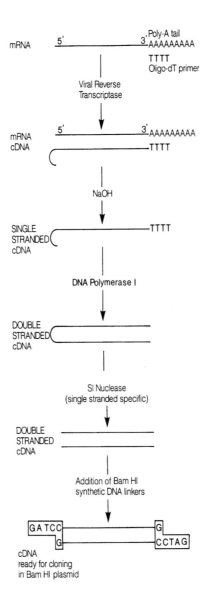

Figure 5.3   **Synthesis of cDNA from eukaryotic mRNA**. DNA fragments which contain only the coding regions of eukaryotic genes can be generated *in vitro* from eukaryotic mRNA. In the first step, a chemically synthesized oligo-dT primer is poly-Δ annealed to the 3' tails of the mRNA molecules. Complementary DNA strands (cDNA) are synthesized from deoxynucleotides by the aid of reverse transcriptase. The mRNA templates are removed by hydrolysis with sodium hydroxide to give a population of single-stranded cDNA molecules, which in turn are used as templates for a new round of DNA synthesis using DNA polymerase resulting in double-stranded cDNA. Single-stranded loops are removed with S1 nuclease. In order to construct a cDNA library, synthetic linkers which contain a suitable restriction endonuclease site (e.g. for BamHI) may be added to the ends of the double-standed DNA molecules. The resulting preparation is cleaved with the restriction enzyme and cloned into a DNA vector (e.g. pBR322) as shown in Figure 5.1.

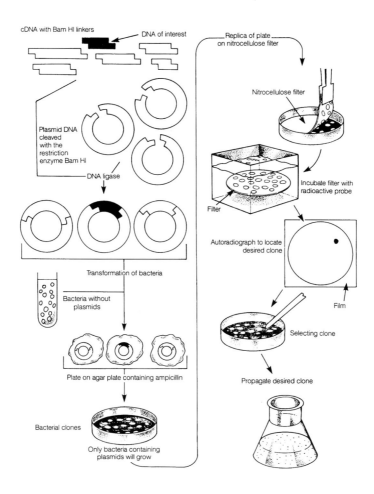

Figure 5.4   Generation of a cDNA library and identification of a specific clone by the aid of the DNA hybridization technique.

of the cDNA molecules generated by reverse transcription corresponds to the protein of interest. Cloning of the complete cDNA population results in a so-called tissue-specific cDNA library. From this library, the clones that contain the desired cDNA (often less than one per ten thousand) must be identified and isolated before analysis. This can sometimes be a formidable task, and the employed method depend on the cDNA in question. A standard identification procedure is the DNA hybridization technique shown in Figure 5.4. This method requires some knowledge about the sequence of the cDNA, e.g. a partial amino acid sequence of the encoded protein. This sequence can be used to design a synthetic radioactive DNA probe which is able to bind (hybridize) to the desired cDNA through base pairing, thus giving rise to a signal from this clone.

If no sequence information is available, other methods must be used which usually depend on expressing the protein encoded by the cDNA. In these cases, the cloning vector must contain signals which allow for expression of the cDNA insert (see Section 5.3). Although it is not always possible to produce eukaryotic proteins that maintain their biological activities in *E. coli*, it is usually possible to make a protein which share antigenic determinants with the native protein. Therefore, an identification procedure based on antibody screening of a cDNA expression library can be used if a specific antibody is available. The method is similar to the hybridization technique outlined in Figure 5.4, except that an antibody is used instead of a DNA probe.

In some cases the biological activity of a protein may be the only way to identify the cDNA clone encoding it. Thus, it becomes necessary to use host cells which preserve this activity. An obvious choice is mammalian cells grown in culture, and many different mammalian host-vector systems now exist for such purposes. Other host cells, notably frog oocytes, have also proven very versatile in their ability to express complex functional proteins, such as mammalian membrane receptors or ion channels.

5.2.3 PCR cloning

Recently, the polymerase chain reaction (PCR) has become very important as a cloning tool. The PCR technique is based on enzymatic *in vitro* amplification of a specific DNA. Figure 5.5 shows how a specific sequence, often called the target or template DNA, can be amplified from a population of single stranded cDNA.

Repeated rounds of DNA synthesis are catalyzed by a thermostable DNA polymerase in a suitable buffer containing the cDNA template, a specific set of two short synthetic DNA primers and a mixture of the four deoxynucleotides. The primer set is designed so that one primer can bind near one end of the cDNA and the other can bind near the other end of the complementary strand. When the first primer anneals to its target, it creates a starting point for the DNA polymerase and a complementary copy of the template is made. By heating the reaction mixture, the two complementary strands are separated, and targets for both primers are thereby exposed. When the temperature is lowered, both primers can anneal to their respective targets and both strands can now be copied by DNA polymerase. Each consecutive cycle consists of the same series of strand separation, primer annealing and DNA polymerization, and after around 20 cycles the target may be amplified more than a million fold.

Some knowledge about the sequence of the template DNA is needed in order to design primers which are able to bind to the target. In addition to using protein sequence data as described previously, other types of data can also be used for primer design. Thus, the sequences now available for a vast number of genes have made it clear that genes coding for particular functions have evolved as gene families which exhibit substantial sequence homology. Primers designed to recognize conserved regions from such a gene family may readily amplify cDNA for new members of the gene family. This procedure has proven enormously successful and has expanded the knowledge of gene families rapidly.

5.3 EXPRESSION OF RECOMBINANT PROTEINS

Production of recombinant proteins and peptides to be used as pharmaceuticals requires efficient expression systems where proteins with the correct structure and function

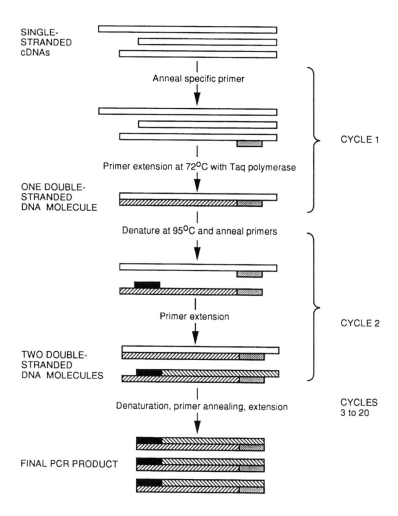

Figure 5.5 **Amplification of specific DNA from single-stranded cDNA by the polymerase chain reaction (PCR).** The black and grey bars represent primers complementary to opposite DNA strands. The hatched bars are amplified DNA.

are made. In this section, some requirements for expression will be outlined together with a discussion of the relative merits and drawbacks of different host-vector expression systems.

5.3.1 Transcription, translation and protein modifications

The first step in gene expression is transcription into RNA (Fig. 5.2). Transcription is initiated with the binding of the enzyme RNA polymerase to a specific DNA sequence at the beginning of the coding region, the so-called promoter. Many different promoters and other elements that influence transcription efficiency have been characterized in both pro- and eukaryotes. Promoters are most often species-specific, and in higher organisms

Table 5.1   Examples of post-translational protein modifications.

Modification	Occurrence
Cleavage of peptide bonds (maturation)	Pro- and eukaryotes
Formation of disulphide bonds	
Phosphorylation of tyrosine, serine or threonine	
N-linked glycosylation of asparagine	Eukaryotes
O-linked glycosylation of threonine or serine	
Hydroxylation of proline or lysine	
Myristylation of N-terminal glycine	
Prenylation of cysteine	
γ-Carboxylation of glutamic acid	Higher eukaryotes
Amidation of C-terminal glycine	
Sulphation of tyrosine	

also tissue-specific. In procaryotes, the RNA produced by transcription (called the primary transcription product) is used without any major modifications as mRNA to direct protein synthesis. In eukaryotes, mRNA is generated from the primary transcription products by complex enzymatic processing steps which remove intron regions.

The next step in gene expression is translation of the mRNA into a protein. The basic translation mechanisms are identical in pro- and eukaryotes. Thus, the codon for translation initiation is universal and leads to translation products containing methionine at their N-terminus. The N-terminal methionine is, however, often removed already during protein elongation by a ribosome-associated methionyl amino peptidase. Proteins destined for secretion from cells are synthesized with a so-called signal peptide of 20–30 amino acids at their N-terminus. The signal sequence mediates contact between the membrane and the nascent protein, and it is often cleaved off during translocation over the membrane before the protein is fully synthesized. Compared to prokaryotes, eukaryotes have a very complex pathway for secretion of proteins, and many essential modifications of proteins occur in the secretory pathway. Therefore, a eukaryotic maturation of primary translation product to a protein with correct secondary and tertiary structure may be problematic in prokaryoles. To overcome this problem, several efficient eukaryotic expression systems have been developed in addition to the "classical" *E. coli* systems. Examples of post-translational protein modifications in pro- and eukaryotes are shown in Table 5.1.

5.3.2 *E. coli* as production host

Since 1977, when a human protein (somatostatin) for the first time was expressed in *E. coli* in a functional form, an overwhelming number of eukaryotic genes have been expressed in this organism. The bacterium is incapable of performing many of the post-translational modifications that occur in mammalian cells and is therefore most suitable for production of proteins with no or limited modifications. However, its ease of handling and the accumulated data on its safety as a production organism has maintained *E. coli* as an important host even for proteins which may not be completely matured in this organism. A number of approved recombinant pharmaceuticals are produced in *E. coli*, e.g. growth hormone, insulin, interferon-α and interleukin 2. These proteins are made as secreted proteins in man,

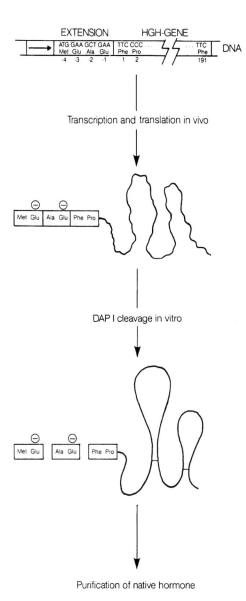

Figure 5.6   **Production of authentic human growth hormone (HGH) in** *E. coli*. The hormone is expressed from a synthetic gene as a fusion protein consisting of four amino acids fused to the N-terminus of the native 191 amino acid peptide hormone. Treatment of the expressed fusion protein with the enzyme dipeptidyl aminopeptidase I (DAP I) results in sequential removal of dipeptides from the N-terminus. DAP I is unable to cleave after a proline residue. Consequently, the processing stops after removal of the four amino acid extension which results in HGH with the correct N-terminus.

where they are subject to limited post-translational modifications such as cleavage of peptide bonds and formation of disulphide bridges. In order to obtain correctly formed proteins in *E. coli* various ingenious methods have been devised. It has in some cases been necessary to perform the final maturation *in vitro* . An example of this is shown in Figure 5.6.

Intensive work has been performed aiming at optimising the signals involved in expression in *E. coli*. For high production levels are used promoters from highly transcribed bacterial genes, or synthetic promoters. Both constitutive and regulated promoters are used. Regulated promoters can be turned on or off by altering the growth environment (temperature, added chemicals etc.) and are often used for production of recombinant products that are harmful to the cell. Examples of such promoters are the *lac* promoter from the β-galactocidase operon, or the bacteriophage λ promoters P_L and P_R. The advantage of these promoters is that synthesis of recombinant proteins can be delayed until the cell density has reached a high level where a short protein production phase suffices.

5.3.3 Yeast as production host

Yeasts are fungi which grow predominantly as single cells. As a small eukaryote, yeast performs many post-translational modifications which also occur in humans. This makes it useful for production of peptides and proteins of medium complexity, while proteins with very complex structures may need to be made in higher organisms. The long tradition of using yeast for food production contribute significantly to its acceptability as a producer of pharmaceutical proteins.

The term yeast is for many molecular biologists almost synonymous with *Saccharomyces cerevisiae* (baker's yeast), which has been studied extensively at the genetic and molecular level. In the future, other yeast species, e.g. *Pichia pastoris*, *Hansenula polymorpha* and *Yarrowia lipolytica*, may also become useful for production purposes. However, only *S. cerevisiae* produced drugs have so far been approved for human use (e.g. insulin and a Hepatitis B vaccine).

Like *E. coli*, *S. cerevisiae* contains a natural plasmid (2-micron DNA) which can be used as vector when equipped with a selectable marker. Instead of using a gene conferring resistance to an antibiotic, a yeast gene which complements a mutated gene in the host genome is usually used for plasmid selection. This principle is preferable to antibiotic selection in large-scale work.

As a eukaryote, yeast possesses a secretory pathway which resembles that of mammalian cells. It is often an advantage to produce recombinant proteins from yeast in a secreted form for the dual reason that secreted proteins may be subjected to desired post-translational modifications in the secretory pathway and are easier to purify. However, undesirable changes may occur during passage through the secretory pathway, e.g. incorrect N- and O-linked glycosylation. Since the glycosyl side chains made in yeast and humans are different, yeast-produced glycoproteins may be immunogenic in man. Thus, glycoproteins are generally not suitable for production in yeast.

5.3.4 Expression of complex proteins in mammalian cells

Mammalian systems are the obvious choice for production of glycoproteins or proteins with other complex post-translational modifications. Some of the modifications (e.g. sulphation,

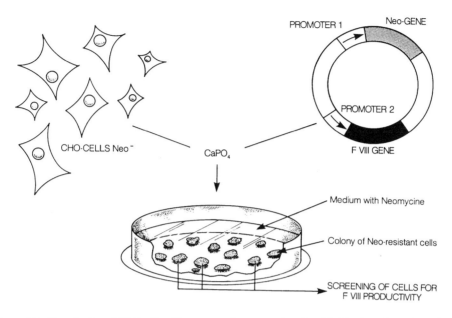

Figure 5.7 **Transfection of CHO cells with a mammalian expression plasmid**. The plasmid contains a cDNA for coagulation factor VIII (F VIII) and the neomycin resistance gene (Neo). The plasmid is transfected into CHO cells which are made permeable by treatment with calcium phosphate. Only cells containing the plasmid are able to grow in the presence of neomycin. Individual neomycin resistant clones may give different F VIII expression levels, usually due to a variable number of F VIII genes. Clones with high expression are found by screening.

amidation and γ-carboxylation) are often essential for the biological activity of the proteins. For example, the activity of a number of blood coagulation factors (Factors II, VII, IX and X) is completely dependent on γ-carboxylation of glutamic acid, a modification which only occurs in higher eukaryotes.

Many different mammalian host-vector systems have become available for expression of recombinant proteins. Examples of immortalized mammalian cell lines, which can be grown in culture and therefore are suitable as host cells, are CHO (Chinese Hamster Ovary), BHK (Baby Hamster Kidney), COS (african green monkey kidney) and HeLa (human epitheloid carcinoma) cells. Mammalian viruses which replicate autonomously in cells can be used as vectors for recombinant DNA, but it is also possible to perpetuate introduced DNA in mammalian cells without an autonomously replicating vector, because exogenous DNA integrates into mammalian chromosomes with a low, but often sufficient frequency. Viruses which have been modified to be particularly useful as vectors include SV40 (Simian Virus), Epstein-Barr virus and retroviruses. The two former are self-replicating while the latter mediates cellular uptake and integration into the genome with significantly increased efficiency compared to DNA constructs without retroviral elements (see Section 5.7). To allow easy isolation of cells in which recombinant DNA has been taken up, a selectable marker gene such as resistance to the cytotoxic drug neomycin is introduced into the vector (Fig. 5.7). The promoters used for gene expression in mammalian cells are often strong viral promoters such as the SV40 and CMV (cytomegalovirus) promoters.

It is important to realize that post-translational modifications may not be completely identical to those seen in the native protein, even when mammalian cells are used for production. In the body, proteins are produced in organs composed of specialized cells, and it has become increasingly clear that differences exist in the processing capabilities of different tissues. Also, immortalized cell lines may very well have diverged from their progenitors not only in their growth characteristics but also in other ways. Proteins with aberrant post-translational modification may be recognized as "non-self" by the immune system and therefore be useless or even dangerous. Therefore, careful characterization of recombinant proteins produced from mammalian cells and from microbial sources is equally important.

From an economical point of view, mammalian cell culture systems are less attractive than microbial systems. The slow growth rate, moderate expression levels, complex medium requirements and the need for advanced cultivation equipment are the main reasons for the relatively high cost of producing biologicals from mammalian cell lines.

5.3.5 Expression in transgenic animals

An alternative to the expression of recombinant proteins in mammalian cell cultures is to use so-called transgenic animals (see also Section 5.6). Transgenic animals can be generated by injection of a foreign gene into fertilized eggs by *in vitro* micromanipulation. The injected foreign gene integrates into a chromosome in the egg, normally at random locations. The eggs are then implanted into the oviduct of a foster mother which after a normal period of pregnancy will give birth to transgenic progeny with the foreign gene incorporated permanently into the genome of all cells.

When using transgenic animals as producers of recombinant proteins it is important that expression of the transgene is regulated. The reason is that the compound usually is biologically active and therefore should be produced and stored in organs or compartments where it does not affect the animal. The most attractive transgenic production systems employ mammary gland specific regulatory elements that target accumulation of the protein to the milk of the animal. Transgenic sheep have been made which express substantial levels of recombinant proteins in the milk, e.g. tissue plasminogen activator, α1-antitrypsin and coagulation Factor IX. None of the proteins produced by transgenic animals have, however, yet been marketed as pharmaceuticals.

5.3.6 Recombinant protein expression in insect cells

Insect cell expression systems have lately become very popular, especially for small-scale production of mammalian recombinant proteins. High expression levels of active proteins can usually be obtained much faster than in mammalian cells, which is a key attraction of the systems.

Most vectors are based on a lytic insect virus belonging to the Baculovirus family, and the foreign cDNA is inserted in the viral genome without interfering with the lytic life cycle of the virus. Protein production thus occurs during a lytic infection of insect cells with recombinant viruses, and usually less than a week is needed from infection to maximal product yield. The fact that baculoviruses are non-infectious to vertebrates and their promoters inactive in mammalian cells gives insect systems a potential advantage over

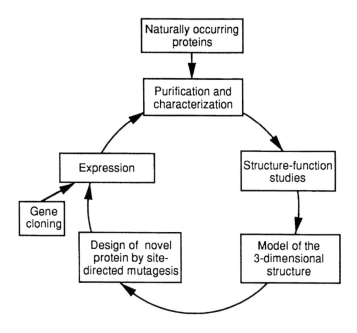

Figure 5.8   The protein engineering and design cycle.

other systems when expressing oncogenes or other genes that are harmful to mammals. Thus, baculovirus has been used for expression of a HIV protein (gp160) which is at present in phase III clinical trial as a recombinant AIDS vaccine.

However, at present the insect system is mainly used when only limited amounts of a recombinant protein are required for characterization or when a recombinant protein is used as a tool in drug design rather than as a drug in its own right (see Section 5.5).

5.4 PROTEIN DESIGN

Recombinant DNA technology makes it feasible to produce not only natural proteins, but also to design and produce new types of protein molecules. New proteins can be broadly classed in two categories: 1) natural protein variants harbouring replacements, insertions and deletions of small numbers of amino acids, and 2) chimeric proteins with domains from different proteins. These approaches have been very useful in structure-function studies of enzymes and receptors, e.g. in determining which part of the protein is responsible for binding of substrate or ligand. A third category comprising proteins designed from scratch is also conceivable, but is at present at a very preliminary level.

For a rational approach to the design of new protein pharmaceuticals, a so-called "protein engineering and design cycle" is usually set up (Fig. 5.8). Design cycles are a familiar

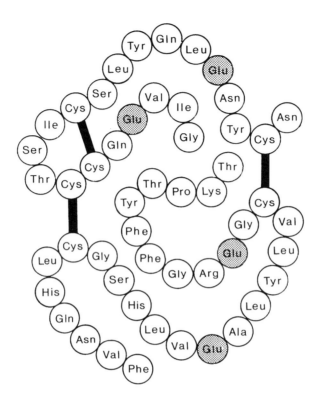

Figure 5.9 **Structure of the insulin molecule**. The four negatively charged glutamic acid residues (Glu) are marked. By site-directed mutagenesis, the codons for Glu (GAA) can be changed to e.g. the codon CAA for the neutral glutamine residue (Gln) resulting in an insulin variant with a higher isoelectric point.

concept in the pharmaceutical industry where the knowledge gained by testing the chemical, physical and biological characteristics of a so-called lead compound is used to design a modified version of the lead, which is again tested etc. until a satisfactory compound is found.

5.4.1 Protein variants

Protein variants can be generated by a genetic engineering method called site-directed mutagenesis. Using this method, it is possible to change, delete or insert one or a few nucleotides within a coding region. Expression of a mutated gene will result in a protein variant with a specific amino acid alteration, the function of which is then tested in various ways. Engineering small changes in proteins can have a variety of objectives, such as changing the solubility or stability properties or the affinity for substrates or receptors.

As an example, extensive work has been performed to design insulin molecules with improved characteristics. The insulin molecule contains four glutamic acid residues, and by changing one or more of these to the neutral amino acid glutamine the isoelectric point is shifted towards a higher pH thus giving an insulin variant with a lower solubility at the physiological pH around 7.3 (Fig. 5.9). Such insulin variants might constitute improved alternatives to existing slow-release formulations made by complexing native insulin with protamine or zinc ions. Similarly, other amino acid substitutions might lead to new quick-acting insulin preparations. As anticipated, many variants have proven undesirable at various stages in clinical or preclinical test programs, for instance because of altered affinity for the receptors for insulin and the related hormone insulin-like growth factor. Another major problem for the clinical application of analogues is the risk of adverse reactions due to immunogenicity or altered physiological functions of degradation products. These risks are very serious for a pharmaceutical like insulin which is administered daily for years, and extensive test programs for adverse reactions are therefore necessary. However, a couple of insulin analogues are now in phase III clinical trial, and seem very promising as improved therapeutics.

5.4.2 Protein chimeras

Chimeric proteins are made by fusing the coding region for one protein (or protein domain) with that of another followed by expression of the combined coding regions. The successful generation of a functional chimeric protein usually requires that structure-function relationships of the two starting proteins are well known, so that active domains will be maintained within the new protein. Conversely, the chimeric approach can also be used as a means to discover which regions of a protein are important for its activity.

A chimeric protein approach might for instance be employed for the production of so-called humanized monoclonal antibodies, which could become very important pharma-ceuticals. The so-called hybridoma technique, based on the selection, immortalization and proliferation of individual antibody forming B-cells, has been very successful for production of murine monoclonal antibodies. However, in spite of major efforts, it has been difficult to establish similar production methods for human monoclonal antibodies. Instead, with access to cloned antibody genes of both human and murine origin, "humanized" antibodies can be made by expression of a chimeric antibody gene in a suitable host. In mice antibodies with a required specificity can readily be obtained by immunisation with an antigen and the corresponding cDNA isolated. By combining the coding region corresponding to the variable region from such a murine antibody with the constant region from a human antibody, one can generate a chimeric antibody with the antigenic specificity of the murine antibody, but which is tolerated by the human immune system.

Such humanized antibodies may have numerous therapeutic applications, either alone or coupled to other biologically active substances. For example, they might be used in the elimination of toxic substances such as bacterially derived endotoxins, or as regulators of the humoral immune response by binding of excess levels of cytokines (interleukin 1, tumour necrosis factor etc.). In cancer therapy, antibodies might be able to mediate selective destruction of tumour cells, not only via normal immunological mechanisms, but also via targeted toxin delivery. Thus, a tumour-cell specific antibody fused to parts of a cellular toxin, such as diphtheria toxin, might selectively interact with and destroy tumour cells. This so-called "magic bullet" approach is not limited to antibody-toxin fusions; chimeras between toxins and protein ligands for cell-type specific receptors is another possibility for targeted delivery.

5.5 GENE TECHNOLOGY IN NON-PEPTIDE AND PEPTIDE DRUG DISCOVERY

Some of the most common targets for drugs are enzymes, receptors, ion channels and active transport complexes. All these targets are proteins, and as such they can be isolated by cloning and expression of their corresponding genes. This has had a profound effect on non-peptide drug discovery and development, because access to pure targets allows examination of drug-target interactions that previously was not possible. The following overview of the impact of gene technology on the development of drugs interacting with membrane receptors is intended as an example. In general, any protein with a significant role in physiological processes can become a target for drug development in a similar manner.

5.5.1 Membrane receptors as targets for drug discovery

Over the years, pharmacological characterization of membrane receptors have led to a classification based on either their function or their type of ligand (for examples and a detailed discussion of the receptor concept, see Chapter 6). The cloning and characterization of a large number of membrane receptors has added structural information to the pharmacological data, and has also allowed localization of receptors in various organs and tissues. This has revealed that many of the receptors previously classified as single entities in fact consists of families of related receptors. Receptor subtypes within a certain family share structural as well as functional features, such as interaction with the same ligands. However, the separate expression and pharmacological characterization of cloned receptor subtypes has in many cases shown that the affinity for ligands may vary between different subtypes. This is a very important finding, because it opens up the possibility of finding selective drugs that exclusively — or at least preferentially — interact with a single receptor subtype. Since a significant degree of tissue specificity has been observed in the distribution of receptor subtypes, a subtype-specific drug would have a higher specificity, and hence fewer side-effects, than drugs interacting with several receptor subtypes.

With this possibility in mind, the classical method in drug discovery based on screening of huge collections of pure chemical substances or complex biological extracts is now extensively applied to purified receptor preparations. The assays used for screening are either based on whole cells expressing the cloned target receptor or on a crudely purified receptor preparation from a recombinant source. Since a screening can easily comprise thousands of different substances, a judicious design of the screening assay is worth spending some time on, an area where gene technology again may contribute. These screening programs are likely to produce significant new advances in drug development.

Another object for receptor-based screening programs is a search for non-peptide analogues of peptide hormones. Peptide hormones have the disadvantage of only being available as pharmaceuticals in injection formulations, since peptides are broken down (digested) in the stomach if taken orally. Thus, the goal for these programs is to find stable analogues which can be taken orally or as inhalation preparations. Once a promising lead compound has been found, a lead optimization project can be set up in a design cycle that in principle resembles the one shown in Figure 5.8.

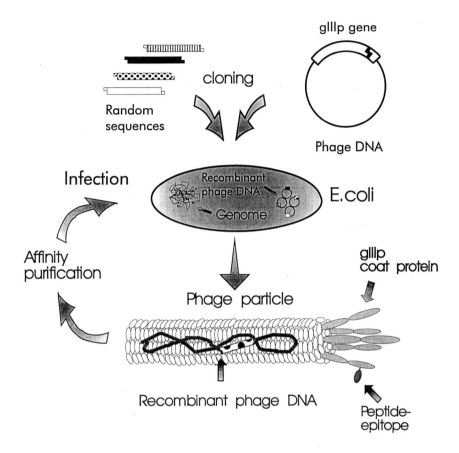

Figure 5.10 **Phage-display of peptide epitopes**. Cloning of random DNA sequences in frame with the coding region for a phage coat protein (gIIIp) results in the formation of phage particles each displaying one new peptide epitope on the surface. Phage particles displaying an epitope for a specific target (e.g. a receptor or an enzyme) can be isolated by affinity purification and amplified by re-infection of *E. coli*. (Figure courtesy of J. Engberg).

5.5.2 Epitope display libraries

As a complement to the libraries of chemical entities and natural biological extracts, "genetic" epitope libraries can be used as a source for new pharmacologically active substances. An example of a genetic epitope library is the so-called phage display system for peptides and proteins (Fig. 5.10). A phage is a bacterial virus which can be used as a cloning vector in bacteria (just as animal viruses can be used as cloning vectors in mammalian cells). Some of the coat proteins of phages can accommodate foreign sequences in certain positions without destroying their normal function. By cloning random nucleotide sequences in frame with the coding region of these proteins, a library of phages each displaying a unique peptide or protein sequence on the surface will be generated. The phage library, which can comprise more than 10^9 different peptide epitopes, can be subjected to affinity purification procedures using immobilized purified receptors (or any other target), and selected phages can be amplified by re-infection of *E. coli*. If necessary, selection and amplification can be repeated until a pure phage clone is obtained. The sequence of the selected peptide is deduced from the sequence of the DNA encapsidated in the phage particle, and this sequence can then be used in various design cycle set-ups.

Genetic libraries with DNA or RNA epitopes can also be constructed; here, amplification is accomplished by tagging the random sequences with known sequences that can be used for PCR. In both cases, the beauty of the set-up is that an enormous repertoire of epitopes can be analyzed as a mixture, because those few that interact with the target can be selected and amplified. When working with non-genetic substance libraries, selective amplification is not possible, and each substance must therefore be analyzed separately by screening.

5.6 TRANSGENIC ANIMALS AS DISEASE MODELS

As mentioned previously, transgenic animals can be used to produce pharmaceutically active proteins. However, transgenic animals are likely to become more important as models for human diseases than for production. Only a limited number of animal disease models were available before the advent of the transgenic techniques. These were either generated spontaneously or established with great experimental difficulty. However, with the methods that now exist for introducing or inactivating genes in experimental animals, much more efficient and direct ways of generating disease models have become available. Transgenic mice are normally used as disease models because they are easy to generate and breed.

The simplest transgenic mouse model expresses a foreign gene in an unregulated manner, i.e. in most or all of its organs. However, for some purposes it may be necessary to limit expression to specific organs, and in this case tissue-specific regulatory elements must be used. There is no absolute requirement for the foreign gene to be inserted at a specific locus on a chromosome, and as described previously such animals can be generated by injection of the foreign gene into a fertilized egg.

A more sophisticated transgenic model is one where a specific gene has been inactivated, a so-called knock-out mouse. The inactivation is accomplished by an elegant, but time-consuming technique called targeted gene replacement (Fig. 5.11). Briefly, a cloned version of the gene is interrupted by the insertion of a gene coding for a selectable marker, usually one conferring resistance to the drug neomycin. The interrupted gene is introduced into embryonic stem cells grown in culture and cells that have taken up the DNA are selected by growth in neomycin-containing medium. In some rare instances, the gene has not integrated at random locations in the genome, but has actually switched place with its normal counterpart as a result of homologous recombination. Since this event is very rare, a method to select the cells where this has happened has also been devised. Another selectable marker gene, this time one which confers sensitivity to an extraneous agent (usually the *Herpes Simplex* thymidine kinase gene which confers sensitivity to the drug ganciclovir), is placed in the vector adjacent to the interrupted gene. Cells which have taken up the whole vector by a random integration event will, in addition to the neomycin gene, contain the thymidine kinase gene and therefore be sensitive to ganciclovir. Only those cells in which homologous gene integration has occurred will contain the neomycin gene

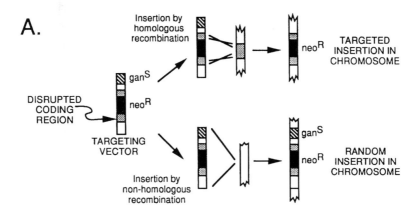

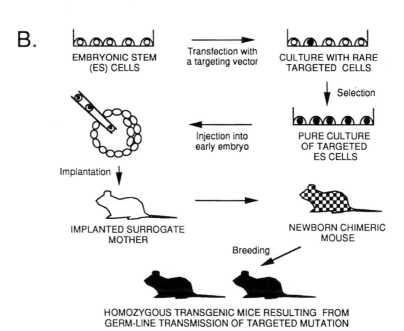

Figure 5.11 **Generation of a knock-out mouse by targeted gene replacement**. **A**: Homologous and non-homologous insertion of an inactivated gene into a chromosome. Neo^R (resistance to neomycin) and gan^S (sensitivity to ganciclovir) are the selectable markers used to distinguish between the two situations. **B**: Transfection of embryonic stem cells with a targeting vector containing the inactivated gene, followed by generation of chimeric mice by injection of the targeted stem cells into early embryos. Mice homozygous for the gene disruption are generated from the chimera by breeding. Easy identification of mice descending from the targeted stem cells can be obtained by using stem cells and early embryos from mouse lines with different fur colour.

alone, and therefore be resistant to both neomycin and ganciclovir. Approximately one cell in a million treated has the desired gene replacement, but this low replacement frequency suffices since these cells can be selected and propagated. The embryonic stem cells are then inserted into early embryos, which are allowed to develop into so-called chimeric mice, in which some of the cells descend from the stem cells harbouring the gene replacement. It now remains to find those mice that carry the interrupted gene in their germ line cells. These mice are used for breeding so that progeny homozygous for the interrupted gene can be obtained. Altogether, the process of generating a knock-out mouse takes about a year from start to finish. If desired, the method can of course also be used to replace a spontaneously mutated gene with a wild type gene.

In a "simple" knock-out mouse the target gene is inactivated in all cells of the animal, and in several cases this has been found to be lethal. Therefore, even more sophisticated models where target genes are conditionally turned on or off in predetermined organs have recently been developed. These systems make use of various thoroughly characterized regulating mechanisms, and the end result is transgenic mice containing a number of foreign genes with a finely orchestrated interplay.

Transgenic mouse models now exist for a number of diseases, both monogenic and polygenic. An example of the former is cystic fibrosis (CF), which has been shown to be caused by a defect in the gene encoding a large membrane protein, the CF transmembrane conductance regulator. Simple knock-out of this gene results in a mouse with symptoms similar to those found in humans, namely accumulation of mucus in the lungs. This model has been used to test various therapeutic approaches, including somatic gene therapy (see Section 5.7). This approach seems very promising, and has recently entered clinical trials. However, another CF therapeutic has already successfully passed phase III clinical trial. It is a recombinant human DNase I, an enzyme which degrades DNA. The therapy is effective, because DNA makes up a large proportion of the mucus in the lungs of the patients and is responsible for its high viscosity.

Examples of polygenic diseases for which transgenic models exist are cancer and atherosclerosis. Atherosclerosis is a complex disease which has both genetic and lifestyle causes. In both cases, a high content of various lipids in the blood seems to be a determining factor. A number of lipid transport proteins are known, and to test their influence on the development of atherosclerosis, transgenic mice either over-expressing or lacking these proteins have been made. The results obtained correlate well with human epidemiological survey results, and augurs well for the usefulness of the transgenic models. By the aid of these models, it has been shown that certain transporters, such as cholesteryl ester transfer protein (CETP), promote atherosclerosis when overexpressed. Inhibitors of these transporters might be useful as therapeutics. If such inhibitors are found by screening in a suitable *in vitro* assay, they can be tested for *in vivo* efficacy in the transgenic mouse prior to testing in humans. The great advantage of the transgenic models is thus that various hypotheses for both disease etiology and intervention can be tested.

5.7 GENE THERAPY

In the transgenic animals described above, the foreign genes were indiscriminately inserted into all cells, including the germ line cells. However, foreign genes can also be introduced into whole animals in such a way that only specific body cells (somatic cells), and not the germ cells, are affected. For ethical as well as medical reasons, only the latter possibility, the so-called somatic gene therapy, is relevant in humans. Somatic gene therapy holds great promise for successful treatment of genetic diseases as well as many other diseases, and some good results have been obtained already. At present, more than a hundred clinical applications of somatic gene transfer into patients are under investigation.

In order for somatic gene therapy to work, efficient gene delivery systems are necessary, especially if the gene transfer is to be done *in situ*. In some cases, cells (e.g. blood cells) can be taken out of the body and transfected while cultivated *in vitro* . Here, propagation and selection of transfected cells is in principle possible, but since long-term cultivation of the isolated cells may not be feasible in practice, it is very important also here that a sufficient fraction of the cells have been transfected.

To obtain efficient gene delivery replication-defective retroviral vectors may be used. Such viral DNA constructs generally behave like non-viral DNA, but if taken up by a mammalian cell containing genes for the retroviral coat proteins it can be packaged into a viral particle. So-called packaging cell lines have been specifically designed for this purpose. The recombinant viral particles generated from these cells possess normal retroviral ability to infect other cells. Viral infection of cells is much more efficient than standard DNA transformation methods, and in addition the retrovirus mediated integration of DNA into chromosomes is more efficient than spontaneous integration. However, for safety reasons it is very important that the receiving cells are unable to generate new viral particles, because this might lead to spreading of recombinant viruses. Retroviral systems are widely used in current gene therapy protocols for fatal diseases such as cancer, and it is a serious concern to ensure that the procedures do not lead to any spread of retrovirus to other organs (particularly not to the germ cells) or to other persons.

In order to avoid the potential dangers of the retroviral systems, a number of other gene delivery systems are being investigated. Some build on the use of other types of viruses, and thus have potential risks similar to those of retroviruses. Others use totally different approaches, such as "packaging" of DNA into liposomes which can be taken up by cells via efficient endocytotic mechanisms, or fusion of DNA to a ligand for a cellular uptake receptor.

It has been debated whether gene therapy constitutes a procedure, a device or a drug. However, from a regulatory point of view, the consensus seems to be that the materials for gene therapy (including the therapeutic gene and the vector) should be classified as "medicinal products from biotechnology" and be treated as drugs. It is predicted that production of gene/vector constructs will eventually become commercial, and, as for any other drug, strict criteria for production processes and quality control must therefore be enforced.

Although human gene therapy was initially viewed as a means to correct inherited diseases with monogenic causes, there is no doubt that gene therapy for more common diseases such as AIDS, cancer and neurodegenerative diseases will be just as important. A large number of the current gene therapy protocols have cancer cells as targets, and include attempts to overproduce proteins such as tumour necrosis factor, interferon and interleukins (all of which seem to be able to promote selective immunological destruction of the targeted cells), as well as attempts to block the production of factors such as insulin-like growth factor I (which seems to promote cancer growth). As yet, gene therapy for AIDS has not reached

Table 5.2   Recombinant protein drugs on the market.

Product	Category	Indication	Introduction
Insulin	Hormone	Diabetes	1982
Growth hormone	Hormone	Growth defects	1985
Interferon-α	Cytokine	Cancer therapy	1986
Interferon-γ	Cytokine	Cancer therapy	1990
Interleukin 2	Cytokine	Cancer therapy	1989
Granulocyte colony-stimulating factor (G-CSF)	Cytokine	Leucopenia	1991
Granulocyte-macrophage colony-stimulating factor (GM-CSF)	Cytokine	Leucopenia	1991
Erythropoetin	Cytokine	Anaemia	1989
Plasminogen activator	Antithrombotic	Thrombosis	1987
Factor VIII	Coagulation factor	Haemophilia A	1989
α1-antitrypsin	Enzyme inhibitor	α1-antitrypsin deficiency	1992
DNase I	Enzyme	Cystic fibrosis	1994
Hepatitis B subunit vaccine	Vaccine	Hepatitis prevention	1988

clinical trials, but laboratory studies have proven that the approach may work in principle. Examples of monogenic diseases with ongoing human gene therapy trials include cystic fibrosis and a severe immunological disorder caused by deficiency of the enzyme adenosine deaminase (ADA).

5.8 RECOMBINANT DNA DERIVED PRODUCTS ON THE MARKET — AND IN THE PIPELINE

Table 5.2 lists the recombinant proteins which to our knowledge have been marketed as drugs at the time of writing. Only a few of these drugs were previously produced by non-recombinant means, and only one (insulin) was available in ample amounts. As can be seen, they represent a broad variety of biological substances spanning from hormones and cytokines over enzymes and blood coagulation regulators to vaccines.

According to various sources, there are at present around 150 new proteins in advanced clinical trials, and around a hundred of these represent truly novel pharmaceutical substances with no precedent in medical therapy. A large number of them belong to the cytokine families, but hormones, antithrombotic proteins, antibodies and vaccines are also represented. Some of the proteins are modified versions of natural ones, or designed chimeric proteins.

It is estimated that around 2,000 gene technology-based drugs, comprising both proteins and non-proteins, are in early stages of development. In the non-protein drug area, so-called antisense molecules constitute a promising new therapeutic possibility. Antisense molecules are short RNA or DNA molecules (or modified versions hereof) which are complementary to a target mRNA. Because of the base complementarity, the antisense molecules can bind to their targets and inhibit translation into protein. To be efficient *in vivo*, the antisense molecules must be able to enter cells and be reasonably stable, characteristics which have so far been only partially met. Presently, the antisense approach is most actively pursued within antiviral research, but it may have applications in many different disease areas if successful. Antisense therapy mimics the effect of gene disruption, and would thus be an alternative to gene therapy where inactivation of a gene is the desired goal. As mentioned previously, gene therapy constitutes another non-protein therapeutic avenue, which is expected to lead to significant new drug developments — and perhaps in the long run replace protein (and other) therapeutics completely. This is, however, quite speculative. But it is indisputable that the basic scientific discovery of gene splicing has had an impressive effect on drug development within a remarkably short time span. The impact is not likely to diminish within the foreseeable future.

FURTHER READING

Ausubel, F.M., Brent, R., Kingston, R.E., Moore, D.D., Seidman, J.G., Smith, J.A. and Struhl, K.A. (1989) *Current protocols in molecular biology.* J. Wiley & Sons.

Barinaga, M. (1994) Knock-out mice: round two. *Science*, **265**, 26–28.

Blundell, T.L. (1994) Problems and solutions in protein engineering — towards rational design. *Tibtech*, **12**, 145–148.

Bristow, A.F. (1993) Recombinant-DNA-derived insulin analogues as potentially useful therapeutic agents. *Tibtech*, **11**, 301–305.

Capecchi, M.R. (1994) Targeted gene replacement. *Scientific American*. March issue, 52–59.

Cortese, R., Felice, F., Galfre, G., Luzzago, A., Monaci, P. and Nicosia, A. (1994) Epitope discovery using peptide libraries displayed on phage. *Tibtech*, **12**, 262–267.

Creighton, T.E. (1993) *Proteins: Structures and Molecular Properties.* 2nd edition. New York: W.H. Freeman & Co.

Culver, K.W. and Blaese, R.M. (1994) Gene therapy for cancer. *Trends in Genetics*, **10**(5), 174–178.

Dalbøge, H., Dahl, H.H.M., Pedersen, J., Hansen, J.W. and Christensen, T. (1987) A novel enzymatic method for production of authentic human growth hormone from an *E. coli* produced hGH-precursor. *Biotechnology*, **5**, 161–164.

Dougall, W.C., Peterson, N.C. and Greene, M.I. (1994) Antibody-structure-based design of pharmacological agents. *Tibtech*, **12**, 372–379.

Hodgson, J. (1993) Expression systems: A User's guide. *Biotechnology*, **11**, 887–893.

Hutton, I. (1994) *Pharma. Projects.* United Kingdom: PJB publications.

McCormick, D.K. (1993) Biotechnology 10th anniversary section. *Biotechnology*, **11**(3), S9–S46.

Meager, A. and Griffiths, E. (1994) Human somatic gene therapy. *Tibtech*, **12**, 108–113.

Sambrook, J., Fritsch, E.F. and Maniatis, T. (1989) *Molecular cloning. A Laboratory Manual*, 2nd edition. New York: Cold Spring Harbor Laboratory Press.

6. RECEPTORS

CLAUS BRAESTRUP

CONTENTS

6.1 INTRODUCTION

All drugs have a target within the living organism. The target is known for the vast majority of drugs; only a few stubborn groups of molecules, such as volatile anaesthetics, maintain elusive mechanisms of action. Drug research and drug development are usually not entertained without prior knowledge of presumed mechanisms of action, preferentially related to a precise well-defined target. When the target is known there are good chances of predicting beneficial effects and the non-occurrence of certain side effects. There are numerous kinds of targets for drugs, the most common ones being enzymes, receptors, ion channels, and active transport complexes. Drugs acting directly on DNA or RNA are remarkably scarce (see Chapter 17). Enzymes, receptors, ion channels, and transport complexes (see Chapters 8 and 10) have in common their protein nature and the fact that they possess distinctive sites or targets within the molecule, or complex of molecules, which recognize and bind the physiological substrate or drugs. Enzymes, channels, receptors, and transport complexes differentiate in function rather than in fundamental biochemical nature.

The concept of receptors stems back to the turn of the century. In 1906 Langley coined the phrase 'specific receptive substances' for a site in the myoneural junction as the specific site of action for nicotine and curare by postulating: 'The mutual antagonism of nicotine and curari on the muscle can only satisfactorily be explained by supposing that both combine with the receptive substance. It receives the stimulus and by transmitting it causes contraction'. This phrasing covers the activation of receptors by agonists, to which class most natural messengers belong, and the receptor/effector coupling. Implicitly it also covers the existence of antagonists which have affinity in common with the agonist but lack the capacity to activate the receptors. Erlich, coming from the different research field of chemotherapeutics, reached similar insight at about the same time as Langley. Based on the resistance and susceptibility of bacteria to dye chemotherapeutics, Erlich postulated 'corpora non agunt nisi fixata' (it doesn't work if it doesn't bind), the first simple formulation of the 'lock-&-key' model for receptors.

The receptor concept being quite broad at first boiled down to a very narrow scope in the 1930's and 1950's when many of the theoretical developments by Clark, Ariëns, and Stephenson were based on experimental studies using agonists and antagonists to neurotransmitter receptors on organs in simple organ baths. However, in the 1980's, deeper knowledge of the biochemistry of a number of biochemical processes led to the understanding that 'receptor like' systems were operating in a broad sense which provided the basis for the present broad receptor concept. Table 6.1 shows various classes of receptors. Uptake "receptors" are not receptors but are often treated as such.

Table 6.1   Classes of receptors.

Activator Modality
Neurotransmitter
Hormone
Drug
Taste/Odour
Toxin
Immune
Light
(Uptake)

See text for further details.

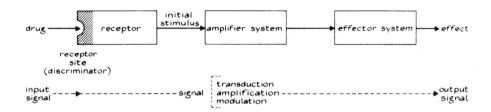

Figure 6.1   Main steps in the pharmacodynamic phase of action of bioactive agents. In its broad term, the receptor comprises the initial amplifier system. (From Ariëns *et al.*, p. 35 in Receptors, a Comprehensive Treatise, Ed. O'Brien, Plenum, 1979).

6.1.1 Receptor definition

Due to changing concepts, receptors are not unambiguously defined. The following definition is consistent with current thinking: 'A receptor is a macromolecule or a macromolecular complex which binds agonists with high structural selectivity, and with the consequence that a characteristic effect occurs'.

Note that two aspects are contained in this receptor definition. A selective binding, the receptor recognizes its ligand in the midst of myriads of molecules and binds it. As the second aspect, binding must be followed by consequence — something is triggered, a conformational shift in the receptor ligand complex is the first step in a chain of events leading to response. Receptors in their full context therefore include the ligand recognition site as well as the initial stimulus generating mechanism (see Fig. 6.1).

6.1.2 Classification

Receptors are classified according to the nature of their ligand, i.e. a chemical substance which binds to the receptor (see Table 6.1).

Neurotransmitter receptors are found throughout the central and the peripheral nervous system. They are receptors for signal molecules, neurotransmitters, which are released by nerve endings with the role of transmitting electric signals from a neurone over the synaptic cleft. Once diffused over the synapse, neurotransmitters are met by receptors either on other neurones or on effector organs. Neurotransmitters may also function as neuromodulators. Each nerve cell may have numerous types of receptors on the surface, some of which serve in fine tuning of the intrinsic activity of the neurone, their electric set point, their rhythm of spontaneous activity, their sensitivity to other stimuli, etc. Some of these receptors are modulatory rather than signal transmitting. Neurotransmitter receptors can also be expressed where neurotransmission may be absent, for example on blood platelets or in organs without neuronal input. Neurotransmitter and modulatory receptors remain important targets in medicinal chemistry; examples of receptor types and important reference ligands are shown in Table 6.2.

In principle, hormone receptors differ from neurotransmitter receptors only by the hormonal nature of the ligand. Some molecules function both as neurotransmitters and as

Table 6.2 Selected neurotransmitter subtypes and reference agonists and antagonists.

Receptor	Agonist	Antagonist
α_1	Methoxamine	Prazosin
α_2	Clonidine	Idazoxan
β_1	Xamoterol	Atenolol
β_2	Proceterol	ICI 118,551
β_3	BRL 37344	—
5-HT$_{1a}$	8-OH-DPAT	WAY 100135
5-HT$_2$	α-Methyl-5-HT	Ritanserin
5-HT$_3$	2-Methyl-5-HT	Ondansetron
Histamine H$_1$	2-Methylhistamine	Mepyramine
Histamine H$_2$	Dimaprit	Ranitidine
Histamine H$_3$	N-Methylhistamine	Thioperamide
Dopamine D$_1$	Fenoldopam	SCH 23390
Dopamine D$_2$	LY 171555	Spiroperidol
GABA$_A$	Muscimol	Bicuculline
GABA$_B$	Baclofen	Saclofen
Glycine$_A$	Glycine*	Strychnine
Glycine$_B$	D-Serine	7-Chlorokynurenic acid
NMDA	NMDA	D-AP5
AMPA	AMPA	NBQX
Muscarine M$_1$	Bethanecol	Pirenzepine
Muscarine M$_2$	Bethanecol	AF-DX 116
Muscarine M$_3$	Bethanecol	Hexahydrosiladifenol
Muscarine M$_4$	Bethanecol	Tropicamide
Nicotine	Nicotine	Hexamethonium
Adenosine A$_1$	PIA	DPCPX
Adenosine A$_2$	CGS 21680	KF 17837
Opiate μ	Morphine	Naloxone
δ	DPDPE	Naltrindole
κ	U 69593	Nor-binaltorphimine

*non-selective.

For further information, see *Trends Pharmacol. Sci.*, **15**, Suppl. 3, 1994: Receptor and Ion Channel Nomenclature Supplement.

hormones, for example the adrenergic β-receptor on fat cells may be classified as a hormone receptor although these receptors are similar to the neurotransmitter adrenergic receptors on neurones. On the other hand, hormones are often of peptide nature, and peptide receptors usually have much more complicated ligand receptor interaction patterns and structure activity relations. Furthermore, peptide receptors are less accessible to medicinal chemistry (see also Chapter 14).

Taste and smell receptors respond to selective taste and smell molecules with receptors in the tongue or nasal mucosa. These receptors have not yet been in focus in medicinal chemistry.

Selective recognition and binding sites for drugs are called drug receptors when drug binding results in the occurrence of the characteristic drug effects. The physiological function of the recognition site of a drug receptor is in principle unknown, otherwise the receptor would be characterized according to the physiological function. Drug receptors may "advance" to becoming physiological receptors be it neurotransmitter or hormone receptors, if and when their function is clarified. This occurred for the opiate receptors in the mid 1970's when endorphines and enkephalins were discovered and found to be the natural ligands to the already known opiate receptors. Drug receptors may also turn out to be enzymes, ion channels, uptake carriers, etc.

The concept of immune receptors emerged from the realization that antibodies are not designed by acute demands in the organism but that antibodies rather preexist in millions of different forms each of which fits a certain antigen. Antibodies each have their specific predetermined recognition property, and they circulate in the body as receptors which recognize and bind their antigen with high structural selectivity and with the effect that the cascade of immunological defense mechanisms is activated. In addition to the antibodies of the various Ig classes a number of other receptors exist in the immune system; the T-cell receptor is biochemically similar to the immunoglobulins and in addition there are receptors for the various cytokines and monokines. The recognition sites of the immune receptors are not open to classical medicinal chemistry — biotechnological approaches prevail (see Chapter 5).

Active uptake carriers are not receptors. However, medicinal chemistry of neurotransmitter uptake sites is similar to medicinal chemistry of receptors (see Chapter 10), and the biological models used to screen and further investigate uptake sites and receptors are also very similar. Therefore, uptake sites are sometimes erroneously referred to as uptake receptors. Drug receptors may, however, be located on uptake carriers.

6.2 RECEPTOR STRUCTURE AND FUNCTION

Neurotransmitter receptors belong to two major families: ion channel gating receptors and second messenger system coupled receptors.

Ion channels are pores in the cell membrane which, when open, allow small inorganic ions to pass through, following the electrochemical gradient (see Chapter 8). Ion channels can be opened by a variety of mechanisms among which receptor gating and voltage gating are most common.

6.2.1 Receptor gated ion channels

The nicotinic acetylcholine receptor is the most thoroughly studied ion channel gating receptor. In the 1970's advantage was taken of the easy availability of nicotinic receptors in the electroplaques of *Torpedo californica* for the characterization and purification, and in the 1980's the nicotinic receptor represented the first ion channel receptor to be cloned and made available for site directed mutagenesis (see Chapter 5). The nicotinic acetylcholine receptor is a complex of proteins, it is a pentameric protein $\alpha_2\beta\gamma\delta$ made up of four types of subunits arranged around a central ion channel (see Fig. 6.2).

The primary structures (amino acid sequence) of all four subunits have been determined by means of recombinant DNA methods. The subunits span the lipid cell membrane; when two acetylcholine molecules (one molecule is not sufficient) combine each with one of the two α-subunits, the ion channel in the middle of the receptor complex opens for a few milliseconds allowing thousands of sodium ions to pass the otherwise impermeable cell membrane resulting in chemical synaptic transmission from nerve to muscle or such

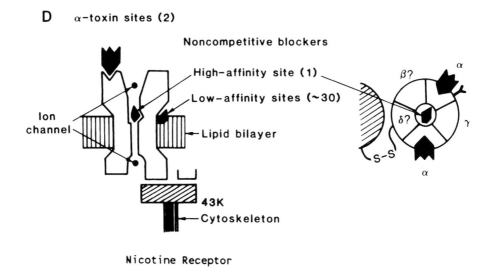

Figure 6.2 Nicotinic acetylcholine receptor. Schematic distribution of the binding sites for pharmacologically active ligands on the light-form pentamer. (Left) (i) The two primary sites for acetylcholine and snake venom α-toxins have an apical location on the α subunits; (ii) the unique high-affinity site for non-competitive blockers is located in or near the ion channel; (iii) multiple low-affinity sites for non-competitive blockers are distributed at the lipid-protein interface; (iv) association with the peripheral protein (43 K) on the cytoplasmic face immobilizes the receptor molecules in the membrane by cross-linking with the cytoskeleton. (Right) The top view of the pentamer shows the arrangement of the subunits around the central ion channel. Localization of the β and δ subunits in the rosette are still debated. The proposed differences in glycosylation state of the two primary acetylcholine binding sites on the α subunits is schematically represented by a Y. The chains link the two light forms of a heavy-form dimer in a flexible manner (From Changeux *et al.*, *Science*, **225**, 1335, 1984).

other location where nicotinergic neurotransmission occurs. The four subunits of the nicotinic receptor are not identical, but they share a high level of homology; in average, 40% of the amino acids are identical while many more show conservative substitution indicating that they are substituted by single base mutations. Furthermore, the subunits from different species show great similarity. The human and calf α-subunits, like that of *Torpedo californica*, have 437 amino acids and show 81% and 80% identity with the α-subunit of *Torpedo*. The structure of the acetylcholine receptor protein is thus exceptionally well conserved throughout the vertebrate phylum. The presumed transmembrane topography of a single subunit is shown in Figure 6.3. Detailed recognition points for acetylcholine on the α-subunit have not been identified — methionine in position 192 is probably involved.

Several subunits from two other ion channel gating receptors, the 4-aminobutanoic acid$_A$ (GABA$_A$) and the glycine$_A$ receptors have been cloned and show homology both internally (high homology), to each other, and also to the nicotinic receptor. These findings strongly suggest that ion channel gating receptors are products of a single ancestral gene and that they belong to one single gene superfamily. Individual recognition properties have evolved for the neurotransmitters and also for the ion selectivity; GABA, for example, does not activate nicotinic receptors. The ion selectivity is determined by the nature of the amino acids lining

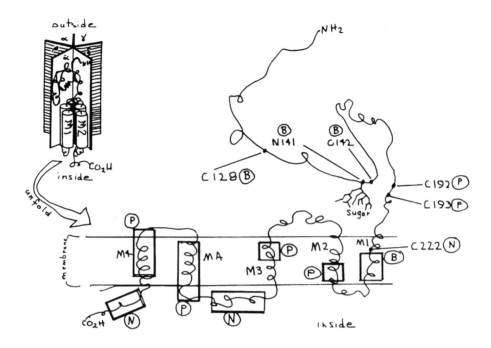

Figure 6.3   Two schemes of the proposed structure of the α subunit of the nicotinic acetylcholine receptor in a membrane. On the top left it is shown forming an ion channel. The larger scheme illustrates the disposition of parts of the protein chain relative to the membrane, and the positions and effects of a variety of deliberate amino-acid substitutions or delegations. N, no effect; P, acetylcholine binding but no gating; B, no binding, no gating. (From Stevens, *Nature*, **313**, 350, 1985).

the wall of the internal pore. The general theme in structure of receptor gated ion channels may explain why several drugs act on clusters of receptors. Tubocurare, for example, acts on both nicotinic and GABA$_A$ receptors, strychnine acts on glycine$_A$ receptors, but has also appreciable affinity for GABA$_A$ receptors.

Within the nicotinic, the GABA$_A$, and the glutamate receptor complexes, a number of allosteric receptor sites exist (see also Section 6.3.2).

6.2.2 Second messenger linked receptors

For a number of receptors, the immediate effect of receptor activation is the formation of a second messenger — a biochemically active small molecule which can produce intracellular changes such as participating in phosphorylation (cAMP) or mobilizing intracellular calcium ions (phosphatidyl inositol). The best known gene superfamily within the second messenger linked receptors is the G-protein coupled receptor superfamily. These receptors all activate (or inhibit) GTP binding proteins (G-proteins), which then in turn activate (or inhibit) adenylate cyclases, phosphatidyl bisphosphate hydrolases or the activity of certain ion channels (see Chapter 8). A great variety of receptors, more than 70, belong

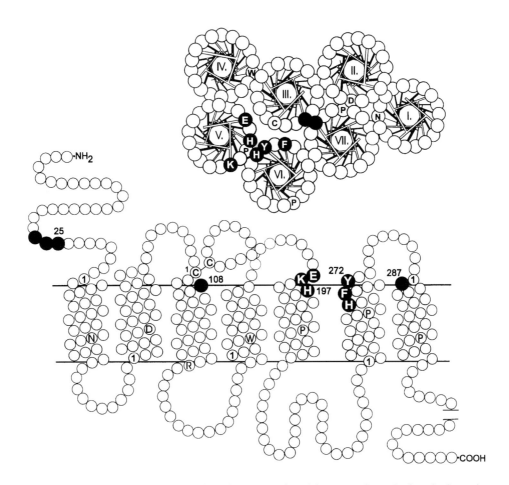

Figure 6.4 The "magnificent seven". A schematic representation of the proposed organization of a G-protein coupled receptor protein within the plasma membrane. A helical wheel (upper panel) and a serpentine (lower panel) diagram of the human NK-1 receptor. *Upper panel*, the helical wheel diagram shows the outer portions of the helices in an outside-inward view of a model of the NK-1 receptor based on the projection map of bovine rhodopsin. Helices have been rotated to optimize inward orientation of presumed ligand contact sites in multiple 7TM receptors. A generic numbering based on alignments of TM fingerprint residues is also indicated. Thus, for example, E78 (Glu^{78}) will have the generic number GluII:10 and corresponds to the normally highly conserved AspII:10. *Lower panel*, in the serpentine diagram, "fingerprint" residues in each transmembrane segment have been pointed out (N in TM-I, C and R in TM-III, W in TM-IV, etc.). Residues suggested to be involved in the binding of the natural peptide agonist, substance P, are shown in black on gray. Residues suggested to be involved in the binding of the non-peptide antagonists CP96,345 are shown in white on black. (Redrawn from Rosenkilde *et al.*, *J. Biol. Chem.*, **269**, 28160, 1994).

to the G-protein coupling family, including α_1 adrenergic receptors; β_1 and β_2 adrenergic receptors; serotonin$_{1A}$ (5-HT$_{1A}$), 5-HT$_{1C}$, 5-HT$_2$ receptors; M$_1$ muscarinic acetylcholine receptors; D$_1$ and D$_2$ dopamine receptors; neurokinin (NK) peptide receptors; and light receptors (rhodopsin). Figure 6.4 shows what is believed to be a general characteristic of the G-protein coupled receptors. The most striking feature is that each of them contains seven

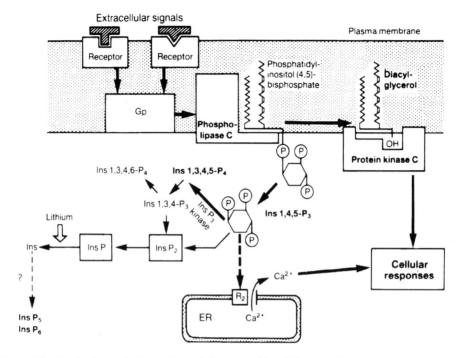

Figure 6.5   Signal pathways for G-protein coupled receptors. Ligands interact with receptors in the upper/outer part. Signals are passed through the lipid bilayer by G-proteins which activate (+) or inhibit (−) enzymes which form second messenger, cAMP, cGMP (not shown), IP$_3$ or diacylglycerol, which in turn affect intracellular phosphorylation, Ca^{++} mobilization, or other. (From Altman and Michell, *Nature*, **331**, 119, 1988).

stretches of 20–28 hydrophobic amino acids which likely represent membrane spanning regions. For this reason, they are generally referred to as the Seven Trans Membrane Receptors (7-TM receptors). Amino acid homology generally occurs in these regions. Other regions that are less, but still reasonably well conserved are the first two cytoplasmic loops from the *N*-Terminus. Proposed extracellular domains, the putative third cytoplasmic loop, and the putative cytoplasmic carboxyterminal are all quite divergent. Another feature shared within the G-protein coupled superfamily is the existence of one or more potential sites for *N*-glycosylation near the amino terminus and potential site of regulatory phosphorylation on cytoplasmic domains. The precise localizations of the ligand recognizing region (or regions) and the G-protein binding domain are unknown. The former may be related to membrane spanning helices II, III, and VII, while the latter may attach to the cytoplasmic region. Figure 6.5 illustrates the flows of events for G-protein coupled receptors after activation by ligands. The G-protein itself is also a family of proteins, which are composed of three subunits: α, β, and γ.

6.2.3 Insulin receptors and other growth factor receptors

Receptors for peptides, be it neurotransmitters, modulators, antigens, cytokines, hormones, or growth factors can be grouped in families and subfamilies according to the various degrees of similarity of their primary structure. The insulin hormone receptor, as an example of a peptide receptor, is an integral membrane glycoprotein (apparent relative molecular mass 350,000–400,000) composed of two α-subunits (apparent M_r 120,000–130,000) and two β-subunits linked by disulphide bonds. Photoaffinity labelling as well as affinity cross linking have shown that insulin interacts with the α-subunit. In intact cells, insulin stimulates the phosphorylation of the β-subunit on serine and tyrosine residues. The insulin receptor exhibits insulin-dependent tyrosine kinase activity. The protein kinase activity catalyzes phosphorylation of both the β-subunit (autophosphorylation) and exogenous peptides and proteins. Phosphorylation is believed to represent the "effect" of insulin receptor interaction. Phosphorylation sets a cascade of kinases in motion which phosphorylate further proteins, first insulin receptor substrate 1 (IRS-1), and eventually stimulate a great number of cellular events, the transport of glucose, amino acids, and ions; the metabolism of glucose, lipids, and proteins; and cell growth.

When insulin binds to insulin receptors, the ligand-saturated receptor migrates into "coated pits" which internalize insulin and the receptors rendering the insulin receptor intracellularly available. The internalized insulin receptor recycles to the cell membrane while insulin is metabolized. As is general for peptide receptors, antagonists are not easily available. Antagonists to insulin receptors are not known, and agonists occur only among closely related insulin analogues. Exceptions are antibodies to insulin receptors, which in certain cases exert weak agonist activity. For one peptide receptor in particular, the opiate receptor, many agonists and antagonists of various chemical classes exist.

The insulin receptor and the closely related receptor for insulin-like growth factor 1 (IGF-1) are classified as a subfamily of the large family of transmembrane tyrosine-specific protein kinases. Other subfamilies are represented by the receptors for epidermal growth factor (EGF), nerve growth factor (NFG), platelet derived growth factor (PDGF), macrophage colony stimulating factor (M-CSF), fibroblast growth factor (FGF) and vascular endothelial growth factor (VEGF). These receptors are allosteric enzymes which dimerize upon interaction with their respective ligands and phosphorylate each other on specific tyrosine residues. This crossphosphorylation is referred to as autophosphorylation because it occurs within the receptor dimer. Phosphorylated tyrosines and their adjacent amino acids serve as high affinity docking into other proteins which are activated themselves by phosphorylation on tyrosine and assemble into a transient intracellular phosphorylation network that transduces signals from the cell surface to the nucleus.

6.2.4 The steroid, retinoid and thyroid receptor superfamily

Three classes of steroid hormones have been described: the adrenal steroids (including cortisol and aldosterone), the sex steroids (progesterone, estrogens, and androgens), and vitamin D_3. Retinoids are vitamin A-derived hormones, the thyroid hormones are iodine-containing tyrosine derivatives. Retinoids and thyroid hormones are chemically quite distinct from steroid hormones, which have cholesterol as a common precursor.

The biological effects of these classes of hormones are mediated by intracellular receptors, soluble proteins of high binding affinity but low capacity with a K_D-range for their respective ligands in the nanomolar to picomolar range. Most of these binding proteins are localized in the cell nucleus even in the absence of ligand, with the exception of the glucocorticoid receptor which is also detected in the cytosol.

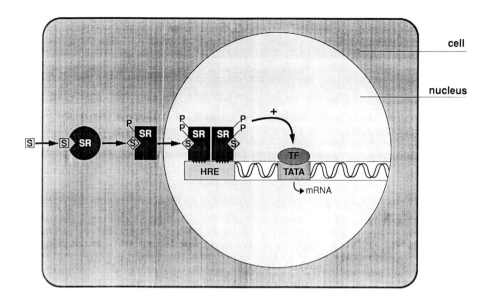

Figure 6.6   The nuclear Receptor Superfamily. (Adapted from Power, Conneely and O'Malley. *Trends Pharmacol. Sci.*, **13**, 318, 1992) (see text for details).

The expression and cloning of the human corticoid receptor (hGR) in the mid 1980's provided the first complete structure of a steroid receptor and revealed a segment with astonishing relatedness to the viral oncogene, erb A. Characterization of the erb A protooncogene product led to its startling identification as the thyroid hormone receptor. This was a critical advance in the establishment of a steroid and thyroid receptor gene superfamily.

The steroid hormone receptors (SHR), including the vitamin D_3 receptor, are encoded by single genes leading to six individual receptors, the retinoid receptors are encoded by six genes that fall into two subclasses, the classical retinoic acid receptors (RARs), α, β, γ, and the retinoid X receptors (RXRs), α, β, γ. Thyroid hormone receptors α and β are encoded by two genes.

The members of the superfamily of nuclear receptors act as ligand responsive transcription factors (LTFs): hormones diffuse from the extracellular milieu into the cell where they recognize their receptor and combine with the hormone binding region. Binding of the hormonal ligand results in a conformational change of the receptor protein which leads to dimerization. The activated receptor dimer binds with high affinity to a specific enhancer sequence (HRE = hormone responsive element) in the promoter of hormonally regulated genes. Ligand binding and DNA binding of the complex are accompanied by step by step phosphorylation of the receptor (see Fig. 6.6). Binding of the receptor dimer to the HRE causes recruitment of and interaction with other essential transcription factors to form a functional transcription initiation complex that is recognized by DNA polymerase II.

Specificity of the biological response to this class of hormones within a particular cell type is accomplished by a combination of several factors: the binding specificity of a ligand to its receptor, recognition of a specific HRE on the DNA by the ligand activated receptor protein, cooperation with other nuclear receptors on the promoter of a responsive gene, and interaction with other (cell specific) transcription factors (TFs).

Recently, it was detected that the activity of nuclear receptors may be modulated by other second messenger pathways which mediate signals of membrane bound receptors ('crosstalk' of signal transduction pathways). Phosphorylation of the nuclear receptor or of (adapter-) proteins involved in formation of the transcription initiation complex are discussed as possible mechanisms of receptor 'cross-talk'.

Receptor agonists and antagonists for all classical SHRs have been synthesized. Antagonists to this class of receptors bind to the hormone binding domain and either inhibit receptor dimerization or DNA binding.

The number of proteins exhibiting the domain structure of the nuclear receptor super-family far exceeds the steroid hormone, retinoid and thyroid receptor family. Proteins without known ligands, the so-called 'orphan' receptors are found within this gene family. About 50 'orphan receptors' have been identified in the nuclear receptor superfamily.

6.3 AGONISTS AND ANTAGONISTS

6.3.1 Agonists and partial agonists

Enzymologists distinguish between substrates (metabolites), which are converted by enzymes to products, and antimetabolites (blockers), which interact with the enzyme recognition site but are not converted (see Chapter 11). A similar differentiation exist in pharmacology between *agonists*, which are agents capable of activating the receptors and thereby eliciting effects (also called stimulus), and specific competitive *antagonists* or receptor blockers. The antagonists share with the agonists a certain, often higher, affinity for the receptor, but lack the capacity for receptor activation; they lack what is called "efficacy" (Stephenson) or "intrinsic activity" (Ariëns). Ariëns and Stephenson assigned values to intrinsic activity (α: between 0 for a competitive antagonist and 1 for a full agonist) and efficacy (e: between 0 and large positive values). Absolute values, however, cannot be determined, only values relative to reference agonists. While affinity values are easily determined by affinity binding experiments, efficacy measures, except for pure antagonists, are less easily achieved. Nevertheless, efficacy is of crucial importance in drug research.

An agonist with efficacy less than a full agonist is called a partial agonist (see Chapter 1). A partial agonist produces less effect than the maximal effect produced by a full agonist, even when it occupies and saturates all receptors. It follows that a partial agonist will always occupy more receptors than a full agonist when both elicit the same response. It is generally assumed that natural physiological agonists possess full efficacy, in principle, however, superagonists having efficacies higher than the classical full agonist may exist. For drug receptors, full agonists can in principle not be defined; history rather than theory determines that for example diazepam is considered a full agonist to benzodiazepine receptors.

The nature of partial agonism is not understood. Presumably, partial agonists produce less pronounced conformational shifts, when binding to the receptor, than full agonists, but still more than a competitive antagonist. It is important to realize that the degree of partial agonism, the apparent efficacy, is dependent on the assay procedure (or experimental model). Some assays need very low stimulus to yield a full response, and almost all agonists appear full agonists in such systems; other assays need strong stimulus — only very efficacious agonists show effect, while weak partial (low efficacy) agonists even may perform like pure competitive antagonists. Variable efficacy may, therefore, erroneously be assigned to each single agonist.

6.3.2 Inverse agonists and allosteric coupling

In a series of investigations of chemicals of various structure, which all had in common a high affinity for the recognition site of benzodiazepine receptors, it was discovered that certain groups of compounds did not elicit the classical sedative, anticonvulsant, and anxiolytic effects characteristic of benzodiazepines, but rather exactly the opposite: they produced activation, convulsions, and anxiety. This was the first example of a receptor function, which was capable of producing an effect in two opposite directions depending on the nature of the ligand binding to the recognition site. The benzodiazepine receptor is a drug receptor located on one or more of the 4 or 5 subunits which form the $GABA_A$ receptor coupled chloride ion channel normally located on the outer cell membrane of neurones.

In this complex, the benzodiazepine receptor is functionally similar to allosteric sites in enzymes, which are sites distinct from the catalytic site (which could be likened to the $GABA_A$ receptor recognition site). A compound that binds to the allosteric site in enzymes is named an effector. At constant enzyme and substrate concentrations, the binding of negative effectors reduces the reaction rate of enzymes (allosteric inhibition); the binding of positive effectors increases the reaction rate (allosteric activation). If the allosteric effector is the substrate molecule itself, the effector is said to be homotropic; if the effector is a molecule other than the substrate, the effector is said to be heterotropic. Thus, by analogy to enzyme biochemistry, benzodiazepines correspond to positive heterotropic effectors; they enhance GABA neurotransmission indirectly. Likewise, DMCM (**6.1**) and β-CCM, two convulsant benzodiazepine receptor ligands, would correspond to negative heterotropic effectors. The pharmacological term for a positive effector is an agonist (agonist = drug that produces a response). However, also the agents with negative efficacy (negative effectors) produce responses and are therefore agonists. The term inverse agonist is used to signify that the response is opposite to that of already known agonists. Partial agonists and partial inverse agonists are all part of this scheme. Receptor antagonists inhibit responses both to partial and full agonists and to inverse agonists by occupying the receptor recognition sites thereby precluding access of the agonists.

Figure 6.7 illustrates the effect of an agonist, partial agonist, antagonist, partial inverse agonist, and inverse agonist at the benzodiazepine receptor as measured in a biochemical assay on the allosterically coupled TBPS binding site, a binding site for a certain class of cage convulsants, which is also located on the $GABA_A$/benzodiazepine receptor chloride channel complex. There are allosteric sites on many receptor complexes including nicotinic receptors, NMDA receptors (see Chapter 9), calcium channels (see Chapter 8), serotonin uptake carriers, G-proteins, and others. Allosteric receptor complexes offer numerous targets for drug research.

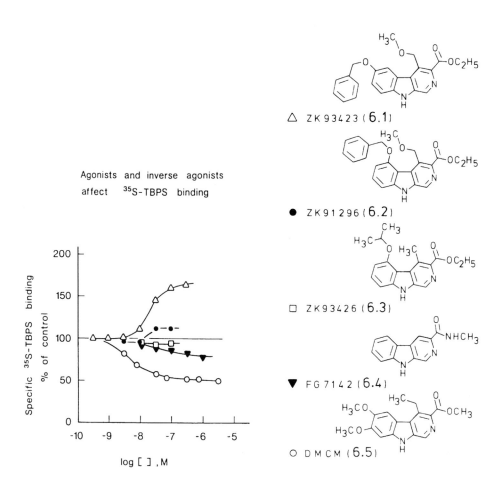

Figure 6.7   Agonists and inverse agonists affect allosterically coupled receptors. TBPS, tert.butylbicyclo-phosphorothionat binds to the chloride gating domain of the GABA$_A$/Benzodiazepine receptor chloride channel. Benzodiazepine receptor ligands with positive (ZK 93423, ZK 91296) and negative (FG 7142 and DMCM) efficacy enhance and reduce, respectively ^{35}S-TBPS binding *in vitro*. EC$_{50}$ values for benzodiazepine receptor binding are $(3 \times 10^{-9} - 10^{-7}$ M). ZK 93426 is a benzodiazepine receptor antagonist. (From Braestrup & Nielsen p. 180 in Benzodiazepine/GABA Receptors and Chloride Channels: Structural and Functional Properties, Eds. Olsen and Venter 1986, Alan B. Liss, Inc.).

6.4 RECEPTOR MODEL SYSTEMS

6.4.1 Organ bath techniques

A variety of techniques are available for monitoring chemicals interacting with receptors. Organ bath techniques are useful for determining ligand receptor interactions coupled with effects.

The classical preparation, guinea pig ileum, is versatile, one single set-up can be applied to a number of receptors. The preparation consists of strips of guinea pig ileum stretched in an organ bath and connected to a pressure transducer; receptor antagonists are investigated in relation to appropriate agonists, and agonists are investigated in the presence of appropriate antagonists to block the function of non-relevant receptors. The guinea pig ileum is a powerful tool in studying the receptor function.

6.4.2 High affinity binding

High affinity receptor binding techniques are particularly useful in the initial phases of medicinal chemistry structure-activity studies. At this stage, information about efficacy is often of less importance than information about receptor affinity and selectivity (see however Section 6.4.3). Screening for lead compounds and for optimizing structure/activity is efficiently and reliably performed by means of radioligand binding techniques once the specific target is selected.

6.4.2.1 Procedures for high affinity binding

Most receptors are membrane bound; they are anchored in the lipophilic cell membrane by lipophilic sequences in their primary protein structure (see for example Figure 6.3). The tissue used for binding experiments usually is a crude membrane preparation from an appropriate organ, which is an organ with high concentrations of the receptor. Selectivity in the receptor binding assay is not based on the purity of the receptor preparation, which may be highly contaminated by other receptors, but rather on the selectivity of the radioligand used to tag the receptor. An alternative is the expression of well defined receptor classes and types by recombinant techniques in immortal cell lines; in this approach receptor selectivity is achieved by the preferential expression of the specific gene for a particular receptor (see Section 6.4.3). This approach is useful for studying receptor subtypes. Radioligands with high specific activity (necessary for measurement of receptors with affinities in the nanomolar range) and with high selectivity for particular receptors and receptor subtypes are easily available from commercial sources. Tritium is favoured for small organic radioligands due to the ease of radiosynthesis, high specific activity ($\approx$25–100 Ci/mmol) and lack of effect on binding properties. Iodine is preferred for peptide ligands due to the ease of introducing iodine into phenol rings. ^{125}I (2,000 Ci/mmol) reaches even higher specific activity than tritium, but due to the size it may change ligand properties. The binding reaction between radioligand and receptor is performed in buffers at 0–37°C, and the amount of binding (total) to membranes and membrane bound receptors is usually determined by filtrating the membrane suspension through glass fiber filters under reduced pressure. Glass fiber filters function as adsorbants rather than filters — breakthroughs occur at high tissue load. Total binding is binding to receptors plus binding elsewhere such as adsorption to lipids etc. Binding to receptors and to other saturable sites is usually referred to as 'specific' or 'displaceable'; non-specific binding is binding that cannot be displaced by a large surplus of unlabelled ligands for the particular receptor under study. Specific binding is total binding less non-specific binding.

Binding experiments can be used to determine the number of receptors in a given preparation, $B_{\max}$, the affinity of the radioligand for the receptor, the K_D-value, and the affinity of any other unlabelled substances for the receptor, expressed as the K_I-value for that substance.

The following reaction takes place in the assay

$$L + R \underset{k_{-1}}{\overset{k_1}{\rightleftharpoons}} LR \tag{6.1}$$

where L is radioligand, R is the receptor, LR is ligand bound receptor (also called B for bound ligand), k_1 is the association rate constant, the second order rate constant for the binding (association) reaction, and k_{-1} is the dissociation rate constant for the first order dissociation reaction.

At equilibrium this reaction follows the classical law of mass action for enzyme substrate interaction. If we define F = free ligand L, B_{max} = total number of receptor binding sites $(R + RL)$, and $K_D = k_{-1}/k_1$ then

$$B = \frac{B_{max} F}{F + K_D} \tag{6.2}$$

which transforms to

$$B/F = \frac{-1}{K_D} B + \frac{B_{max}}{K_D} \tag{6.3}$$

which is the Scatchard equation. Thus, knowledge of the concentration of ligand, bound and free, at equilibrium and at various concentrations of ligand allows the determination of both the equilibrium binding constant (K_D) and the maximum number of binding sites (B_{max}). In Scatchard plots, corresponding values for B/F on the ordinate are plotted against the concentration of B on the abscissa; the slope of the resulting linear plot equals $\alpha = -1/K_D$ while the intercept on the abscissa equals B_{max}.

Note the similarity between equation (6.2) and the Michaelis Menten equation; the Michaelis Menten constant, K_m, corresponds to K_D which is also the concentration of radioligand which occupies 50% of the available receptors. Equation (6.3) can be transformed to linear plots in several ways. Lineweaver-Burk plots can be applied (see Chapter 11), but Scatchard plots are preferred due to their greater sensitivity; even small deviations from simple mass action, such as for example multiple sites or cooperativity, or small changes in K_D or B_{max}, are detectable.

6.4.2.2 Competition

Determination of B_{max} and K_D values for ligand-receptor interaction is used to characterize the assays with reference to the literature, if available. Competition experiments are performed to characterize new compounds. Addition of a new compound (I for inhibitor) to binding assays results in the following two reactions.

$$L + R \rightleftharpoons LR$$

$$I + R \rightleftharpoons IR$$

$$L + I + R \overset{K_D, K_I}{\rightleftharpoons} LR + IR \tag{6.4}$$

Where L is the radioligand, R is the receptor, K_D is the affinity constant for the radioligand, K_I is the affinity constant for the inhibitor. With negligible concentrations of I, equation (6.4) becomes equal to equation (6.1); with a large surplus of I, all of the receptors are occupied by I and the amount of LR approaches zero. The IC$_{50}$ concentration of I is that particular concentration which inhibits by 50% the specific radioligand binding. The IC$_{50}$ value is dependent on the nature of the inhibitor, the properties of the receptor, and the concentration of the radioligand. The affinity constant for I, K_I, however, is a constant for I in relation to the receptor and can be determined by the Cheng Prusov equation

$$K_I = \text{IC}_{50}/(1 + [L]/K_D) \tag{6.5}$$

where $[L]$ is the free concentration of radioligand, and K_D is the dissociation constant for the radioligand.

6.4.2.3 Schild analysis

Receptor binding studies fundamentally yield measures of drug affinity and receptor selectivity. Efficacy, however, a measure of the drug's ability to cause conformational shifts in the receptor complex and thereby effects, is available in many transactivation assays (see Section 6.4.3) and for affinity binding studies in certain restricted cases of coupled allosteric receptors. For allosteric receptors, binding of an agonist to one receptor site causes conformational shifts in a second allosterically coupled site which may either increase or decrease the affinity of the second site for its radioligand.

Let $R_A - R_B$ be allosterically coupled receptors for A and B, respectively,

$$
\begin{array}{ccc}
R_A - R_B + A & \rightleftharpoons & AR_A - R_B^* \\
+ & & + \\
B & & B \\
\updownarrow K_B & & \updownarrow K_B^* \\
R_A - R_B B & & AR_A - R_B^* B
\end{array}
\tag{6.6}
$$

occupation of R_A by A changes the affinity of R_B for B. K_B and K_B^* are the dissociation constants for R_B and R_B^*, respectively; $K_B \neq K_B^*$. The EC$_{50}$ value for the agonist A, the concentration causing half maximal effect, is easily determined from dose response curves (see Fig. 6.8). Addition of antagonists to the assay displaces dose response curves of the agonist to the right. The affinity of antagonists can be deduced from this kind of experiments by Schild analyses. Schild analyses also apply to the determination of antagonist affinity in transactivation assays.

A Schild analysis of pitrazepine (a GABA$_A$ antagonist) acting on an allosterically coupled GABA$_A$ receptor is shown in Figure 6.8. Let muscimol, a GABA$_A$ agonist (see Chapter 10), act on R_A and let ^{35}S-TBPS bind to the allosterically coupled chloride channel R_B. Occupation of the GABA$_A$ receptor by muscimol will reduce the affinity of R_B for ^{35}S-TBPS. Muscimol causes half of its maximal inhibition of ^{35}S-TBPS binding at 1.6 μM (Fig. 6.8), however, the affinity constant of muscimol for the GABA receptor does not exactly equal 1.6 μM nor can the agonist affinity be determined from experiments of this

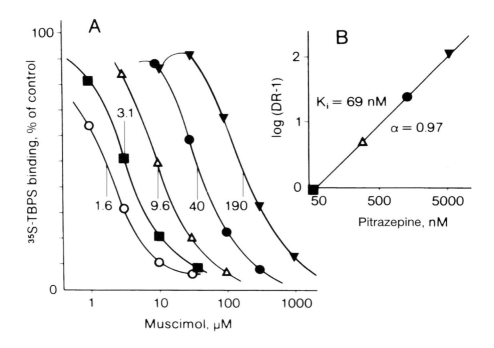

Figure 6.8 Schild Analysis. Inhibition of ^{35}S-TBPS binding by the GABA$_A$ agonist muscimol and antagonism by pitrazepine. Dose-response curves for muscimol were made in duplicate in the presence of various concentrations of pitrazepine (○, 0 nM; ■, 63 nM; △, 320 nM; ●, 1600 nM; ▼, 6400 nM). See text for further information. (From Braestrup & Nielsen, *Eur. J. Pharmacol.*, **118**, 115, 1985).

kind because occupation does not necessarily equal response. It is unknown whether 10 or 90% GABA$_A$ receptors need be occupied to give 50% response on ^{35}S-TBPS binding. While agonist affinity cannot be determined from such experiments, affinities of antagonists can be accurately determined by Schild analyses. In these experiments, dose response curves for agonists are determined in the presence of various predetermined concentrations of the antagonist. Competitive antagonists will cause a rightward parallel shift in the agonist dose response curves. When both agonist and antagonist interact competitively with R_A, the inhibition will follow the following equation

$$\log(DR - 1) = -\log[I] + \log K_I \qquad (6.7)$$

DR is called the dose ratio, which is the concentration of agonist giving a particular response in the presence of inhibitor divided by the concentration of agonist that gives the same response in the absence of inhibitor, a dose ratio of 10, for example, corresponds to a ten-fold rightward shift in the dose response curve for agonist in the presence of antagonist; [*I*] is the concentration of inhibitor, K_I is the affinity constant for the inhibitor.

Affinity constants for inhibitors are determined by the intercept on the abscissa, the slope of the inhibition curves equals 1 in the case of competitive inhibition. A slope less than 1 occurs for non-competitive inhibition. Figure 6.8 shows that pitrazepine is an apparently competitive inhibitor of $GABA_A$ receptors and that the K_I value is 69 nM.

Schild analyses are very powerful tools for allosterically coupled receptors, for receptors coupled to second messengers such as adenylate cyclase enzymes, and for recombinant cell lines (transactivation assays).

6.4.3 Recombinant cell lines

Recombinant DNA techniques have substantially enlarged the ability to characterize receptors and to develop discovery projects based on mechanism of action. Recombinant baculovirus infected insect cells, for example, are used for high level expression of functionally active receptor molecules, because this expression system utilizes most of the protein modification and processing steps present in higher eucaryotic cells. Besides the provision of recombinant receptors for binding studies, recombinant DNA technology can also provide screening organisms with inherent receptor subtype specificity. Genetically engineered yeast cells and recombinant animal cell lines are increasingly used to design *in vitro* models and screening tools. Molecular pharmacology is an integral part of pharmaceutical research and drug discovery.

In general, recombinant DNA molecules (receptor gene plus appropriate promoters) are constructed and transfected (introduced) into the appropriate cellular background in order to (over-)express the desired receptor or even a set of target-molecules, which are needed to restore a whole signalling cascade associated with a given (patho-)physiological process.

Studies concerning steroid hormones provide some of the best characterized examples for the latter approach. Both, transiently and stably transfected recombinant cell line models are used as tools for the evaluation of steroid hormone action. Steroid hormone receptors (see Section 6.2.4) belong to a superfamily of ligand dependent transcription factors and exert their regulatory activity through binding to hormone responsive elements (HRE's) found in the regulatory region (promoter) of certain genes. Receptor activation occurs upon hormone binding and the dimerized receptors bind to the HRE's with high selectivity to activate gene transcription.

Functional analysis of steroid hormone action *in vitro* requires the availability of the appropriate hormone receptor and an easily detectable reporter gene product, which is finally synthesized following transactivation, i.e. binding of the hormone loaded receptor to a hormone responsive promoter in front of the reporter gene (i.e. CAT: chloramphenicol acetyl transferase or firefly luciferase, see Figure 6.9). The results of this *in vitro* experiment can be used to characterize the efficacy of a compound and the affinity of antagonists.

6.4.4 Other receptor models

The number of available models for monitoring receptors far exceeds the scope of this chapter. In principle, any measurable effect of a receptor interaction is applicable for medicinal chemistry. The measures range from social behaviour in animals to spin changes in receptor molecules upon binding, as measured by NMR. Electrophysiological changes in single neurones or single ion channels are popular and useful techniques using either 'natural' cells or recombinant cells. Electrophysiological techniques are becoming

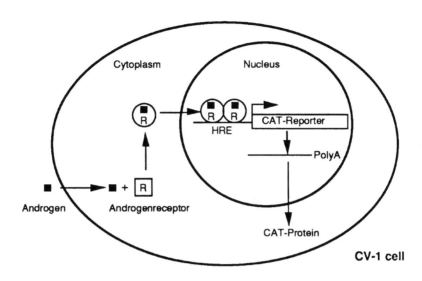

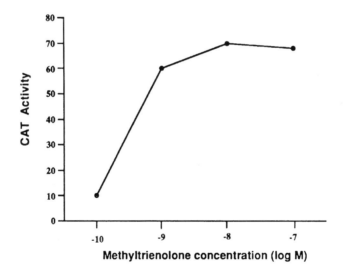

Figure 6.9   Genetically engineered cells to measure androgen activity. *Top*, the gene for the human androgen receptor was introduced into CV-1 kidney cells by lipofection. The androgen receptor responsive element was inserted in front of the chloramphenicol acetyl transferase (CAT) gene and likewise introduced. Addition of androgenic compounds, such as methyltrienolone, leads to stimulation of the hormone responsive element (HRE) and transcription of the CAT gene. The CAT enzyme produced is measured in lysates. *Bottom*, example of dose response curve. Reportergenes other than CAT, such as luciferase, urokinase are applicable.

increasingly powerful in combination with the expression of particular receptors in frog oocytes or other cells by microinjection or transfection of mRNA. Oocytes are easily accessible to intracellular recordings, due to their large size.

6.5 MULTIPLE RECEPTORS

The concept of multiple receptors emerged mainly from the adrenergic receptors as stimulated by symphathomimetics. In 1948, Ahlquist compared the relative potencies on different tissues of a number of sympathomimetics including noradrenaline, adrenaline and isoprenaline. He found that the order of potency on those smooth muscles that respond with contraction was, adrenaline > noradrenaline > isoprenaline, whereas on those smooth muscles that responded with relaxation the order of potency was isoprenaline > adrenaline > noradrenaline. The order of potency for stimulation of the heart was similar to that for relaxation of smooth muscle. In order to explain these findings, he postulated that there are two types of receptors which he designated α-receptors and β-receptors. Effector cells with α-receptors (or α-adrenoreceptors) have a high sensitivity to adrenaline and noradrenaline but are practically insensitive to isoprenaline, whereas those with β-receptors have a higher sensitivity to isoprenaline than other catecholamines and are usually more sensitive to adrenaline than to noradrenaline. Further subclassification followed (α_1, α_2, β_1, β_2, etc.). Ahlquist's approach to receptor subclassification based on differential pharmacological responses is widely used. Later, in the 1970's high affinity ligand binding methods proved useful for receptor subclassification (for example high- and low-affinity $GABA_A$ receptors, benzodiazepine receptors type I and type II etc.). Receptor subclassification again gained momentum by the advent of recombinant DNA techniques by the discovery of multiple distinct but highly homologous genes which coded for the same receptor types. Early examples are genes coding for 5 muscarinic subtypes ($m_1 - m_5$) (see Chapter 10), nicotinic receptors, and $GABA_A$ receptors. The number of subtypes for nicotinic and $GABA_A$ receptors are expanded by their assembling of 4–5 subunits which of course increase the diversity and obscure the significance. Genetically defined receptors are easily expressed with high purity in stable cell lines, and this gives a new multitude of potential targets for structure activity studies and drug research (see Section 6.4.3).

Receptor classification by recombinant techniques does not always follow classification following pharmacological criteria. For example, within the serotonin receptor family, it seems that $5\text{-}HT_1$, $5\text{-}HT_2$ receptors and their subclasses belong to the G-protein receptor superfamily while $5\text{-}HT_3$ receptors belong to the ligand gated ion channel superfamily.

FURTHER READING

Andersen, P.H., Gingrich, J.A., Bates, M.D., Dearry, A., Falardeau, P., Senogles, S.E. and Caron, M. (1990) Dopamine receptor subtypes: beyond the D_1/D_2 classification. *Trends Pharmacol. Sci.*, **11**, 231–236.
Ariëns, E.J., Beld, A.J., Rodrigues de Miranda, J.F. and Simonis, A.M. (1979) The Pharmacon-Receptor-Effector Concept. A basis for understanding the transmission of information in biological systems. In *The Receptors. A Comprehensive Treatise*, edited by R.D. O'Brien, pp. 33–91, New York and London, Plenum Press.
Braestrup, C. and Nielsen, M. (1986) Benzodiazepine receptor binding *in vivo* and efficacy. In *Benzodiazepine/GABA Receptors and Chloride Channels: Structural and Functional Properties*, edited by R.W. Olsen and J.C. Venter, pp. 167–184, New York: Alan R. Liss, Inc.

Changeux, J.-P. Devillers-Thiéry, A. and Chemouilli, P. (1984) Acetylcholine receptor: an allosteric protein. *Science*, **225**, 1335–1345.

Hubbard, S., Wei, L., Ellis, L. and Hendrickson, W. (1994) Crystal structure of the tyrosine kinase domain of the insulin receptor. *Nature*, **372**, 746–754.

Lefkowitz, R.J. and Caron, M.G. (1988) Adrenergic receptors. Models for the study of receptors coupled to guanine nucleotide regulatory proteins. *J. Biol. Chem.*, **263**, 4993–4996.

Rosenkilde, M., Cahir, M., Gether, U., Hiorth, U. and Schwartz, T. (1994) Mutations along transmembrane segment II of the NK-1 receptor affect substance P competition with non-peptide antagonists but not substance P binding. *J. Biol. Chem.*, **269**, 28160–28164.

Schofield, P.R., Darlison, M.G., Fujita, N., Burt, D.R., Stephenson, F.A., Rodriguez, H., Rhee, L.M., Ramachandran, J., Reale, V., Glencorse, T.A., Seeburg, P.H. and Barnard, E.A. (1987) Sequence and functional expression of the GABA$_A$ receptor shows a ligand-gated receptor superfamily. *Nature*, **328**, 221–227.

Tsai, M.-J. and O'Malley, B.W. (1994) Molecular mechanisms of action of steroid/thyroid receptor superfamily members. *Annual Rev. Biochem.*, **63**, 451–486.

7. RADIOTRACERS: SYNTHESIS AND USE IN IMAGING

CHRISTER HALLDIN and THOMAS HÖGBERG

CONTENTS

7.1 INTRODUCTION

Molecules labelled with radioactive isotopes (radionuclides) have been used extensively to study transformations and distributions of endogenous compounds and pharmaceuticals, since it allows for detection of very low levels of materials. Thus, it is a useful technique to track transformed compounds with a common origin without the need for development of specific analytical methods for each of the constituents. Recently, this field has entered a new area with the development of techniques to measure and display radioactivity in three dimensions by computerised tomography.

The chapter illustrates the synthesis of radioactive compounds. It is divided in sections depending upon the half-life of the radionuclides used, since this will have a profound influence on the synthetic strategy. It is not a comprehensive treatment, but it will give the reader some insight into this special discipline of organic chemistry. The second part of the chapter illustrates the use of different types of imaging.

Compounds radiolabelled with long-lived radionuclides such as ^{14}C, ^{3}H and ^{125}I are commonly used in *in vitro* imaging autoradiographic studies. Several imaging techniques are available for the *in vivo* visualization of morphology or biochemical processes in the human body, i.e. X-ray CT (Computed Tomography), MRI (Magnetic Resonance Imaging), SPECT (Single Photon Emission Computed Tomography) and PET (Positron Emission Tomography). X-ray CT provides anatomical information based on the differential absorption of X-rays by tissue. MRI uses magnetic and radiofrequency fields to afford anatomical information based on the proton relaxation properties and proton density of tissue. SPECT is used to visualize and measure the relative concentration of radioactivity in tissue after injection of compounds labelled with a relatively short-lived single photon emitting radionuclide such as ^{123}I. PET has been widely used to visualize and quantify different biochemical processes such as metabolic processes and receptor densities. The PET technique utilizes radiotracers labelled with relatively short-lived positron emitting radionuclides such as ^{18}F or ^{76}Br or ultrashort-lived radionuclides such as ^{11}C, ^{13}N and ^{15}O. With this technique, minute amounts of radiotracers can be used due to the very high specific radioactivity obtainable by the short-lived radionuclides.

Biochemical changes can be determined by PET and SPECT in order to monitor pathological conditions in living humans even before any anatomical defects occur. This has a great diagnostic value and gives new information about disease states and their potential therapeutic treatments. Radiolabelling of endogenous compounds such as glucose, amino acids and acetate have been used in studies on metabolism and synthesis of various human tissues such as tumor, cardiac and brain tissue. Receptor selective radioligands which display a high affinity for the receptor and a minimal metabolic degradation are used to probe receptor status. Imaging of CNS receptors in the human brain is a rapidly expanding area which previously was restricted to postmortem binding studies. While both PET and SPECT can detect radiotracer distribution the SPECT technique is more readily available than PET. PET requires a cyclotron to generate the radionuclides in close connection to the radiochemistry laboratory and the PET camera. However, the PET technique offers several advantages such as the ability to measure the concentration of the tracer quantitatively, a greater sensitivity, a higher resolution and chemically more diverse radiotracers.

7.2 NUCLEAR CHEMISTRY

An array of precursors and compounds labelled with the long-lived radionuclides ^{14}C, ^{3}H and ^{125}I are commercially available. These radiolabelled compounds have been used for a long time in biochemical and pharmaceutical research, e.g. metabolic, receptor binding

Table 7.1 Preparation and some physical properties of commonly used radionuclides.

Nuclide	Half-life	Reaction[a]	Mode of decay	Maximum specific radioactivity (Ci/mmol)
^{11}C	20 min	$^{14}N(p,\alpha)^{11}C$	β^+ (100%)	9.2×10^6
^{15}O	2 min	$^{14}N(d,n)^{15}O$	β^+ (100%)	9.1×10^7
^{13}N	10 min	$^{16}O(p,\alpha)^{13}N$	β^+ (100%)	1.9×10^7
^{18}F	110 min	$^{18}O(p,n)^{18}F$	β^+ (97%)	1.7×10^6
^{76}Br	16 hr	$^{75}As(d,n)^{76}Br$	β^+ (57%)	1.9×10^5
^{123}I	13 hr	$^{121}Sb(\alpha,2n)^{123}I$	E.C. (100%)	2.4×10^5
^{125}I	60 days	$^{124}Xe(n,\gamma)^{125}I$	E.C. (100%)	2.2×10^3
^{3}H	12 years	$^{6}Li(n,\alpha)^{3}H$	β^- (100%)	29
^{14}C	5730 years	$^{14}N(n,p)^{14}C$	β^- (100%)	6.2×10^{-2}

[a]The nuclear reactions indicate the target isotope and the bombarding particle, e.g. $^{14}N(d,n)^{15}O$: nitrogen-14 produce, upon bombardment with one deuteron, oxygen-15 and eject a neutron. d = deuteron; n = neutron; p = proton; α = alpha particle.

and autoradiographic studies. SPECT uses γ-emitting radionuclides such as ^{123}I, ^{99m}Tc, ^{67}Ga and ^{111}In. The former radionuclide is commercially available and can be produced by the $^{121}Sb(\alpha,2n)^{123}I$ reaction (Table 7.1), i.e. by bombardment of α-particles on a target containing the stable isotope ^{121}Sb to produce the radionuclide ^{123}I and two neutrons. Iodine-123 has a half-life of 13 hours and can easily be incorporated with a sufficient level of radioactivity into several types of organic molecules such as receptor radioligands. The transportation of ^{123}I from the cyclotron to the laboratory/hospital should be rapid and the experimental logistics effective. Compounds labelled with the short-lived PET radionuclides ^{18}F and ^{76}Br (half-lives 110 min and 16 hours) and the ultrashort-lived ^{11}C, ^{13}N and ^{15}O (half-lives 20, 10 and 2 minutes) are not commercially available and must be prepared in the vicinity of a cyclotron, even if ^{76}Br potentially should be able to handle in a similar fashion as ^{123}I.

In a PET facility, the cyclotron, the radiochemistry laboratory and the PET camera constitute the three main operative units. Today, most centers employing PET are using low or medium energy sized cyclotrons to produce one or more of the positron-emitting radionuclides: ^{11}C, ^{13}N, ^{15}O and ^{18}F. The ultrashort half-lives of ^{11}C, ^{13}N and ^{15}O, implies that they must be produced immediately prior to use by an adjacent cyclotron. They are formed by means of nuclear reactions that occur on bombardment of target mediums with charged particles (Table 7.1). The production of $^{11}CO_2$ is demonstrated in Figure 7.1 as an example of this special type of chemistry. The irradiated materials can be either in a solid, liquid or gaseous state. Radiochemical yields are dependent on factors including target shape, design of target foil and efficiency of target cooling. The amount of radioactivity that can be obtained is regulated by the energy of the accelerated particles and the beam current imposed on target.

Labelling of a compound without affecting its biochemical properties is possible by exchange of stable atoms present in the parent molecule. For instance, carbon-12 (^{12}C) or oxygen-16 (^{16}O) is replaced with the corresponding positron emitting radionuclides ^{11}C or ^{15}O. The small kinetic isotope effect that may occur is considered negligible for most

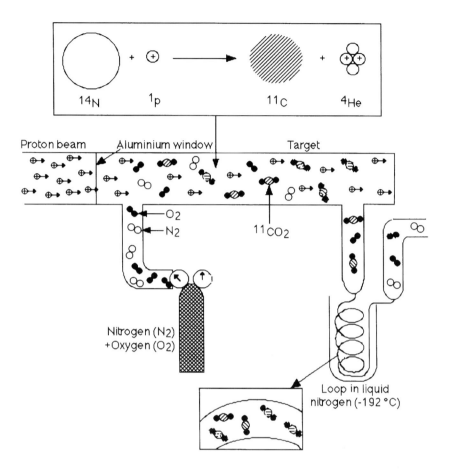

Figure 7.1   The production of ^{11}C via the nuclear reaction $^{14}N(p,\alpha)^{11}C$. ^{11}C is produced by proton bombardment of N_2 which is reacting with trace amounts of O_2 to give $^{11}CO_2$. The prepared $^{11}CO_2$ is trapped in a loop cooled with liquid nitrogen until further use.

applications. The ultrashort half-lives of especially ^{11}C or ^{15}O make them advantageous for sequential investigations with short time intervals in the same individual (animal or human), thereby allowing the subject to be its own control. The use of radionuclides with relatively longer half-lives such as ^{18}F or ^{76}Br provides an opportunity to follow the radioactivity from the radiolabelled compound for a longer period of time, but leads to use of analogues rather than of natural compounds.

The specific radioactivity is defined as the ratio of radioactivity per mole of the labelled compound with a maximum specific radioactivity inversely related to the physical half-lives of the radionuclide. The maximum theoretically possible specific radioactivity for ^{11}C is 10^7 Ci/mmol (Table 7.1), but due to the difficulties of completely eliminating external sources of ^{12}C this high specific radioactivity is never obtained. A specific radioactivity higher than 500 Ci/mmol (18.5 GBq/μmol), is sufficient for most of the radioligands in use in PET investigations of receptors.

7.3 LONG-LIVED RADIONUCLIDES

Access to ^{14}C-, ^{3}H- or ^{125}I-labelled precursors or common compounds for biological work can in most cases be obtained from commercial sources. This is especially the case for ^{14}C- and ^{3}H-labelled materials with the longest half-life. The simpler the structure the lower the price, i.e. in many situations it is preferable to make the target structure via a lengthy sequence from very simple compounds. For example, [^{14}C]CH$_3$I, [^{14}C]BaCO$_3$, [^{14}C]KCN, [^{3}H]H$_2$ and [^{3}H]CH$_3$I are commonly used sources for the introduction of these long-lived radionuclides. Some representative examples of the synthesis of labelled compounds will be given to show what the effect of considerations such as price, availability and half-life will have on the synthetic strategy.

7.3.1 ^{14}C-labelled compounds

Studies of metabolism and disposition of drugs in animals are preferably made with ^{14}C-labelled derivatives in order to avoid exchange of labile tritium for hydrogens *in vivo* (cf. Section 7.3.2), which is a common problem with tritium-labelling, and to give more easily identified metabolites. However, synthetic limitations or the low obtainable specific radioactivity may necessitate other labelling protocols especially with tritium as discussed in 7.3.2. Depending upon the structure, the radiolabel should be introduced in the part of the structure that will provide most of the expected metabolites in radioactive form. One should for example avoid synthetically attractive choices like methylation of a heteroatom (e.g. N-^{14}CH$_3$), which is likely to be lost via P450 mediated α-oxidation to form radioactive formaldehyde instead of the radioactive desmethyl metabolite needed for the identification work.

NNC 756 (**7.8**) is a potent dopamine D$_1$ receptor ligand, which was needed in radiolabelled form for studies on the distribution and metabolic fate. The obvious way to label the nitrogen with ^{14}CH$_3$ was not used for reasons outlined above. Instead, the label was introduced in the ring via a six step sequence shown in Scheme 7.1. The radioactive precursor (**7.1**) was made with tetrafluoroborate as counteranion and reacted with 7-benzofurancarbaldehyde to produce the epoxide (**7.2**), which was reacted with N-methyl-3-chloro-4-methoxyphenethylamine. Opening of the epoxide produced two compounds (**7.3**) and (**7.4**) in a ratio of 9:1, with the desired isomer (**7.3**) in excess. Separation by reversed-phase chromatography and acid catalysed ring closure with sulphuric acid in trifluoroacetic acid of (**7.3**) gave (**7.5**), which was resolved as dibenzoyl-D-tartrate (DBDT) salt to yield (**7.6**). Demethylation with boron tribromide gave optically pure (**7.7**). Finally, the hydrogenation over Rh/C gave [^{14}C]NNC 756 ([^{14}C]**7.8**) with a specific radioactivity of 24 mCi/mmol and an enantiomeric purity of >97%.

7.3.2 ^{3}H-labelled compounds

Tritium is the most commonly used radionuclide for radiolabelling in biology and medicine. Often the introduction of tritium is made at a late stage in the sequence via exchange or synthetic techniques, which are associated with certain limitations:

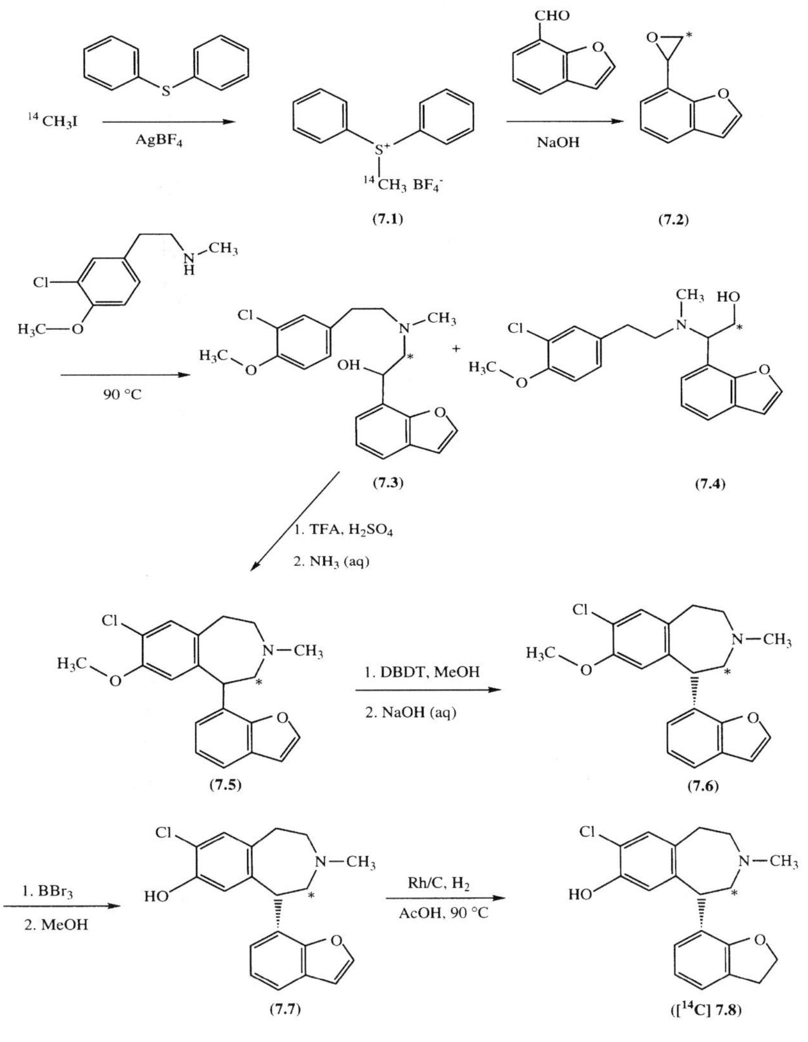

Scheme 7.1

(i)   exchange reactions with tritiated water or acetic acid (CH$_3$COOT) under acid, base or metal-catalysed conditions often produce compounds with a low specific radioactivity

(ii)   hydrogenation reactions are restricted by the availability of multiple C–C bond precursors and the required chemoselectivity in the reactions (e.g. interference from reactions with other multiple bonds and halogens)

(iii) hydrogenolysis of aryl-halogen derivatives (especially Ar-I and Ar-Br) has similar selectivity problems as hydrogenation

(iv)   methylation reactions require a desmethyl precursor and an applicable structure

(v)   hydride reductions are limited by the availability and quality of commercial hydride reagents, i.e. [^{3}H]NaBH$_3$ has often a lower specific activity than theoretically possible.

Since the frequent loss of tritium as tritated water renders the data more difficult to interpret, non-specific equilibration and exchange of labile hydrogens for tritium is less suitable when the tracer will be used for *in vivo* work. Besides, the degree of labelling with tritium in the different positions is usually not known, which can be of importance in studies where metabolic transformations may occur (cf. Section 7.3.1). The development of transition metal catalysed exchange reactions with tritium gas in which heteroatoms (oxygen and nitrogen) in the target structure can coordinate to the metal and promote insertion of tritium in a C–H bond offers a possibility to introduce tritium in positions that are not equally prone to uncatalysed loss of tritium.

Reduction of olefins will lead to a well defined regiochemistry even if the stereochemistry could be characterised to a lesser degree. The choice of catalyst will have a large effect on the obtained specific radioactivity, since hydrogen adsorbed on many catalysts will equilibrate with tritium if the reaction is too slow. Alternatively, hydrogenolysis of halogen derivatives can be applied to ascertain a well defined labelling. Many studies of receptor binding, especially at low affinity binding sites, require high degree of specific radioactivity which translates into two tritium atoms per molecule.

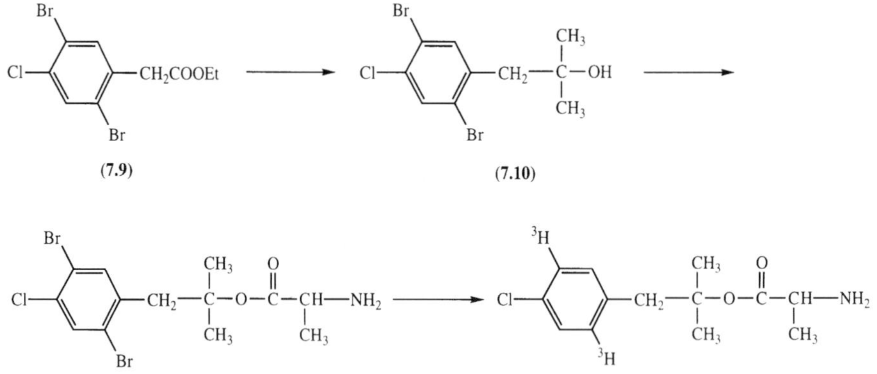

Scheme 7.2

Alaproclate (**7.12**) was developed as a selective synaptic serotonin uptake inhibitor. It also possessed affinity for other unknown receptor sites which prompted the preparation of a derivative with two tritium atoms in positions resistant to metabolic attack (Scheme 7.2). The 2,5-dibromo-4-chlorophenylacetate ester (**7.9**), prepared from 4-chlorotoluene, was subjected to a Grignard reaction with methyl magnesium iodide to give (**7.10**). The alanine ester (**7.11**) was obtained by acylation of (**7.10**) with 2-bromopropionyl bromide followed by amination. After optimisation of the conditions, the two bromine atoms could selectively be hydrogenolyzed with tritium gas over Pd/C as catalyst in DMF and one equivalent triethylamine. The positions of the tritium atoms in ([^{3}H]**7.12**) can be established by ^{3}H-NMR, which shows *ortho* and *meta* ^{1}H–^{3}H couplings in a fully coupled spectrum and the expected *para* substitution of the tritium atoms as two uncoupled peaks of equal intensity in a proton decoupled spectrum.

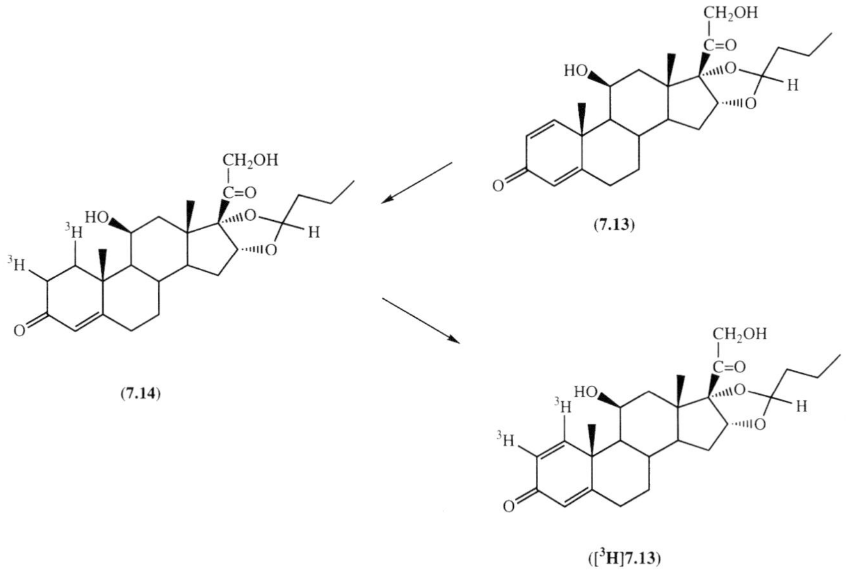

Scheme 7.3

The glucocorticosteroid budesonide (**7.13**) is used in the treatment of asthma, rhinitis and inflammatory bowel diseases. It has been made in tritiated form by an efficient reductive and oxidative sequence (Scheme 7.3). Thus hydrogenation with tritium gas of budesonide gives the corresponding 1,2-ditritio derivative (**7.14**). The following oxidation provides [^{3}H]budesonide containing different levels of tritium in the 1- and 2-positions. In the case of (**7.14**), the hydrogens in the α-position are labile due to the possibility of enolisation, which will lead to loss of tritium, in contrast to ([^{3}H]**7.13**) which is not subject to a facile tritium-hydrogen exchange.

7.3.3 ^{125}I-labelled compounds

In order to obtain higher specific radioactivity, than is possible with ^{3}H, the radionuclide ^{125}I can be used in applicable cases, which is especially advantageous for autoradiographic studies. The gamma emitting radionuclide ^{125}I has a half-life of 60 days which enables work during a reasonable time span. Tritium ligands can be made with a specific radioactivity up to 29 Ci/mmol per tritium, compared to 2200 Ci/mmol for ^{125}I-labelled ligands. One reason for the high specific radioactivity of ^{125}I is that the preparation is carrier-free with no dilution of stable iodine. For the development of ^{123}I-labelled radioligands for SPECT (see Sections 7.4.1 and 7.6.2), the use of ^{125}I-labelled radioligands provides essential initial information about the binding properties of the ligand *in vitro* and *in vivo* in animals.

It is common to make nonspecific labelling of proteins with this radionuclide. Several types of radioligands for use in receptor binding studies have been designed with ^{125}I substituents. The synthetic work with iodine is, however, more demanding with respect to safety aspects than synthesis with tritium.

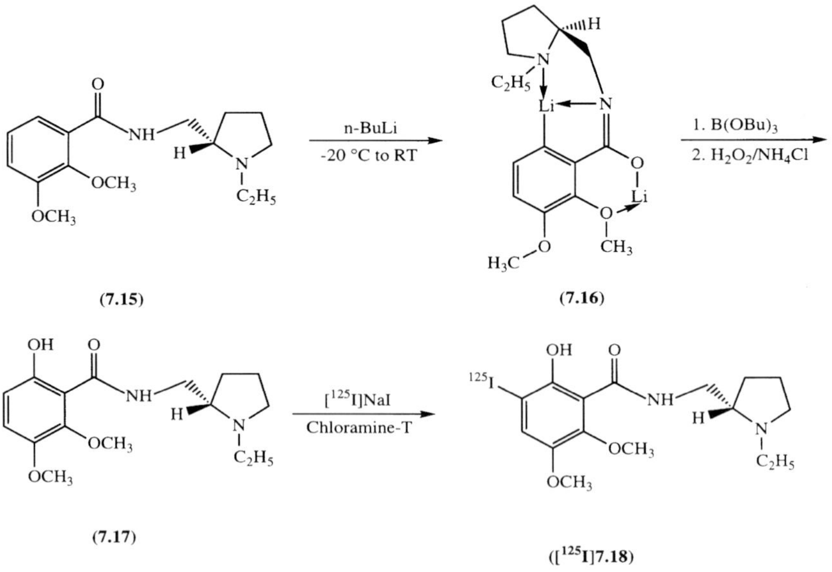

Scheme 7.4

NCQ 298 (**7.18**) is a highly selective and potent ligand, developed in our laboratories, for labelling of dopamine D_2 receptors. The regiospecific synthesis of $[^{125}I]NCQ$ 298 ($[^{125}I]$**7.18**) from the dimethoxy compound (**7.15**) is shown in Scheme 7.4. The desiodo compound (**7.17**) is made by *ortho*-lithiation of the benzamide to produce the doubly chelated intermediate (**7.16**), which is reacted with tributyl borate and oxidized with hydrogen peroxide. Carrier-free ^{125}I was oxidized by chloramine-T in dilute hydrochloric acid and reacted with (**7.17**) to produce the radioligand ($[^{125}I]$**7.18**) in high radiochemical yield and purity. Notably, the direct halogenation reaction proceeds with full regiocontrol.

On the other hand, if the 2,3-dimethoxybenzamide (**7.15**) is iodinated or brominated (see Section 7.4.2) a mixture of halogenated isomers will be formed. In order to achieve a regioselective introduction, one can for example use the *ipso*-directing effect of silicon or use a halogen-metal exchange reaction by starting with the corresponding trialkyltin-derivative (**7.22**), as exemplified in Scheme 7.6 in the synthesis of $[^{76}Br]FLB$ 457.

7.4 SHORT-LIVED RADIONUCLIDES

7.4.1 ^{123}I-labelled compounds

The most widely used gamma emitting radionuclides in SPECT are ^{99m}Tc and ^{123}I. A number of successful ligands labelled with ^{123}I for SPECT imaging of various receptors have been developed during the past 10 years. Introduction of ^{123}I is usually carried out in a similar way as for ^{125}I, i.e. by electrophilic substitution of an electron-rich aromatic ring by reaction with $[^{123}I]$NaI in the presence of oxidation agents such as chloramine-T or peracetic acid. The nuclide ^{99m}Tc is often chelated to the molecule, which can be a suitable tagging technique for studies of e.g. formulations of pharmaceuticals or vascular perfusion (e.g. $[^{99m}$Tc]hexamethylpropyleneamine oxime) ($[^{99m}$Tc] HMPAO ($[^{99m}$Tc]**7.21**)).

($[^{99m}$Tc]**7.21**)

An example of preparation of a ^{123}I SPECT tracer is given by the cocaine analogue $[^{123}I]\beta$-CIT ($[^{123}I]$**7.19**) (Scheme 7.5), which has been used for examination of Parkinson's disease as demonstrated in Section 7.6.2. The introduction of iodine-123 in the phenyl ring, which is not electron-rich enough to permit an efficient direct oxidative iodination analogous to the one used in the synthesis of ($[^{125}I]$**7.18**), requires a different strategy. Thus, a trimethyltin precursor (**7.20**) was made by a palladium catalysed reaction using hexamethylditin in the presence of palladium-tetrakis-triphenylphosphine of the parent iodo compound (**7.19**) as shown in Scheme 7.5. This reaction is an efficient chemoselective way (note the ester and tertiary amine functions) to set up the molecule for a mild iodostannylation reaction. The trimethyltin precursor (**7.20**) is treated with no-carrier-added (no dilution with stable iodine) $[^{123}I]$NaI to form $[^{123}I]\beta$-CIT ($[^{123}I]$**7.19**) with high specific radioactivity (usually > 12000 Ci/mmol). When using this labelling method careful purification of the trimethyltin precursor must be performed to ensure a precursor which is free from unlabelled (^{127}I)β-CIT. Presence of carrier β-CIT will reduce the specific radioactivity of the final product and may also result in undesired pharmacological effects for the patient. The advantages of the iodostannylation method are a rapid reaction, high yield, mild radioiodination conditions and a regiospecific incorporation of the iodine. Alternatively, one can use a Cu(I) assisted reaction starting from the corresponding bromo precursor or a method based on direct iodination of the desiodo precursor at oxidative conditions. An advantage with the latter method is facile access to the precursor and elimination of the risk for unlabelled β-CIT in the final solution. Disadvantages are, however, that the direct iodination is not regiospecific, requires heating and results in lower yields.

7.4.2 ^{76}Br-labelled compounds

The positron emitting radionuclide ^{76}Br has a half-life of 16 hours, which makes it possible to follow the radioligand distribution for more than 24 hours, if the biological half-life of

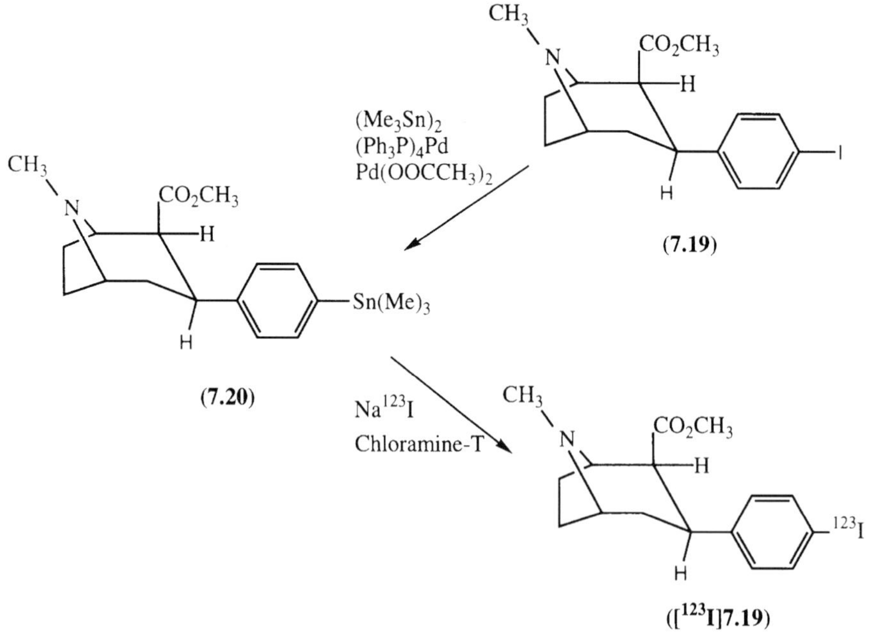

Scheme 7.5

the compound is long enough. However, the limited access to [76]Br and the relatively high doses of radiation to target organs, when [76]Br is injected into the body, are disadvantages compared to other PET radionuclides with shorter half-lives. Several substituted benzamides and salicylamides developed at the Astra laboratories have high affinity and selectivity for central dopamine D_2 receptors. These properties and a low level of non-specific binding are reasons for their suitability as radioligands for PET.

One recently developed ligand, FLB 457 (**7.23**) has an extremely high affinity for the dopamine D_2 receptors, which makes it possible to also study regions containing low densities of receptors outside the striatum. This ligand has also been prepared in carbon-11 labelled form by a reaction analogous to the one described for raclopride ([^{11}C]**7.41**) in Section 7.5.1. Scheme 7.6 shows the preparation of the bromine-76 labelled benzamide FLB 457 ([[76]Br]**7.23**) as well as the corresponding salicylamide FLB 463 ([[76]Br]**7.24**). In the former case, a bromostannylation reaction of the tributyltin derivative (**7.22**) is required in order to establish full regiocontrol, whereas the bromination of (**7.17**) provides only one regioisomer (cf. the synthesis of the corresponding iodo derivative ([^{125}I]**7.18**)).

7.4.3 ^{18}F-labelled compounds

Compared to ^{11}C, the half-life of 110 minutes of ^{18}F allows for a relatively long synthesis and transportation of the radiotracer over moderate distances as well as studies of relatively slow biological processes. The labelling of radiotracers with radioactive halogen nuclides

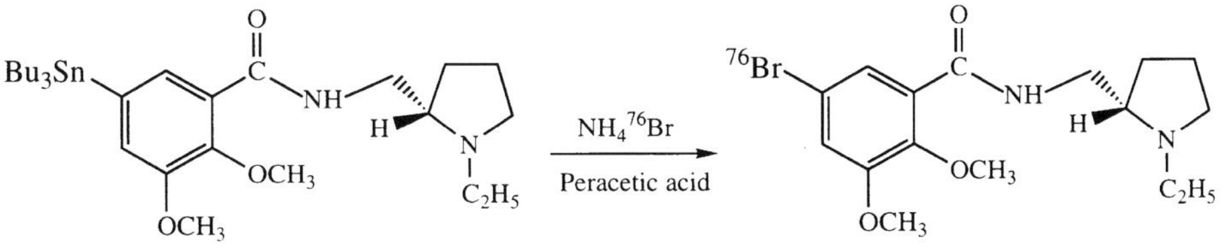

(7.22)   ([^{76}Br]**7.23**)

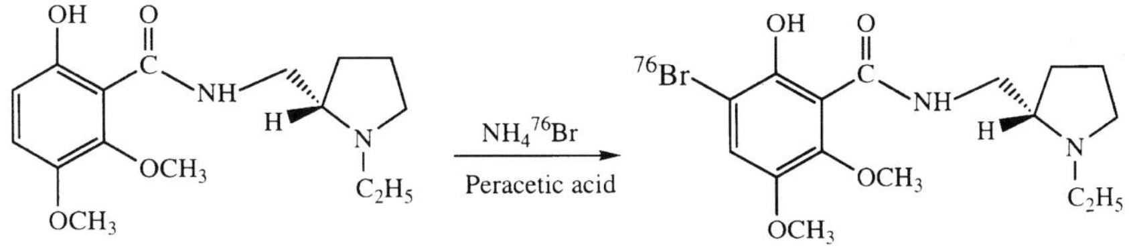

(7.17)   ([^{76}Br]**7.24**)

Scheme 7.6

usually implies synthesis of analogues rather than of the natural molecules. However, the small size of fluorine makes it possible to replace a hydrogen in many cases without distorting the properties. Accordingly, ^{18}F is a widely used tag in PET of naturally occurring molecules and therapeutic agents. However, the unique electronic properties of fluorine may lead to compounds with deviating properties, which must be investigated prior to the use. For example, a profound influence on the pK_a of amines substituted with fluorine in α- or β-position has been shown to affect the binding affinities of ligands. There are also possibilities to take advantage of the slightly altered properties inflicted by fluorine incorporation in the design of the tracer, e.g. in the most extensively used tracer 2-[^{18}F]fluoro-2-deoxyglucose ([^{18}F]FDG) ([^{18}F]**7.25**). [^{18}F]FDG has been widely used in

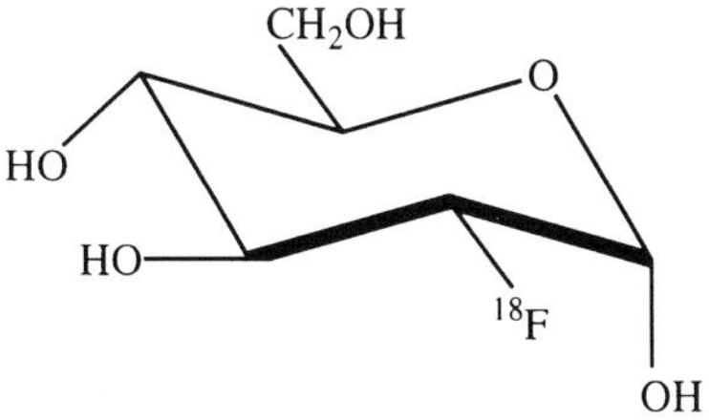

([^{18}F]**7.25**)

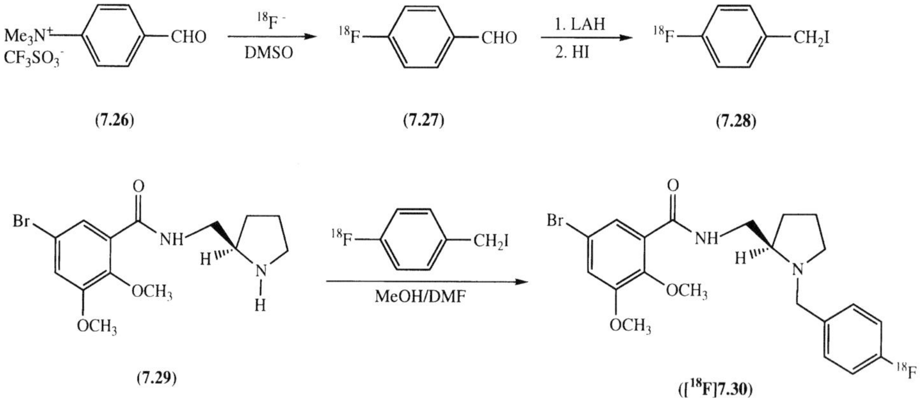

Scheme 7.7

metabolic studies of the brain and the heart. After intravenous administration, $[^{18}F]$FDG is phosphorylated to FDG-6-phosphate mediated by hexokinase. Because FDG-6-phosphate is not a substrate for glycolysis and does not undergo further metabolism, it remains trapped in the cell over the course of several hours. $[^{18}F]$FDG is usually prepared from $[^{18}F]$fluoride which can be produced from $^{18}O(p,n)^{18}F$ using $H_2^{18}O$ as target (Table 7.1). $[^{18}F]$Fluoride can be separated by an anion-exchange column and allowed to react with 1,3,4,6-tetra-O-acetyl-2-O-trifluoromethanesulphonyl-β-D-mannopyranose in the presence of an aminopolyether such as Kryptofix[2.2.2] to enhance the nucleophilicity of fluoride to yield $[^{18}F]$FDG in about 50% total yield.

Another example of fluorine labelling is the preparation of $[^{18}F]$NCQ 115 ($[^{18}F]$**7.30**) (Scheme 7.7) which is a selective dopamine D_2 receptor antagonist. Notably, the affinity of this N-benzyl pyrrolidine (**7.30**) for the receptor resides in the opposite stereoisomer compared to the other mentioned benzamides with N-ethyl pyrrolidine side chains, e.g. (**7.18**), (**7.23**) and (**7.24**). NCQ 115 has a fluorine in a synthetically accessible position in the parent compound and was therefore suggested as a potential ^{18}F-labelled radioligand for PET. $[^{18}F]$4-Fluorobenzyl iodide (**7.28**) was prepared in a 3-step synthesis from potassium $[^{18}F]$fluoride. The first critical step relies upon a nucleophilic displacement of the quaternary anilinium group which proceeds with regiocontrol due to the influence of the electron-withdrawing aldehyde para-substituent. The nucleophilicity of the fluoride ion is enhanced by using the aminopolyether cryptand Kryptofix[2.2.2] to complex the potassium counterion. N-4-Fluorobenzylation of the corresponding secondary pyrrolidine precursor (**7.29**) was performed giving ($[^{18}F]$**7.30**) with a total synthesis time of 90 minutes including purification with semi-preparative HPLC (Scheme 7.7).

7.5 ULTRASHORT-LIVED RADIONUCLIDES

In the preparation of compounds labelled with radionuclides such as ^{11}C, ^{13}N or ^{15}O (half-lives 20, 10 and 2 minutes) a series of requirements related to the ultrashort half-life

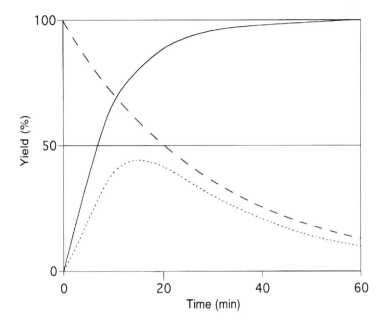

Figure 7.2   The radiochemical yield of a hypothetical ^{11}C-reaction as a function of time (dotted line). Dashed line: the decay curve of the radionuclide. Solid line: the chemical yield of the reaction.

of the radionuclide must be considered. When optimizing the radiochemical yield of a reaction, influence of conventional parameters such as substrate and reagent concentrations, temperature, pH and solvent compositions are considered. However, the most critical parameter in the synthesis of these ultrashort-lived tracers is time. Even if a reaction is completed within two half-lives of the radionuclide, it may be favourable to stop the reaction earlier since the radioactivity decay has also to be considered (Figure 7.2).

7.5.1 ^{11}C-labelled compounds

The radioactivity must be introduced by readily accessible radiolabelled precursors. Examples of ^{11}C-labelled precursors that can either be produced directly in the target or obtained via rapid on-line reactions starting from ^{11}CO$_2$ are shown in Scheme 7.8. The most widely used labelled ^{11}C-labelled precursor today is [^{11}C]methyl iodide. Recently, a more reactive precursor [^{11}C]methyl triflate was shown to give higher yields in the synthesis of some commonly used PET radioligands.

The labelling reactions must occur rapidly and in high yields. The complete procedure, from the production of the labelled precursor to the delivery of the purified labelled compound should not exceed more than three half-lives of the radionuclide. A typical total synthesis time for a ^{11}C-labelled radioligand including purification is 30 minutes. The principal strategy is to introduce the labelled precursor as late as possible, followed by

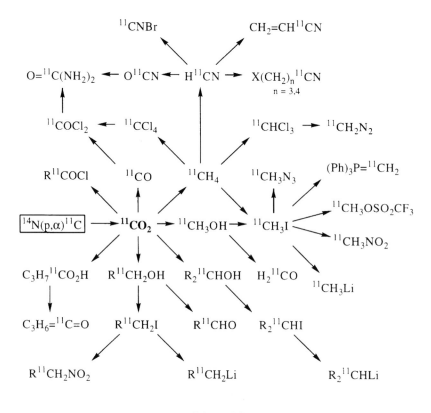

Scheme 7.8

none or just a few additional reactions before the final purification. In addition, handling of high levels of radioactivity on a routine basis requires an automated/remote-controlled experimental set-up installed in a lead-shielded hot-cell to ensure maximal radiation protection. On-line and one-pot reactions shorten the total synthesis time and reduce radioactivity losses.

The stoichiometry of a radiolabelling reaction differs from that of an ordinary chemical synthesis. The amount of the radionuclide produced in the cyclotron is in the nanomolar range. With such small amounts, all other substrates or reactants used are necessarily in large excess. This condition will favour a fast incorporation of the labelled precursor. However, because of the small amounts of the labelled precursor a general problem is that even small amounts of impurities might disturb the reaction. The various steps for the synthesis and PET-application of a radiotracer are presented in Figure 7.3. Efficient PET investigations require an unusually high degree of interdisciplinary collaboration and coordination set in a very tight time frame. Thus, PET centres have been established to optimise all steps in this sequence of events and to be cost-effective units. At the end of 1994 the number of PET research centers has reached more than 120 compared to only about 30 centers ten years ago.

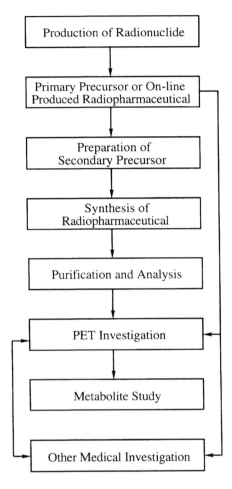

Figure 7.3   Various steps involved before and during medical investigations using positron-emitting radionuclides.

   An example of a multi-step synthesis that can be performed with ^{11}C is the seven-step synthesis of optically enriched L-[3-^{11}C]phenylalanine ([^{11}C]**7.34**) from [^{11}C]carbon dioxide via [^{11}C]benzaldehyde (**7.32**) (Scheme 7.9). The labelled benzaldehyde was prepared by a selective oxidation of [^{11}C]benzylalcohol (**7.31**). The three steps from [^{11}C]CO$_2$ to (**7.32**) were accomplished within 5 minutes. [^{11}C]Benzaldehyde was condensed with a 2-phenyl-5-oxazolone to give the [α-^{11}C]-4-benzylidene-2-phenyl-5-oxazolone which was opened by sodium hydroxide in ethanol to give the amide protected α-aminocinnamic acid (**7.33**). Asymmetric catalytical hydrogenation was performed using a chiral Wilkinson catalyst to obtain the L-form of the amino acid ([^{11}C]**7.34**) in 80% e.e. The total synthesis time for this seven-step synthesis was 50 minutes including HPLC purification.

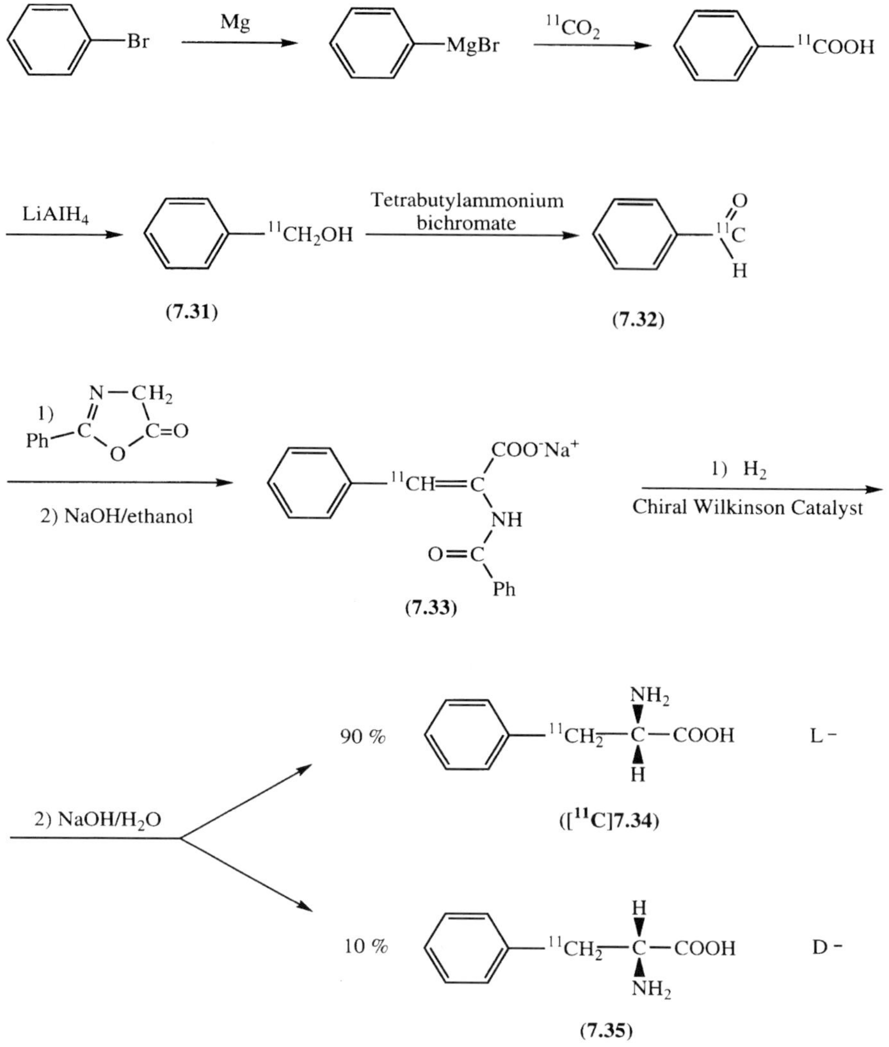

(7.31)   (7.32)

(7.33)

90 %   ([^{11}C]7.34)   L –

2) NaOH/H$_2$O

10 %   (7.35)   D –

Scheme 7.9

Many analogues of norepinephrine have been radiolabelled for investigation of presynaptic binding sites of the heart. In order to investigate the sympathetic nerve terminal and the noradrenaline metabolism it may be of advantage to use the endogenous transmitter norepinephrine itself and not an analogue. A synthetic approach has been developed for the preparation of racemic [^{11}C]norepinephrine ([^{11}C]7.39) starting from [^{11}C]nitromethane (7.36) (Scheme 7.10). In the first step, piperonal is reacted with [^{11}C]nitromethane with the mild base tetrabutylammonium fluoride (TBAF) as catalyst to give 80–90% of the

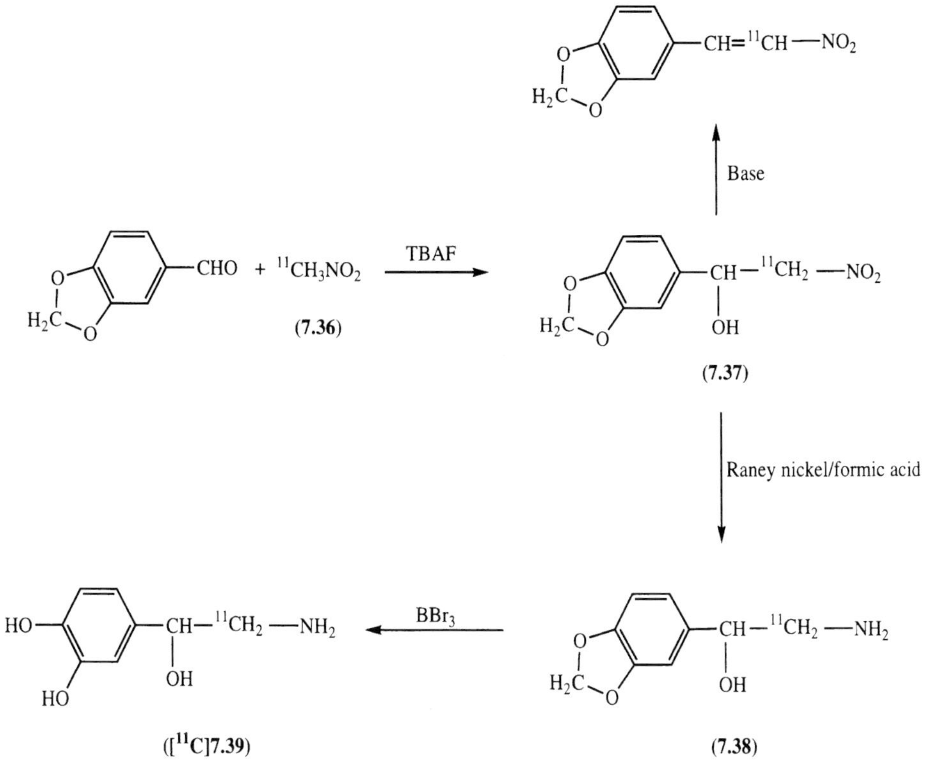

Scheme 7.10

initial condensation product (**7.37**). Usual bases employed in Knovenagel reactions, such as sodium hydroxide or secondary amines, lead to the nitrostyrene derivative after dehydration of (**7.37**). Reduction of the nitro group is accomplished with Raney nickel/formic acid to give (**7.38**), which is deprotected with boron tribromide.

The salicylamide [^{11}C]raclopride ([^{11}C]**7.41**) is the most extensively used PET radioligand for the quantitative examination of dopamine D_2 receptors in striatum by PET. Both enantiomers, [^{11}C]raclopride ([^{11}C]**7.41**) and the inactive isomer [^{11}C]**7.43**, have been labelled with ^{11}C by O-methylation with [^{11}C]methyl iodide from the corresponding desmethyl precursors (Scheme 7.11). Both enantiomerically pure precursors were obtained by resolving 2-aminomethyl-1-ethylpyrrolidine by fractional crystallization of the ditartrates. The enantiomeric excess of both enantiomers was over 99.8% according to gas chromatographic analysis of the diastereomeric O-methylmandelic amides. Coupling of the resolved pyrrolidine amines with 3,5-dichloro-2,6-dimethoxybenzoyl chloride followed by bisdemethylation gave the enantiomerically pure and symmetrical precursors (**7.40**) and (**7.42**). The O-methylation with [^{11}C]methyl iodide was performed by use of 5 M NaOH as the base in dimethylsulphoxide (DMSO) (Scheme 7.11).

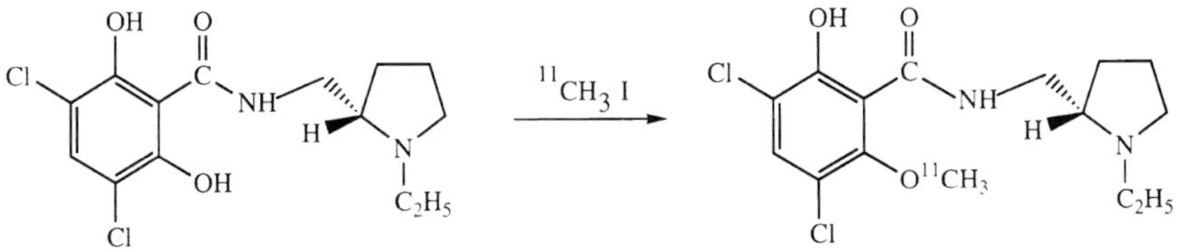

(7.40)

([^{11}C]7.41)

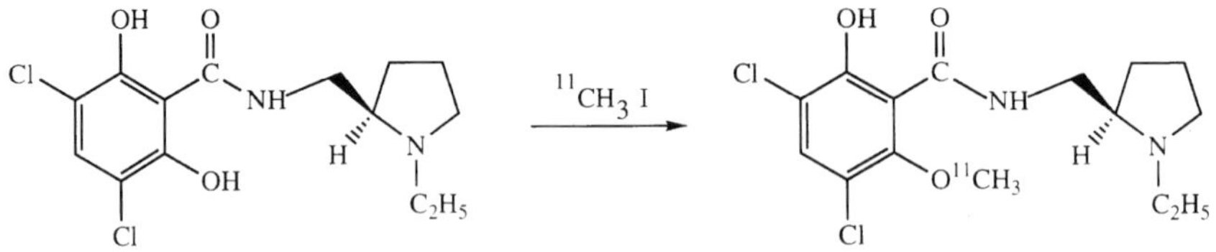

(7.42)

([^{11}C]7.43)

Scheme 7.11

7.5.2 ^{13}N-labelled compounds

The half-life of 10 minutes of ^{13}N limits the reaction time available and gives an unusual challenge for the development of synthesis methods and strategy for its incorporation into suitable PET tracers. Both synthetic and enzymatic approaches have been applied to the preparation of ^{13}N labelled radiotracers. Nitrogen-13 can be produced by the ^{16}O(p,α)^{13}N reaction. [^{13}N]NH$_3$ is a blood flow tracer, which can be produced by reduction of [^{13}N]nitrate and nitrite in the presence of a mixture of NaOH and TiCl$_3$, with a radiochemical purity greater than 99%. An alternative method is the deuteron irradiation of methane from which [^{13}N]ammonia is collected in an acidic water solution.

A number of enzymatically synthesized L-[^{13}N]amino acids, such as alanine, leucine, aspartic acid, valine, tyrosine and phenylalanine, have been reported. The general reaction used is glumatic acid dehydrogenase catalyzed formation of L-[^{13}N]amino acids from [^{13}N]NH$_3$ and an α-keto acid. Alternatively, [^{13}N]glutamic acid is synthesized and the ^{13}N amino group is transferred to an α-keto acid in a transaminase reaction catalyzed by glutamate-pyruvate or glutamate-oxaloacetate transferase. A variety of ^{13}N-labelled tracers has thus been synthesized, but the half-life limits the number of tracers used routinely today.

7.5.3 ^{15}O-labelled compounds

Preparation of oxygen-15 tracers for PET provides the ultimate challenge in organic synthesis due to the ultrashort half-life of 2 minutes. Despite the short half-life of ^{15}O the following tracers are used routinely worldwide today:

(i) $[^{15}O]O_2$ is produced by the $^{14}N(d,n)^{15}O$ or $^{15}N(p,n)^{15}O$ reaction. $[^{15}O]O_2$ has been used to determine blood flow, oxygen extraction fraction and oxygen metabolism after administration to patients by inhalation

(ii) $[^{15}O]CO_2$ is produced by passing $[^{15}O]O_2$ over activated charcoal heated at 400 °C to 600 °C

(iii) $[^{15}O]H_2O$ is prepared by bubbling $[^{15}O]CO_2$ into water or by direct action of $[^{15}O]O_2$ with hydrogen. Cerebral blood flow is measured routinely with $[^{15}O]H_2O$

(iv) $[^{15}O]$butanol, a new tracer for blood flow, is produced by the reaction between tri-n-butyl borane and $[^{15}O]O_2$. The yield is high, and more than 100 mCi of $[^{15}O]$butanol can be prepared with intervals of 10 minutes.

7.6 IMAGING TECHNIQUES

7.6.1 Autoradiography

The use of radioligands in autoradiographic imaging studies of small animals can give valuable information on distribution, density and kinetics. Slices of the human post mortem brain can also be incubated with radioligands in order to map the distribution of different receptors. For autoradiography the brain is cryosectioned using a cryomicrotome into 100 μm whole hemisphere sections. The tissue sections are transferred to glass plates, put into specially designed incubation chambers and incubated with radiolabelled compounds. The sections are then put into X-ray cassettes together with beta radiation sensitive film for exposure 4 days for ^{125}I labelled compounds and 4 weeks for ^3H-labelled compounds. The films are developed and fixed using conventional techniques. The autoradiograms can be analyzed using computerized densitometry and with a high resolution video camera. Also ^{11}C- and ^{18}F-labelled compounds can be used with exposure times of only 1–4 hours. Because of the differences in the range of the radiation, higher resolution is obtained with radioligands labelled with ^3H (0.0072 mm in H_2O) and ^{125}I than with ^{11}C (4.12 mm in H_2O) or ^{18}F.

An example of an autoradiogram of a whole hemisphere section of a human brain post mortem is given in Figure 7.4. It illustrates the binding of the highly selective and potent dopamine D_2 receptor radioligand $[^{125}I]NCQ$ 298 ($[^{125}I]$**7.18**). The image of the whole hemisphere demonstrates a high uptake of radioactivity in the basal ganglia (caudate nucleus and putamen) a region known to have a high density of dopamine D_2 receptors.

7.6.2 SPECT

The most common SPECT systems consists of a gamma camera with one or three NaI detector heads mounted on a gantry, an on-line computer for acquisition and processing of data, and a display system. The detector head rotates around the axis of the patient at small angle increments (3°–10°) for 180° or 360° angular sampling. The data are collected at each angular position and normally stored in the computer for later reconstruction of the images of the planes of interest. Multi-head gamma cameras collect data in several projections simultaneously and reduce the time of imaging. The best SPECT cameras of today have a resolution of 5–6 mm.

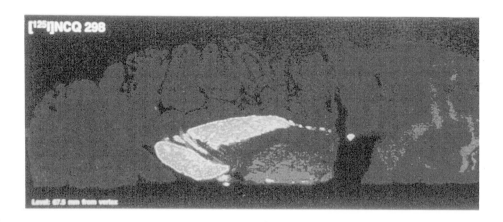

Figure 7.4 $[^{125}I]$NCQ 298 ($[^{125}I]$**7.18**) binding to dopamine D_2 receptors in a post-mortem human brain using whole hemisphere autoradiography. The figure was kindly provided by Dr Håkan Hall, Karolinska Institutet, Sweden. (See Color Plate I.)

SPECT radiopharmaceuticals are used for detecting radioactivity in the whole body. For brain imaging, there exists a large number of tracers for monitoring blood-brain-barrier transport, cerebral perfusion, receptor binding and binding to monoclonal antibodies. A perfusion tracer which is widely used for detection of a number of diseases is $[^{99m}Tc]$hexamethylpropyleneamine oxime ($[^{99m}Tc]$HMPAO, $[^{99m}Tc]$**7.21**).

The SPECT tracer $[^{123}I]\beta$-CIT ($[^{123}I]$**7.19**) is an analogue to cocaine with a high affinity for the dopamine transporter ($K_d = 0.11$ nM). This recently developed radioligand has proven to be useful for studies of Parkinson's disease. Figure 7.5 shows a 52 year old control subject (upper images) and a 55 year old patient with Parkinson's disease (lower images). The patient had recieved no medication before this study. A reduced uptake of $[^{123}I]\beta$-CIT was demonstrated in the Parkinson's patient in a brain region normally having a high density of dopamine transporters (localized by arrows). This finding is of high diagnostic value in the examination of Parkinson's patients.

7.6.3 PET

The influence of the biological system on the radioligand *in vivo* cannot easily be simulated *in vitro*. Several conditions such as protein binding in plasma and the extracellular fluids, radioligand metabolism and ligand transport across the blood brain barrier cannot be explored *in vitro*. By use of imaging techniques such as PET, *in vivo* visualization of biochemical processes can be performed in the human body.

While SPECT is more readily available than PET, the PET technique offers advantages such as the ability to measure the concentration of the tracer quantitatively, a greater sensitivity, a higher resolution and more diverse types of radiotracers. The use of short-lived radionuclides and PET gives a low radiation dose to the subject. In addition repeated investigations can be performed within short time intervals.

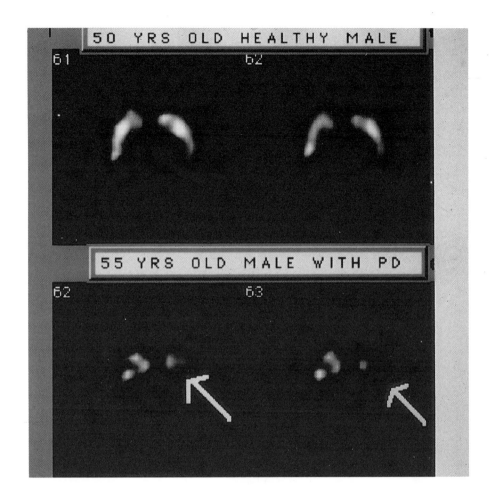

Figure 7.5 SPECT images taken 21 hours after injection of $[^{123}I]\beta$-CIT ($[^{123}I]$**7.19**) in a healthy male (top) and a patient with Parkinson's disease (bottom). The images demonstrate highly reduced uptake in the patient with Parkinson's disease (arrow). The figure was kindly provided by Dr Jyrki Kuikka, Kuopio University Hospital, Finland. (See Color Plate II.)

The principles of the PET technique is demonstrated in Figure 7.6. Positron emitting radionuclides disintegrate and emit positrons (positively charged electrons, β^+), that interact with the corresponding anti-particle, an electron (β^-) after travelling in tissue for 1–2 mm. The mass of the two particles is converted to gamma (γ) radiation (annihilation) and two 511 keV photons are emitted simultaneously in opposite directions. The rays emitted are detected externally by a ring of scintillation detectors placed around the subject. The two γ-signals have to be registered by two coincidence coupled detectors within a time window to be counted as originating from the same disintegration. The last generation of PET-systems is used for data acquisition and image reconstruction of 47 slices in

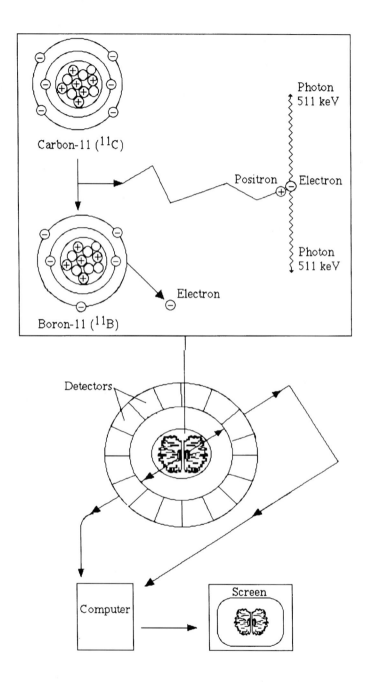

Figure 7.6   The positron-emitting radionuclide ^{11}C decays to form a positron, which annihilates with an electron. The resulting gamma energy, two photons travelling in opposite directions, can be detected externally by a ring of scintillation detectors placed around the subject in the PET camera.

the 3D mode with a spatial resolution of 3–4 mm where 2 mm is the maximum theoretical resolution.

Several PET radiopharmaceuticals are today used as standard tools for investigations of various disease states and control of treatment effects with drugs. The following examples can be mentioned:

(i)   2-[^{18}F]fluoro-2-deoxyglucose ([^{18}F]FDG, ([^{18}F]**7.25**) is the most frequently used tracer. It measures the glucose metabolism in tumors, heart and especially brain in various disease conditions

(ii) [1-^{11}C]acetate, which enters the Krebs tricarboxylic acid cycle at the last possible step by binding to coenzyme-A, can be used as a tracer to reflect the oxygen consumption in the heart. It is prepared from methylmagnesium bromide and [^{11}C]CO$_2$

(iii) [^{13}N]ammonia is a precursor that can be incorporated into biomolecules. However, it is a readily diffusible tracer and it enters tissues and metabolic processes, which will reflect the regional blood flow

(iv) L-[^{11}C]methionine reflects the amino acid utilisation, i.e. transport, protein synthesis, transmethylation and other metabolic processes. It can be easily prepared from the sulfide anion of L-homocysteine and [^{11}C]CH$_3$I

(v)   n-[^{15}O]butanol and [^{15}O]H$_2$O are used to study blood flow in the brain and other organs. The partition coefficient of n-[^{15}O]butanol is 1.0, which is an advantage compared to [^{15}O]H$_2$O.

(vi) [^{11}C]raclopride ([^{11}C]**7.41**) is a selective antagonist for the dopamine D$_2$ receptors that has been used to measure the receptor occupancy in patients treated with different antipsychotics. The preparation is shown in Scheme 7.11.

Besides [^{11}C]raclopride ([^{11}C]**7.41**), a large number of receptor radioligands have been developed during the past ten years. Selective radioligands are prepared and widely used in PET for visualization of dopamine, benzodiazepine, muscarinic and serotonin receptors.

Several PET radioligands have been developed for the presynaptic norepinephrine uptake system in the heart. Most of them are, however, analogues labelled with either ^{18}F or ^{76}Br. Recently, the endogenous compound itself, [^{11}C]norepinephrine ([^{11}C]**7.39**), has been synthesized and evaluated in the monkey with PET. Figure 7.7 shows two PET experiments in the monkey heart. The first experiment is a control study (left). In the second pretreatment experiment (right), the selective norepinephrine uptake inhibitor desipramine was given 30 minutes before injection of [^{11}C]norepinephrine. The results demonstrate that a major part of the radioactivity visualized by PET results from neuronal uptake of racemic ([^{11}C]**7.39**) in the monkey heart.

The preparation and PET examination of radiolabelled stereoisomers are important in radioligand development. Stereospecificity has been demonstrated for drug binding to plasma proteins to a moderate degree. Active transport across membranes is also stereospecific, whereas passive diffusion is primarily related to lipophilicity, which is identical for enantiomers. Stereospecificity is a basic criterion for specific binding to a receptor, an enzyme or a transport mechanism. The active enantiomer (sometimes called eutomer) with specific binding should have a higher accumulation in a target region *in vivo* than the inactive enantiomer (distomer). Comparative PET studies with enantiomers have been suggested as a method to differentiate specific from nonspecific binding, which is the key problem in quantitative determination of receptor binding. The usefulness of this method has been

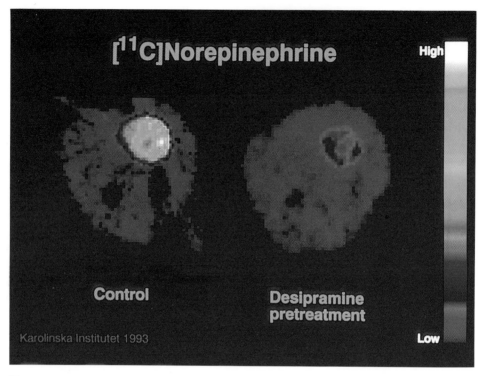

Figure 7.7   PET images showing distribution of radioactivity in the chest of a monkey after injection of [^{11}C]norepinephrine ([^{11}C]**7.39**) in a control experiment (left) and a pretreatment experiment with desipramine (right). The figure was kindly provided by Dr Lars Farde, Karolinska Institutet, Sweden. (See Color Plate III.)

demonstrated by PET for several enantiomeric pairs and is exemplified here with the dopamine D$_2$ receptor antagonist [^{11}C]raclopride ([^{11}C]**7.41**) and its inactive enantiomer ([^{11}C]**7.43**).

Enantiomers have identical physicochemical properties, such as partion coefficient, in a symmetrical environment. In general, if there is no involvement of chiral transport processes across the blood-brain barrier, then the identical partition coefficient of the enantiomers will result in an identical distribution ratio (radioactivity in brain/radioactivity in plasma). Accordingly, it may be possible in PET studies to use the measured brain radioactivity after the injection of an inactive enantiomer as an estimate of the background concentration of radioactivity obtained after the injection of an active enantiomer (Figure 7.8). In radioligand binding experiments *in vitro*, the background level is reduced by simply washing away the free radioligand before the radioactivity is measured. This cannot be accomplished in *in vivo* experiments with PET, because the free radioligand concentration adds to the non-specific binding and increases the background.

After the injection of ([^{11}C]**7.41**), there was a high accumulation of radioactivity in the dopamine-rich basal ganglia, whereas the concentration of radioactivity in any other regions could not be differentiated reliably from the background level (Figure 7.9). After the injection of ([^{11}C]**7.43**), there was no such accumulation of radioactivity. Thus, the binding of [^{11}C]**7.41**) is stereoselective.

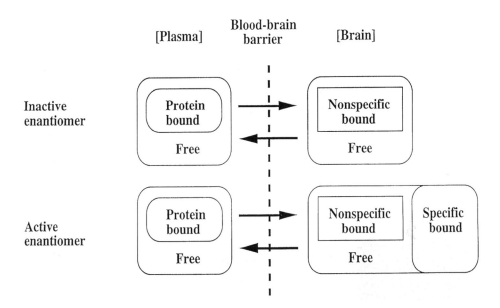

Figure 7.8   Compartments for the distribution of enantiomers.

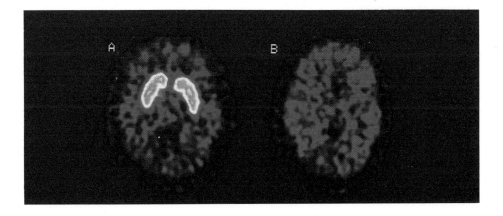

Figure 7.9   PET images showing distribution of radioactivity in the brain after injection of [^{11}C]raclopride ([^{11}C]**7.41**) (A) and the inactive enantiomer ([^{11}C]**7.43**) (B). The figure was kindly provided by Dr Lars Farde, Karolinska Institutet, Sweden. (See Color Plate IV.)

It is generally assumed that the antipsychotic effect of neuroleptic drugs is mediated by blockade of dopamine receptors. By the use of this *in vivo* technique it is possible to relate clinical drug effects to receptor binding data obtained in the same living subjects. New information of relevance for the identification of tentative target regions for the antipsychotic drug effect may be found by a regional examination of radioligand binding *in vivo* in the human brain.

FURTHER READING

Fowler, J.S. and Wolf, A. (1986) Positron emitter-labelled compounds: priorities and problems. In *Positron Emission Tomography and Autoradiography: Principles and Applications for the Brain and Heart*, edited by M. Phelps, J. Mazziotta and H. Schelbert, pp. 391–450. New York: Raven Press.

Saha, G.B. (1993) *Physics and Radiobiology of Nuclear Medicine*. 1st ed. New York: Springer-Verlag.

Coenen, H.H., Moerlein, S.M. and Stöcklin, G. (1983) No-carrier-added radiolabelling methods with heavy halogens. *Radiochemica Acta*, **34**, 47–68.

Coenen, H.H. (1986) Radiohalogenation methods: an overview. In *Progress in Radiopharmacy*, edited by P.H. Cox, S.J. Mather, C.B. Sampson, and C.R. Lazarus, pp. 196–220. Dordrecht: Kluwer Academic Publishers.

Stöcklin, G. and Pike, V.W. Eds. (1993) *Radiopharmaceuticals for Positron Emission Tomography. Methodological Aspects*. Dordrecht: Kluwer Academic Publishers.

Stöcklin, G. (1992) Tracers for metabolic imaging of brain and heart. Radiochemistry and radiopharmacology. *Eur. J. Nucl. Med.*, **19**, 527–551.

Halldin, C. (1991) Radioligands for dopamine receptor PET studies: benzamides and ligands for dopamine D_1-receptors. In *Brain Dopaminergic Systems: Imaging with Positron Tomography*, edited hy J.C. Baron, D. Comar, L. Farde, J.L. Martinot and B. Mazoyer, pp. 23–38. Dordrecht: Kluwer Academic Publishers.

Högberg, T. (1993) The development of dopamine D_2-receptor selective antagonists. *Drug Design and Discovery*, **9**, 333–357.

Halldin, C. and Nilsson, S.-O. (1992) Carbon-11 radiopharmaceuticals — radiopharmacy aspects. In *Progress in Radiopharmacy*, edited by P.A. Schubiger and G. Westera, pp. 115–129. Dordrecht: Kluwer Academic Publishers.

Maziere, B. and Delforge, J. (1994) Contribution of positron emission tomography to pharmacokinetic studies. In *Pharmacokinetics of Drugs*, edited by P.G. Welling and L.P. Balant, pp. 455–480. New York: Springer-Verlag.

Saha, G.B., MacIntyre, W.J. and Raymundo, T.G. (1994) Radiopharmaceuticals for brain imaging. *Seminars in Nuclear Medicine*, **24**, 324–349.

Farde, L., Hall, H., Ehrin, E. and Sedvall, G. (1986) Quantitative analysis of dopamine D_2 receptor binding in the living human brain by positron emission tomography. *Science*, **231**, 258–261.

Bengtsson, S., Gawell, L., Högberg, T. and Sahlberg, C. (1985) Synthesis and ^{3}H NMR of ^{3}H alaproclate of high specific activity. *J. Labelled Compd. Radiopharm.*, **22**, 427–435.

Foged, C., Hansen, L. and Halldin, C. (1993) ^{14}C-Labelling of NNC 756, a new dopamine D_1 antagonist. *J. Labelled Compd. Radiopharm.*, **33**, 747–757.

Maziere, B., Coenen, H.H., Halldin, C., Någren, K. and Pike, V.W. (1992) PET radioligands for dopamine receptors and re-uptake sites: chemistry and biochemistry. *Nucl. Med. Biol.*, **19**, 497–512.

Halldin, C. (1995) Dopamine Receptor Radioligands. *Med. Chem. Res.*, **5**, 127–149.

Kung, H.F. (1990) Radiopharmaceuticals for CNS receptor imaging with SPECT. *Nucl. Med. Biol.*, **17**, 85–92.

Högberg, T., Ström, P., Hall, H., Köhler, C., Halldin, C. and Farde, L. (1990) Synthesis of [^{123}I], [^{125}I]- and unlabelled (S)-3-iodo-5,6-dimethoxy-N-((1-ethyl-2-pyrrolidinyl)methyl) salicylamide (NCQ 298), selective ligands for the study of dopamine D_2 receptors. *Acta Pharm. Nord.*, **1**, 53–60.

Hall, H., Högberg, T., Halldin, C., Köhler, C., Ström, P., Ross, S.B., Larsson, S.A. and Farde, L. (1991) NCQ 298, A new selective iodinated salicylamide ligand for the labelling of dopamine D_2 receptors. *Psychopharmacology*, **103**, 6–18.

Halldin, C., Högberg, T. and Farde, L. (1994) Fluorine-18 labelled NCQ 115, a selective dopamine D_2 receptor ligand. Preparation and positron emission tomography. *Nucl. Med. Biol.*, **21**, 627–631.

Någren, K., Schoeps, K.-O., Halldin, C., Swahn, C.-G. and Farde, L. (1994) Selective synthesis of racemic 1-^{11}C-labelled norepinephrine, octopamine and phenethylamine and *in vivo* study of [1-^{11}C]norepinephrine in the heart with PET. *Appl. Radiat. Isot.*, **45**, 515–521.

Farde, L., Halldin, C., Någren, K., Suhara, T., Karlsson, P., Schoeps, K.-O., Swahn, C.-G. and Bone, D. (1994) PET shows high specific [^{11}C]norepinephrine binding in the primate heart. *Eur. J. Nucl. Med.*, **21**, 345–347.

Halldin, C. and Långström, B. (1985) Asymmetric synthesis of L-[3-^{11}C]phenylalanine using chiral hydrogenation catalysts. *Int. J Appl. Radiat. Isot.*, **35**, 945–948.

Loch, C., Halldin, C., Bottleander, M., Swahn, C.-G., Moresco, R.-M., Maziere, M., Farde, L. and Maziere, B. (1994) Preparation and evaluation of [^{76}Br]FLB 457, [^{76}Br]FLB 463 and [^{76}Br]NCQ 115, three selective benzamides for mapping dopamine D_2 receptors with PET. *J. Labelled Compd. Radiopharm.*, **35**, 437–438.

Långström, B., Antoni, G., Gullberg, P., Halldin, C., Malmorg, P., Någren, K., Rimland, A. and Svärd, H. (1987) Synthesis of L- and D-[methyl-^{11}C]methionine. *J. Nucl. Med.*, **28**, 1037–1040.

Halldin, C., Suhara, T., Farde, L. and Sedvall, G. (1995) Preparation and examination of labelled stereoisomers *in vivo* by PET. In *Chemist's Views of Imaging Centers*, edited by A.M. Emran. pp. 497–511. New York: Plenum.

Aquilonius, S.-M., Eckernäs, S.-Å. and Gillberg, P.-G. (1983) Large section cryomicrotomy in human neuroanatomy and neurochemistry. In *Brain Microdissection Techniques*, edited by A.C. Cuello, pp. 155–170. New York: Wiley.

Hall, H., Sedvall, G., Magnusson, O., Kopp, J., Halldin, C. and Farde, L. (1994) Distribution of D_1- and D_2-dopamine receptors, dopamine and its metabolites in the human brain. *Neuropsychopharmacology*, **11**, 245–256.

Kuikka, J., Bergström, K., Vanninen, E., Laulumaa, V., Hartikainen, P. and Länsimies, E. (1993) Initial experience with single-photon emission tomography using iodine-123 labelled 2β-carbomethoxy-3β-(4-iodophenyl)tropane in human brain. *Eur. J. Nucl. Med.*, **20**, 783–786.

Halldin, C., Farde, L., Högberg, T., Hall, H., Ström, P., Ohlberger, A. and Solin, O. (1991) A comparative PET-studies of five carbon-11 or fluorine-18 labelled salicylamides. Preparation and *in vitro* dopamine D_2 receptor binding. *Nucl. Med. Biol.*, **18**, 871–881.

Farde, L., Pauli, S., Hall, H., Eriksson, L., Halldin, C., Högberg, T., Nilsson, L., Sjögren, I. and Stone-Elander, S. (1988) Stereoselective binding of [^{11}C]raclopride in living human brain — a search for extrastriatal central D_2-dopamine receptors by PET. *Psychopharmacology*, **94**, 471–478.

8. ION CHANNELS

DAVID J. TRIGGLE

CONTENTS

8.1 INTRODUCTION

8.1.1 Ion channels and cellular function

The cell is not a silent place. The constant noise from ions moving through the ion channels of the cell is an integral component of the music of life. Ion channels serve as one of the mechanisms by which excitable cells respond to informational inputs. Ion channels permit, under physiologic conditions, the orderly movements of ions across cellular membranes — both extra- and intracellular. Under pathologic conditions ion channels contribute to disorderly movements of ions and the death of the cell.

8.1.2 Ion channels as membrane effectors

Excitable cells respond to a variety of informational inputs, chemical and physical, including neurotransmitters, hormones, pheromones, and heat, light and pressure. These informational inputs are coupled to cellular response through transducing processes that include enzyme activation, substrate internalization and ion channel opening and closing (Fig. 8.1). Ion channels serve as one class of biological effectors. They function to permeate ions including the physiologic cations Na^+, K^+, Ca^{2+}, and Mg^{2+} and the anion Cl^- in response to cell stimuli. The resultant ion current may itself be the end consequence as in the maintenance of membrane potential and its discharge in electric fish. More commonly, the ion current is coupled to other events, including the alteration of cellular sensitivity to other stimuli and the major processes of excitation-contraction and stimulus-secretion coupling. In the latter examples there is a dual function for calcium since it serves both a current carrying role as a permeant ion and simultaneously fulfills a chemical messenger function coupling cell excitation to these calcium-dependent events.

The cell maintains an asymmetric distribution of ions across its membranes. Na^+, Ca^{2+} and Cl^- are maintained at low intracellular levels and K^+ at a high intracellular level relative to the extracellular environment. The asymmetric environment is maintained because cell membranes are selectively permeable to ions and because the cell membranes maintain ion pumps, including Na^+, K^+-ATPase and Ca^{2+}-ATPases, that function to maintain the ion gradients in the face of constant rundown through leakage and to restore them subsequent to dissipation by channel activating stimuli.

The lipid bilayer of the cell is essentially impermeable to ions and ion channels (or an equivalent function) are, therefore, necessary components of the cell membrane and likely arose early during cellular evolution. Uncontrolled movements of ions represent lethal signals to cells. Ion channels must, therefore, be regulated species and the processes of regulation are critical to the understanding of the physiologic and pharmacologic control of channel activity.

8.1.3 Ion channels and ion distribution

The relationship between ion concentrations, membrane potential and ion chemical and electrical gradients is depicted in Figure 8.2. At a typical resting cellular potential of 70 mV (by convention negative interior) both electrical and concentration gradients combine to provide a net inward driving force for Na^+ entry of 120 mV. When the membrane potential

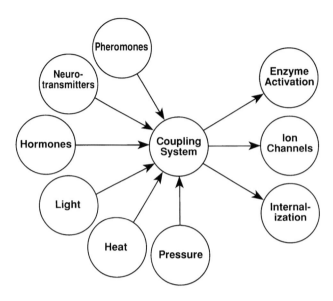

Figure 8.1   Ion channels as one of several mechanisms by which informational inputs are translated through intermediate coupling devices into cellular responses.

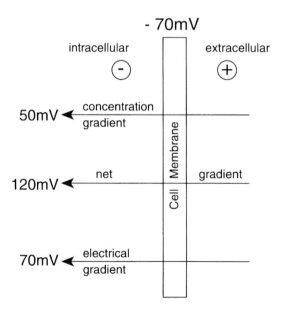

Figure 8.2   Ion movements across a cell membrane are determined by the net product of concentration and electrical gradients. In the example depicted at −70 mV both concentration and electrical gradients favor Na$^+$ entry into the cell. If the membrane potential were set at the equilibrium potential for Na$^+$, $\approx$ +50 mV (depending on ion concentrations), then the gradients would balance and there would be no net movement of Na$^+$.

Table 8.1   Ionic concentrations and ionic equilibrium potentials in excitable cells.

Ion	$[X]_{ext}$ mM	$[X]_{int}$ mM	Equil. Pot. mV (approx.)
Na^+	145	12	+70
K^+	4	155	−90
Ca^{2+}	1.5	$<10^{-4}$	$>+120$
Cl^-	123	4	−90

is maintained at the equilibrium potential for Na^+ (positive interior) the inwardly directed concentration gradient is now exactly opposed by the outwardly directed electrical gradient and there is no net movement of ions. A comparison of the equilibrium potentials for Na^+, K^+, Ca^{2+} and Cl^- is presented in Table 8.1. Quite generally, the opening of Na^+ and Ca^{2+} channels will dissipate membrane potential to mediate excitation, whilst the opening of K^+ and Cl^- channels will elevate or maintain membrane potential to mediate inhibitory responses. Conversely, the closing of K^+ or Cl^- channels will be disinhibitory in nature, leading to cell excitation. When two or more channel classes are opened together the resultant membrane potential will represent the sum of both events.

There are important implications of these ion movements to considerations of drug action. Drugs that open Ca^{2+} or Na^+ channels will tend to depolarize cells and will be excitatory in character while drugs that open K^+ or Cl^- channels will tend to hyperpolarize cells and to be inhibitory in nature. A similar, but opposite relationship, will apply to antagonists at these channels (Fig. 8.3). The control of ion channels must not be viewed in isolation, but rather should be seen as a linked event whereby the activity of one channel category influences the activity of others. Thus, the influx of Ca^{2+} through Ca^{2+} channels can activate Ca^{2+}-dependent K^+ channels. A further example is depicted in Figure 8.4 where, in an insulin secreting pancreatic β-cell, there exist both ATP-sensitive K^+ channels and voltage-gated Ca^{2+} channels. When the ATP level is elevated in response to elevated glucose or amino acid concentrations the K^+ channel closes; the subsequent depolarization activates the Ca^{2+} channel and the resultant Ca^{2+} influx promotes insulin release.

8.1.4 Activation and inactivation of ion channels

Axonal nerve impulse conduction (Fig. 8.5) indicates the association between different ionic processes. Depolarization of a nerve axon by maintenance of a step depolarization results in the rapid activation of Na^+ channels to permit an inward current carried by Na^+ ions and a later outward current carried by K^+ ions. Figure 8.5 illustrates several important properties of ion channels. According to their class, channels may open rapidly or slowly and they may stay open or rapidly close even in the presence of a maintained stimulus. Thus the rates of activation and inactivation are clearly important molecular determinants of channel function. Figure 8.5 also illustrates the principle of the voltage clamp whereby the maintenance of a constant level of membrane potential ("clamp") permits the magnitudes, directions and kinetics of ion currents to be measured. This may be achieved at the macroscopic level where large numbers of channels may be studied (tissue, whole cell), with a few channels

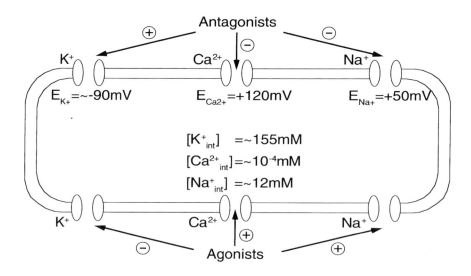

Figure 8.3   The equilibrium potentials for Na⁺, K⁺ and Ca²⁺ and the effects of drugs that open or close selectively these channels. (See text for additional details). (+) Indicates excitatory effects and (−) inhibitory effects on the cell.

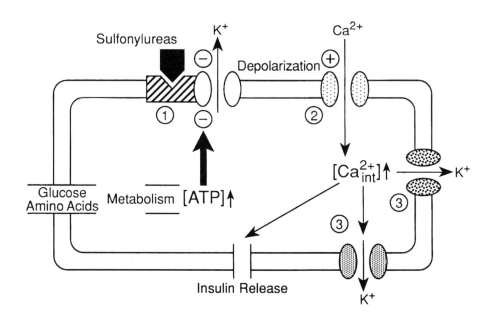

Figure 8.4   Ion channels frequently function in cooperative fashion. In this insulin-secreting pancreatic β-cell ATP derived from metabolic sources blocks K⁺-ATP channels (1) thus depolarizing the cell. This K⁺ channel is the target site for type II antidiabetic sulfonylureas. Depolarization activates Ca²⁺ channels (2) that cause via a Ca²⁺-dependent process the release of insulin. The elevation of Ca²⁺ also activates Ca²⁺-dependent K⁺ channels (3) to restore membrane potential. Thus, the net balance of electrical activity in the cell will be determined by the combined activities of the three types of ion channels.

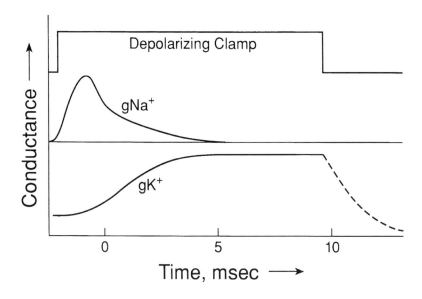

Figure 8.5   Schematic representation of Na$^+$ and K$^+$ conductance changes during a period of maintained depolarization (clamp). The Na$^+$ conductance [gNa$^+$] activates and inactivates rapidly while the K$^+$ conductance [gK$^+$] activates more slowly and does not inactivate during the period of the clamp.

or even with single ion channels as in patch-clamp techniques that study small patches of native or reconstituted membranes (Fig. 8.6).

8.2 ION CHANNELS AND THEIR PROPERTIES

8.2.1 Ion channels as efficient and regulated species

They discriminate ions on the basis of type — cations versus anions — on the basis of charge — monovalent versus divalent — and on the basis of size-according to ionic radius. Channels permeate ions very efficiently at rates $> 10^7$ ion/sec, that approach diffusion controlled limits. Enzymes and carriers operate at orders of magnitude lower efficiency. Thus to charge a membrane of capacity 1 μF/cm^2 by 100 mV requires the transfer of some 6000 ions per square micrometer and with a channel of conductance 20 pS this can be accomplished in 0.5 msec. Because of this efficiency many ion channels are minor components of excitable cells. Channels are also regulated species, regulated most frequently by chemical or electrical potential. Accordingly, ion channels must be accorded a certain minimal organizational structure (Fig. 8.7). It is helpful to regard ion channels analogously to allosteric enzymes, functioning to accelerate ion transit across an essentially impermeable membrane barrier.

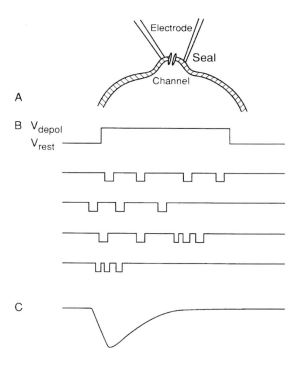

Figure 8.6   The principle of the voltage clamp. (A) In this version a small piece of membrane containing a single open channel is clamped between two electrodes. (B) The opening and closing of single channels is observed as an all-or-none stochastic process and the sum of these openings is shown under (C).

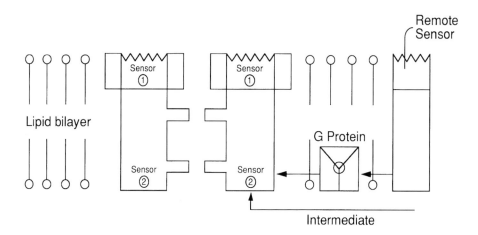

Figure 8.7   The fundamental architecture of ion channels depicting sensors (integral and remote), gates in the middle of the channel pore and both G protein and cytoplasmic routes for messenger modulation of the channel.

Table 8.2   Summary of channel classes.

Voltage-gated channels	Ligand-gated channels
Na^+	γ-Aminobutyric acid
K^+	Glycine
Ca^{2+}	n-AChR
	cyclic-GMP (vision)
	Excitatory amino acids

8.2.2 The structure of ion channels

The structure depicted in Figure 8.7 includes sensors that serve as regulatory components and that are responsive to chemical or physical stimuli, gates that open or close in response to such stimuli, a pore through which ions pass and a "selectivity filter" that confers upon the channel its ionic selectivity. The ionic selectivity of a channel may occur by two limiting, and very different, mechanisms. The channel may select for a desired ion by specific binding or may select against ions by steric factors (molecular sieving). Increasingly, evidence is accumulating that channels discriminate ions according to their specific binding characteristics. That size alone cannot determine permeation through this channel is also evident from the very high Ca^{2+}:Na^+ permeability ratio of approximately 1000, although the bare radii of the two cations are very similar (Na^+, 0.95 Å and Ca^{2+}, 0.99 Å) and the radius of hydrated Ca^{2+} is larger than hydrated Na^+. However, it is also clear that tight binding of an ion within a channel is not compatible with the very high permeation rates that exist. Accordingly, it is likely that channels have multiple ion binding sites and that multiple occupancy of these sites facilitates ion transit, perhaps by mutual ion repulsion.

8.3 THE CLASSIFICATION OF ION CHANNELS

8.3.1 Criteria for ion channel classification

Ion channels may be classified according to a variety of criteria. The nature of the permeant ion serves as one scheme to designate Cl^-, Na^+, K^+ or Ca^{2+} channels. Although appropriately descriptive this classification is very broad, since it is now clear that multiple classes of channels exist for single ions. Additionally, few channels are completely selective for a single ionic species. Channels may be classified according to the nature of the regulatory signal — as potential-dependent channels, activated by changes in membrane potential, and receptor-operated channels that are activated by chemical signals. This primary classification generates two major channel families (Table 8.2), a classification that is confirmed by structural studies (Section 8.6.1). The former class is principally sensitive to changes in membrane potential over defined ranges and the latter to changes in chemical potential through drug-receptor interactions. Receptor-operated channels may, however, exist according to several distinct models in which the chemical sensor is an integral or remote component (Fig. 8.7). Thus, in Figure 8.8a, which represents the nicotinic acetylcholine receptor (nAChR) channel complex (and related proteins of the same family)

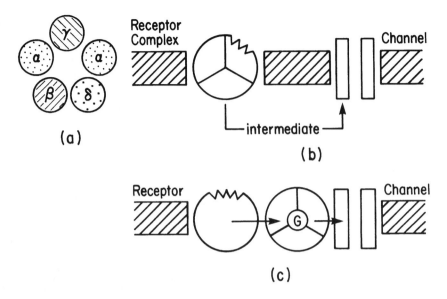

Figure 8.8   Schematic arrangements of ligand-gated ion channels depicting: (a) An oligomeric association of subunits which contain both the ligand binding site and the channel machinery. (b) A separate assembly where the ligand binding site and channel are linked through an intermediate (soluble) messenger. (c) A separate assembly where the ligand binding site and the channel are coupled through an intermediate guanine nucleotide (G) binding protein.

the channel and receptor functions are clearly part of the same protein association, whereas in Figures 8.8b and 8.8c the receptor and channel functions are clearly distinct.

The distinction between receptor-operated and potential-dependent channels is also not absolute. All channels exhibit chemical sensitivity and voltage-dependent channels are well characterized to be modulated by endogenous chemical signals. Thus, the cardiac Ca^{2+} channel is a potential-dependent channel, yet its probability of opening is modulated by the β-adrenoceptor linked adenylate cyclase pathway (kinase A) which phosphorylates the channel. Thus, the total current is given by:

$$I = N_f P_o i$$

where N_f is the total number of functional channels, P_o is the opening probability (zero to one) and i is the unitary current. Phosphorylation serves to increase the probability of channel opening at a particular membrane potential. Since, however, the number of functional channels is given by:

$$N_f = N_t P_f$$

where N_t is the total number of channels and P_f is the probability that the channel is available, it is possible that chemical modulation may also increase the number of channels available.

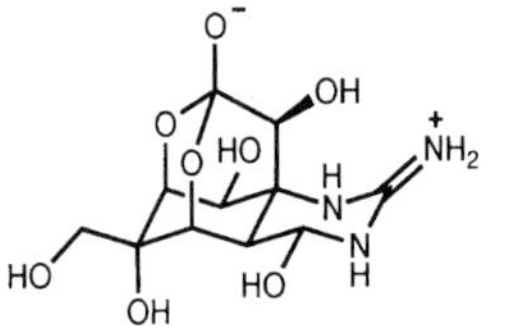

Figure 8.9 Drugs that interact with ion channels: Tetrodotoxin (**8.1**) (Na$^+$) and tetraethylammonium (**8.2**) (K$^+$). Nifedipine (**8.3**), verapamil (**8.4**) and diltiazem (**8.5**) represents the first-generation Ca^{2+} channel antagonists. These drugs interact potently and selectively at the L-type voltage-gated Ca^{2+} channel to define their clinical roles.

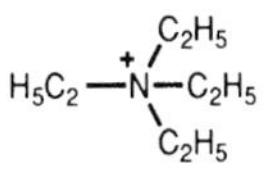

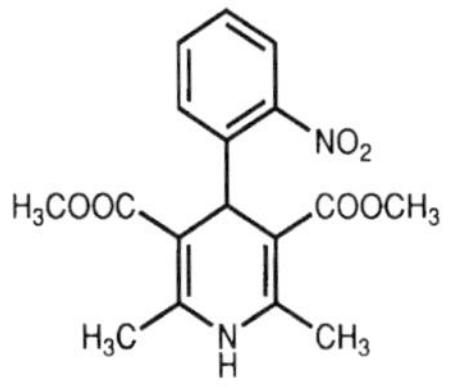

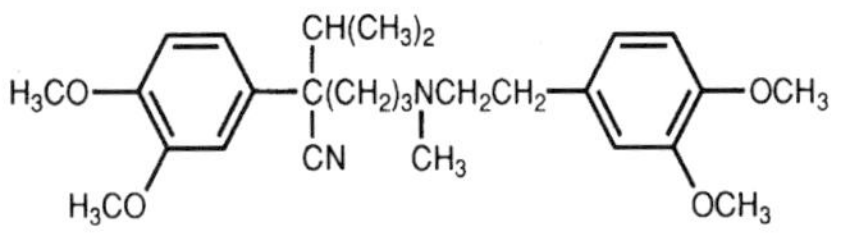

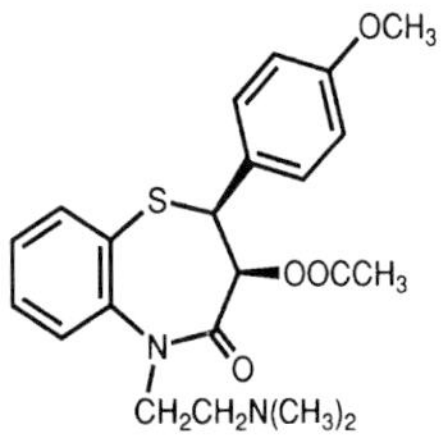

8.3.2 Ion channel classification by electrophysiologic criteria

Channels are also classified according to their electrophysiologic characteristics — conductance (current carried) and kinetics and completeness of activation and inactivation. Such distinctions can be seen clearly in the currents of Figure 8.5 where the Na$^+$ current activates rapidly and inactivates rapidly and completely, whereas the K$^+$ current activates slowly and fails to inactivate over the timescale depicted.

8.3.3 Ion channel classification by drug action

Ion channels may also be classified according to drugs with which they interact. This classification scheme is obviously in place for the ligand-gated ion channels such as the nicotinic acetylcholine receptor, but it is also very applicable to the voltage-gated channels. Thus, the Na$^+$ and K$^+$ currents of Figure 8.5 are discriminated by tetrodotoxin (**8.1**) and tetraethylammonium (**8.2**) (Fig. 8.9), which serve as inhibitors of Na$^+$ and K$^+$ channels, respectively. The 1,4-dihydropyridine nifedipine (**8.3**) blocks voltage-gated Ca^{2+} channels. Naturally occurring toxins and synthetic agents continue to be of major use both to the provision of a pharmacologic classification of ion channels and to the generation of therapeutic agents. Thus, lidocaine, procaine and related compounds owe their local anesthetic and antiarrhythmic properties to their selective interactions with Na$^+$ channels. Similarly, the heterogeneous groups of agents depicted in the lower part of Figure 8.9, including the 1,4-dihydropyridine nifedipine (**8.3**), the phenylalkylamine verapamil (**8.4**) and the benzothiazepine diltiazem (**8.5**) are used as molecular tools for characterization and

Table 8.3   Therapeutic uses of calcium-channel antagonists.

	Antagonists		
Uses	Verapamil (Class I)[*]	Nifedipine (Class II)	Diltiazem (Class III)
Angina:			
exertional	+++	+++	+++
Prinzmetal's	+++	+++	+++
variant	+++	+++	+++
Paroxysmal supraventricular tachyarrhythmias	+++	−	+++
Atrial fibrillation & flutter	++	−	++
Hypertension	++	+++	+
Hypertrophic cardiomyopathy	+	−	−
Raynaud's phenomenon	++	++	++
Cardioplegia	+	+	+
Cerebral vasospasm (posthemorrhage)	−	+[**]	−

[*]Provisional and preliminary classification by World Health Organization.

[**]Refers to nimodipine (Section 8.5.3).

+++, very common use; ++, common use; +, less common use; −, not used.

Table 8.4   Classification of voltage-gated calcium channels[*].

	Channel class			
Property	L	T	N	P
Conductance (pS)	25	8	12–20	10–12
Activation threshold	high	low	high	moderate
Inactivation rate	slow	fast	moderate	rapid
Permeation	$Ba^{2+} > Ca^{2+}$	$Ba^{2+} = Ca^{2+}$	$Ba^{2+} > Ca^{2+}$	$Ba^{2+} > Ca^{2+}$
Function	E-Coupling in cardiovascular system, smooth muscle, endocrine cells and some neurons	Cardiac SA node: neuronal spiking, repetitive spike activity in neurons and endocrine cells	Neuronal only neurotransmitter release	
Pharmacologic sensitivity 1,4-Dihydropyridines (Activators/antagonists) Phenylalkylamines Benzothiazepines	Sensitive	Insensitive	Insensitive	Insensitive
ω-Conotoxin	Sensitive? (some)	Insensitive	Sensitive	Insensitive
Octanol, amiloride	Insensitive?	Sensitive	Insensitive	?
Funnel web spider toxin	Insensitive	Insensitive	Insensitive	Sensitive

[*]This classification, presented particularly from a pharmacologic perspective, is oversimplified. At least one other class of channel exists that is pharmacologically insensitive to the agents listed here.

Table 8.5 Classification of potassium channels.

Class*	Type	Pharmacologic sensitivity		Properties
		Conductance pS	Antagonists/ Activators**	
A. Voltage gated	K_V delayed rectifier	5–60	TEA, 4-AP, LA, 9-AA, PCP, scorpion toxin	Activated with delay; slow inactivating
K_{VR}	-rapid	—	Dofetilide, sotalol quinidine, tedisamil	Rapid activating component of cardiac delayed
K_{VS}	-slow			Very slow activating component of cardiac delayed rectifier
K_A	transient outward	<1–20	4-AP, quinidine THA, PCP DTX, MCDP	Activated by depolarization after period of hyperpolarization
K_{IR}	inward rectifier (anomalous)	5–30	TEA, gaboon viper venom	Conductance greatest at hyperpolarized potentials
B. Ca^{2+}-activated				
BK_{Ca2+}		100–250	TEA, CBTX, noxiustoxin, iberatoxin	Activated by Ca^{2+}_{int}
IK_{Ca2+}		19–50	TEA, quinine CBTX	Activated by Ca^{2+}_{int}
SK_{Ca2+}		6–40	Quinine, 9-AA apamin	Activated by Ca^{2+}_{int}
C. Receptor-coupled				
K_{ACH}		7–50	4-AP, TEA, quinine	G-protein linked
D. Other				
K_{ATP}		5–90	Glibenclamide; tolbutamide; cromakalim, diazoxide	Inhibited by ATP (intracellular) channel activated on metabolic depletion.

*K_{VR} — rapid delayed rectifier; K_{VS} — slow delayed rectifier; K_A — A-type channel; K_{IR} — inward rectifier; BK_{Ca2+} — "big" conductance; IK_{Ca2+} — "intermediate" conductance; SK_{Ca2+} — "small" conductance; K_{ACH} — activated by muscarinic ligands; K_{ATP} — ATP-sensitive.

**TEA, tetraethylammonium; 4-AP, 4-aminopyridine; LA, local anesthetics; 9-AA, 9-aminoacridine; PCP, phencyclidine; THA, tetrahydroaminoacridine; DTX, dendrotoxin; MCDP, mast cell degenerating peptide; CBTX, charybdotoxin.

classification of the voltage-gated Ca^{2+} channel. These agents are also major cardiovascular therapeutic drugs (Table 8.3).

In practice, all of these properties are used to provide a classification of ion channels. This is illustrated in Table 8.4 for the voltage-gated Ca^{2+} channel family. K^+ channels are a particularly diverse group as is illustrated in Table 8.5. The application of molecular biology techniques to receptors and ion channels has added a particularly fundamental base — classification according to primary structure. These techniques (Section 8.6) have revealed that ion channels fall into a limited number of families and that within each family substantial homology exists. Additionally, it is clear that ion channels of apparently fundamentally different characteristics exhibit considerable similarities in their proposed membrane topologies. One of the most important questions now to be solved is that of relating ion channel function to ion channel structure and to generate self-consistent models of channel gating processes.

8.4 ION CHANNELS AS PHARMACOLOGIC RECEPTORS

8.4.1 Receptor properties of ion channels

The pharmacologic specificity of ion channels indicates that they may be considered as pharmacologic receptors. It may then be anticipated that:

1. Channels should exist as homologous protein families
2. Channels should possess specific drug binding sites which exhibit defined structural requirements, including stereoselectivity, for ligands
3. Both activator and antagonist drugs should exist
4. Ion channels may be associated with guanine nucleotide binding (G) proteins that couple many receptor and effector systems
5. Ion channels should be regulated by drug and hormone influence and by pathological state.

These expectations have been realized for a number of ion channels, including the voltage-gated Ca^{2+} channel where drug interactions have been studied with particular intensity. However, ion channels do exhibit a number of specific properties of ligand binding that reflect uniquely their fundamental properties.

8.4.2 State-dependent interactions of ion channels

Ion channels exist in a number of states or families of states where they are resting and activatable, open and permeant and, in the case of voltage-gated channels, inactivated following the activation process (Fig. 8.10). Each of these states represents a different channel conformation and, in principle, a different conformation of, or access pathway to the drug binding site. In the scheme of Figure 8.10 a drug may exhibit a higher affinity for the inactivated state of a channel and will thus serve as an antagonist. Similarly, an agent may stabilize a channel in the open state and function as a channel activator or agonist. Furthermore, alternative pathways for drug access to a binding site may exist. A hydrophilic agent with preferential affinity for the inactivated channel state may access this state preferentially through the open channel conformation (pathway A, Fig. 8.10), whereas a hydrophobic species that partitions extensively into the membrane may access the site through the lipid bilayer pathway of the membrane (pathway B, Fig. 8.10). Similar considerations dictate the pathways by which these drugs leave their channel binding sites. According to this modulated receptor hypothesis:

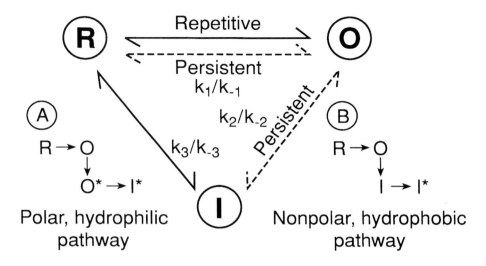

Figure 8.10   The "modulated-receptor" mechanism of drug action at ion channels. Drugs may bind to or access preferentially binding sites in the channel during resting, open or inactivated states. These sites may offer different affinities and hence drug potency will vary with equilibrium between channel states as determined by physiologic or pathologic stimulus. Repetitive depolarization defines a frequency-dependent process: persistent depolarization defines a maintained state of depolarization. As example one may note cardiac and vascular smooth muscle, respectively.

1. Different channel states have different affinities for drugs
2. Drugs may exhibit quantitatively and qualitatively different structure-activity relationships for different channel states
3. Drugs stabilize different channel states
4. Drugs alter the kinetics of channel state interconversion

These considerations apply both to voltage-gated and ligand-gated ion channels and examples of drugs that exhibit state-dependent binding are readily available for both channel classes. If drug binding is considered at two states, A and B, characterized by dissociation constants K_A and K_B, then K_{app}, the observed dissociation constant, will be given by:

$$K_{app} = 1/[h/K_A] + [1 - h/K_B]$$

where h is the fraction of the channel in state A and $1 - h$ is the fraction of the channel in state B.

These state-dependent interactions are illustrated in a number of ways. The local anesthetic lidocaine demonstrates enhanced affinity, by a factor of several hundred-fold, in its selective interactions for the depolarized (inactivated) state of the Na^+ channel (Fig. 8.11). Access to and from binding sites associated with the ion channel will also control drug-receptor interactions. Interaction of local anesthetics with Na^+ channels reveals a clear dependence of potency upon stimulation frequency (Fig. 8.12). This frequency-dependent property is consistent with a process whereby drug binding requires

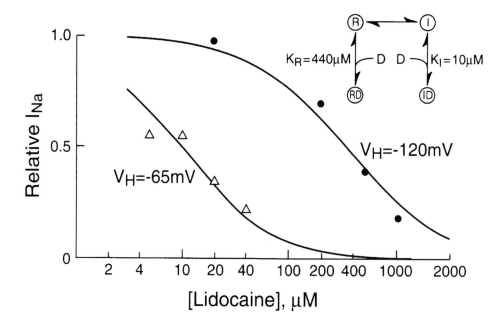

Figure 8.11   Voltage-dependent binding of lidocaine at the Na$^+$ channel. Dose-response curves for lidocaine inhibition of Na$^+$ current (I_{Na+}) at holding potentials of −120 mV and −65 mV [From Bean, Cohen and Tsien, (1983) *J. Gen. Physiol.*, **8**, 613–642].

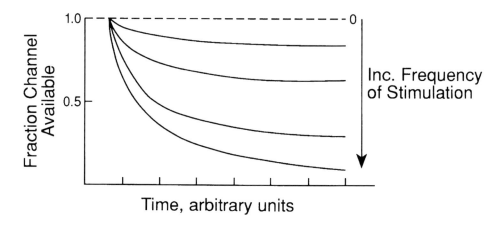

Figure 8.12   Schematic representation of drug with frequency-dependent inhibition of ion channel function. At a fixed concentration of drug and with the depicted increased frequency of stimulation there is an increased inhibition of channel function.

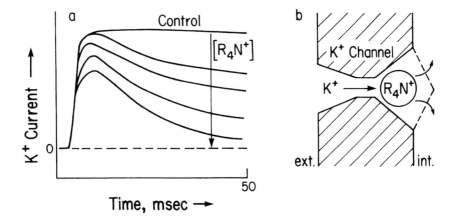

Figure 8.13 (a) Time-dependent blockade of K^+ current by quaternary ammonium ion. The extent of block is dependent upon time and progressively increases with duration of channel opening. This suggests that the blocking drug accesses a binding site via an open channel state. (b) Schematic representation of a quaternary ammonium ion K^+ channel blocker being trapped in the pore after channel closure. K^+ ion movements and channel opening will serve to displace the blocker.

channel opening, whereas drug dissociation can occur during stimulus-free intervals. Thus with increasing frequency of stimulation drug progressively accumulates at the binding sites to block channel function.

Quaternary ammonium ions block K^+ channels and reveal further complexities in channel-drug interactions (Fig. 8.13). Quaternary ammonium ions applied intracellularly to nerve fibers will enter and block the channel only during the open state. The channel may close with drug trapped at the binding site from which it cannot escape until the channel is reopened.

Similarly, drugs that function as non-competitive antagonists in ligand-gated channels may interact at sites associated with the channel rather than the receptor component of the receptor-channel complex. At the nicotinic acetylcholine receptor the quaternary ammonium local anesthetic QX 222 (**8.6**) preferentially interacts with the open channel state, and at the N-methyl-D-aspartate class of excitatory amino acid receptors the agents phencyclidine (**8.7**) and MK-801 (**8.8**) (Fig. 8.14) bind also with highest affinity to the open channel state (see Chapter 9).

These state-dependent aspects of drug interactions at ion channels are important from three perspectives. They are important in the determination of selectivity of action. Thus properties of voltage- and frequency-dependent interactions of local anesthetics underscore their general utility as Class I antiarrhythmic agents, whereby the efficacy of the drug is in principle enhanced by pathologic electrophysiologic conditions.

The state-dependent interactions also serve as valuable molecular probes of channel structure and function by revealing subtleties of interactions and access pathways. Finally, these interactions are important to the determination of structure-activity relationships of drugs active at ion channels.

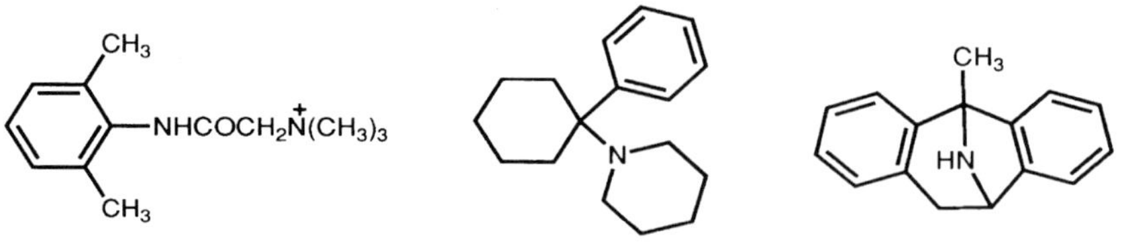

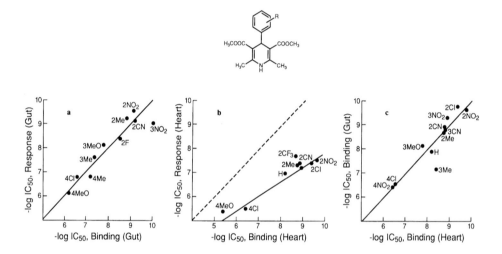

(8.6)   (8.7)   (8.8)

Figure 8.14   Structural formulae of drugs that show selective interactions with the open state of the Na^+ channel [QX-222 (**8.6**)] or the ligand-gated NMDA channel [PCP (**8.7**) and MK-801 (**8.8**)].

Figure 8.15   Comparison of the binding and pharmacologic affinities of a series of 1,4-dihydropyridines in smooth and cardiac muscle. The 1,4-dihydropyridines are all analogs of nifedipine (**8.4**) with the indicated phenyl ring substituents. Binding and pharmacologic affinities were measured in, a: intestinal smooth muscle, b: cardiac muscle. A comparison of binding affinities in the two preparations is depicted in panel c. The filled line represents the lines of regression and the dashed line 1:1 equivalence.

8.4.3 Structure-activity relationships and state-dependent properties

The interpretation of structure-activity relationships for channel active drugs is complex since it may depend significantly upon the choice of experimental conditions. These conditions may be best controlled during electrophysiologic studies. Such studies may not generate large structure-activity relationships, but they can establish the fundamental modes of interaction of lead compounds. Accordingly, comparisons of drug activities under different experimental conditions or in different preparations must be interpreted with care. Differences in activity may indicate the existence of channel subtypes, but may be equally consistent with the existence of state-dependent interactions. The comparisons of

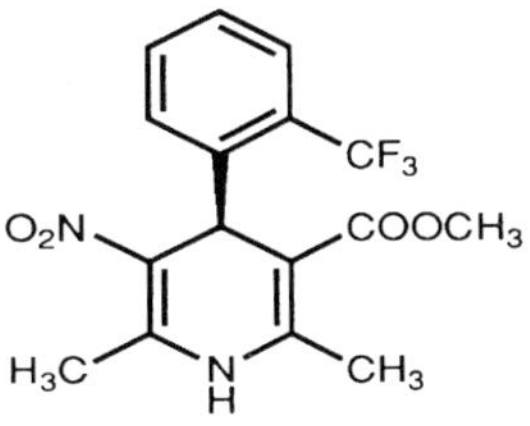

(8.9) (*S*)-form, Activator 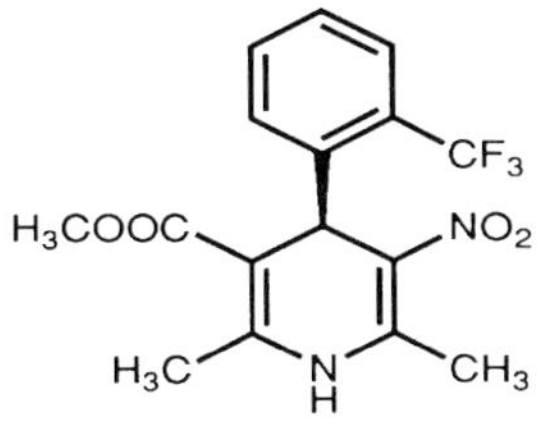   **(8.10)** (*R*)-form, Antagonist

Figure 8.16   The enantiomers of 1,4-dihydropyridines that show activator (*S*) and antagonist (*R*) properties.

Local Anesthetic Stereoselectivity

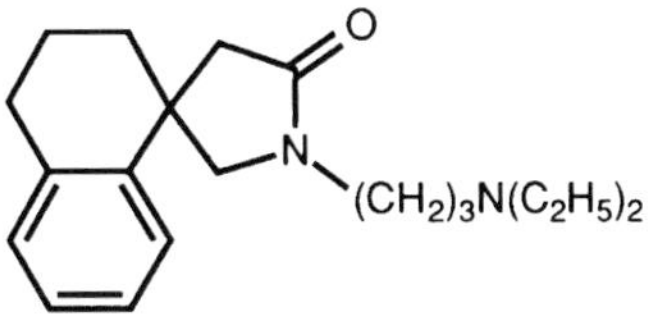

	Enantiomeric Ratio	
Tonic block	Phasic block	Phasic block
	0 mV	+80 mV
1.0	5.0	14

(8.11)

Figure 8.17   The stereoselectivity of a chiral local anesthetic according to stimulus mode. Tonic block describes the Na$^+$ channel under resting condition and phasic block describes the Na$^+$ channel under two states of progressively increased depolarization.

pharmacologic and radioligand binding activities of a series of 1,4-dihydropyridine Ca^{2+} channel antagonists of the nifedipine class depicted in Figure 8.15 is illustrative of this issue. Clearly, the higher pharmacologic activity of this series in smooth muscle relative to cardiac muscle may indicate receptor subtypes with different affinities. However, the equal binding affinities of the same compounds revealed in the radioligand binding data obtained from depolarized membrane preparations are consistent with the existence of voltage-dependent binding. Thus binding affinity increases with increasing and maintained depolarization: this will be the situation with smooth muscle where maintained depolarization, rather than the repetitive depolarization observed for cardiac muscle, is the stimulus mode.

A further example, also from the 1,4-dihydropyridine class, derives from the enantiomeric pair of Figure 8.16. In this series the (*S*)- and (*R*)-enantiomers show activator and antagonist properties, respectively. However, if the (*S*)-enantiomer interact with channels in a depolarized state it may function as an antagonist species. A further example is presented in Figure 8.17 where the stereoselectivity of a local anesthetic varies according to stimulus mode, increasing under those conditions that favor the inactivated state of the Na$^+$ channel. Thus, state-dependent interactions may generate both quantitative and qualitative changes in structure-activity relationships.

Table 8.6   Classification of drug action at voltage-gated Na^+ channels.

Receptor site	Drugs	Channel response
1	Tetrodotoxin	Inhibition of permeation
	Saxitoxin	
	ω-Conotoxin	
2	Veratridine	Persistent activation
	Batrachotoxin	
	Aconitine	
	Grayanotoxin	
3	α-Scorpion toxin [North African]	Inhibit activation
		Enhance persistent activation
	Sea Anenome toxin	
4	β-Scorpion toxin [North American]	Shift activation
5	Ptychodiscus brevis toxin [red tide]	Repetitive firing
	Ciguatoxin	Persistent activation

Data from Catterall (1989).

8.5 DRUGS ACTING AT SPECIFIC ION CHANNELS

8.5.1 Multiple sites for drug action

A major characteristic of drug action at ion channels is the existence of multiple binding sites for different classes of drugs. These sites are frequently linked one to the other and to the functional machinery of the channel by complex allosteric interactions. Thus, binding of a drug to one site may not only alter ion permeation, but may also alter simultaneously the binding of drugs at other discrete sites associated with the channel. Useful examples are provided by the Na^+, Ca^{2+} and K^+ channels as representative of voltage-gated channels and the K^+-ATP and NMDA receptor as examples of ligand gated channels.

8.5.2 Drug action at Na^+ channels

At least five major classes of drugs interact at the Na^+ channel where they mediate a number of discrete responses (Table 8.6). The guanidinium toxins, tetrodotoxin (**8.1**) and the closely related saxitoxin are generally assumed to block the ion permeation pathway proper of the Na^+ channel and it is possible that the guanidinium group itself interacts with carboxyl residues of the channel. However, the chemistry of these and related toxins has not encouraged the synthesis of analogs and structure-activity data are scarce. It seems clear, however, that both the guanidinium function and hydroxyl groups are necessary for effective interactions. In contrast, the other groups of Na^+ channel drugs exhibit more complex interactions with their properties being profoundly state-dependent. Veratridine (**8.13**) and the lipid-soluble alkaloid toxins (Fig. 8.18) have the common property of causing Na^+ channels to open and to remain open at rest. Although these agents may not interact via a single process, consistent with their very different chemical structures, the net consequence of their interaction is to produce a state of persistent activation of the Na^+ channel. This appears to be achieved by a selective binding and stabilization of the open channel state.

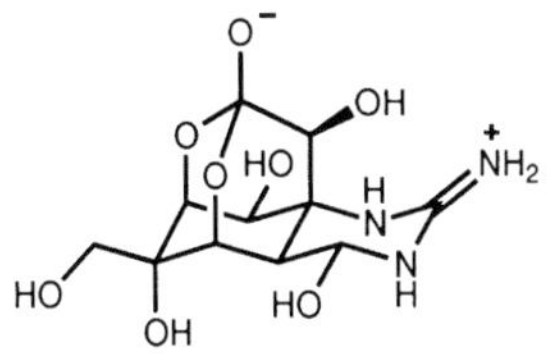

(8.1) 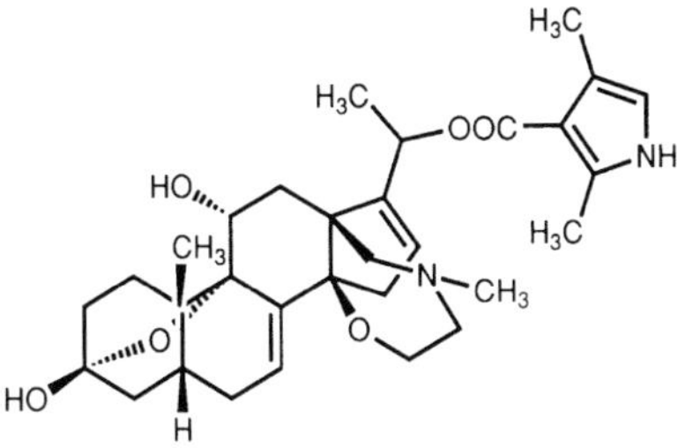   (8.12)

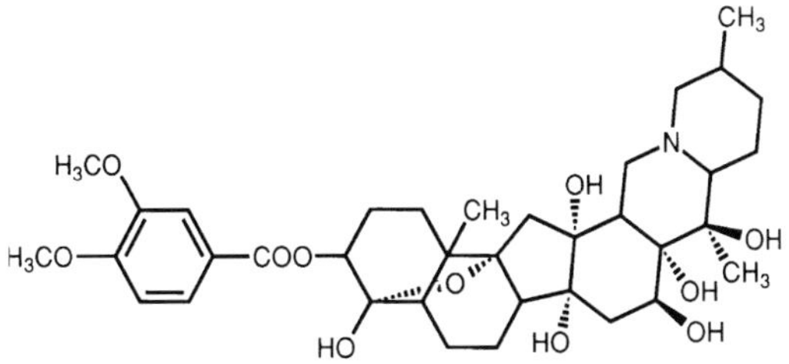

(8.13) 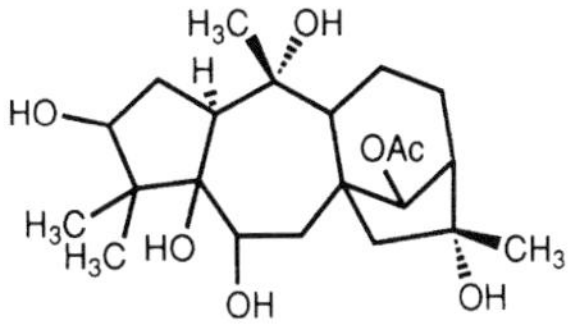   (8.14)

Figure 8.18   Structural formulae of toxins interacting at the Na$^+$ channel, tetrodotoxin (**8.1**), batrachotoxin (**8.12**), veratridine (**8.13**) and grayanotoxin (**8.14**).

Thus, drug modified channels are activated at membrane potentials far more negative than unmodified channels and these activated channels fail to inactivate.

A variety of peptide toxins also interact at Na$^+$ channels and are derived from scorpions, sea anemones and fish-hunting cone snails. The toxins from sea anemones and scorpions are small proteins with 46–50 and 60–70 amino acid residues, respectively, and the ω-conotoxins from cone snails are significantly smaller with 22 residues. They all contain several disulfide bridges, three each for conus and sea anemone toxins and four for the scorpion toxins, which renders their structure both compact and rigid. However, the toxins interact via different mechanisms at the Na$^+$ channel. The conotoxins appear to act similarly to tetrodotoxin, whilst the scorpion and anemone toxins exhibit more complex interactions. The latter two shift activation curves to more negative membrane potentials, facilitating Na$^+$ channel opening, and inhibit channel inactivation. Although the pharmacology of the Na$^+$ channel has been dominated by naturally occurring alkaloids and toxins, increasing attention is being paid to the pyrethroid insecticides, synthetic analogs of the pyrethrin neurotoxins isolated from Chysanathemums. These agents (Fig. 8.19) interact with Na$^+$ channels in a manner similar to that of veratridine and they bind preferentially to the open channel state.

8.5.3 Drug action at Ca^{2+} channels

In marked contrast to the situation with the Na$^+$ channel, the pharmacology of the Ca^{2+} channel has been dominated by synthetic agents of the 1,4-dihydropyridine,

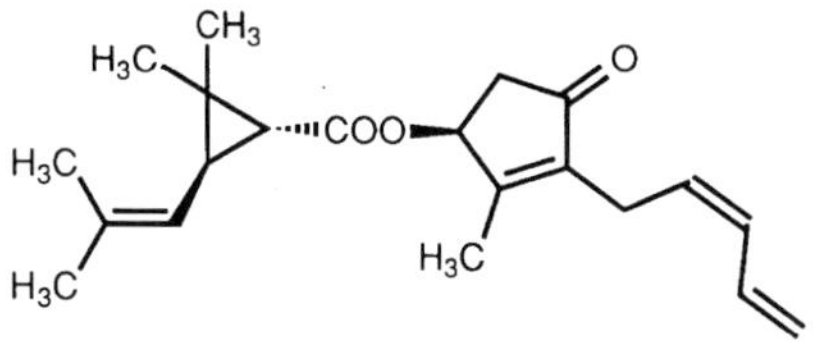

(8.15)

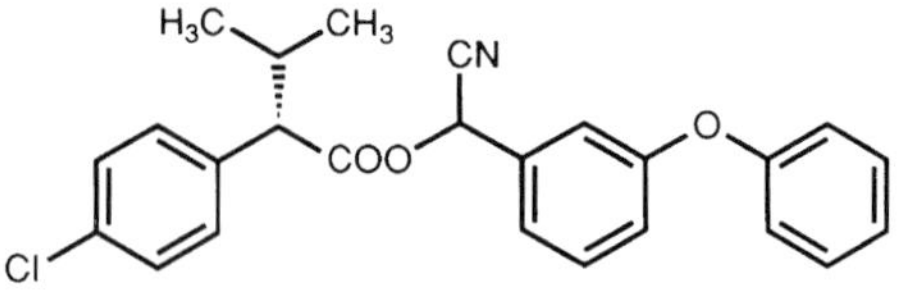

(8.16)

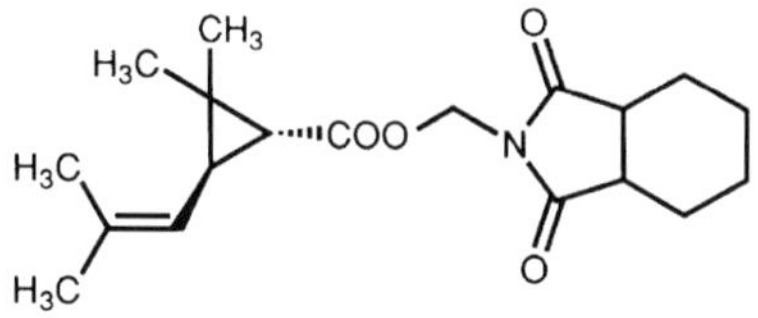

(8.17)

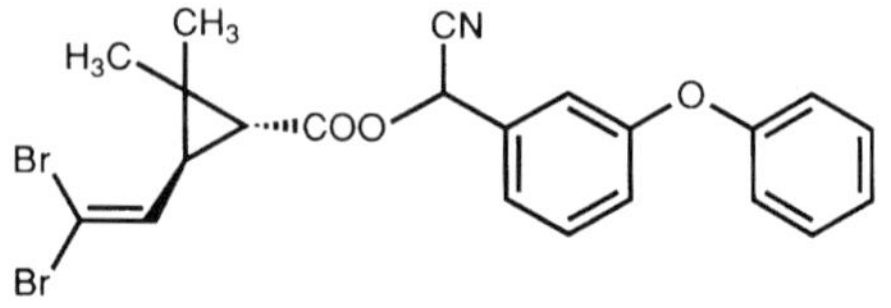

(8.18)

Figure 8.19   Some pyrethrins active at the Na$^+$ channel, pyrethrin I (**8.15**), fenvalerate (**8.16**) and analogues.

phenylalkylamine and benzothiazepine classes (Fig. 8.9). These agents have served simultaneously as molecular probes of the Ca^{2+} channel and as valuable drugs employed in a variety of cardiovascular disorders (Table 8.3). Although these drugs inhibit Ca^{2+} current through the L class of voltage-gated Ca^{2+} channels, they do so by interaction at discrete sites. This is consistent with their chemical heterogeneity and no single all-encompassing structure-activity correlation can be described. The arrangement of these sites is shown schematically in Figure 8.20 which depicts a set of allosteric linkages. Quite generally, these agents exhibit state-dependent interactions associating preferentially with the inactivated state of the channel. Thus, under depolarizing conditions, which favor the equilibrium between the open and inactivated channel states (Fig. 8.10) the activity of these agents is enhanced. However, verapamil (**8.4**) and diltiazem (**8.5**), which are protonated species at physiological pH, exhibit frequency-dependent interactions, whereas the neutral nifedipine (**8.3**) exhibits voltage-dependent interactions. This difference in mechanisms may reflect hydrophilic and hydrophobic access pathways for these drugs and may also underlie their different therapeutic indications with verapamil being an effective antiarrhythmic agent and nifedipine lacking such properties (Table 8.3). 1,4-Dihydropyridine interactions at the Ca^{2+} channel can initiate both antagonist and activator responses and the 1,4-dihydropyridine structure embraces both antagonist and activator ligands.

Consistent with the view of ion channels as pharmacologic receptors each of the discrete binding sites at the Ca^{2+} channel can be described by structure-activity relationships. These have been best investigated for the 1,4-dihydropyridines and are summarized in Figure 8.21. In a QSAR approach to 1,4-dihydropyridine interactions, activity in a series of nifedipine analogs bearing substituents in the phenyl ring could be described by:

$$\log 1/IC_{50} = 0.62\pi + 1.96\sigma m - 0.44 L\text{meta} - 3.26 B_1\text{para} - 1.51 L\text{meta}' + 14.23$$

$$n = 46, r = 0.90, s = 0.67, F = 33.93$$

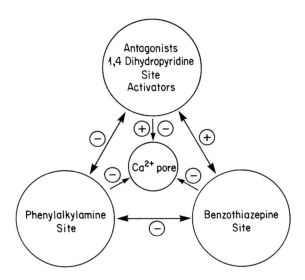

Figure 8.20 Representation of three primary pharmacologic receptors at the voltage-gated Ca^{2+} channel depicting their linkage to the permeation and gating machinery of the channel and the allosteric linkages between the discrete receptor sites (+, stimulating; −, antagonizing).

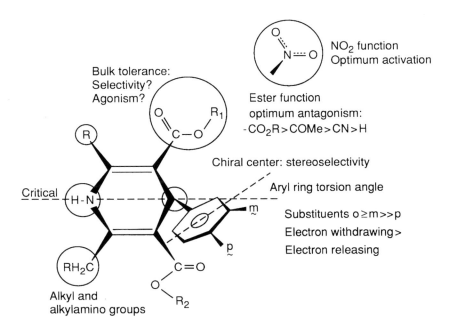

Figure 8.21 The structure-activity relationships of 1,4-dihydropyridine activators and antagonists.

where σm is the electronic parameter, π a hydrophobicity index and L and B_1 are steric parameters. The stereochemical requirements for interaction of the 1,4-dihydropyridines have been examined through several techniques including the synthesis of rigid analogs, the determination of solid state and solution conformations and the application of computing techniques. There is general agreement that the requirements for optimum activity include a flattened boat conformation of the 1,4-dihydropyridine ring and a pseudoaxial aryl ring oriented orthogonally to the 1,4-dihydropyridine ring with the aryl substituents oriented away (antiperiplanar) from the 1,4-dihydropyridine ring (Fig. 8.21). Additionally, in selected 1,4-dihydropyridines there is a remarkable enantiomeric discrimination of biological activity whereby the (S)- and (R)-enantiomers exhibit potent activator and antagonist properties respectively (Fig. 8.16). Because the interactions of the (S)- and (R)-enantiomers are differently modulated by membrane potential the properties of the (S)-enantiomer undergo a transition from activator at polarized membrane potentials to antagonist at depolarized states. Such agents may be regarded as molecular chameleons of the Ca^{2+} channel.

The 1,4-dihydropyridine series of antagonists also provides a useful example of how first- and second-generation drugs may differ. Second-generation 1,4-dihydropyridines, including nimodipine, nitrendipine, felodipine and amlodipine interact at the 1,4-dihydropyridine receptor of the L-type voltage-gated channel (Fig. 8.22), but exhibit specific original vascular selectivity.

K^+ channels are a remarkably diverse group with corresponding diverse pharmacology (Table 8.5). From the clinical perspective particular attention has been directed to the K^+-ATP channel where both activators and antagonists exist (Fig. 8.23). The type II antidiabetic sulfonylureas, including the first- and second-generation tolbutamide (**8.19**) and glibenclamide (**8.20**), function as antagonists, whilst a diverse collection of molecules, including cromakalim (**8.21**), nicorandil (**8.22**) and pinacidil (**8.23**), function as activators (Fig. 8.23). The latter class of agents have attracted particular attention because of their potential cardiovascular (hypertension, angina), noncardiovascular (asthma, urinary incontinence) and central nervous system (anticonvulsant, anti-neurodegenerative) therapeutic roles.

The ion channels thus far discussed represent multiple drug receptors — multiple drug binding sites regulating channel function. The ligand-gated channels for excitatory (glutamic acid) and inhibitory [glycine and γ-aminobutyric acid (GABA)] present a similar situation with multiple discrete activator and antagonist sites (Chapters 9 and 10).

8.6 STRUCTURE AND FUNCTION OF ION CHANNELS

8.6.1 Families of ion channels

Structural studies indicate that there are at least two major families of ion channels. This structural classification into the voltage-gated and ligand-gated families parallels the functional classification previously established. Biochemical and molecular biologic studies have permitted the determination of the sequences of the Na^+, K^+ and Ca^{2+} voltage-gated channels and of the n-AChR, $GABA_A$, glycine and ATP ligand-gated channels. The major issue is now to generate from these sequences detailed models of channel organization and

Ca²⁺ Antagonist Classification

	Vasodilation	Contractility	A-V Conduction
Verapamil	++	+++	+++
Diltiazem	++	++	++
1,4-Dihydropyridines			
Nifedipine	+++	+	0
Nicardipine			
Isradipine			
Amlodipine			
Felodipine	++++	0	0

Figure 8.22 The classification of first and second generation Ca²⁺ channel antagonists in terms of vascular:cardiac selectivity. The actions of the drugs in producing vasodilation, depression of cardiac contractility and depression of cardiac conduction provide an index of selectivity. 0 to ++++ indicates increasing activity. All 1,4-dihydropyridines are more vascular selective than verapamil or diltiazem and the second generation 1,4-dihydropyridines are more vascular-selective than nifedipine.

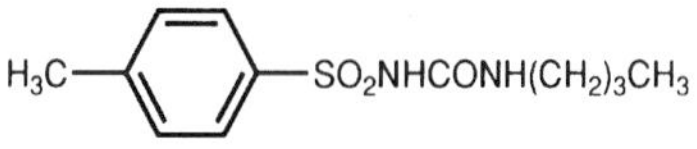

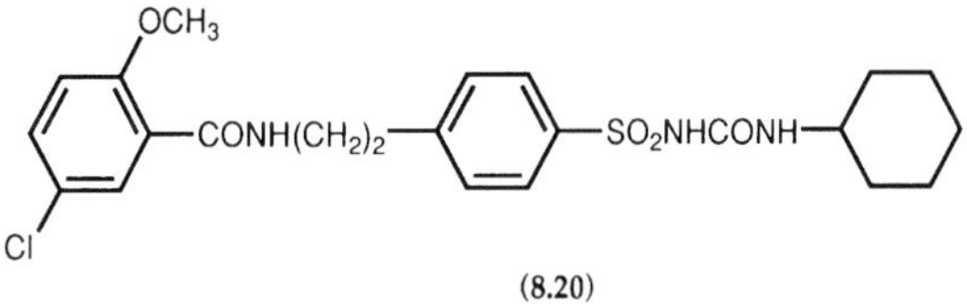

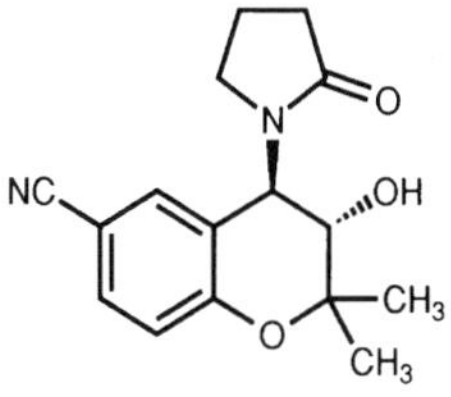

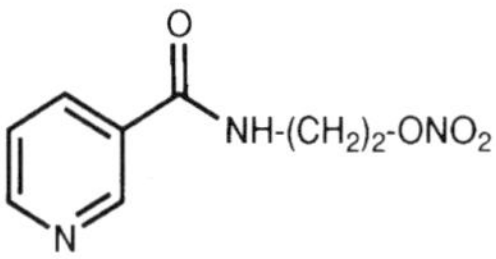

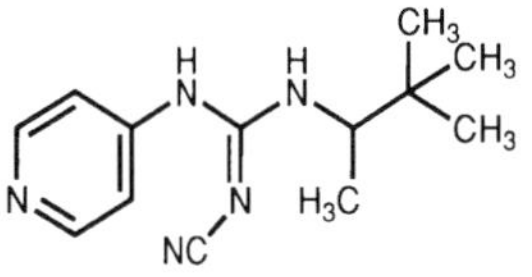

Figure 8.23 Drugs active at the K⁺-ATP channel (see also Fig. 8.4). Antagonists; tolbutamide (**8.19**) and glibenclamide (**8.20**). Activators; cromakalim (**8.21**), nicorandil (**8.22**) and pinacidil (**8.23**).

to correlate structure and function including the definition of the sites and mechanisms of drug action.

Each of these major channel families is internally homologous, but both families share fundamental structural and topologic similarities. This common structural plan consists of an approximately symmetric disposition of homologous subunits or domains surrounding a central pore. The ligand-gated channels are composed of a set of subunits of molecular weight approximately 45–60 kDa which, though substantially homologous, bear specialized functions including the receptor and regulatory drug binding sites. Complete expression of ligand-gated channel function requires the participation of all subunits. Voltage-gated channels are also subunit structures, but the principal channel functions are associated with the major subunit of molecular weight approximately 200 kDA which is made up of four homologous domains. An exception to this arrangement of voltage-gated channels is provided by the K^+ channel, which is composed of a single polypeptide containing one domain homologous to those of the larger Na^+ and Ca^{2+} channels. A comparison of the major organizational features of these two channel families is provided in Figure 8.24. Hydropathy profiles indicate that each of the subunits of the ligand-gated channels or the domains of the voltage-gated channels have a number of transmembrane helices, four and six for the two classes respectively, and that these transmembrane components, which are highly homologous within families, contain the functional and gating machinery of the ion channels.

The smaller size of the K^+ channel suggests that it may be ancestral to other channels. Consistent with this argument there are more variations on the K^+ channel structural theme than on other ion channels. This thematic diversity is illustrated in Figure 8.25.

Quite generally ion channels show remarkable structural conservation across major evolutionary periods — Drosophila to man. This is an eloquent testimony both to the cellular importance of ion channels and to the fitness of molecular design once achieved.

8.6.2 Structure-function correlations

Increasingly, knowledge of the sequences of ion channels and of their components makes it possible to assign specific structural motifs to defined functions including the sites of drug action. A detailed exposition of these findings is outside the scope of this text, but two illustrative examples may be helpful.

The GABA gated Cl^- channel is a heteromeric organization of homologous subunits. This pentameric association is derived from five classes of subunits — α, β, γ, δ and ρ. Functional receptors may be homomeric or heteromeric, but the pharmacological and biophysical properties depend critically upon the subunit composition. Thus, homomeric receptors respond to GABA, the physiologic ligand, the presence of the γ-subunit together with α- and β-subunits is critical for the expression of benzodiazepine activity. Thus, in the absence of the γ-subunit the characteristic potentiation of GABA inhibition by benzodiazepines such as diazepam is not observed. Additionally, the pharmacology of the heteromeric assembly may depend quantitatively upon the nature of individual subunits. Thus, the GABA receptor containing the α_6-subunit, which is found only in cerebellar granule cells, has a very low affinity for benzodiazepine agonists such as diazepam, but a high affinity for benzodiazepine antagonists such as Ro 15-4513 (Chapter 10).

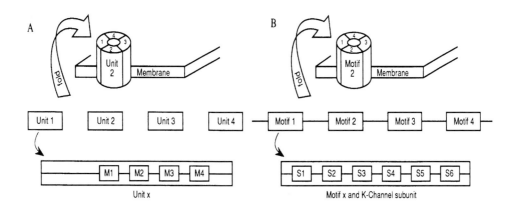

Figure 8.24   Schematic representation of the organizational features of ligand- and voltage-gated ion channels. A. Ligand-gated channels are depicted as composed of several subunits each with four [M1–M4] transmembrane helices. B. Voltage-gated channels are depicted as composed of four similar domains (motifs 1–4) each possessing six transmembrane helices (S_1–S_6) of which S_4 represents the voltage-sensor. This model is operative for Na^+ and Ca^{2+} channels, but K^+ channels represent a single domain that forms tetramers to generate a functional channel (see Fig. 8.25). Reproduced with permission from Stevens, (1987) *Nature*, **328**, 198. Copyright 1987, Macmillan Journals.

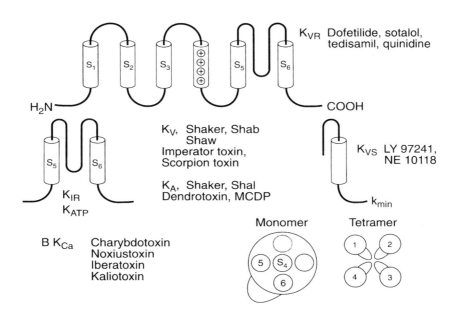

Figure 8.25 K^+ channels present a considerable variety of structures and properties (Table 8.5). These are illustrated here for several basic channel types — K_V, K_A, K_{IR}, K_{ATP} and BK_{Ca} together with a proposed model of tetrameric organization to form a functional channel. At least three principal structural classes exist defined by the number of transmembrane segments — 6, 2 or 1. Illustrated are arrangements of known channel types to structural class and pharmacologic sensitivity. The terms "Shaker, Shab, Shaw and Shal" define the channel clones as isolated from "Drosophila".

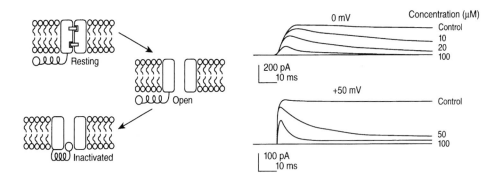

Figure 8.26 Schematic representation of inactivation mode of K$^+$ channel. Left: the N-terminal segment serves as a "ball-and-chain" to inactivate the open channel. Right: intracellular addition of free segments of the N-terminal peptide at the concentrations indicated can produce inactivation of a non-inactivating channel (see B. Hille for further details).

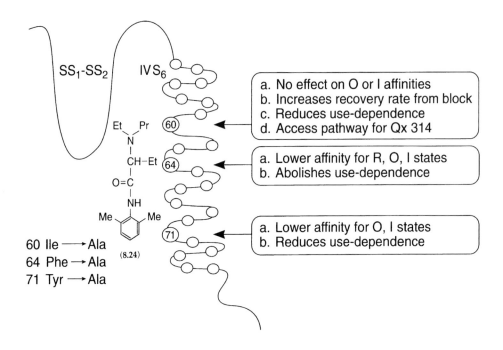

Figure 8.27 Structure-activity relationships in Na$^+$ channel for interaction with the local anesthetic etidocaine (**8.24**). Mutations by alanine replacement at the positions 60, 64 and 71 indicated in transmembrane helix S$_6$ of domain IV (adjacent to pore-forming region SS$_1$–SS$_2$) produced the indicated effects in channel function; resting (R), open (O) and inactivated (I) states. Data from Ragsdale, McPhee, Scheuer and Catterall, (1994) *Science*, **265**, 1724.

Voltage-gated ion channels present a similar transmembrane profile, but have six transmembrane helices designated S1 to S6 (Fig. 10.24). The S4 helix has a common sequence in all voltage-gated channels being composed of positively charged lysine and arginine residues separated by two nonpolar functions. Each helix thus carries five or six positive charges and may well serve as the voltage sensor for these channels. As the membrane depolarizes, this helix unscrews by breaking and remaking hydrogen bonds to adjacent helices and thus effectively transfers one gating charge. Progressive replacement of these positive charges by neutral residues shifts the voltage-dependence of the channel activation process. Other sequences of these channels can be identified with other functions. The intracellular sequence linking domains III and IV of the Na^+ channel is likely critical to channel inactivation since in its absence Na^+ channels fail to inactivate following opening. Similarly, the Ca^{2+} N-channel terminus is believed also to act as an inactivation particle, binding to the open intracellular mouth of the channel and causing inactivation (Fig. 8.26).

Local anesthetics interact at the Na^+ channel in state-dependent fashion. The binding site and some of the molecular determinants defining voltage- and frequency-dependent interactions have now been defined by the process of site-directed mutagenesis. These determinants are outlined in Figure 8.27.

8.7 FUTURE DEVELOPMENTS

Ion channels represent both a major challenge and a major opportunity to the discipline of medicinal chemistry. They are a major challenge because of the conformational changes integral to channel function, the ability to classify drug action and because determination of structure-activity relationships is more difficult than in other receptors. The opportunities arise because these difficulties are being realized at the very time that molecular biology is making available detailed information about channel structure and function. Additionally, ion channels represent a major opportunity because they serve as major integrating loci of the cell where many different signals are integrated to modulate the health and welfare of the cell. Ion channel drugs will become increasingly important as we move the science of Medicinal Chemistry to the Twenty-First Century.

FURTHER READING

Anderson, O.S. and Koeppe, R.E. (1992) Molecular Determinants of Channel Functions. *Physiol. Revs.*, **72**, S89–S158.

Brown, A.M. (1993) Functional Bases for Interpreting Amino Acid Sequences of Voltage–dependent K^+ channels. *Ann. Rev. Biophys. Biomol. Struct.*, **22**, 173–198.

Catterall, W.A. (1988) Structure and Function of Voltage-Sensitive Ion Channels. *Science*, **242**, 50–61.

Catterall, W.A. (1992) Cellular and Molecular Biology of Voltage-gated Sodium Channels. *Physiol. Revs.*, **72**, S15–S48.

Cook, N.S. (Ed.) (1990) *Potassium Channels*. Halsted Press, UK.

Hille, B. (1992) *Ionic Channels in Excitable Membranes.*, 2nd Ed., Sinauer Assoc., Sunderland, MA.

McDonough, S. and Lester, H.A. (1994) Overview of the Relationship Between Structure and Function In Ion Channels. *Drug Dev. Res.*, **33**, 190–202.

Nichols, C.G. and Gross, J. (1994) Spotlight on ATP-sensitive Potassium Channels. *Cardiovas. Res.*, **28**, 725–931.

North, R.A. (Ed.) (1994) *Ligand- and Voltage-gated Ion Channels*. CRC Press, Boca Raton, FL.

Rampe, D. (1994) Ion Channels. *Drug. Dev. Res.*, **33**, 189–372.

Trends in Pharmacological Sciences (1994) Receptor and Ion Channel Nomenclature Supplement.

Triggle, D.J. (1990) Drugs Acting on Ion Channels In Membrane. In *Comprehensive Medicinal Chemistry*, edited by C. Hansch, J.C. Emmett, P.D. Kennewell, C.A. Ramsden, P.G. Sammes and J.B. Taylor. Vol. 3, pp. 647–1099, Pergamon Press, Oxford, UK.

Triggle, D.J. and Langs, D.A. (1990) Ligand-gated and Voltage-gated Ion Channels. *Ann. Rep. Med. Chem.*, **25**, 225–234.

9. EXCITATORY AMINO ACID RECEPTORS

ULF MADSEN

CONTENTS

9.1 GLUTAMIC ACID: EXCITATORY AMINO ACID AND EXCITOTOXIN

(S)-Glutamic acid (Glu) and a number of other endogenous acidic amino acids show excitatory effects when applied on central neurones. These excitatory amino acids also show neurotoxic properties when administered locally either at high concentrations for short periods or at lower concentrations for longer periods of time. This combination of neuroexcitatory activity and neurotoxic properties have been termed "excitotoxicity" and seems to be a general phenomenon for excitatory amino acids.

9.1.1 Neurotransmitter role of glutamic acid

Glu is ubiquitously distributed in the central nervous system (CNS) in high concentrations, where it functions as the major excitatory neurotransmitter. In addition Glu participates in many metabolic processes and it is a precursor for the inhibitory neurotransmitter γ-aminobutyric acid (GABA) (see Chapter 10). The high concentrations of Glu found in the CNS made it difficult to accept a transmitter role of Glu. Specific release and uptake mechanisms have, however, been identified and characterized, and these mechanisms can explain how the concentration-levels of Glu in the synaptic cleft is regulated. These highly efficient systems control the synaptic activity and prevent the above mentioned neurotoxicity of Glu in the normal mature brain. It is still unclear to what extent other acidic amino acids, such as (S)-aspartic acid or (S)-homocysteic acid, serve as endogenous neurotransmitters. Glu receptors are present in high numbers on most neurones in the CNS, reflecting its importance for many different physiological functions, such as learning and memory. Glu receptors play an important role in the synaptic plasticity associated with these mechanisms, and these aspects open interesting therapeutic possibilities for Glu receptor agonists or other agents enhancing synaptic excitatory activity. Such agents may be used for improving learning and memory functions, in certain pathological situations (see Section 9.5).

9.1.2 Excitatory amino acids and neurodegenerative disorders

In certain neurodegenerative disorders such as Alzheimer's disease, Huntington's chorea and epilepsy hyperactivity of Glu probably is a factor of importance. The pattern of neurodegeneration is different for these diseases and involves different neurotransmitter systems and different brain regions. The primary causes are unknown, but genetic factors may play a decisive role. The possible role of Glu receptors in such diseases opens up the possibility for therapeutic application of agents capable of blocking the activity at Glu synapses. This may, at least, slow down the progress of these very severe chronic disorders. The question is whether such an intervention can be performed without unwanted side-effects. A general blockade of excitatory amino acid receptors may cause severe adverse effects due to the many physiological functions of Glu receptors. The question is, whether agents can be developed which selectively interact with the receptors involved in the neurodegenerative processes.

Extensive neurodegeneration can also be observed in the brain after ischemic insults such as stroke or cardiac arrest. In such acute situations, an immediate treatment with Glu antagonists may be of beneficial value, and the concern towards side-effects will be less strict for a short term treatment compared to chronic administration. In animal models of ischemia, various Glu receptor antagonists have shown promising neuroprotective properties.

In Alzheimer's disease an especially complicated neuropathological pattern is observed. Brain tissue from Alzheimer patients is characterized by deposits of β-amyloid protein and extensive degeneration of especially cholinergic neurones. Hyperactivity of glutamatergic neurones are believed to be involved in the development of this degeneration. In some brain areas, neurodegeneration of glutamatergic neurones have also been observed. The cause for this degeneration is not known, but this reduction of Glu neuronal function possibly plays an important role in relation to the learning and memory deficits observed in Alzheimer patients. This dual role of Glu neurones, involving both hypo- and hyperactivity, is illustrated in Figure 9.1. A Glu antagonist, capable of preventing the neurotoxicity due to Glu hyperactivity (Fig. 9.1b), may simultaneously aggravate the hypoactivity observed in other brain areas (Fig. 9.1c). On the other hand, a Glu agonist, administered in order to restore activity in the latter situation, may enhance the neurotoxicity observed in the hyperactivity situation. A possible therapeutic solution, at least in theory, may be the use of a partial agonist. With an appropriately balanced agonist/antagonist profile, a partial Glu agonist may partially block the hyperactivity in certain brain areas, whereas a certain level of activity may be maintained in areas of hypoactivity due to the reduced intrinsic activity of a partial agonist itself. It is not known whether such a strategy can be exploited therapeutically, but it does focus pharmacological attention on partial agonists (see Section 9.5).

Abnormal excitatory amino acid neurotransmission may also play a role in schizophrenia. One characteristic of schizophrenia seems to be hypoactivity at some Glu receptors, suggesting that Glu agonists, partial agonists, or agents capable of enhancing activity in Glu synapses may have therapeutic interest in this psychiatric disease.

9.2 CLASSIFICATION OF EXCITATORY AMINO ACID RECEPTORS

9.2.1 Receptor multiplicity

The receptors for excitatory amino acids are at present subdivided into four classes (Fig. 9.2) comprising both receptor-operated ion channels and G-protein coupled receptors. Three types of ionotropic receptors have been identified, named N-methyl-D-aspartic acid (NMDA), 2-amino-3-(3-hydroxy-5-methyl-4-isoxazolyl)propionic acid (AMPA) and kainic acid (Kain) receptors. The fourth class is a very large and heterogeneous group of receptors named metabotropic receptors (G-protein coupled receptors). All four receptor types are activated by Glu (**9.1**), and the three ionotropic receptors are named after selective agonists. This pharmacological classification is based on these and other selective agonists, supported by a number of selective antagonists. As far as antagonists is concerned there has been, and still is, an unfilled need for more selective agents. The knowledge about the metabotropic receptors has developed tremendously during the last couple of years as the result of extensive molecular biological studies.

Figure 9.2 illustrates the number of subunits cloned within each class of receptors. At present, five NMDA receptor subunits, named NR1 and NR2A–NR2D, four AMPA-preferring subunits, named GluR1–4, and five Kain preferring subunits, named GluR5–7, KA1 and KA2, have been identified. The stoichiometry of the subunits forming the receptor

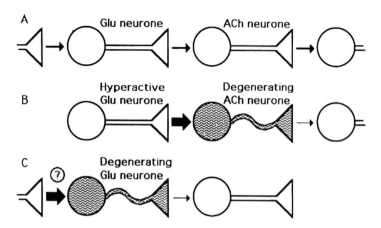

Figure 9.1   Schematic illustration of the interaction between a glutamatergic (Glu) and a cholinergic (ACh) neurone. (A); normal condition, (B); hyperactive and (C); hypoactive Glu neurones, the two latter representing situations in Alzheimer's disease.

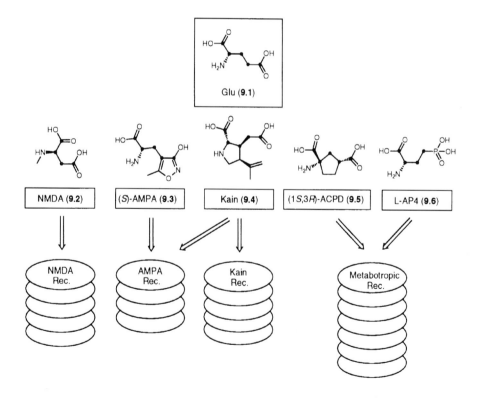

Figure 9.2   Schematic illustration of the multiplicity of excitatory amino acid receptors and the structure of Glu (**9.1**) and a number of selective agonists.

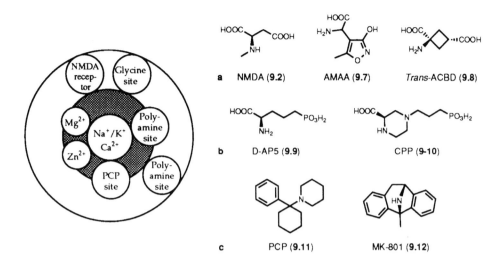

Figure 9.3 Schematic illustration of the NMDA receptor complex and structures of some examples of selective (a) agonists, (b) competitive antagonists and (c) non-competitive antagonists.

complexes is still not clarified, but it is believed to be pentameric structures, possibly of heteromeric nature. For the metabotropic receptors each circle in Figure 9.2 represents a single receptor protein (mGluR1–7). The subdivision of metabotropic receptors is based on structural differences and differences in pharmacology and second messenger coupling.

In the following sections (9.2.2–9.2.5) some of the characteristics of the four receptor classes will be briefly covered. Some of the more important ligands, which has been used for pharmacological characterization, will be described. More detailed structure-activity studies are discussed in Sections 9.3 and 9.4 for NMDA and AMPA receptor ligands.

9.2.2 The NMDA receptor complex

The NMDA receptors have been characterized extensively and have been shown to be a receptor complex comprising a number of different binding sites (Fig. 9.3), which can be manipulated pharmacologically. The NMDA receptor ion channel fluxes Na^+, K^+ and Ca^{2+} ions. Ca^{2+} ions have important intracellular functions as a second messenger, and Ca^{2+} also is implicated in the neurotoxicity observed after excessive receptor stimulation. NMDA (**9.2**), (*RS*)-2-amino-2-(3-hydroxy-5-methyl-4-isoxazolyl)acetic acid (AMAA, **9.7**) and *trans*-1-aminocyclobutane-1,3-dicarboxylic acid (*trans*-ACBD, **9.8**) (Fig. 9.3a) are potent and selective agonists at the NMDA receptor. A great number of competitive NMDA receptor antagonists have been developed, most of which are analogues of (*R*)-2-amino-5-phosphonovaleric acid (D-AP5, **9.9**) or (*R*)-4-(3-phosphonopropyl)-2-piperazinylcarboxylic acid (CPP, **9.10**) (Fig. 9.3b).

Glycine has been shown to be a co-agonist at the NMDA receptor. Thus, in order to get a response at the NMDA receptors, both the NMDA receptor site and the glycine site have to be activated simultaneously by an agonist. Electrophysiological studies seem to indicate that in most cases a high extracelluar glycine concentration, perhaps a saturating concentration, is normally found in the synapse. Thus, release and uptake of Glu seem to be the determining factors for triggering excitatory responses at NMDA receptors, whereas a more slow change in the glycine concentration may modulate the level of activity at these receptors. It should be noted though that the question about the physiological concentration of glycine at NMDA receptors has not been fully clarified.

Apart from a strict requirement for both Glu and glycine to activate the NMDA receptors, another unusual factor is observed for this ligand gated ion channel. At normal resting potentials, the NMDA receptors are blocked by Mg^{2+}, probably binding to a site within the ion channel. When the neurone is partially depolarised, e.g. by activation of other ionotropic Glu receptors on the same neurone, the Mg^{2+} blockade is released, and the NMDA receptor ion channel can be activated to give further depolarisation. Thus, in some respects the NMDA receptors seem to function as an amplification system working only at a certain level of activity of the neurones.

A site for non-competitive NMDA antagonists has been characterized, most often referred to as the phencyclidine (PCP, **9.11**) site. The action of PCP, dizocilpine (MK-801, **9.12**) (Fig. 9.3c) and other non-competitive NMDA antagonists are use-dependent, meaning that repeated activation of the NMDA receptors by an agonist is needed to obtain effective antagonist activity of these antagonists. The interpretation of this phenomenon has been that these agents require access to the open ion channel in order to exert their use-dependent antagonism. The mechanism of use-dependency seems very interesting in relation to the treatment of neurodegenerative disorders. In principle, such non-competitive antagonists should elicit therapeutically useful antagonism at synapses with hyperactivity, as observed in the neurodegenerative situations, whereas less efficient antagonism are to be expected at synapses with normal synaptic activity. This would be expected to lead to reduced side-effects of non-competitive NMDA antagonists as compared to competitive antagonists. Unfortunately and unexpectedly, the non-competitive antagonists, so far studied, show severe psychotomimetic side-effects, which have prevented therapeutic applications.

Other binding sites, including two different sites for polyamines and a site for Zn^{2+}, have also been identified at the NMDA receptor complex, but these sites will not be further described here.

9.2.3 AMPA receptor ligands

Originally, the AMPA receptors were named Quis receptors after the naturally occurring compound quisqualic acid (Quis, **9.13**). Quite early it was however realized, that Quis is a non-selective Glu receptor agonist. Quis receptors were named AMPA receptors on the basis of the very potent and specific agonist activity of (*S*)-AMPA (**9.3**). Tritiated AMPA is used as the standard ligand for AMPA receptor binding studies. The excitatory activity elicited by Quis and AMPA could not be antagonized by NMDA antagonists, whereas Glu diethyl ester (GDEE, **9.14**) blocked the effects of these agonists. GDEE is, however, a poor antagonist due to chemical instability and a low potency, and, furthermore, the antagonist effects could not be reproduced in all systems. The subsequently discovered compound 6-cyano-7-nitroquinoxaline-2,3-dione (CNQX, **9.15**), showed improved potency and selectivity, but it did also elicit potent antagonist activity at Kain receptors. There are

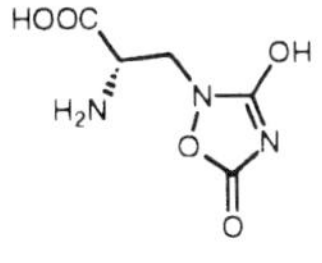

Quis (**9.13**) 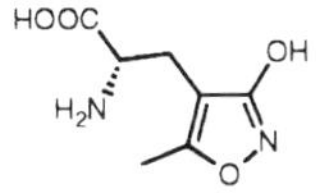   (*S*)-AMPA (**9.3**)

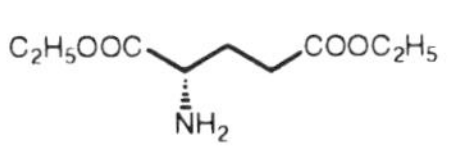

GDEE (**9.14**) 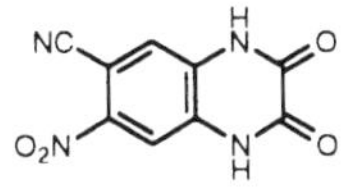   CNQX (**9.15**) 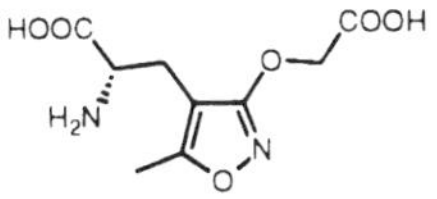   (*S*)-AMOA (**9.16**) 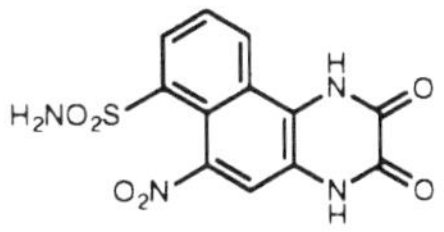   NBQX (**9.17**)

Figure 9.4   Structure of the agonists Quis (**9.13**) and (*S*)-AMPA (**9.3**), and of some competitive antagonists (**9.14–9.17**).

still difficulties in separating the pharmacology of AMPA and Kain receptors. Therefore, the two receptors are often collectively named non-NMDA receptors as opposed to the NMDA receptors. Two more recent compounds, the isoxazole (*S*)-2-amino-3-[3-(carboxymethoxy)-5-methyl-4-isoxazolyl]propionic acid [(*S*)-AMOA, **9.16**], derived from AMPA, and the quinoxalinedione 2,3-dihydroxy-6-nitro-7-sulfamoylbenzo(*f*)quinoxaline (NBQX, **9.17**), derived from CNQX, do show some selectivity towards AMPA receptors. The AMPA receptors mediate fast excitatory activity, and AMPA antagonists have shown neuroprotective properties in animal models. It is as yet unknown, whether such antagonists can be administered to man without severe side-effects.

Recently molecular cloning studies have shown the AMPA receptors, as other ionotropic receptor classes, to consist of subunits with different but related amino acid sequences. Like the NMDA receptors, the AMPA receptors probably are pentameric structures, but the stoichiometry is not known, and subtype-selective agents are not known either. It still is unknown, whether special subtypes of receptors are involved in the disorders described earlier, and whether subtype-selective agents will be of therapeutic utility. In agreement with the previous discussion, AMPA receptors may have particular therapeutic interest (see also Section 9.5).

9.2.4 Kainic acid receptor ligands

Studies using molecular cloning techniques have shown AMPA and Kain receptors to be closely related at the molecular level. Furthermore, these receptors show similar pharmacology, and only a limited number of selective Kain agonists are known. Most of these agonists are naturally occurring compounds like Kain (**9.4**) itself (Fig. 9.5). Examples of such kainoids are domoic acid (**9.18**) and acromelic acid (**9.19**), and the synthetic cyclopropane-analogue *trans*-MCG (**9.20**) also shows selective Kain receptor agonism. Saturation of the isopropenyl side-chain of Kain leads to almost complete loss of agonist activity, whereas dihydro-Kain (**9.21**) show weak inhibitory activity towards Glu uptake. The structure-activity relationship for compounds active as Kain agonists seem to indicate

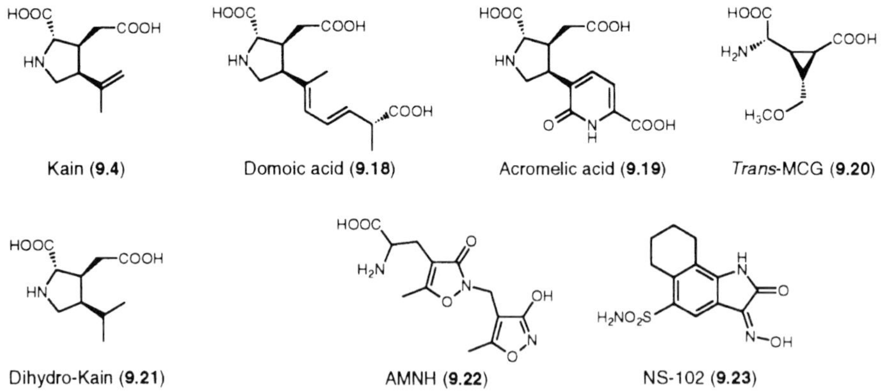

Kain (**9.4**)   Domoic acid (**9.18**)   Acromelic acid (**9.19**)   *Trans*-MCG (**9.20**)

Dihydro-Kain (**9.21**)   AMNH (**9.22**)   NS-102 (**9.23**)

Figure 9.5   Structure of some Kain receptor agonists (**9.4** and **9.18–9.20**), of a Glu uptake inhibitor (**9.21**), and of two Kain antagonists (**9.22** and **9.23**).

that an unsaturated or another electron rich substituent is necessary for potent activity at Kain receptors.

Only a few antagonists at Kain receptors have been developed, generally showing poor selectivity. CNQX (**9.15**) show approximately equipotent antagonism towards AMPA and Kain responses. AMNH (**9.22**) seem to be a selective but fairly weak Kain receptor blocker, whereas NS-102 (**9.23**) has been reported to be somewhat more active.

9.2.5 Metabotropic receptor ligands

Metabotropic receptors are coupled to second messenger systems through membrane bound G-proteins and are not directly coupled to ion channels. Thus, the responses obtained through such receptors are slower than ionotropic receptor responses. Originally, the metabotropic receptors were pharmacologically divided into two classes, the first activated by the three agonists (1*S*,3*R*)-1-amino-1,3-cyclopentanedicarboxylic acid [(1*S*,3*R*)-ACPD, **9.5**], Quis (**9.13**) and ibotenic acid (Ibo, **9.24**), and the second class sensitive to (*S*)-2-amino-4-phosphonobutyric acid (L-AP4, **9.6**). Of the former class, only (1*S*,3*R*)-ACPD proved fairly selective. In different brain regions, the order of potency of these four agonists varied significantly, suggesting the existence of different subtypes. Receptors sensitive to L-AP4 are found especially in schaffer-collateral fibres. Excitatory activity mediated by these receptors can be blocked by L-AP4. These receptors are presumably located presynaptic and may act as autoreceptors. L-AP4-sensitive metabotropic receptors are also found in the retina. Molecular cloning studies have shown these two groups of L-AP4-sensitive receptors to be structurally related, though coupled to different second messenger systems. Seven metabotropic receptor clones (mGluR1–7) have, so far been characterized. These receptor subtypes are characterized by different G-protein coupling and second messenger systems. Some of the metabotropic receptors are coupled to phosphoinositol metabolism and intracellular Ca^{2+} mobilisation (mGluR1 and 5), whereas others are negatively coupled

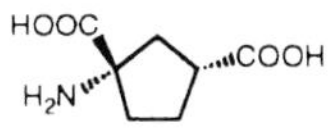

(1*S*,3*R*)-ACPD (**9.5**)

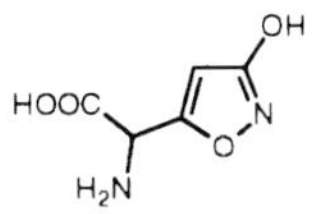

Ibo (**9.24**)

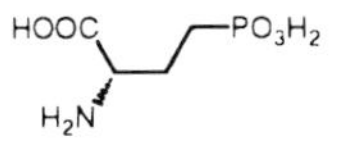

L-AP4 (**9.6**)

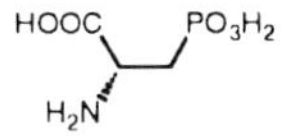

L-AP3 (**9.25**)

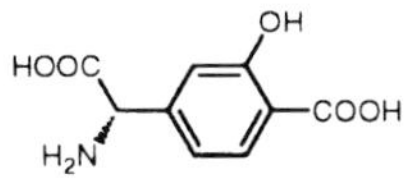

4C3HPG (**9.26**)

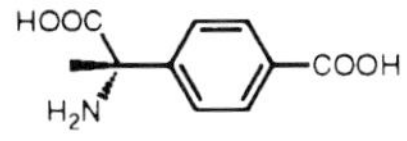

MCPG (**9.27**)

Figure 9.6 Structure of three metabotropic agonists (**9.5**, **9.24** and **9.6**) and of three antagonists (**9.25–9.27**).

to the formation of cyclic AMP (mGluR2–4, 6 and 7). The metabotropic receptors can indirectly affect ion channels and studies in animal models have shown both neuroprotective and neurotoxic properties of metabotropic agonists. This may reflect that some metabotropic receptors are presynaptically located, whereas other subtypes are postsynaptic in nature.

At present, many medicinal chemistry groups are involved in the development of ligands selective for the different metabotropic receptors. Some of the antagonists, so far available, are shown in Figure 9.6 (Formulas **9.25–9.27**). Both agonists and antagonist show more or less different pharmacology at different mGluRs. Along with the development of selective ligands, the physiological functions of the metabotropic receptors are being investigated. The overall goal of these studies is the development of novel therapeutic agents for the treatment of diseases in the CNS (see Section 9.1.2).

9.3 IBOTENIC ACID: A NATURALLY OCCURRING EXCITOTOXIN

Many naturally occurring acidic amino acids have shown activity at excitatory amino acid receptors and are currently used as pharmacological tools. Furthermore, such compounds have been extensively used as lead structures in the search for new and better ligands. The *Amanita muscaria* constituent ibotenic acid (Ibo, **9.24**) shows potent activity at both NMDA and certain metabotropic receptor subtypes, and it is a weak agonist at non-NMDA receptors. It is used as a pharmacological and neurotoxic tool, although chemical instability limits the utility of Ibo in experimental pharmacology.

9.3.1 Ibotenic acid as a lead structure

It is believed that Glu (**9.1**) interacts with the different Glu receptors in different conformations, suggesting that development of Glu analogues with restricted conformations may lead to compounds with selective actions. Ibo (**9.24**) is a conformationally restricted analogue of Glu in which the 3-hydroxy-isoxazole moiety functions as a bioisostere to the

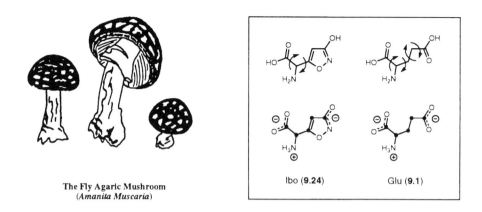

The Fly Agaric Mushroom
(*Amanita Muscaria*)

Figure 9.7   Illustration of the structural flexibility of Ibo (isolated from the fly agaric mushroom) and of Glu and delocalization of the three charges existing at physiological pH (pKa values: Glu, 2.2, 4.3 and 10.0; Ibo, 3.0, 5.0 and 8.2).

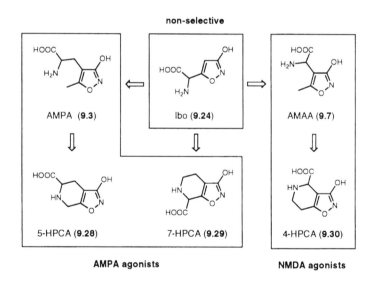

Figure 9.8   Examples of mono- and bicyclic analogues developed using Ibo as a lead structure.

distal carboxyl group of Glu (Fig. 9.7). In Figure 9.8 a number of compounds designed and synthesized using Ibo as a lead structure are illustrated. These compounds show a high degree of receptor selectivity and, with the exception of the bicyclic Ibo analogue 7-HPCA (**9.29**), do not possess the chemical instability elicited by Ibo itself. The two compounds, AMAA (**9.7**) and AMPA (**9.3**), described previously, show potent and specific agonist action at NMDA and AMPA receptors, respectively. In order to obtain further information about the conformational requirements for receptor activation, bicyclic analogues of AMPA, Ibo and AMAA were synthesized. The three structures, named 5-HPCA (**9.28**), 7-HPCA (**9.29**) and 4-HPCA (**9.30**) are rigid structures with very low conformational flexibility. The AMPA analogue, 5-HPCA, proved to be a selective AMPA agonist like its parent compound, though with somewhat lower potency. This may reflect that the conformations attainable by 5-HPCA are close to the receptor active conformation of AMPA and Glu at AMPA receptors. These aspects will be discussed further in Section 9.5.2.

The bicyclic analogue 4-HPCA is a very weak NMDA agonist, approximately 100 times weaker than AMAA on cortical neurones. 4-HPCA does, however, show potent neurotoxic action in spite of this low agonist activity. The structure-activity relationships for 4- and 5-HPCA will be further discussed in Section 9.4.

9.3.2 Conformational studies of ibotenic acid

Quite surprisingly 7-HPCA (**9.29**), the bicyclic analogue of Ibo (**9.24**), proved to be a selective AMPA agonist, slightly more potent than 5-HPCA (**9.28**). This is in contrast to the activity of the parent molecule Ibo, being primarily a potent NMDA receptor agonist. This observation prompted an investigation of the conformational flexibility for Ibo. Semi-empirical molecular orbital calculations using AM1 were performed for Ibo, revealing the variation in potential energy as a function of rotation around the torsional angel, as illustrated in Figure 9.9. The rotation around τ (Fig. 9.9) is of major importance for the possible conformations accessible to Ibo. The energy-curve shows a global minimum around $30°$ and an energy-barrier around $-160°$. X-ray analysis of Ibo have shown a conformation in the crystalline state very close to the global minimum identified by the calculations, whereas the conformation of 7-HPCA identified by X-ray analysis is very different. The X-ray structure of 7-HPCA has the carboxylate group in a pseudo-equatorial position, as depicted in Figure 9.9. The conformation of Ibo corresponding to the one found for 7-HPCA in the crystalline state is close to the energy-barrier, indicating that it is energetically unfavourable for Ibo to adopt this conformation. These results indicate that Ibo, when interacting with the NMDA receptors, exist in a conformation significantly different from the conformation reflected by 7-HPCA, which elicits AMPA agonist activity.

The group of closely related compounds shown in Figure 9.8 illustrates the dramatic changes in receptor pharmacology, which can be obtained by relatively small structural changes of the Ibo structure.

9.4 NMDA AND AMPA RECEPTOR LIGANDS

9.4.1 AMAA: a selective NMDA receptor ligand

Originally, the NMDA agonist AMAA (**9.7**) was found to be a very weak agonist at spinal cord neurones, tested by *in vivo* electrophoretic experiments on cat spinal neurones. Later, AMAA was tested *in vitro* on rat cortical neurones as shown in Figure 9.10. This shows AMAA to be a potent and specific NMDA agonist, slightly more potent than NMDA itself. These results indicate regional and perhaps species dependent differences in the

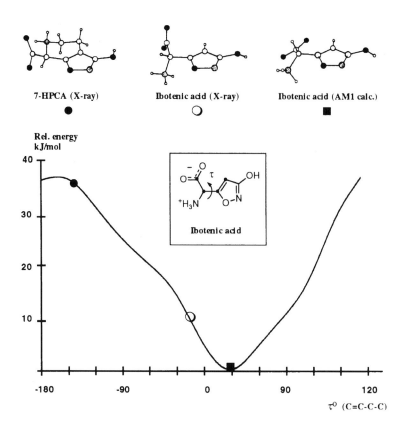

Figure 9.9 Potential energy curve of Ibo zwitterion as a function of the torsion angle τ, obtained by AM1 calculations. A global minimum is observed at ca. 30° and the solid state conformation is found close to this, with a relative energy ca. 10 kJ/mol above. The energy of the Ibo conformation similar to that found for the bicyclic analogue 7-HPCA is close to the energy barrier for rotation (ca. 37 kJ/mol above the global minimum).

pharmacology of NMDA receptors. This may be related to different subtypes of NMDA receptors as identified by cloning studies, though this has not been clarified yet. The bicyclic AMAA-analogue 4-HPCA (**9.30**) is, as described, a very weak NMDA receptor agonist. This weak activity for 4-HPCA may be due to the conformation of the aspartic acid backbone present in 4-HPCA. This conformation may be significantly different from the conformation of AMAA during its interaction with the NMDA receptors.

Another explanation may be that a certain degree of molecular flexibility is necessary for potent NMDA receptor agonist activity. This has been proposed to be the case for other NMDA agonists, though this is difficult to prove.

9.4.2 AMPA analogues

The two bicyclic Glu analogues 5-HPCA (**9.28**) and 7-HPCA (**9.29**), are rigid structures, and their activity indicates that such structural modifications of AMPA are acceptable as far

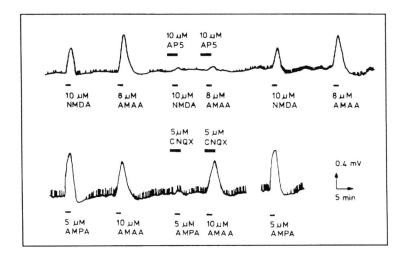

Figure 9.10   Recordings from rat cortical slice neurones depolarized by administration of NMDA (**9.2**), AMAA (**9.7**) or AMPA (**9.3**) and antagonism of these by the NMDA antagonist AP5 (**9.9**) (top) or the non-NMDA antagonist CNQX (**9.15**) (bottom) and recovery.

as AMPA receptor agonism is concerned. Thus, conformational flexibility does not seem to be a necessity for activation of AMPA receptors, in contrast to what has been suggested for NMDA receptor activation.

Another factor to consider is the acidity of the functional groups of AMPA analogues. The pKa values of especially the distal acidic group is highly variable and can be influenced by designing different derivatives, as for example Trifluoro-AMPA (**9.31**). An electronegative substituent in the 5-position of the isoxazole ring of AMPA analogues has significant influence on the pKa value of the 3-hydroxy group. The pKa values for the 3-hydroxy-isoxazole moiety of AMPA and Trifluoro-AMPA, are 4.8 and 3.4, respectively. When tested in binding studies and electrophysiological experiments the two compounds showed very similar potencies as AMPA receptor agonists. AMPA and Trifluoro-AMPA showed IC_{50} values of 0.04 and 0.08 μM in the [^{3}H]AMPA binding assay, respectively, and EC_{50} values of 3.5 and 2.3 μM, respectively, in electrophysiological experiments. This indicates that the large increase of acidity found for Trifluoro-AMPA does not significantly influence the biological activity. It should be noted that the volume a trifluoromethyl group is fairly similar to that of the methyl group.

The bromomethyl analogue, ABPA (**9.32**), was designed in order to investigate whether the chemically reactive bromomethyl group would react irreversibly with the AMPA receptors. When tested in binding studies and in different *in vitro* and *in vivo* electrophysiological experiments, no indications of irreversible effects were detected. ABPA was shown to be a very potent agonist, which suggests that when ABPA is interacting with the AMPA receptors no nucleophile is present in a position enabling it to react with the bromomethyl group. The rather large bromoatom obviously can be tolerated in this position of the ligand, with only minor effect on the potency.

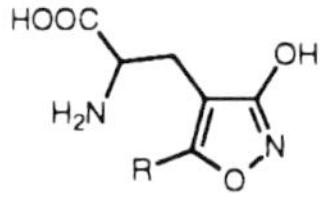

R	EC$_{50}$ (µM)	R	EC$_{50}$ (µM)	R	EC$_{50}$ (µM)
CH$_3$– (9.3)	3.5	CH$_3$–CH$_2$– (9.33)	2.3	CH$_3$–CH$_2$–CH$_2$, CH$_3$–CH$_2$–CH$_2$ CH– (9.36)	>1000
CF$_3$– (9.31)	2.3	CH$_3$–CH$_2$–CH$_2$–CH$_2$– (9.34)	30	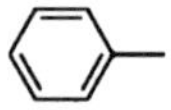 (9.37)	400
Br–CH$_2$– (9.32)	13	CH$_3$ CH$_3$–C– CH$_3$ (9.35)	48	HO–CH$_2$– (9.38)	110

Figure 9.11 AMPA analogues with different substituents and their depolarizing activity (EC$_{50}$ values) determined in the rat cortical slice preparation.

The tolerance for bulk in the 5-position of the isoxazole ring for AMPA analogues has been further investigated by synthesizing a number of other analogues with different substituents. A number of these analogues are shown in Figure 9.11. Ethyl-AMPA (9.33) is equipotent with AMPA (9.3), whereas Butyl-AMPA (9.34) shows some loss of activity. Similarly the very large and bulky *tert*-butyl group, present in ATPA (9.35), reduces the activity to some extent, but like Butyl-AMPA, ATPA still shows considerable potency. Introduction of the more bulky 1-propylbutyl substituent (compound 9.36), results in a complete loss of activity.

The compound APPA (9.37) having a phenyl substituent, shows a different pharmacological profile. APPA is a very weak compound, approximately 100 times less potent compared to AMPA. APPA actually is a partial agonist with an intrinsic activity of approximately 60% of that of AMPA (see also Section 9.5). These structure-activity studies, seem to indicate that there is a limited capacity for bulky substituents in the 5-position of the isoxazole ring in AMPA analogues. Another interesting observation is that the hydroxymethyl analogue of AMPA, HO-Me-AMPA (9.38), is significantly weaker than AMPA (Fig. 9.11). This decrease in activity is unlikely to be due to the steric bulk of the hydroxymethyl group, but may indicate that polar substituent are less well tolerated than lipophilic substituents. An alternative explanation could be a conformational effect of the hydroxymethyl substituent on the amino acid side-chain, perhaps due to intramolecular hydrogen bonding. The results of these structure-activity studies suggest the presence of a cavity at the AMPA receptor, which can accommodate lipophilic substituents at a certain size.

9.4.3 Conformational studies on AMPA analogues

The preferred conformation of the bicyclic AMPA analogue, 5-HPCA (9.28), in aqueous solution has been determined by ^{1}H NMR spectroscopy. The coupling constants deduced

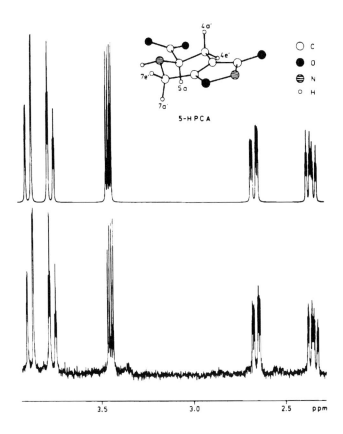

Figure 9.12   Perspective drawing of the preferred conformation of the dianionic form of 5-HPCA (pH ca. 10) as deduced from the 500 MHz ^{1}H NMR spectrum (bottom) and the computer simulated spectrum (top). Coupling constants for H_{5a}: $J_{4a'5a} = 10.1$ Hz and $J_{4e'5a} = 4.8$ Hz.

from the spectrum (Fig. 9.12) showed the six-membered ring to be preferentially in a half-chair conformation, and the carboxylate group to be in an equatorial position. 5-HPCA is a ringclosed analogue of AMPA, but the amino acid side-chain of AMPA is unlikely to be in a conformation similar to that represented by 5-HPCA. The 5-methyl group in AMPA imposes some steric hindrance, and the bulky *tert*-butyl group of ATPA (**9.35**) greatly influences the conformation of the amino acid side-chain. In 4-AHCP (**9.39**), a bicyclic homologue of AMPA, the amino acid moiety, obviously is placed in a position very different from that observed in 5-HPCA. These considerations, supported by modelling studies, have suggested the receptor active conformation of AMPA to be different from the conformation represented by 5-HPCA. This is illustrated in Figure 9.13, showing the interaction of the three ionized groups of the agonists with complementary ionized groups at the receptor protein. This simple model, which also comprises the proposed lipophilic cavity, illustrates some important features to be considered in the design of AMPA receptor agonists.

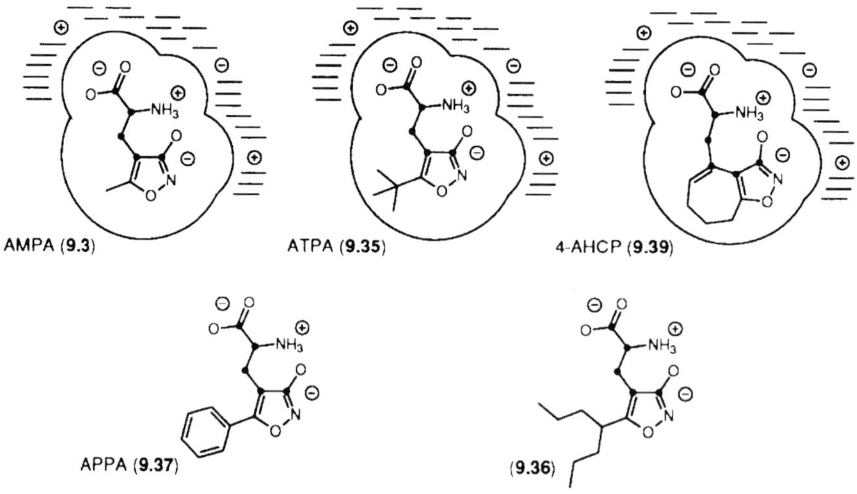

Figure 9.13   Schematic illustration of the binding of some AMPA agonists to a hypothetical pharmacophore model assumed to contain a cavity capable of accommodating relatively bulky substituents on the agonist molecules. Below is shown two structures with very bulky substituents and very weak (APPA, **9.37**) or no activity (compound **9.36**).

9.4.4 Stereoselectivity of AMPA and NMDA receptor agonists

The molecules of Glu and most other Glu analogues contain one chiral centre, consistent with the existence of a pair of enantiomers. Normally, one enantiomer of a biologically active compound carries the activity, whereas the other enantiomer is weak or inactive. This is the case for AMPA and a number of AMPA agonists, where the *S*-form is active. In the case of NMDA agonists the *R*-enantiomers (corresponding to the D-forms), are often the active molecular species. But, there are several exceptions to this rule, and the NMDA receptors does generally show low stereoselectivity as compared to the AMPA receptors.

It is important to realize that the above mentioned examples, where one enantiomer is active and the other one weak or inactive do not represent a general rule. There are many exceptions, for example of enantiomeric compounds showing completely different biological effects mediated by the same or different receptors. Enantiomeric compounds may, for example, show agonist and antagonist activity, respectively, at the same receptor. This is illustrated in the subsequent section, which also describes a new pharmacological principle.

9.5 FUNCTIONAL PARTIAL AGONISM

The partial agonism described for racemic APPA (**9.37**) (Section 9.4.2) greatly stimulated the interest in this compound and a resolution procedure was developed to furnish the

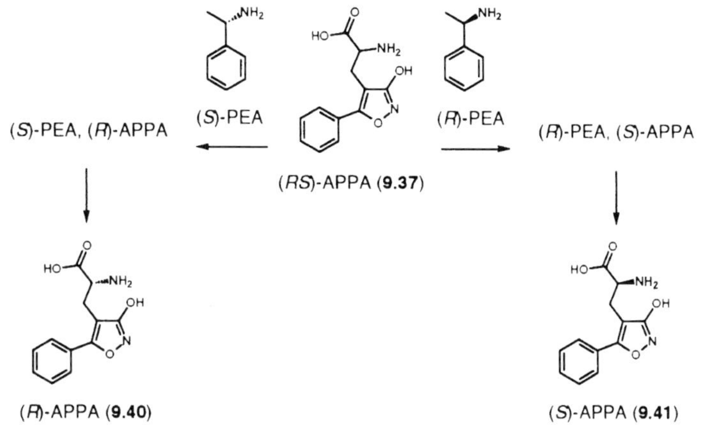

Figure 9.14 Resolution procedure for APPA (**9.37**) using (*S*)- and (*R*)-phenylethylamine (PEA) to give diastereomeric salts. Upon acidification (*R*)-APPA (**9.40**) or (*S*)-APPA (**9.41**) are liberated, respectively.

two enantiomers. Resolution was accomplished by diastereomeric salt formation using racemic APPA and (*R*)- or (*S*)-phenylethylamine (PEA) (Fig. 9.14). When (*RS*)-APPA was mixed with (*S*)-PEA and recrystallized from ethanol, the diastereomeric salt consisting of (*R*)-APPA and (*S*)-PEA precipitated and could be purified by repeated recrystallization, affording (*R*)-APPA (**9.40**) after liberation from the salt. Analogously, (*S*)-APPA (**9.41**) was obtained using (*R*)-PEA for the salt formation.

In contrast to the racemate, originally characterized as a partial agonist, (*S*)-APPA (**9.41**) proved to be a full agonist at AMPA receptors, slightly more potent than the racemate (Fig. 9.15A). (*R*)-APPA (**9.41**) had no intrinsic activity at AMPA receptors when applied alone, but when co-applied with AMPA or (*S*)-APPA it antagonised the excitation evoked by these agonists. The dose-response curves of these two AMPA agonists could be shifted to the right in a parallel fashion, indicating that (*R*)-APPA was a competitive AMPA receptor antagonist. These results reveal that the original partial agonism observed for (*RS*)-APPA was due to the interaction of a full agonist [(*S*)-APPA] and a competitive antagonist [(*R*)-APPA]. Subsequently, dose-response curves were obtained using different ratios of (*R*)- and (*S*)-APPA. This is shown in Figure 9.15B for (*S*)-APPA alone and for increasing ratios of (*S*)-APPA/(*R*)-APPA [(1:1) (racemic APPA), (1:2) and (1:3)]. It is seen that with an increasing ratio, the maximum response is depressed. The curves have not been extended further due to the rather low potency of the enantiomers. The figure illustrates the principle of "functional partial agonism". This principle implicates that, in theory, any desired level of intrinsic activity can be obtained when mixing an agonist and a competitive antagonist in a fixed molar ratio. Functional partial agonism can be achieved using any pair of agonist and competitive antagonist. Furthermore, this principle can be applied not only to AMPA receptor ligands, but also to ligands of other ionotropic Glu receptors or other ionotropic neurotransmitter systems in general. The maximal activity attainable will depend on the relative potency of the two agents. It is important to notice the difference between these experiments using agonists and competitive antagonists, to achieve

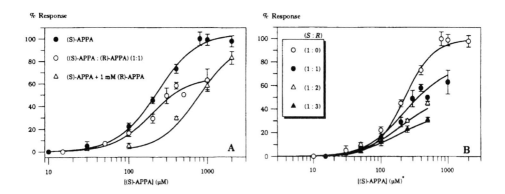

Figure 9.15   Dose-response curves from the rat cortical slice preparation. (A) (*S*)-APPA (**9.41**), (*RS*)-APPA (**9.37**) and parallel shift of the (*S*)-APPA (**9.40**) curve with 1 mM (*R*)-APPA. (B) Curves obtained with fixed molar ratios of (*S*)- and (*R*)-APPA; 1:0, 1:1 (racemate), 1:2 and 1:3. *The X-axis represents the concentration of (*S*)-APPA and the concentration of (*R*)-APPA, which is 0, 1, 2 or 3 times the concentration of (*S*)-APPA in the four different experiments.

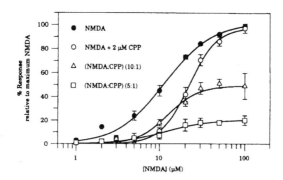

Figure 9.16   Dose-response curves from the rat cortical slice preparation. Curves obtained with NMDA (**9.2**), fixed molar ratios of NMDA and CPP (**9.10**) (10:1 and 5:1) and rightward shift of the NMDA curve with 2 μM CPP.

functional partial agonism, and the conventional pharmacological experiment designed to demonstrate competitive antagonism. In the latter case, a dose response-curve for the agonist is determined in the presence of a fixed concentration of a competitive antagonist, which will shift the dose response curve for the agonist to the right in a parallel fashion. In contrast to this, functional partial agonism is established using fixed molar ratios of the two components, i.e. the curves are obtained using increasing doses of fixed ratios of agonist and antagonist.

Another example of the principle of functional partial agonism is shown in Figure 9.16 using NMDA (**9.2**) and the competitive NMDA antagonist CPP (**9.10**). The high potency of these two compounds makes it possible to obtain full curves. Again, the figure shows the possibility of reaching any level of activity between 0 and 1, by choosing appropriate ratios of agonist and competitive antagonist.

Partial agonists may be therapeutically interesting in relation to Alzheimer's disease as described in Section 9.1.2 and may also prove to have therapeutic applicability in other disorders. For *in vivo* studies of functional partial agonism, a number of factors will have to be very carefully considered. First of all, the level of efficacy desired for the disease in question is not known and will have to be determined. If the two compounds, the agonist and the appropriate competitive antagonist, are administered systemically it is important to make sure that both compounds actually reach the site of action in the necessary concentrations. This means that absorption, metabolism, penetration and other factors will have to be established for both compounds. At this point, the principle of functional partial agonism has been introduced — the future will show the applicability.

FURTHER READING

Ebert, B., Lenz, S., Brehm, L., Bregnedal, P., Hansen, J.J., Frederiksen, K., Bøgesø, K.P. and Krogsgaard-Larsen, P. (1994) Resolution, absolute stereochemistry, and pharmacology of the (*S*)-(+)- and (*R*)-(−)-isomers of the apparent partial AMPA receptor agonist (*R,S*)-2-amino-3-(3-hydroxy-5-phenylisoxazol-4-yl)propionic acid [(*R,S*)-APPA]. *J. Med. Chem.*, **37**, 878–884.

Hollmann, M. and Heinemann, S. (1994) Cloned glutamate receptors. *Annu. Rev. Neurosci.*, **17**, 31–108.

Johansen, T.N., Frydenvang, K., Ebert, B., Krogsgaard-Larsen, P. and Madsen, U. (1994) Synthesis and structure-activity studies on acidic amino acids and related diacids as NMDA receptor ligands. *J. Med. Chem.*, **37**, 3252–3262.

Krogsgaard-Larsen, P. and Hansen, J.J. (eds.) (1992) *Excitatory amino acid receptors — design of agonists and antagonists.* London: Ellis Horwood.

Krogsgaard-Larsen, P., Ebert, B., Johansen, T.N., Bischoff, F. and Madsen, U. (in press) Excitatory amino acid agonists, partial agonists, antagonists and modulators: Design and therapeutic prospects. In *Excitatory amino acids and synaptic transmission*, edited by H. Wheal and A. Thomson A, 2. ed.

Madsen, U., Ferkany, J.W., Jones, B.E., Ebert, B., Johansen, T.N., Holm, T. and Krogsgaard-Larsen, P. (1990) NMDA receptor agonists derived from ibotenic acid. Preparation, neuroexcitation and neurotoxicity. *Eur. J. Pharmacol. Mol. Pharmacol. Sect.*, **189**, 381–391.

Madsen, U., Ebert, B. and Krogsgaard-Larsen, P. (1994) Modulation of AMPA receptor function in relation to glutamatergic abnormalities in Alzheimer's disease. *Biomed. & Pharmacother.*, **48**, 312–318.

Meldrum, B. and Garthwaite, J. (1990) Excitatory amino acid neurotoxicity and neurodegenerative disease. *Trends Pharmacol. Sci.*, **11**, 379–387.

Monaghan, D.T., Bridges, R.J. and Cotman, C.W. (1989) The excitatory amino acid receptors: their classes, pharmacology, and distinct properties in the function of the central nervous system. *Ann. Rev. Pharmacol. Toxicol.*, **29**, 365–402.

Nakanishi, S. and Masu, M. (1994) Molecular diversity and functions of glutamate receptors. *Annu. Rev. Biophys. Biomol. Struct.*, **23**, 319–348.

Nielsen, E.Ø., Madsen, U., Schaumburg, K., Brehm, L. and Krogsgaard-Larsen, P. (1986) Studies on receptor-active conformations of excitatory amino acid agonists and antagonists. *Eur. J. Med. Chem. — Chim. Ther.*, **21**, 433–437.

Watkins, J.C., Krogsgaard-Larsen, P. and Honoré, T. (1990) Structure-activity relationships in the development of excitatory amino acid receptor agonists and competitive antagonists. *Trends Pharmacol. Sci.*, **11**, 25–33.

10. SYNAPTIC MECHANISMS AS PHARMACOLOGICAL TARGETS: GABA, ACETYLCHOLINE AND HISTAMINE

POVL KROGSGAARD-LARSEN and BENTE FRØLUND

CONTENTS

10.1 SYNAPTIC PROCESSES AND MECHANISMS

The synapses are key elements in the interneuronal communication in the peripheral and the central nervous system (CNS). In the CNS, each neurone has been estimated to have synaptic contact with several thousand other neurones, making the structure and function of the CNS extremely complex.

Each neurotransmitter system operates through a characteristic set of synaptic processes and mechanisms (Fig. 10.1) with distinct requirements for activation and regulation. In principle, each of these steps in the neurotransmission process is susceptible to specific pharmacological intervention. Synaptic functions may be facilitated by stimulation of the neurotransmitter biosynthesis, for example by administration of a biochemical precursor, or by inhibition of the metabolism/degradation pathway(s). There are several examples of therapeutically successful inhibitors of enzymes catalysing intra- or extracellular metabolic processes. Similarly, it has been shown in a number of cases that neurotransmitter function can be stimulated in a therapeutically beneficial manner via inhibition of neuronal uptake (transport) systems. It is possible that transport mechanisms in synaptic storage vesicles (Fig. 10.1) also are potential sites for effective pharmacological intervention. Autoreceptors normally play a key role in regulating the release of certain neurotransmitters, making this class of presynaptic receptors therapeutically interesting.

Pharmacological stimulation or inhibition of the above mentioned synaptic mechanisms are, however, likely to affect the function of the entire neurotransmitter system. Activation of neurotransmitter receptors (see Chapter 6) may, in principle, represent the most direct and selective approach to stimulation of a particular neurotransmitter system. Furthermore, activation of distinct subtypes of receptors operated by the neurotransmitter concerned may open up the prospect of highly selective pharmacological intervention. This principle may apply to pre- as well as postsynaptic receptors and also to ion channels associated with or independent of receptors (Fig. 10.1) (see Chapter 8).

Direct activation of receptors by full agonists may result in rapid receptor desensitization (insensitive to activation). Partial agonists (see Chapter 1) are much less liable to induce receptor desensitization and may therefore be particularly interesting for neurotransmitter replacement therapies. Whereas desensitization may be a more or less pronounced problem associated with pharmacological or therapeutic use of receptor agonists, receptor antagonists, which in many cases have proved useful therapeutic agents, may inherently cause receptor supersensitivity. The presence of allosteric binding sites at certain receptor complexes, which may function as physiological modulatory mechanisms, offer unique prospects of selective and flexible pharmacological manipulation of the receptor complex concerned (see subsequent section and Chapter 9). Whilst some receptors are associated with ion channels, others are coupled to second messenger systems (see Chapter 6). Key steps in such enzyme-regulated multistep intracellular systems (Fig. 10.1) may represent future targets for therapeutic interventions.

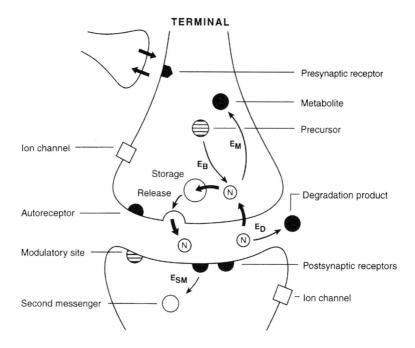

Figure 10.1   Generalized schematic illustration of processes and mechanisms associated with an axosomatic synapse in the CNS. E, enzymes; N, neurotransmitter.

There is an urgent need for novel psychoactive drugs with specific actions. This demand is particularly pronounced in the field of neurodegenerative diseases, where effective drugs are not yet available, even for symptomatic treatments. In light of the overwhelming complexity of the structure and function of the CNS, these aspects represent major challenges for medicinal chemists.

10.2 NEURODEGENERATIVE DISEASES

Neurodegenerative diseases are characterized by progressive loss of certain types of neurones in different regions of the CNS. It is generally accepted that degeneration of dopamine neurones is a key factor in Parkinson's disease, whereas degenerative loss of central acetylcholine and glutamic acid neurones is a dominating characteristic of Alzheimer's disease (see Chapter 9). In the former neurological disorder, dopamine neurones in the basal ganglia are degenerating, whereas cortical and hippocampal acetylcholine neurones are particularly vulnerable in the brains of Alzheimer patients.

The primary cause(s) of degenerative diseases, including ischemic and seizure-related brain damages, are far from being fully elucidated. Several factors may play important roles in the etiology of these diseases, including free radical processes and, perhaps, autoimmune mechanisms. Studies in recent years have, however, been focused on the role of the central excitatory amino acid neurotransmitter, glutamic acid, in the processes causing neurone injury and, ultimately, death. The view that hyperactivity of central glutamic acid neurones is an important causative factor in neurodegenerative processes ("excitotoxicity") is supported by *in vitro* and *in vivo* studies in a variety of model systems (see Chapter 9).

10.3 THE GABA SYSTEM

Dysfunctions of the central inhibitory 4-aminobutanoic acid (GABA) (**10.1**) neurotransmitter system seem to play important roles in certain diseases. Analyses of brain tissue samples from sites near seizure foci in epileptic patients or in animals made epileptic have revealed severe impairments of the GABA system. The low levels in GABA nerve terminals of the GABA-synthesizing enzyme, (*S*)-glutamate decarboxylase (GAD) (Fig. 10.3), and the reduced GABA uptake capacity measured in different models of epilepsy probably reflect degeneration of GABA neurones. Pharmacological evidence from animal studies supports the view that impairments of the GABA-mediated neurotransmission is a major factor underlying epileptic phenomena.

Low levels of GABA and GAD have also been measured in postmortem brain tissue from patients dying with Huntington's chorea, and neurochemical studies have disclosed abnormalities of GABA receptors in certain regions of brains of choreic patients. There is evidence for GABA dysfunctions in schizophrenia and tardive dyskinesia, and a GABAergic contribution to the symptoms in parkinsonian and depressed patients has been proposed.

These aspects have focused interest on the various processes and mechanisms associated with GABA-mediated neurotransmission in the CNS as potential targets for clinically useful drugs.

10.3.1 GABA: complex molecule with multiple functions

A considerable degree of flexibility is a trait of the molecule of GABA, and molecular orbital calculations have disclosed a relatively high degree of delocalization of the positive as well as the negative charges of GABA (Fig. 10.2). These molecular characteristics probably are essential for the entire synaptic activity of GABA, and there is strong evidence supporting the view that GABA adopts dissimilar active conformations at different synaptic recognition sites. Although the molecule of GABA is achiral, the prochiral hydrogen atoms at each carbon atom of the GABA backbone become mutually different during the interaction of GABA with the chiral biomolecules of the different GABA synaptic mechanisms. GABA itself obviously is not suitable for molecular pharmacological studies. Synthesis and structure-activity studies of GABA analogues, in which the conformational and electronic parameters have been systematically changed, and model compounds containing chiral centres with established absolute stereochemistry have, however, shed much light on the molecular pharmacology of the GABA synaptic mechanisms.

10.3.2 Chiral analogues and bioisosteres of GABA

The degree of stereoselectivity of the GABA transport mechanisms has been compared with that of the $GABA_A$ receptors/binding sites using the (*S*)- and (*R*)-forms of chiral GABA

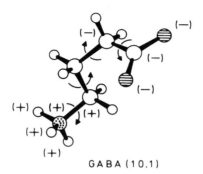

GABA (10.1)

Figure 10.2   Structure, conformational flexibility, and approximate charge distribution of the molecule of GABA (**10.1**).

analogues as test compounds. The (S)- and (R)-forms of the flexible GABA analogue 4-aminopentanoic acid (**10.2**) are equally effective at GABA$_A$ receptor sites, and both interact with the neuronal as well as the glial GABA uptake systems. The (R)-form of homo-β-proline (**10.3**) proved to be more than an order of magnitude more potent than its (S)-enantiomer as an inhibitor of GABA$_A$ receptor binding, whereas the enantiomeric forms of this cyclic, but relatively flexible, GABA analogue were approximately equieffective as inhibitors of neuronal GABA uptake. Conformational immobilization of the C2-C3 bonds of the enantiomers of **10.2** to give (S)- and (R)-trans-4-aminopent-2-enoic acid (**10.4**) has quite dramatic effect on the pharmacological profiles. Thus, the (S)-form of this conformationally restricted GABA analogue specifically binds to and activates GABA$_A$ receptors, whereas its (R)-isomer interacts with neuronal and glial GABA uptake without showing detectable affinity for GABA$_A$ receptor sites.

GABA (**10.1**)

(S)-   (R)-   (S)-   (R)-

(**10.2**)   (**10.3**)

(S)-   (R)-

(**10.4**)

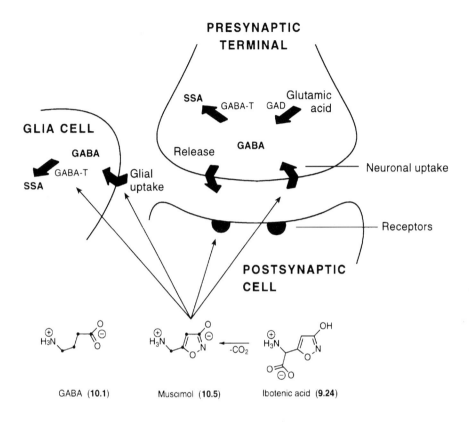

Figure 10.3 Schematic illustration of the biochemical pathways, transport mechanisms, and receptors at a GABA-operated axo-somatic synapse. GAD: (*S*)-glutamate decarboxylase; GABA-T: GABA: 2-oxoglutarate aminotransferase; SSA: succinic acid semi-aldehyde. The interaction with various GABA synaptic mechanisms of the heterocyclic GABA analogue muscimol (**10.5**), which is formed in the fly agaric mushroom *Amanita muscaria* by decarboxylation of ibotenic acid (see Chapter 9), is illustrated.

These stereostructure-activity studies have disclosed that the degree of stereoselectivity of GABA synaptic mechanisms depends on the conformational mobility of the chiral GABA analogues tested. Thus, enantiomers of semi-rigid, but not very flexible, chiral GABA analogues show markedly different pharmacological profiles.

Studies on chiral analogues of muscimol (**10.5**), a 3-isoxazolol bioisostere of GABA isolated from the mushroom *Amanita muscaria*, have supported this structure-activity relationship (Fig. 10.3). Thus, (*S*)-**10.7** shows a thirty times higher affinity for GABA$_A$ receptors than its (*R*)-enantiomer. Whereas neither (*S*)- nor (*R*)-**10.7** bind detectably to GABA uptake mechanisms, the (*S*)-form of dihydromuscimol (DHM, **10.8**) is an extremely potent and highly selective GABA$_A$ agonist and (*R*)-**10.8** a selective inhibitor of GABA uptake. It is evident that (*S*)-**10.8** can adopt conformation(s) reflecting the active conformation of GABA at GABA$_A$ receptors.

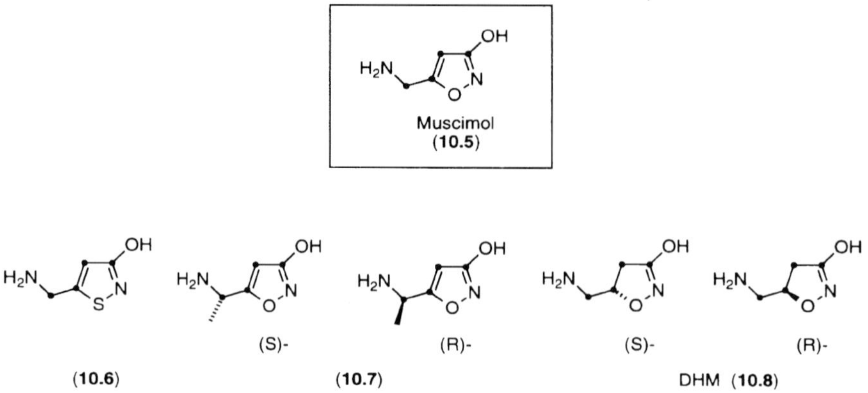
Muscimol
(10.5)
(S)-
(R)-
(S)-
(R)-
(10.6)
(10.7)
DHM (10.8)

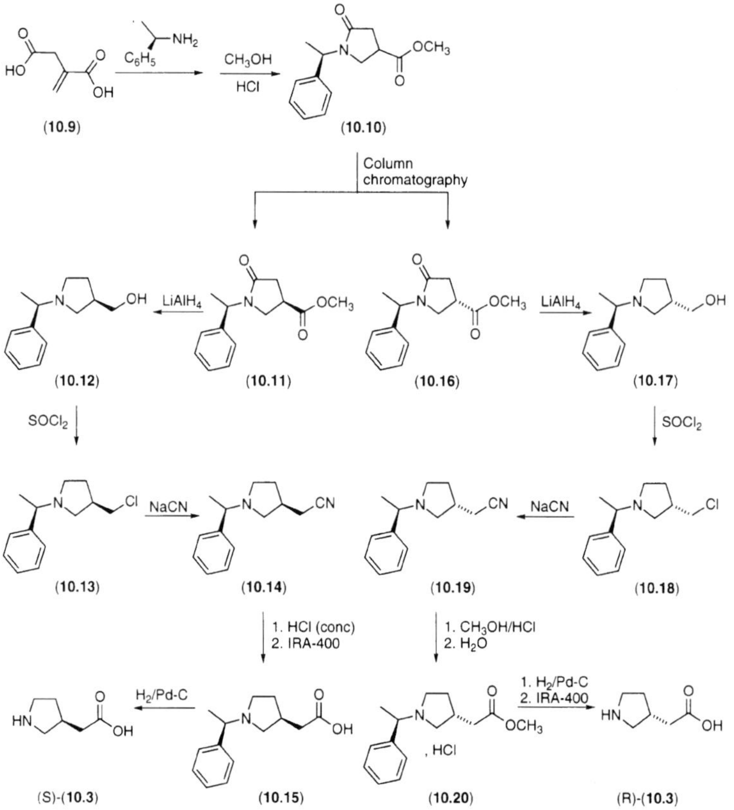
(10.9)
(10.10)
Column chromatography
LiAlH4
SOCl2
NaCN
(10.11)
(10.12)
(10.13)
(10.14)
(10.15)
(10.16)
(10.17)
(10.18)
(10.19)
(10.20)
1. HCl (conc)
2. IRA-400
1. CH3OH/HCl
2. H2O
H2/Pd-C
1. H2/Pd-C
2. IRA-400
(S)-(10.3)
(R)-(10.3)

Scheme 10.1

The syntheses of (*S*)- and (*R*)-**10.3** are outlined in Scheme 10.1. A conjugate addition/cyclization reaction between itaconic acid (**10.9**) and (*R*)-1-phenylethylamine and subsequent esterification gave the mixture (**10.10**) of the diastereomeric compounds **10.11** and **10.16**, which were separated by conventional column chromatography. The absolute configuration of methyl (3*S*)-1-[(*R*)-1-phenylethyl]-5-oxo-3-pyrrolidinecarboxylate (**10.16**) was determined by X-ray crystallography. This analysis also revealed the absolute stereochemistry of **10.11**. Through slightly different series of stereoconservative reactions **10.16** and **10.11** were converted into (*R*)-**10.3** and (*S*)-**10.3**, respectively. At different steps both series of reactions involved treatment with the strongly basic ion exchange resin, IRA-400.

The resolution and determination of the absolute configuration of (*S*)- and (*R*)-**10.8** are shown in Scheme 10.2. From the mixture of diastereomeric cinchonidine salts of *N*-protected racemic DHM (**10.21**), which contains a 2-isoxazolin-3-ol isostere of the carboxyl group, the salt of the (*S*)-form of the substrate crystallized. From these crystals and from the mother liquor partially resolved **10.23** and **10.22**, respectively, were isolated. Both of these enantiomeric compounds, which had melting points higher than that of their racemic form (**10.21**), were obtained in optically pure forms via recrystallizations. The absolute configuration of **10.23**, and thus of (*S*)-**10.8**, was established by chemical correlation to the (*S*)-form of 3-hydroxy-GABA (**10.26**), which has been synthesized stereospecifically from D-arabinose. As shown in Scheme 10.2, **10.23** and (*S*)-**10.26** were transformed into the same product, (**10.24**). Di-tert.butyl pyrocarbonate (DTPC) was used as a reagent for protection of the amino group of (*S*)-**10.26**.

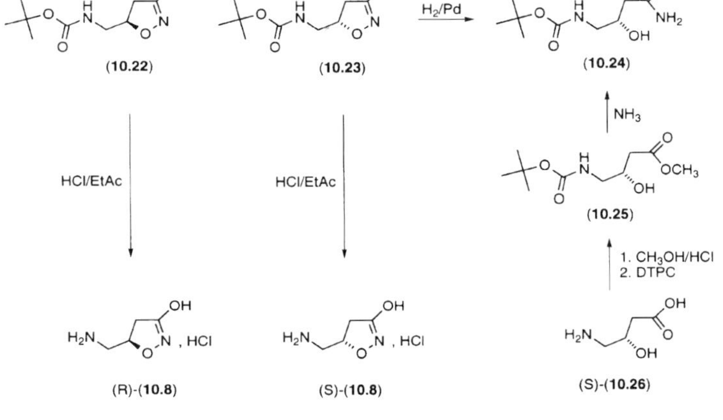

Scheme 10.2

10.3.3 *In vivo* and *in vitro* test systems

The *in vivo* agonistic effects of the GABA analogues described in this chapter were assessed on the basis of microelectrophoretic (iontophoretic) studies on cat spinal interneurones. Extracellular action potentials were recorded by means of the centre barrel of multi-barrel micropipettes, and the compounds were administered electrophoretically from the outer barrels of the micropipettes as cations.

Similarly, microelectrophoretic techniques offer the most direct approach to examination of the effects of GABA uptake inhibitors on GABA synaptic mechanisms *in vivo*. The depressant effect of GABA, administered microelectrophoretically on single central neurones, can be enhanced by GABA uptake inhibitors administered simultaneously using the same technique. This technique, however, does not distinguish between inhibitors of the neuronal and glial uptake systems (Fig. 10.3). Studies of the selectivity of GABA uptake inhibitors with respect to neuronal and glial transport systems are performed using *in vitro* test systems. Primary cultures of neurones and astrocyte cells are normally used as model systems for studies of neuronal and glial GABA transport, respectively.

GABA (**10.1**)   Muscimol (**10.5**)   Thiomuscimol (**10.6**)   THIP (**10.27**)

BMC (**10.28**)   SR 95531 (**10.29**)   (R)-Baclofen (**10.30**)

Cultures of mammalian central neurones have also been used as model systems for electrophysiological studies based on voltage-clamp and patch-clamp techniques. These and other types of electrophysiological studies have provided insight into the mechanisms underlying different synaptic functions.

The affinities of new compounds for receptors are normally measured using receptor binding techniques, where the ability of test compounds to displace radioactively labelled ligands from the receptor sites is a measure of their affinity (see Chapter 6). GABA$_A$ receptor (see Section 10.3.6) affinity of new GABA analogues has been determined using a number of tritium labelled GABA$_A$ agonists and antagonists. In addition to radioactive GABA, tritiated forms of the GABA$_A$ agonists, muscimol (**10.5**), thiomuscimol (**10.6**) and 4,5,6,7-tetrahydro[5,4-*c*]pyridin-3-ol (THIP) (**10.27**) are frequently used as radioligands. The 3-isoxazolol and, in particular, the 3-isothiazolol heterocyclic units are photosensitive.

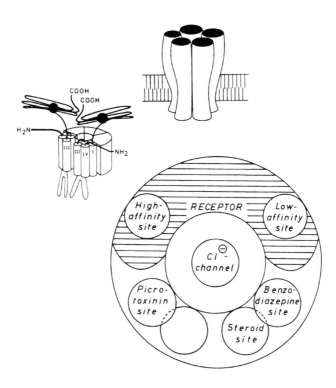

Figure 10.4   A sketch of the pentameric structure of the GABA$_A$ receptor complex and a schematic illustration of this GABA$_A$ receptor complex indicating the multiplicity of GABA binding sites, the chloride ion channel, and additional binding sites which may have physiological modulatory functions. This "pharmacological depiction" of the GABA$_A$ receptor complex does not indicate the localization of the different binding sites on the receptor subunits.

These properties have made radioactive muscimol (**10.5**) and thiomuscimol (**10.6**) useful photolabels for studies of the localization of the GABA recognition site(s) at the GABA$_A$ receptor complex (Fig. 10.4). Furthermore, tritiated forms of the GABA$_A$ antagonists, bicuculline methochloride (BMC) (**10.28**) and SR 95531 (**10.29**) are useful ligands for GABA$_A$ receptor studies, whereas tritiated (R)-baclofen (**10.30**) is a standard ligand for studies of GABA$_B$ receptor affinities (see Section 10.3.6.3). Receptor binding studies using these agonist and antagonist radioligands have consistently shown that the GABA$_A$ receptor contains at least two, perhaps three, recognition sites as demonstrated by Scatchard analyses (see Chapter 6) of receptor binding data.

The physiological relevance of these multiple binding sites is unknown. In general, low or very low affinity receptor sites for neurotransmitters are likely to correspond to functional receptors. In the case of GABA, this view may be supported by the observation that the coupling between the GABA$_A$ receptors and the benzodiazepine (BZD) sites (Fig. 10.4) seems to involve very low affinity GABA receptor sites. Like THIP (**10.27**), the antagonist BMC (**10.28**) interacts preferentially with low-affinity GABA$_A$ receptor sites.

In the presence of physiological concentrations of calcium the selective $GABA_B$ receptor agonist (R)-baclofen (**10.30**) (see Section 10.3.6.3) binds to receptor sites in brain synaptic membranes showing a pharmacological profile distinctly different from those of $GABA_A$ sites.

Different procedures for studies of $GABA_A$ agonist-induced enhancement of BZD binding have been developed (see Section 10.3.6.2). Rat brain synaptic membranes are incubated with the radioactive BZD ligands such as diazepam or flunitrazepam (see Chapter 6) in the presence of the $GABA_A$ agonists under study. The effects of GABAergic compounds on BZD binding are dependent on a variety of factors, notably temperature and concentration of chloride ions in the incubation media, in agreement with the coupling of the $GABA_A$ receptor to a chloride ion channel (Fig. 10.4).

10.3.4 GABA biosynthesis and metabolism

The biochemical pathways underlying the biosynthesis and catabolism of GABA have largely been mapped out and the key enzymes identified and characterized. Although the relative importance of the various biosynthetic routes for GABA has not been determined precisely, it is generally accepted that the major pathway involves decarboxylation of glutamic acid to GABA catalysed by the enzyme GAD (Fig. 10.3).

GABA is released from the presynaptic terminals via a specific release system. This release system, which may be regulated by presynaptic autoreceptors, is, at least partially, dependent on calcium ions.

The initial step of the catabolism of GABA is transformation into succinic acid semi-aldehyde (SSA). This transamination reaction, which is catalysed by GABA: 2-oxoglutarate aminotransferase (GABA-T), takes place within presynaptic GABA terminals and also in surrounding glia cells (Fig. 10.3). Extracellular enzymatic degradation does not seem to play any role in the inactivation of GABA.

Vigabatrin (**10.31**)   (**10.32**)   (**10.33**)   (**10.34**)

(**10.35**)   (**10.36**)   (**10.37**)   (**10.38**)

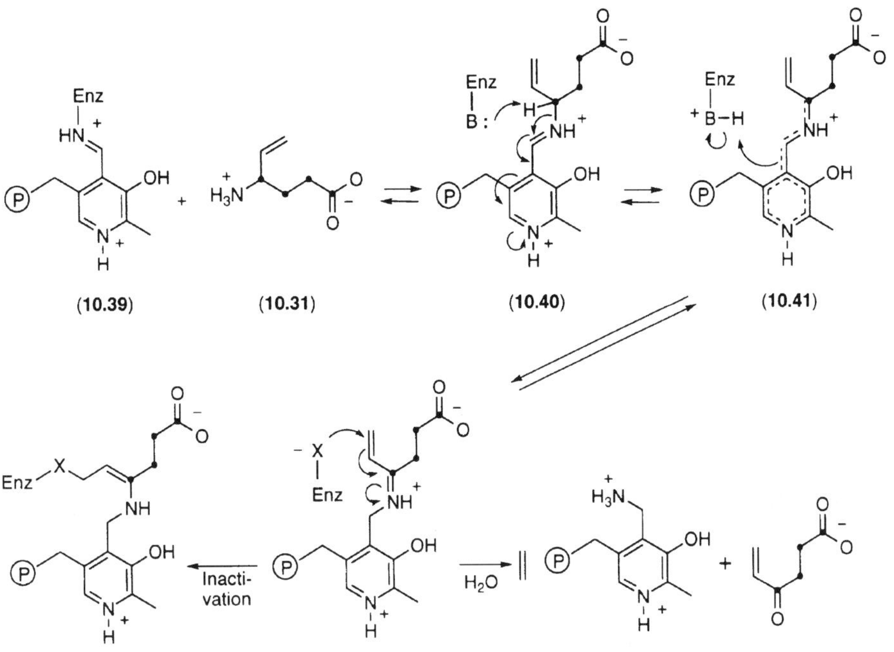

Scheme 10.3

10.3.4.1 Inhibitors of GABA metabolism

A number of mechanism-based inactivators of GABA-T have been developed and shown to inactivate the enzyme *in vitro* and *in vivo* (see Chapter 11). These compounds are typically analogues of GABA, containing appropriate functional groups at C4 of the GABA backbone, which are converted by GABA-T into electrophiles, which react with nucleophilic groups at or near the active site of the enzyme and thereby inactivate the enzyme irreversibly. Although GABA-T, like other pyridoxal phosphate-dependent enzymes (see Chapter 11), does not show strict stereospecificity with respect to inactivation by mechanism-based inactivators (suicide-substrates), such inhibitors do react with the enzyme in a stereoselective manner. Thus, the (*S*)-forms of the GABA-T suicide-substrates 4-aminohex-5-enoic acid (Vigabatrin, **10.31**), 4-aminohex-5-ynoic acid (**10.32**), 4-aminohept-5,6-dienoic acid (**10.33**), and the fluoromethyl derivative (**10.34**) are more active as GABA-T inactivators than the respective (*R*)-isomers. Vigabatrin has clinical interest as an anti-epileptic agent. In this regard it is interesting and fortunate that the active (*S*)-isomer of Vigabatrin (**10.32**) is actively taken up by the neuronal as well as the glial transport mechanisms, whereas the (*R*)-isomer is not transported.

The cyclic GABA analogues gabaculine (**10.35**) and isogabaculine (**10.36**) are also mechanism-based inhibitors of GABA-T, but in contrast to the suicide-substrates **10.32** or **10.33**, the cyclic GABA analogues **10.35** and **10.36** do not alkylate the enzyme. As a result of enzymatic processing by GABA-T these compounds are converted into aromatic pyridoxamine-5-phosphate adducts, which do not desorb from the active site of the enzyme. The GABA-T inhibitor 4-amino-4,5-dihydro-2-furancarboxylic acid (**10.37**) probably inactivates the enzyme by a similar mechanism. 4-Nitro-1-butanamine (**10.38**) is a GABA-T inhibitor, in which the weakly acidic nitromethylene group acts as a "mechanistic" bioisostere of the carboxyl group of GABA (see Scheme 10.4).

The mechanism for inactivation of GABA-T by Vigabatrin (**10.31**) is outlined in Scheme 10.3. As shown, pyridoxal phosphate is present in the active site as a Schiff base (**10.39**) with the terminal amino group of a lysine residue. Transimination with **10.31** generates a new imine (**10.40**), which undergoes rate-determining enzyme-catalysed deprotonation to give the imine **10.42** after reprotonation. In analogy with the transamination reaction on GABA, **10.42** could be hydrolysed to give the SAA analogue **10.44** and pyridoxamine-5-phosphate (**10.43**). However, **10.42** is an electrophile, a Michael acceptor, which undergoes conjugate addition by an active-site nucleophile (X) and produces inactivated enzyme (**10.45**).

The initial steps in the inactivation of GABA-T by the naturally occurring inhibitor, gabaculine (**10.35**) (Scheme 10.4, upper part) are analogous with those described for Vigabatrin (**10.31**) (Scheme 10.3). Gabaculine (**10.35**) is recognized by GABA-T and coupled to pyridoxal phosphate to give the Schiff base **10.46**. Although **10.47**, formed by deprotonation on **10.46**, contains a dihydrobenzene ring showing some electrophilic character, **10.47** is not sufficiently reactive to alkylate GABA-T. As shown in Scheme 10.4, one of the highly activated protons at C-2 in the dihydrobenzene ring of **10.47** is removed. Subsequent reprotonation of the complex by a protonated nucleophile on the enzyme (GABA-T) gives compound **10.48**, which inactivates GABA-T *via* tight, but non-covalent, binding to the active site. A major driving force in the conversion of **10.47** into **10.48** is the aromatization of the dihydrobenzene ring of **10.47**.

The mechanism of action of the GABA-T inhibitor **10.38** is outlined in Scheme 10.4 (lower part). Like gabaculine (**10.35**), **10.38** reacts with pyridoxal phosphate. This reaction produces **10.51**, which inhibits the action of GABA-T in a manner analogues with that described for compound **10.48**. The key step in the formation of **10.51** is the intramolecular nucleophilic reaction between the anionic nitromethylene and iminium groups of **10.50**.

10.3.5 GABA uptake

GABA uptake mechanisms are concerned with the removal of synaptically released GABA as part of the termination of the GABA neurotransmission process (Fig. 10.3), but the precise mechanism of action, including the time course and capacity, of these mechanisms *in vivo* are not fully understood. The involvement of neuronal as well as glial cells in high-affinity GABA uptake has been demonstrated using a variety of different techniques and model systems. Studies of the uptake of GABA into isolated nerve endings (synaptosomes) have revealed the presence of both high- and low-affinity transport systems. GABA uptake data obtained from studies using cultured cells from the mammalian CNS are consistent with heterogeneity not only of neuronal but also of glial transport mechanisms. It has been proposed that facilitated diffusion of GABA into the postsynaptic membrane rather than carrier-mediated transport into terminals and glia cells may constitute the primary event in

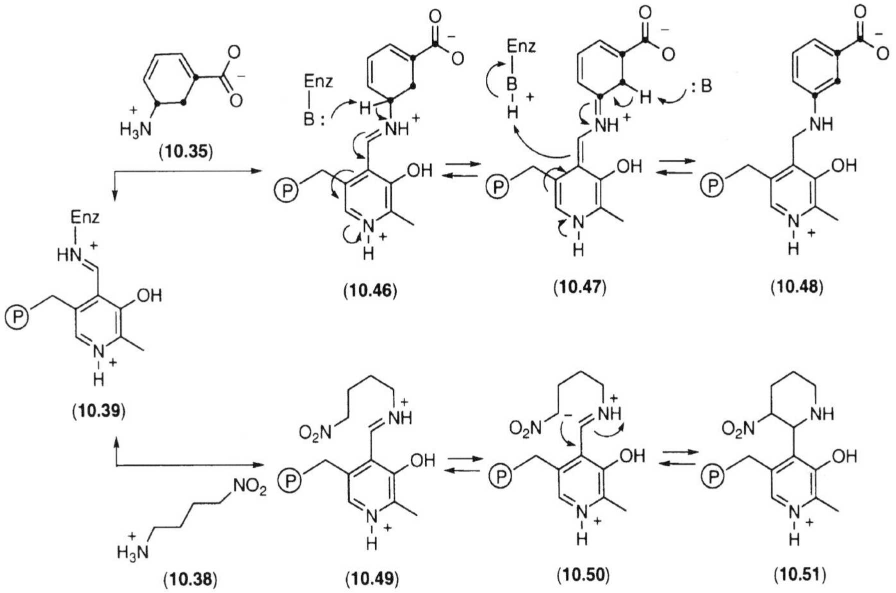

Scheme 10.4

the termination of the synaptic actions of GABA with subsequent transfer of GABA from the postsynaptic cell to nerve terminals and/or glia cells. The amount of GABA accumulated in terminals, but not that taken up by glia cells, is partially re-used as neurotransmitter substance.

10.3.5.1 Inhibitors of GABA uptake

In light of the limited knowledge of the processes underlying the termination of the synaptic action of GABA, it is at present not possible to single out with certainty the transport mechanism most susceptible to pharmacological intervention. It has, however, been established that neuronal and glial GABA uptake mechanisms have dissimilar substrate specificities, which are distinctly different from those of post-synaptic GABA receptors making selective pharmacological studies on GABA uptake possible.

The most logical and realistic strategies for such pharmacological interventions with the purpose of stimulating GABA neurotransmission seem to be:

1. effective blockade of both neuronal and glial GABA uptake in order to enhance the inhibitory effects of synaptically released GABA or, preferentially,

2. selective blockade of glial GABA uptake in order to increase the amount of GABA taken up by the neuronal carrier with subsequent elevation of the GABA concentration in nerve terminals.

Nipecotic acid (**10.52**) is an effective inhibitor of neuronal (N) as well as glial (G) GABA uptake, being twice as potent at the latter system as indicated by an N/G ratio of 0.5. Furthermore, nipecotic acid has been shown to be a substrate for neuronal and glial GABA transport carriers (Fig. 10.3). A number of cyclic amino acids structurally related to nipecotic acid (**10.52**), including 1,2,5,6-tetrahydropyridine-3-carboxylic acid (guvacine) and *cis*-4-hydroxynipecotic acid show a profile very similar to that of **10.52**.

Nipecotic acid

(**10.52**)   (**10.53**)

None of these amino acids are capable of penetrating the blood-brain barrier (BBB). Whereas introduction of small substituents on the amino groups of nipecotic acid (**10.52**) or guvacine results in compounds with decreased affinity for the GABA transport carriers, the *N*-4,4-diphenyl-3-butenyl (*N*-DPB) analogues of these amino acids, such as **10.53**, are much more potent than the parent amino acids. Furthermore, the lipophilic character of the DPB substituent explains why these *N*-DPB substituted GABA uptake inhibitors are pharmacologically active after systemic administration. In animal models these compounds are potent anticonvulsants, and a compound structurally related to **10.53** is being studied clinically as an antiepileptic agent.

The precise mechanisms underlying the interaction of this series of analogues with GABA uptake systems are, as yet, unknown. The relative potencies of these *N*-DPB analogues and of the respective classical amino acid uptake inhibitors, such as nipecotic acid, are, however, very similar. This structure-activity relationship strongly suggests that the amino acid moieties of these *N*-DPB analogues are recognized and bound by GABA transport carriers, with which the parent amino acids interact (see formula for **10.53**).

10.3.6 GABA receptors

Electrophysiological and receptor binding studies (see Section 10.3.3) have been used to detect GABA receptors and to identify subtypes of these receptors. GABA receptors are now divided into two main classes: GABA$_A$ receptors, which are blocked by BMC (**10.28**) and **10.29**, and GABA receptors insensitive to these antagonists, including GABA$_B$ receptors. Both classes of GABA receptors are heterogeneous.

GABA$_A$ receptors are coupled to a chloride ion channel (Fig. 10.4), and activation of these receptors results in a net influx or efflux of chloride ions, depending on the prevailing concentration gradient. The postsynaptic GABA$_A$ receptor, which is a receptor complex

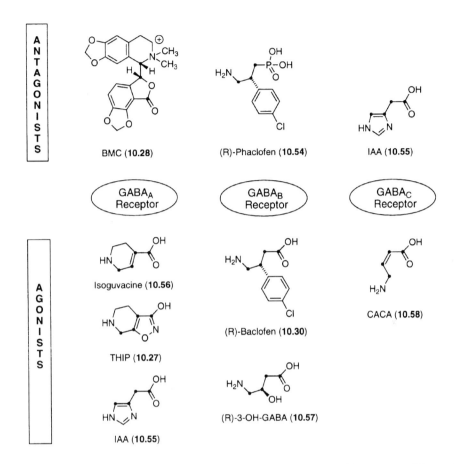

Figure 10.5 Schematic illustration of the different classes of GABA receptors and the structures of the agonists and antagonists normally used for pharmacological characterization of these receptors. Molecular cloning studies have demonstrated a high degree of heterogeneity of GABA$_A$ receptors, and there is pharmacological evidence of the existence of multiple forms of the G protein-coupled GABA$_B$ receptors. Like GABA$_A$ receptors (Fig. 10.4), the as yet incompletely characterized GABA$_C$ receptors belong to the ionotropic receptor superfamily.

containing a number of modulatory sites (Fig. 10.4), regulates the influx of chloride ions in such a way that receptor activation causes hyperpolarization of the cell membrane and, thus, decreased sensitivity of the neurone to excitatory input.

The classification of GABA receptors is outlined in Figure 10.5, which also shows the agonists and antagonists normally used to characterize the different classes of receptors. Whereas BMC (**10.28**) and SR 95531 (**10.29**) are the classical antagonists at GABA$_A$ receptors, isoguvacine (**10.56**) and THIP (**10.27**) are specific GABA$_A$ receptor agonists. Whereas isoguvacine is a full GABA$_A$ agonist, THIP as imidazole-4-acetic acid (IAA) (**10.55**) are very efficacious partial GABA$_A$ agonists.

Whereas (*R*)-baclofen (**10.30**) is the classical GABA$_B$ receptor agonist, the corresponding phosphonic acid analogue, (*R*)-phaclofen (**10.54**) was the first GABA$_B$ antagonist to

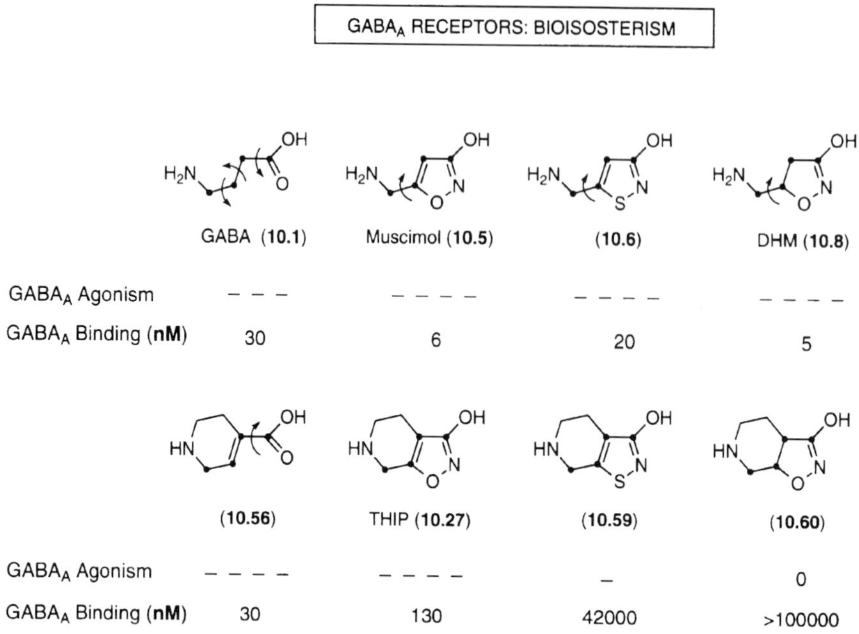

Figure 10.6   Structures and *in vivo* and *in vitro* effects on GABA$_A$ receptors of GABA and a number of mono-
and bicyclic bioisosteres of GABA.

be characterized. The (*R*)-form of 3-hydroxy-GABA (**10.57**) is a GABA$_B$ agonist, but
the stereochemical orientation of the hydroxy group of **10.57** is opposite to that of the
very lipophilic 4-chlorophenyl group of (*R*)-baclofen (**10.30**), suggesting that these two
groups interact with different structural units at the GABA$_B$ recognition site (Fig. 10.5).
Cis-4-aminobut-2-enoic acid (CACA) (**10.58**) is a selective agonist at GABA$_C$ receptors,
and, interestingly, the partial GABA$_A$ agonist, IAA (**10.55**) has recently been shown to be
a potent antagonist at GABA$_C$ receptors.

10.3.6.1 GABA$_A$ agonists, partial agonists and antagonists

Muscimol (**10.5**), thiomuscimol (**10.6**), and DHM (**10.8**) are highly potent GABA$_A$ agonists
(Fig. 10.6). These structure-activity studies indicate that the 3-isoxazolol, the 3-isothiazolol,
and the 2-isoxazolin-3-ol heterocyclic systems are effective bioisosteres of the carboxyl
group of GABA with respect to GABA$_A$ receptors.

Whereas muscimol (**10.5**) interacts more effectively than GABA with GABA$_A$ receptors
in vivo and *in vitro* (Fig. 10.6), it binds much less tightly to GABA$_B$ receptor sites and to
GABA transport mechanisms. Thiomuscimol (**10.6**) does not affect GABA uptake *in vitro*,
but the K$_m$ values for this GABA analogue and for **10.5** as substrates for GABA-T (see
Section 10.3.4) are lower than the K$_m$ value of 1.92 mM for GABA. Thus, the fact that
10.5 as well as **10.6** are metabolized by GABA-T reduces the value of these potent GABA$_A$
agonists for *in vivo* pharmacological studies.

A number of analogues of the specific GABA$_A$ agonist THIP (**10.27**) have been synthesized and tested (Fig. 10.6). These structure-activity studies include analogues, in which the 3-isoxazolol unit of THIP has been replaced by other heterocyclic systems. With the exception of thio-THIP (**10.59**), which is a very weak GABA$_A$ agonist, none of these THIP analogues, including **10.60**, show significant GABA$_A$ receptor affinities, emphasizing the marked structural constraints imposed on agonists for GABA$_A$ receptors.

THIP, which undergoes very limited metabolic decomposition *in vivo*, easily penetrates the BBB (see Section 10.4). It has been studied in healthy volunteers and in different groups of patients. THIP shows non-opioid analgesic effects and anxiolytic effects accompanied by sedative side-effects. Its lack of potent anti-epileptic effects, in spite of anticonvulsant effects in animal models, may to some extent reflect rapid GABA$_A$ receptor desensitization by THIP in man (see Section 10.1).

In general, the availability of antagonists with specific or highly selective effects on receptors is essential for elucidation of the physiological role and pharmacological importance of the receptors concerned, and in many areas of neuropharmacology, antagonists have proved to be extremely useful therapeutic agents (see Chapter 6). The fact that all GABA$_A$ antagonists, so far studied pharmacologically, are convulsants makes it unlikely that such compounds are going to play an important role in future psychotherapy. On the other hand, GABA$_A$ agonists have been shown to aggravate symptoms in certain neurological diseases, and in such cases, GABA$_A$ antagonist therapies may, at least theoretically, be beneficial. In this regard, the low-efficacy partial GABA$_A$ agonist 4-PIOL (**10.61**), which shows a dominating GABA$_A$ antagonist profile on brain tissues *in vitro*, has, in principle, therapeutic interest. The 5-isoxazolol and 3-isothiazolol analogues of 4-PIOL (**10.61**), compounds **10.62** and **10.63**, respectively, also show partial GABA$_A$ agonist profiles, **10.62** being less efficacious than **10.61**, whereas **10.63** is equiefficacious with **10.61**.

4-PIOL (**10.61**)   (**10.62**)   (**10.63**)

10.3.6.2 GABA-benzodiazepine interactions

The coupling between the GABA$_A$ receptor and the associated BZD site can be detected electrophysiologically as a facilitating effect of BZDs on the inhibitory effects of GABA or GABA$_A$ agonists (see Chapter 6). Similarly, BZDs are capable of stimulating the receptor binding of GABA or GABA$_A$ agonists, and the reverse effect, enhancement of BZD binding by GABA$_A$ agonists, is a generally used test system for such GABAergic agents (see Section 10.3.3).

As illustrated in Figure 10.7, there are striking differences between the effects on BZD binding of different structural classes of GABA$_A$ agonists. GABA and the GABA$_A$ agonists **10.5**, **10.6**, and (*S*)-**10.8** are very active activators of BZD binding in the absence or presence of chloride ions and at 0 °C. Other GABA$_A$ agonists such as THIP (**10.27**) or IAA (**10.55**) are much weaker.

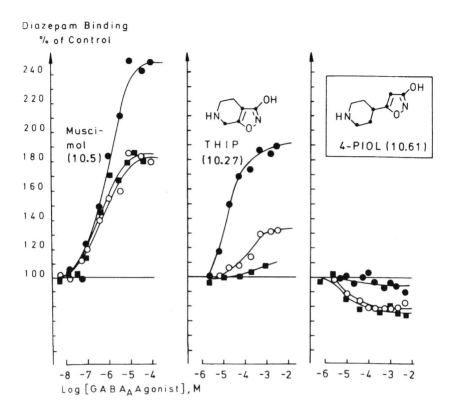

Figure 10.7   Effects on some GABA$_A$ agonists and partial agonists on the binding of radioactive diazepam at 0 °C and in the absence of chloride (■) or at 30 °C in the presence (●) or absence (○) of 150 mM sodium chloride.

10.3.6.3 GABA$_B$ agonists and antagonists

Within the group of GABA receptors insensitive to BMC (**10.28**), the GABA$_B$ receptors have been most extensively studied. These receptors (see Fig. 10.7) are activated by GABA and, in contrast to GABA$_A$ receptors, also by the GABA analogue (*R*)-baclofen (**10.30**). Although relatively little is known about the physiological role of GABA$_B$ receptors, they seem to regulate the release of certain neurotransmitters, including glutamic acid (see Fig. 10.10). GABA$_B$ receptors seem to be predominantly located presynaptically and they affect neurotransmitter release via regulation of a calcium ion channel. Postsynaptically located GABA$_B$ receptors linked to potassium channels have also been described, and neurochemical data have been interpreted in terms of the presence of presynaptic GABA$_B$ receptors, probably autoreceptors, on GABA terminals. Whilst an association between a large population of postsynaptic GABA$_A$ receptors and BZD receptor sites is well documented, it seems unlikely that GABA$_B$ receptors are linked to BZD receptor sites.

(*R*)-Baclofen (**10.30**) is clinically effective in certain types of spasticity. Furthermore, **10.30** has been administered to Huntington's chorea patients for about one year and a half, and during this period these patients showed significantly delayed developments of symptoms as compared with an untreated control group. However, after five years there was no detectable difference between the treated and untreated patients. The initial clinical effects of **10.30** may be the results of inhibition of the release of glutamic acid from hyperactive glutamic acid nerve terminals (see Chapter 9) *via* activation of presynaptic GABA$_B$ receptors.

(R)-Phaclofen (**10.54**)   Saclofen (**10.64**)   2-OH-Saclofen (**10.65**)

CGP-35348 (**10.66**)   CGP-55845 (**10.67**)

There also is a pharmacological and therapeutic interest in GABA$_B$ receptor antagonists. Thus, the *in vitro* release of dopamine, serotonin, and noradrenaline, also seem to be regulated by presynaptically located GABA$_B$ receptors. In principle, administration of GABA$_B$ antagonists would stimulate the release of such neurotransmitters, which may have therapeutic prospects in certain psychiatric diseases.

The phosphonic acid analogue of **10.30**, (*R*)-phaclofen (**10.54**), shows antagonist effects on central as well as peripheral GABA$_B$ receptors. Saclofen (**10.64**) and, in particular, 2-OH-saclofen (**10.65**) are considerably more potent than **10.54**. The phosphinic acids CGP-35348 (**10.66**) and CGP-55845 (**10.67**) are very potent GABA$_B$ receptor antagonists, which are able to cross the BBB. The hydroxy group of **10.67** probably interacts with the same site of the GABA$_B$ receptors as those of **10.57** and **10.65**.

10.4 PHARMACOKINETIC ASPECTS OF GABA ANALOGUES

All compounds so far known with specific actions on GABA synaptic processes have zwitterionic structures, although most of the GABA analogues described in this Chapter are depicted in the unionized forms. Small fractions of neutral amino acids exist as unionized molecules in solution, the ratio between the concentrations of ionized (zwitterionic) and unionized molecules (I/U ratio, zwitterionic constant) being a function of the difference between the pKa I and II values. Thus, a great difference between the pKa values of neutral amino acids is tantamount to high I/U ratios for the compounds.

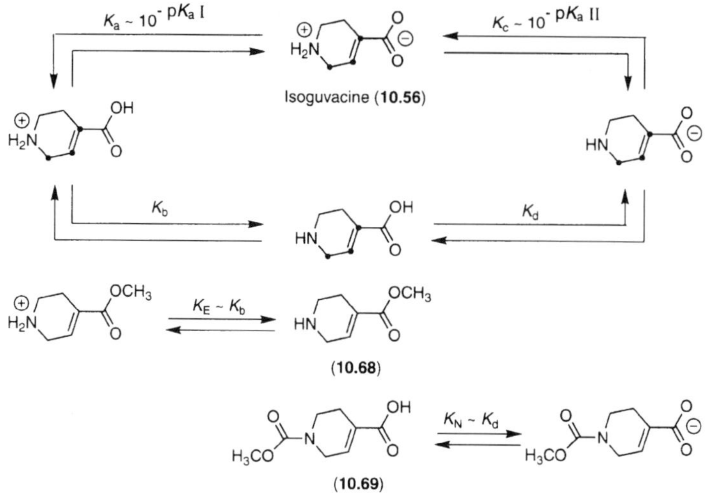

$$\frac{[\text{Zwitterionic isoguvacine}]}{[\text{Unionized isoguvacine}]} = \text{I/U Ratio} = \frac{K_a}{K_b} \sim \frac{K_a}{K_E} = \frac{10^{-3.6}}{10^{-8.9}} = 200000$$

$$= \frac{K_d}{K_c} \sim \frac{K_N}{K_c} = \frac{10^{-4.5}}{10^{-9.8}} = 220000$$

Figure 10.8 The four ionization constants for the neutral amino acid isoguvacine (**10.56**) and an illustration of the determination of the I/U ratio (zwitterionic constant) for **10.56** in aqueous solution using two analogous methods of calculation. In both cases, these calculations are based on the mass-law equations for the respective dissociation steps.

Since amino acids are likely to penetrate the BBB in the unionized form, it is of pharmacological interest to develop analogues of centrally active amino acids with small differences between the pKa values, and thus lower I/U ratios than the parent compounds. The pKa values of isoguvacine (**10.56**) (3.6; 9.8) are comparable with those of GABA (4.0; 10.7), which does not penetrate the BBB (see Fig. 10.9). The calculation of the I/U ratio for **10.56** is illustrated in Figure 10.8. Approximate values of K_a and K_c for **10.56** can be obtained by titration. The values of K_b and K_d for **10.56** have to be estimated indirectly by titration of appropriate derivatives of **10.56**, K_E for isoguvacine methyl ester (**10.68**) and K_N for 1-methoxycarbonyl-1,2,3,6-tetrahydropyridine-4-carboxylic acid (**10.69**) representing approximate values for K_b and K_d, respectively. Using two analogous methods of calculation, I/U ratios of 200 000 and 220 000 for **10.56** are found (Fig. 10.8). Based on similar calculations, I/U ratios of about 1000 have been determined for THIP (**10.27**) (Fig. 10.9). Thus, approximately 0.1% of a dose of **10.27** exists as unionized molecules in aqueous solution, whereas **10.56** is almost completely on the zwitterionic form in solution. These calculations explain why THIP, in contrast to **10.56** or GABA, enters the brain after peripheral administration. In the case of the $GABA_B$ agonist (*R*)-baclofen (**10.30**) the lipophilic character of the 4-chlorophenyl group, rather than a low I/U ratio, explains the ability of **10.30** to penetrate the BBB (see previous section).

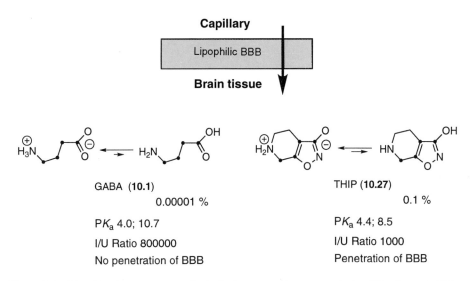

Figure 10.9   The pKa values, percentage of unionized compound in aqueous solution, I/U ratios, and abilities to penetrate the BBB of GABA and the GABA$_A$ agonist THIP (**10.27**).

10.5 CHOLINERGIC SYNAPSES AS THERAPEUTIC TARGETS

There is accumulating evidence of major impairments in central cholinergic neurotransmission in patients with the pathology characteristic of Alzheimer's disease (AD) and senile dementia of the Alzheimer type (SDAT). This cholinergic deficit may be of particular relevance to disturbances in learning and memory in AD/SDAT patients.

Neurochemical examination of biopsy and autopsy brain material from Alzheimer patients has revealed loss of presynaptic marker enzymes, acetyl-CoA:choline-O-acetyltransferase (ChAT) and acetylcholinesterase (AChE), and of presynaptic muscarinic receptor sites of the M_2 subtype (see Fig. 10.10) correlating with dementia score and severity of neurohistopathology. Postsynaptic muscarinic receptor sites which primarily are of the M_1 subtype do, however, to a large extent seem to survive the loss of cholinergic nerve terminals in different brain regions.

These observations form the basis of the "cholinergic hypothesis" of AD and SDAT. The primary cause(s) of these diseases are, however, far from being fully elucidated. A variety of possibilities have been proposed, including: (1) autoimmune reaction, (2) programmed genetic predisposition, (3) environmental factors, (4) viral infections, or (5) multifactorial origins. Although several factors may play a role in the etiology of these diseases, recent studies have been focused on the role of the central excitatory neurotransmitter glutamic acid in the degenerative processes characterizing AD and SDAT (see Chapter 9).

If excitotoxic mechanisms really are responsible for some of the changes in brains of Alzheimer patients, it would be expected that structures containing glutamic acid receptors would be selectively targeted for degeneration, resulting ultimately in loss of such receptors. It actually has been demonstrated that there is a selective loss of cortical and hippocampal glutamic acid receptors in AD.

In light of the well documented loss of cholinergic nerve terminals in certain brain areas of AD/SDAT patients, notably in the cerebral cortex and the hippocampus, there is an obvious need for an acetylcholine (ACh) replacement therapy in these diseases. Ideally, such therapeutic approaches should be selectively targeted at cholinergic synapses in the brain areas containing the degenerating ACh systems.

In principle, cholinergic neurotransmission can be stimulated indirectly via the GABA system, which appears to exert inhibitory control of ACh neurones in different brain areas through $GABA_A$ receptors, which may be located pre- or post-synaptically on ACh neurones (Fig. 10.10). Therapies based on agents with antagonistic actions at $GABA_A$ receptors or at one of the modulatory sites of the $GABA_A$ receptor complex (see Fig. 10.4) should theoretically be applicable in AD/SDAT. In principle, the low-efficacy partial $GABA_A$ agonists, 4-PIOL (**10.61**), **10.62**, or **10.63**, all of which show predominant $GABA_A$ antagonist profiles, have therapeutic interest in these diseases.

Most therapeutic interest in AD/SDAT has, so far, been focused on the processes and mechanisms at muscarinic cholinergic synapses. Administration of biosynthetic precursors for ACh should increase the concentration of ACh in the brain and, consequently, stimulate cholinergic neurotransmission. Such therapies would, however, be expected to stimulate indiscriminately all ACh systems in the brain and, perhaps predominantly, in the periphery with virtually unpredictable pharmacological consequences. These aspects may explain the very limited success, so far, of clinical studies in AD/SDAT on the choline precursor, lecithin.

The heterogeneity of muscarinic ACh receptors in the CNS (see subsequent section) may make it possible to identify a subtype of such receptors, which is of particular pharmacological relevance in AD/SDAT. On the basis of the neurochemical evidence so far available, the postsynaptic M_1 receptors seem to be of primary therapeutic interest (Fig. 10.10). Partial agonists at M_1 receptors probably have less predisposition to cause receptor desensitization than full agonists, making the former type of agonists more interesting from a therapeutic point of view (see Section 10.1). As a result of degeneration of ACh nerve terminals, such agents might be expected to act as agonists at the virtually "empty" and, thus, presumably supersensitive postsynaptic M_1 receptors. In other brain areas, where the muscarinic synapses are normosensitive, partial M_1 agonists may have weak or, ideally, no effects. Antagonists at presynaptic M_2 receptors, which may function as autoreceptors, might be useful drugs at the early stages of AD/SDAT, and compounds with mixed M_1 agonist/M_2 antagonist profiles may prove to be of particular therapeutic interest. Agonists for presynaptically located nicotinic ACh receptors (see subsequent section), which seem to be involved in a positive feedback regulation of ACh release, may also have therapeutic interest.

A fundamental question is, however, whether a muscarinic agonist replacement therapy altogether is a realistic possibility. This question is particularly relevant in light of the findings that $GABA_A$ agonist therapies have failed to improve significantly the symptoms of patients suffering from epilepsy (see Section 10.3.6.1), where GABA neurones seem to be in a state of dysfunction or degeneration. It must, however, be emphasized that there are major differences between $GABA_A$ receptors and muscarinic ACh receptors. Whereas the former class of receptors is of the fast type, which are coupled to ion channels, central muscarinic ACh receptors generally are of the slow type, coupled to second messenger systems (see Fig. 10.1).

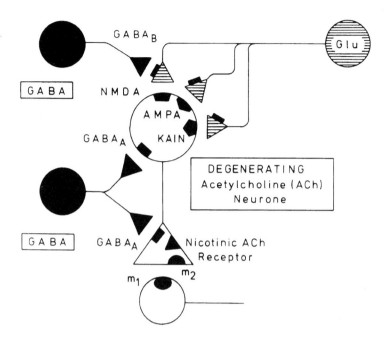

Figure 10.10   Schematic illustration of synaptic contacts between central ACh, glutamic acid (Glu), and GABA neurones and their receptors.

Since hyperactivity of central glutamic acid neurones may be one of the primary cause(s) of the degeneration of ACh neurones in AD/SDAT (see Chapter 9), glutamic acid receptor antagonists have interest as neuroprotective drugs in these diseases. So far, competitive as well as noncompetitive antagonists at the NMDA subtype of glutamic acid receptors have been shown to possess neuroprotective properties in animal models and cell culture systems.

Normal function of central ACh neurones appears to be dependent on stimulation by glutamic acid neurones (Fig. 10.10), and therefore it may be difficult to prevent glutamic acid receptor-mediated degeneration of ACh neurones by glutamic acid antagonists without reducing or, perhaps, blocking the excitatory input from glutamic acid terminals to ACh neurones. Consequently, future therapies in AD/SDAT based on glutamic acid antagonists probably have to be supplemented by concomitant treatment by partial M_1 receptor agonists in order to maintain the function of muscarinic synapses during the treatment with neuroprotective drugs. Thus, partial M_1 receptor agonists may be of major therapeutic interest, not only as drugs for symptomatic treatment of AD/SDAT patients but also as essential components of neuroprotective treatments of such patients.

10.5.1   Muscarinic and nicotinic acetylcholine receptors and ligands

As for other neurotransmitters, multiple receptors exist for ACh in the periphery as well as in the CNS. The ACh receptors are classified into two main groups, the nicotinic and the muscarinic receptors (Fig. 10.11).

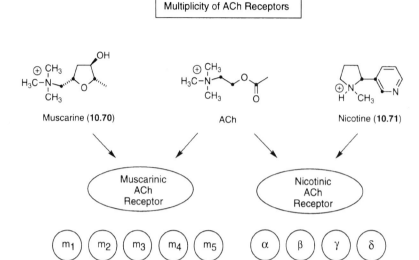

Figure 10.11   Structures of ACh and the classical muscarinic and nicotinic ACh receptor agonists, muscarine (**10.70**) and nicotine (**10.71**), respectively and an indication of the heterogeneity of ACh receptors.

Muscarine (**10.70**), which is also a constituent of *Amanita muscaria* (see Section 10.3.2), to some extent reflects the structure of ACh. The quaternary ammonium group is essential for the interaction of **10.70** with muscarine receptors, and the ether group appears to be strongly involved in the receptor binding of **10.70**. However, the relative importance of the other structure elements of **10.70** for receptor binding and activation has not yet been fully elucidated. The structure of nicotine (**10.71**), on the other hand, is very different from that of ACh, and the molecular basis of the very tight binding of **10.71** to nicotinic ACh receptors is unclear.

Molecular cloning studies have revealed a high degree of heterogeneity of muscarinic receptors (Fig. 10.11). Five subtypes of such receptors ($m_1 - m_5$) have been cloned and expressed in model systems. So far, the correlation between these receptor subtypes, cloned from different tissues, and those identified using classical pharmacological methods ($M_1 - M_3$) is not entirely clear, although $m_1 - m_3$ are generally accepted to have pharmacological characteristics identical with those of $M_1 - M_3$, respectively (Fig. 10.12). There is also pharmacological evidence for heterogeneity of nicotinic ACh receptors (Fig. 10.11), but the mapping of potential subtypes within this class of ACh receptor is at an early stage as compared with the muscarinic receptors.

10.5.2 Muscarinic antagonists

The discovery that the alkaloids atropine (**10.72**) and scopolamine (**10.73**) (Fig. 10.12) block the actions of ACh at muscarinic receptors and produce a number of therapeutically useful actions, including antispasmodic and antiparkinsonian effects, led to an extensive search for

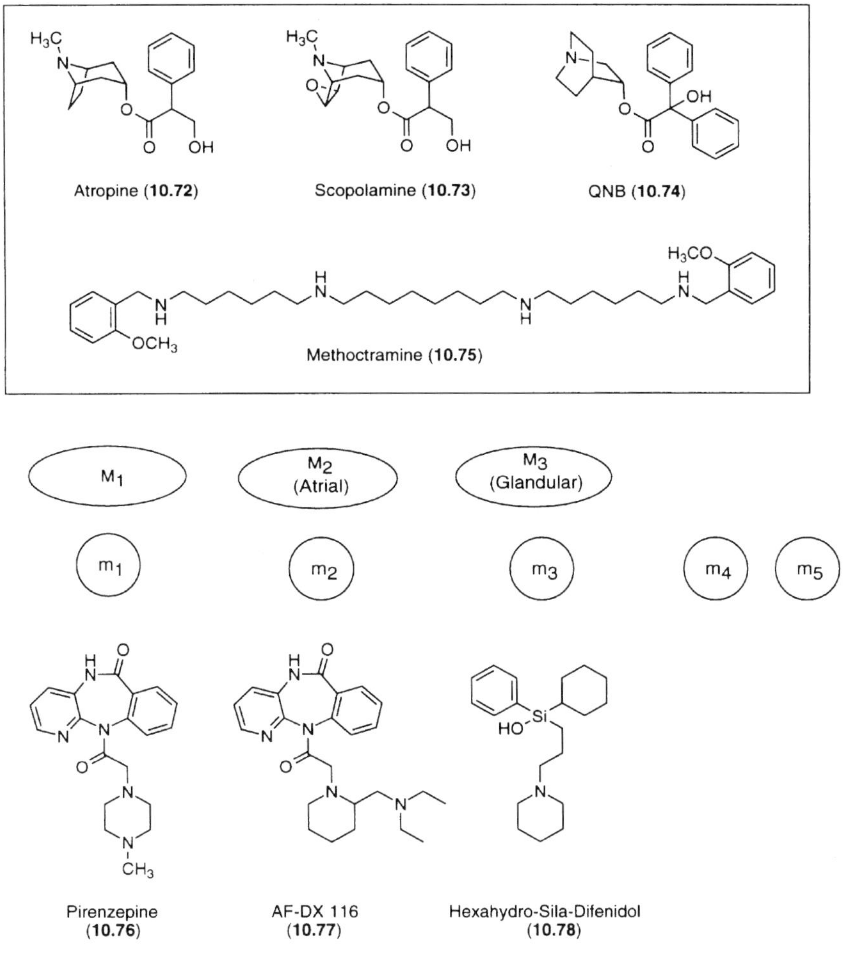

Figure 10.12 Multiplicity of muscarinic ACh receptors and structures of a number of non- and subtype-selective muscarinic antagonists.

synthetic analogues of these natural products. Among various potent synthetic muscarinic receptor antagonists, quinuclidinyl benzilate (QNB, **10.74**) is used as a radioactive ligand for studies of muscarinic receptor sites. Like **10.72** and **10.73**, **10.74** does, however, bind tightly to all subtypes of muscarinic receptors, and this lack of selectivity makes these compounds inapplicable for studies of muscarinic receptor subtypes.

In contrast to these classical muscarinic receptor antagonists, pirenzepine (**10.76**) shows major affinity variations in different tissues. It binds weakly to muscarinic receptors in the heart but interacts strongly with such receptors in the cerebral cortex and sympathetic ganglia, whereas it shows intermediate affinity for receptors in salivary glands and in stomach fundic mucosa. Based on these pharmacological and binding studies, the muscarinic receptors were subdivided into two main classes, M_1 receptors showing high affinity for **10.76** and a heterogeneous class of receptor (M_2) having much lower affinity for **10.76**.

The antagonist **10.76** does not clearly distinguish between the muscarinic receptors classified together as M_2. An analogue of **10.76**, (11-[[2-[(diethylamino)methyl]-1-piperidinyl]acetyl]-5,11-dihydro-6H-pyrido[2,3-b]benzodiazepin-6-one) (AF-DX 116, **10.77**) has, however, been shown to discriminate between M_2 receptor subtypes in peripheral tissues, showing high affinity for the M_2 receptors in the heart (M_2 atrial) and low affinity for the non-M_1 receptors in endocrine glands (M_3 glandular).

Whereas glandular M_3 receptors display low affinity for **10.76** as well as for **10.77**, they are effectively blocked by hexahydrosila-difenidol (**10.78**) and related silicon-containing compounds, which show limited affinity for M_1 and for atrial M_2 receptors. These studies emphasize the different pharmacological characteristics of M_2 and M_3 receptors, and this difference has been supported by the observation that methoctramine (**10.75**) and related polyamines selectively block M_2 receptors (Fig. 10.12).

10.5.3 Muscarinic agonists and partial agonists: bioisosterism and pharmacokinetics

The quaternary structure of ACh (Fig. 10.13) and the rapid hydrolysis of its ester moiety in biological systems make ACh inapplicable for most types of pharmacological experiments and, of course, for clinical studies. Removal of one or more of the N-methyl groups of ACh with the object of obtaining cholinergic compounds capable of penetrating the BBB result in pronounced loss of activity.

Arecoline (**10.79**) which is a constituent of areca nuts, the seeds of *Areca catechu*, is a cyclic "reverse ester" bioisostere of ACh, containing a tertiary amino group. In contrast to the findings for ACh, **10.79** is approximately equipotent with its quaternized analogue, N-methylarecoline, as a muscarinic ACh receptor agonist.

At pH 7.4, **10.79** is partially protonated, and using equation 10.1 the percentage ionization of **10.79** can be calculated to be 71 (Fig. 10.13). Analogously, the percentage of non-ionized acids in aqueous solution can be calculated using this equation. Thus, equation 10.1 can be used to calculate the percentage on acidic form of bases (ionized form) as well as acids (unionized form). Whilst **10.79** is assumed to bind to and activate muscarinic ACh receptors in its protonated form, the presence of a fraction of unionized molecules (29%) allows **10.79** to penetrate the BBB.

$$\% \text{ Ionized} = 100/[1 + \text{antilog (pH} - \text{pKa)}] \qquad (10.1)$$

Compound **10.79**, which actually is a partial agonist at both M_1 and M_2 receptors, has been shown to improve cognitive functions significantly when infused (i.v.) in AD/SDAT patients with presenile dementia, and **10.79** facilitates learning in normal young humans. These effects of **10.79** are, however, shortlived reflecting rapid *in vivo* hydrolysis of the ester group of this compound. Furthermore, the pronounced side-effects of **10.79** probably reflect the ability of this muscarinic agonist to activate peripheral and central M_2 receptors in addition to the desired partial agonist effect on central M_1 receptors.

Bioisosteric replacements of the carboxyl group of GABA analogues by the 3-isoxazolol group or structurally related heterocyclic units with protolytic properties similar to that

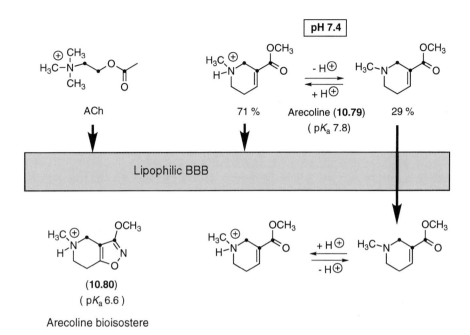

Figure 10.13   Structures of ACh and the muscarinic agonists arecoline (**10.79**) and the isoxazole arecoline bioisostere **10.80**. The ability of **10.79** to penetrate the BBB is illustrated.

of the carboxyl group have led to a number of specific and very potent GABA$_A$ agonists (Fig. 10.6). Similar bioisosteric replacements in the molecule of glutamic acid have led to heterocyclic amino acids with specific actions at subtypes of central glutamic acid receptors (see Chapter 9). These findings prompted the development of the arecoline bioisostere 3-methoxy-5-methyl-4,5,6,7-tetrahydroisoxazolo[4,5-*c*]pyridine (**10.80**) containing the hydrolysis-resistant ester isostere 3-methoxyisoxazole (Fig. 10.13).

Like **10.79**, the isoxazole bioisostere **10.80** interacts potently with central M$_1$ as well as M$_2$ receptors, but the latter compound is a more selective ligand for M$_1$ receptor sites than is **10.79**, and the partial agonist character of **10.80** is more pronounced than that of the lead compound, **10.79**. Compared with **10.79**, the bicyclic bioisostere **10.80** has a lower pKa value (6.6) and a higher log *P* value, and these physico-chemical properties can explain why **10.80** very easily penetrates the BBB.

Compound **10.80** has been used as a "second lead" for the design and development of a number of effective muscarinic agonists showing different degrees of M$_1$ selectivity and pharmacological profiles ranging from antagonists through low-efficacy agonists to full agonists. Like **10.80**, compound **10.87** and 3-methoxy-5,6,7,8-tetrahydro-4*H*-isoxazolo[4,5-*c*]azepine (**10.88**) are partial muscarinic agonists, **10.88** being markedly more potent than **10.80** and **10.87**. The "pharmacological importance" of the *O*-alkyl groups of these compounds is reflected by the observation that the *O*-ethyl analogue (**10.89**) is a competitive muscarinic antagonist, whereas the *O*-isopropyl analogue (**10.90**) shows the characteristics of a non-competitive antagonist.

(10.81)   (10.82)   (10.83)   (10.84)   (10.85)

(10.86)   (10.87)   (10.88)   (10.89)   (10.90)

Oxotremorine (**10.81**) is a very potent partial muscarinic agonist, which shows some selectivity for autoreceptors of the M_2 type. Extensive structural modifications of **10.81** have led to compounds with a broad spectrum of pharmacological effects ranging from full agonists to antagonists at central and/or peripheral muscarinic receptors.

The potent peripheral actions of **10.81**, including the effects on cardiovascular mechanisms, probably reflect its preferential activation of M_2 receptors. Attempts have been made to design analogues of **10.81** with pharmacological profiles relevant to AD/SDAT. One of these analogues (BM5, **10.82**) has been characterized as an M_1 agonist/M_2 antagonist (see Section 10.5). An evaluation of the potential of **10.82** as a therapeutic agent in AD/SDAT must await further behavioural pharmacological studies.

The naturally occurring heterocyclic cholinergic agonist pilocarpine (**10.83**) is widely used as a topical miotic for the control of elevated intraocular pressure associated with glaucoma. The bioavailability of pilocarpine is, however, low, and based on studies in animal models it has been suggested that this compound does not easily penetrate the BBB. Compound **10.83** is a partial muscarinic agonist showing an *in vitro* pharmacological profile very similar to that of arecoline (**10.79**). Impairments of position discrimination learning in animals could be overcome by systemically administered **10.79** as well as **10.83** at doses lower than those producing marked autonomic effects. These observations are interesting in relation to AD/SDAT and have focused behavioural pharmacological interest on prodrugs of **10.83** showing improved bioavailability (see Chapter 13).

The compounds **10.84-10.86** show very high affinity for muscarinic ACh receptors. The 3-amino-1,2,4-oxadiazole **10.84**, which interacts non-selectively with muscarinic ACh receptor subtypes, probably is the most potent muscarinic agonist known. The arecoline (**10.79**) bioisosteres, the 2-ethyltetrazole (**10.86**) and the 3-hexyloxy-1,2,5-thiadiazole (**10.85**) analogues have been reported to preferentially activate M_1 receptors *versus* M_2 receptors. Compound **10.85** is being evaluated clinically as a potential drug for the treatment of AD.

10.5.4 Acetylcholinesterase inhibitors

Inhibitors of AChE allow a build up of ACh at the nerve endings resulting in a prolonged activation of cholinergic receptors. Treatment with such inhibitors has been useful in myastenia gravis, a disease associated with the rapid fatigue of muscles and also in the treatment of glaucoma, where stimulation of the ciliary body improves drainage from the eye and, thus, decreases intraocular pressure.

(10.91)	Physostigmine (10.92)	Tacrine (10.93)
	(pK_a 1.8; 7.9)	(pK_a 10.0)

Two main classes of AChE inhibitors have been developed: (1) irreversible organophosphorus inhibitors, such as dyflos (**10.91**) and (2) carbamoylating, but reversible, inhibitors, such as physostigmine (eserine, **10.92**). The former class of compounds has a long duration of action in the body, and after a single dose of drug the activity of AChE only returns after re-synthesis of the enzyme. Due to dangers of overdosage they are only used therapeutically for the treatment of a limited number of glaucoma patients. A variety of volatile organophosphorus AChE inhibitors have been produced on large scales for use as nerve gasses in war, whereas other less volative compounds of this category have been used as insecticides.

Inhibitors of the latter class including **10.92**, are protonated at physiological pH and are bound at the anionic site of AChE. The relative positions of the ammonium and carbamate groups allow a transfer of the carbamoyl group onto the serine hydroxyl group at the esteratic site of the enzyme (see Chapter 11). The carbamoylated enzyme is hydrolysed to regenerate the enzyme with a half-life of less than one hour. Kinetic studies originally gave the impression that **10.92** and related carbamates were acting as simple reversible competitive inhibitors of AChE.

Inhibitors of AChE, notably **10.92**, have been studied clinically in AD/SDAT. Although treatment of Alzheimer patients with **10.92** have marginally improved learning and memory, these positive effects have been accompanied by unacceptable side-effects. Although amines like **10.92** are capable of penetrating the BBB (see Fig. 10.13), they are likely to enhance the activity at virtually all cholinergic synapses in the periphery and the CNS. Thus, stimulation of all nicotinic and muscarinic ACh receptors may explain the complex therapeutic effect/side-effect profiles observed after administration of **10.92** to AD/SDAT patients.

9-Amino-1,2,3,4-tetrahydroacridine (tacrine, THA, **10.93**) is a non-selective but reversible inhibitor of AChE. In spite of its strongly basic character (pKa 10.0) and, thus, high degree of protonation at physiological pH, **10.93** is capable of penetrating the BBB to some extent probably as a result of the lipophilic character of its phenyl and cycloalkyl ring structures.

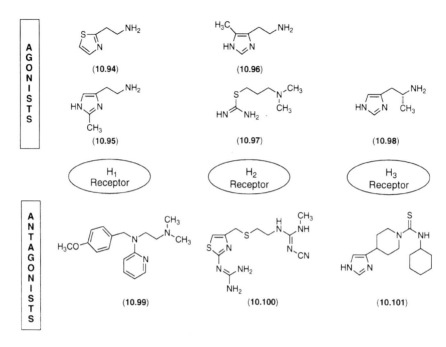

Figure 10.14　Schematic illustration of the multiplicity of histamine receptors and the structures of a number of receptor subtype-selective agonists and antagonists.

Clinical studies of **10.93** in Alzheimer patients have shown improvements in learning and memory, at least in certain groups of patients. These promising effects have been proposed to reflect selective effects of **10.93** on brain AChE. Since **10.93** also has pharmacological effects unrelated to the inhibition of AChE, the mechanism(s) underlying its favourable clinical effects in AD/SDAT are not fully understood.

10.6　HISTAMINE RECEPTORS

Histamine (2-(imidazol-4-yl)ethylamine), which is biosynthesized by decarboxylation of the basic amino acid histidine, is involved as a chemical messenger in a variety of complex biological actions. In mammals it is mainly stored in an inactive bound form in many body tissues, from which it is released by different stimuli and mechanisms. Histamine exerts its biological functions via activation of specific receptors, and during the past 2–3 decades three pharmacologically distinct histamine receptors designated H_1, H_2 and H_3 have been characterized (Fig. 10.14).

　　Activation of H_1 receptors stimulates the contraction of smooth muscles in many organs such as the gut, the uterus, and the bronchi. Contraction of the bronchi leads to restriction of the passage of air into and out of the lungs as in asthma. Stimulation of H_1 receptors on smooth muscles in for example fine blood vessels does, however, cause muscle relaxation, and the resulting vasodilation may result in severe fall in blood pressure. Furthermore, histamine increases the permeability of the capillary walls so that more of the plasma constituents can escape into the tissue space, leading to the formation of oedema. This series of events is manifest in the well-known redness and wheal associated with histamine release, the so-called "triple response". Histamine is also involved in the removal of the products of cell damage during inflammation. Under these circumstances, the liberation of histamine is accompanying the production of antibodies and their interaction with foreign proteins. Under extreme circumstances, however, the effects of histamine can become pathological, leading to exaggerated responses with distressing results, as may occur in some allergic conditions.

A number of selective and very potent antagonists at H_1 receptors are now available. Such compounds, including mepyramine (**10.99**), are structurally very different from histamine. These "antihistamines" are typically developed via lead optimization of accidentally discovered compounds capable of blocking the effects of histamine on the perfused lung or the isolated ileum or trachea from guinea pigs or on human bronchi. A number of these competitive H_1 antagonists are used clinically.

Compounds showing selective agonist activity at subtypes of histamine receptors probably have very limited, if any, therapeutic interest. Nevertheless, such compounds are essential as tools for pharmacological studies of histamine receptors. In order to develop such agonists the molecule of histamine has been subjected to extensive structural modifications. Most of these histamine analogues, in which the imidazole ring and/or the 2-aminoethyl side chain have been alkylated or otherwise structurally modified, show very weak histamine agonist activity. These systematic structural variations of histamine have, however, led to receptor subtype-selective agonists. Thus, 2-methylhistamine (**10.95**) and, in particular, 2-(thiazol-2-yl) ethylamine (**10.94**) are selective agonists at H_1 receptors, though weaker than histamine itself. On the other hand, 5-methylhistamine (**10.96**) selectively activates H_2 receptors. Similarly, S-[3-(N, N-dimethylamino)propyl]isothiourea (dimaprit, **10.97**), in which the imidazole ring of histamine has been bioisosterically replaced by an S-alkylisothiourea group showing similar protolytic properties, is a highly selective H_2 receptor agonist. These two H_2 agonists have been useful tools in connection with the elegant design and development of selective H_2 receptor antagonists such as **10.100** (see Section 10.6.2).

Studies in recent years have established that histamine is acting as a neurotransmitter in the CNS. Whilst H_1 and H_2 receptors seem to be predominantly localized on postsynaptic membranes of central neurones, H_3 receptors appear to function as presynaptic receptors, possibly as histamine autoreceptors. Although H_3 receptors have also been detected in some peripheral organs, this class of histamine receptors exists primarily in the CNS.

The physiological role of the central histamine neurotransmitter system is far from being elucidated, but it has been suggested that it plays a role in cerebral circulation, energy metabolism, and states of wakefulness. These aspects have focused pharmacological interest on agonists as well as antagonists at H_3 receptors. Interestingly, stereoselectivity of agonists is much more pronounced at H_3 receptors than at either H_1 or H_2 receptors, and (R)-α-methylhistamine (**10.98**) has been shown to be a selective and very potent H_3 receptor agonist (Fig. 10.14). Whilst a number of H_2 antagonists interact potently with H_3 receptors, highly selective H_3 antagonists, notably thioperamide (**10.101**), have recently been described. The availability of such compounds is likely to stimulate studies of the precise role of histamine in the CNS.

Histamine   + 2H$^{\oplus}$ (10.102) $-$H$^{\oplus}$ / $+$H$^{\oplus}$ (10.103)

(10.96)   + 2H$^{\oplus}$ (10.104) $-$H$^{\oplus}$ / $+$H$^{\oplus}$ (10.105)

10.6.1 Protolytic properties of histamine

Studies of the protolytic properties of histamine have played an important part in the design of selective H_2 antagonists (see subsequent section) and in the interpretation of structure-activity relationships for subtype-selective histamine receptor agonists. At physiological pH (7.4) the primary amino group (pKa 9.8) of histamine is almost fully ionized, whereas the monobasic imidazole ring (pKa 6.0) is only about 4% protonated (see equation 10.1, Section 10.5.3). Thus, in aqueous solution at physiological pH only ca. 4% of histamine exists as the resonance-stabilized dication **10.102**. The ionized side chain of **10.102** exerts a negative inductive ($-I$) effect on the protonated imidazole ring. This electron-withdrawing effect reduces the electron density at the nearest ring nitrogen atom (N3) and, thus, facilitates the dissociation of a proton from this atom to form the monocation **10.103**, named the N^τ-H tautomer. The methyl group of the H_2 receptor-selective agonist **10.96** exerts a positive inductive ($+I$) effect on the heterocyclic ring. This electron-repelling effect of the methyl group, which increases the electron density at N1, further stabilizes the N1-H bond in **10.104** and, consequently, the N^τ-H tautomer **10.105** after dissociation of a proton from the dication **10.104**.

Based on extensive structure-activity studies of histamine analogues, it is assumed that the monocationic N^τ-H tautomer **10.103** is the active form of histamine at H_1 as well as H_2 receptors. The protonated primary amino group and the lone pair of electrons at N3 in **10.103** are essential for the binding of histamine to H_1 receptors, whereas the protonated primary amino group and the N1-H group are essential molecular components for the binding of **10.103** to H_2 receptors.

10.6.2 H_2 receptor antagonists: design and development

Histamine has a physiological function in regulating the secretion of acid in the stomach where, acting on the H_2 receptor, it stimulates the parietal cells to produce hydrochloric acid. This probably is a protective mechanism, since the acid controls the local bacterial population. Under different conditions, the regulation of acid secretion by histamine or other chemical messengers may run out of control, and under such circumstances excessive acid secretion can lead to the formation of gastric and/or duodenal ulcers.

(10.106)   (10.107)   (10.108)

(10.109)   (10.110)   (10.111)

These aspects prompted the design and development of selective antagonists at H_2 receptors, and this field of drug research represents one of the most active and successful areas in medicinal chemistry. Systematic structural modifications of histamine led to the discovery of burimamide (**10.106**) as a selective but relatively weak H_2 receptor antagonist. The low activity of **10.106** was explained in terms of non-optimal protolytic properties of its imidazole ring, which is substantially more basic (pKa 7.2) than is the ring of histamine. Consequently, the degree of protonation of the imidazole ring of **10.106** is more than an order of magnitude higher than that of histamine at physiological pH. This increased basic character of the ring of **10.106** reflects a $+I$ effect of the alkyl side chain, and, furthermore, this electron-repelling effect favours the dissociation of the proton from N1 in **10.107** by increasing the electron density at N3. Thus, the N^{π}-H tautomer **10.108** will be the dominating neutral form of burimamide. Since burimamide appears to bind to the H_2 receptor in a neutral form, and since the imidazole ring of burimamide is assumed to bind to the site of the H_2 receptor, which binds the imidazole ring of histamine, the N^{π}-H tautomer **10.108** of burimamide was considered nonoptimal for effective receptor binding.

This reasoning prompted modifications of the structure of burimamide in order to obtain compounds, which more closely resembled histamine. Introduction of a sulphur atom into the side chain and a methyl group into position 5 of the ring of burimamide gave metiamide (**10.109**), which showed greater potency and selectivity as an H_2 receptor antagonist than did burimamide. Introduction of the sulphur atom converted the $+I$ effect of the side chain of burimamide into a $-I$ effect, whereas the C5 methyl group exerts a $+I$ effect. As a consequence of these structural modifications, the electron densities at C5-N1 and at C4-N3 in metiamide were, respectively, increased and decreased as compared with burimamide. Thus, the facilitated dissociation of the N3-H proton from protonated metiamide (**10.110**) gives the desired N^{τ}-H tautomer (**10.109**) as the dominating neutral form of metiamide.

Side-effects, such as agranulocytosis, of metiamide (**10.109**) led to the replacement of its thiourea unit by the structurally related cyanoguanidine group to give cimetidine (**10.112**), which is more active than **10.109** as an H_2 antagonist and less toxic. Cimetidine turned out to be a successful drug, and, since its introduction some fifteen years ago, several million patients suffering from diseases caused by unnaturally high gastric secretion of hydrochloric acid have benefited from its therapeutic use. In recent years, a wide variety

Cimetidine (**10.112**)   Ranitidine (**10.113**)

of other H_2 antagonists, notably ranitidine (**10.113**), have been introduced in the human clinic. The structural basis of the proposed interaction of the 2-guanidinothiazole and the 2-dimethylaminomethylfuran groups of **10.100** and **10.113**, respectively, with the imidazole-binding part of the H_2 receptor is under investigation.

FURTHER READING

Olsen, R.W. and Venter, J.C., Eds. (1986) *Benzodiazepine/GABA Receptors and Chloride Channels: Structural and Functional Properties*. New York: Alan R. Liss.

Krogsgaard-Larsen, P., Hjeds, H., Falch, E., Jørgensen, F.S. and Nielsen, L. (1988) Recent advances in GABA agonists, antagonists and uptake inhibitors: structure-activity relationships and therapeutic potential. *Adv. Drug. Res.*, **17**, 381–456.

Nanavati, S.M. and Silverman, R.B. (1989) Design of potential anticonvulsant agents: mechanistic classification of GABA aminotransferase inactivators. *J. Med. Chem.*, **32**, 2413–2421.

Barnard, E.A. and Costa, E., Eds. (1989) *Allosteric Modulation of Amino Acid Receptors: Therapeutic Implications*. New York: Raven Press.

Krogsgaard-Larsen, P. (1990) Amino Acid Receptors. In *Comprehensive Medicinal Chemistry, Vol. 3*, edited by C. Hansch, P.G. Sammes, J.B. Taylor and J.C. Emmett, pp. 493–537. Oxford: Pergamon Press.

Lodge, D., Ed. (1988) *Excitatory Amino Acids in Health and Disease*. Chichester: John Wiley & Sons.

Watkins, J.C., Krogsgaard-Larsen, P. and Honoré, T. (1990) Structure-activity relationships in the development of excitatory amino acid receptor agonists and competitive antagonists. *Trends Pharmacol. Sci.*, **11**, 25–33.

Brown, J.H., Ed. (1989) *The Muscarinic Receptors*. Clifton, New Jersey: The Humana Press.

Wess, J., Buhl, T., Lambrecht, G. and Mutschler, E. (1990) Cholinergic receptors. In *Comprehensive Medicinal Chemistry, Vol. 3*, edited by C. Hansch, P.G. Sammes, J.B. Taylor and J.C. Emmett, pp. 423–491. Oxford: Pergamon Press.

Cooper, D.G., Young, R.C., Durant, G.J. and Ganellin, C.R. (1990) Histamine Receptors. In *Comprehensive Medicinal Chemistry, Vol. 3*, edited by C. Hansch, P.G. Sammes, J.B. Taylor and J.C. Emmett, pp. 323–421. Oxford: Pergamon Press.

Timmerman, H. (1990) Histamine H_3 ligands: just pharmacological tools or potential therapeutic agents? *J. Med. Chem.*, **33**, 4–11.

Fischer, A. and Barak, D. (1994) Progress and perspectives in new muscarinic agonists. *Drug News & Perspectives*, **7**, 453–464.

Krogsgaard-Larsen, P., Frølund, B., Jørgensen, F.S. and Schousboe, A. (1994) $GABA_A$ receptor agonists, partial agonists and antagonists. Design and therapeutic prospects. *J. Med. Chem.*, **37**, 2489–2505.

Frydenvang, K., Hansen, J.J., Krogsgaard-Larsen, P., Mitrovic, A., Tran, H., Drew, C.A. and Johnston, G.A.R. (1994) $GABA_B$ antagonists: resolution, absolute stereochemistry, and pharmacology of (*R*)- and (*S*)-phaclofen. *Chirality*, **6**, 583–589.

11. ENZYMES AND ENZYME INHIBITORS

I. AHNFELT-RØNNE

CONTENTS

11.1 INTRODUCTION

Enzymes are commonly involved in the pathogenesis of diseases. They may, for example, catalyze the production of mediators and modulators of pathophysiological reactions; in such cases, administration of drugs which specifically inhibit the activities of the enzymes may cure the disease or relieve the symptoms. This approach is limited by the fact that few enzymes serve purely pathological functions, but indeed have important functions in the normal, healthy organism. Therefore, inhibition of such enzymes may lead to undesirable effects, so-called action-related side-effects. In other cases, it is possible to avoid such side-effects, because the enzyme target is not in the host but, for example, in microorganisms that have invaded the organism. Penicillin is a bacterial enzyme inhibitor, which does not show direct action-related side-effects, although the intestinal problems that sometimes arise with administration of antibiotics relate to the eradication of the intestinal flora, and are of course, in a very broad sense, an action-related side-effect. In still other cases, disease may ensue from the lack of normal enzyme activity. Since enzymes are proteins encoded by DNA, these conditions sometimes arise as a consequence of hereditary defects, and may be relieved by parenteral administration of the missing or defective enzyme.

In order to understand the involvement of enzymes in disease, and to develop rational therapies to control them, it is necessary to know the mechanism of enzymatic catalysis. The present chapter deals with some aspects of the structure and mechanisms of enzymes, as well as the kinetics of enzyme reactions and enzyme inhibition. The use of enzyme inhibitors as drugs is exemplified by three important clinical disciplines: cardiovascular disease, infectious disease, and inflammation. In the first, the renin-angiotensin system and its inhibitors, and the use of a protease inhibitor, aprotinin, to prevent hyperfibrinolytic bleeding is discussed (Section 11.6.1). The use of sulfonamide antibiotics and β-lactamase inhibitors to treat bacterial infections is described in Section 11.6.2, and the inhibitors of arachidonic acid metabolism in the treatment of inflammatory disease are discussed in Section 11.6.3. The use of enzymes as drugs is not discussed here, but interested readers are referred to literature on e.g. tissue plasminogen activator (tPA) in fibrinolysis, and superoxide dismutase in inflammatory disease as examples of enzyme drugs.

The list of enzyme inhibitors presented in this chapter is by no means exhaustive. The chapter is meant as an introduction to the mechanisms of enzyme catalysis and inhibition; it is the intention to show how the knowledge of the participation of enzymes in disease states has led to significant advances in drug development.

11.2 ENZYME STRUCTURE

Enzymes are proteins serving as highly specific catalysts of biochemical reactions. They are composed of the same amino acids as structural and other non-catalytic proteins, which implies that features of the molecules other than the amino acid constituents as such account for their catalytic properties. This is the sequence of the amino acids, which is referred to as the primary structure, i.e. the order in which the amino acids are assembled to form the polypeptide chain. Enzymes are globular molecules, and the primary structure determines how the amino acid chain can be coiled to form the secondary structure, for example a helix stabilized by hydrogen-bonding (α-helix). The coils are then crumpled to produce a globular molecule of appropriate thickness, and this folding, which also depends on the primary structure, is called the tertiary structure. Finally, single peptide chain units may in some cases be assembled to form clusters of sizes from simple dimers to particulate multi-enzyme systems. The polymerization of peptidic subunits is called the quaternary structure of the enzyme. Globular proteins also include non-enzymatic proteins, but in contrast to other proteins enzymes are characterized by their ability to bind a substrate, e.g. an endogenous compound, a xenobiotic, or a nutritional factor, to a specific site of the enzyme molecule, the active site. The formation of an enzyme-substrate complex is mandatory for the catalysis of the reaction into which the substrate should enter. Finally, in some cases the enzyme does not exert catalytic activity unless combined with a cofactor of non-protein structure. The enzyme-cofactor complex is called a holoenzyme, the cofactor a prosthetic group, and the protein moiety of the holoenzyme an apoenzyme.

Most enzymes have molecular weights (MW) between 30 kDa and 60 kDa. A number of enzymes of known MW are listed in Table 11.1 showing their MW and the number of amino acid residues forming the covalent backbone. The approximate number of amino acids can be calculated by dividing the MW by 120, which is the average weight of amino acids less one molecule of water lost during peptide formation.

The elucidation of the structure of proteins (and, hence, of enzymes) has been possible by the application of two methods: a chemical method developed by Sanger in the early 1950s, and a physical method developed by Perutz, Kendrew and Phillips in the 1960s. Sanger used different, pure peptidases to hydrolyze peptide bonds, thereby degrading polypeptides into small fragments, which could then be analyzed after reaction of the terminal amino group with the reagent 1-fluoro-2,4-dinitrobenzene (Fig. 11.1) and arranged in their original order. By this approach Sanger succeeded in determining the amino acid sequence of insulin (a non-enzymatic hormone protein), and the method was subsequently used to determine the sequence of much larger enzymatic proteins. Perutz and Kendrew introduced X-ray diffraction analysis to study the three-dimensional structure of crystalline proteins, a method which has become particularly useful with the introduction of modern computers. The two methods are complementary in the sense that it is impossible to predict the three-dimensional structure from the primary structure of the protein alone, and it is equally impossible to interpret the X-ray data without knowledge of the amino acid sequence. Enzyme structure analysis by these methods is limited by the demand for isolation of the enzyme in a pure, crystalline form. This has only been achieved in the case of a limited number of enzymes, but future developments in protein purification and structure analysis techniques hold promise of considerable progress in medicinal chemistry laboratories concerned with the design of enzyme inhibitor drugs. Not least the rapidly increasing use of nuclear magnetic resonance (NMR) spectroscopy to study biochemical and pharmacological processes in viable cells and tissues contributes to the optimism regarding the possibility of obtaining detailed information on the structure of the active sites of enzymes. These sites are the targets of enzyme inhibitors.

11.3 MECHANISMS OF ENZYME ACTION

An enzyme is characterized by its substrate specificity, by the chemical reaction it catalyses, and by its cofactor.

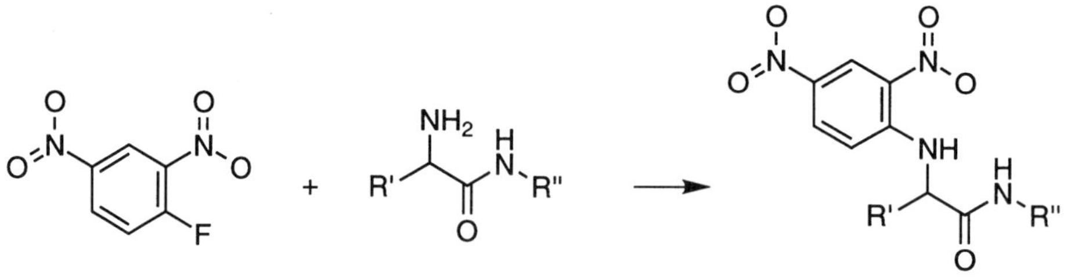

1-Fluoro-2,4-   Amino-terminal   Sanger
dinitrobenzene   end of peptide   product

Figure 11.1   The Sanger reaction.

Table 11.1   Some enzymes of known molecular weight.

Enzyme	Molecular weight (k)	Amino acid residues	Subunits
Lysozyme (egg white)	15	129	1
Papain (papaya latex)	21	172	1
Chymotrypsin (bovine pancreas)	23	241	1
Carboxypeptidase A (bovine pancreas)	37	307	1
Phosphoglycerate kinase (erythrocytes)	50	416	1
Triosephosphate isomerase (rabbit muscle)	56	465	2
Alcohol dehydrogenase (horse liver)	80	~670	2
Creatine kinase (rabbit muscle)	80	~670	2
Hexokinase (yeast)	104	~870	2
Lactate dehydrogenase (bovine heart)	136	~1,100	4
Glucose-6-phosphate dehydrogenase (erythrocytes)	210	~1,750	4
Isocitrate dehydrogenase (bovine heart)	330	~2,750	8
Dihydrolipoamide acetyltranferase (*E. coli*)	960	~8,000	24

11.3.1 Substrates and reactions

It is assumed that the substrate fits the active site of the enzyme as a key fits a lock, but a theory of the exact mechanism of catalysis by any enzyme has not yet been presented which can explain the extraordinary high catalytic efficacy of enzymes, typically resulting in enhancement of chemical reaction rates by 8–10 log scales. Some enzymes show very strict substrate specificity and will not accept even closely related substrate analogues; in particular, many enzymes show stereospecificity. Other enzymes, such as some proteases (e.g. trypsin), have a rather broad range of specificity. Another characteristic feature of some, but not all enzymes, is catalysis of the reverse reaction (reversibility). On the basis of the type of chemical reactions catalyzed, enzymes may conveniently be classified as belonging to one of six groups:

1. Oxido-reductases.
2. Transferases.
3. Hydrolases.
4. Lyases.
5. Isomerases.
6. Ligases.

Within each of these groups subgroups exist. Each enzyme is assigned a number by the International Enzyme Commission (the EC number) and a systematic name, which is based on the nature of the chemical reaction it catalyses. In addition, a great number of enzymes have trivial names, which are more easy to use in daily life. For example, the trivial name of EC 2.7.1.1, ATP:D-hexose 6-phosphotransferase, is simply hexokinase. Representative examples of enzymes, substrates and reactions are shown in Table 11.2.

11.3.2 Cofactors

Many enzymes require a cofactor (or coenzyme) in addition to the substrate before the catalytic activity is present. Cofactors may either be simple metal ions like Zn^{2+}, Mg^{2+}, Mn^{2+}, Fe^{2+}, Fe^{3+}, or Cu^{2+}, or organic molecules. In the latter case, they are called coenzymes. Like the apoenzyme itself, cofactors are not consumed during the catalytic process and may therefore be regarded as part of the catalytic mechanism. The major part of the cofactor act as intermediates carrying electrons, hydrogen atoms or molecular groups (e.g. methyl radicals). The carrier function may be inter-enzymatic, i.e. the coenzyme functions as a substrate for one enzyme by binding a group, which is subsequently utilized by another enzyme in a process which recycles the coenzyme. Alternatively, the cofactor may serve as an intra-enzymatic carrier, in which case it is often firmly bound to the apoenzyme as a prosthetic group.

Two common coenzymes are the nicotinamide adenine dinucleotides, NAD^+ and $NADP^+$. These compounds serve as inter-enzymatic carriers of hydrogen atoms in redox reactions. These coenzymes are ubiquitously present in animal and plant cells, but their main function lies in the respiratory process. Mitochondria reoxidize NADH by means of the respiratory chain, in the reaction called oxidative phosphorylation (equation (1)).

$$2NADH + 2H^+ + 6ADP + O_2 \longrightarrow 2NAD^+ + 8H_2O + 6ATP \qquad (1)$$

The flavoproteins contain either flavinmononucleotide (FMN) or, more commonly, flavin-adenine-dinucleotide (FAD) as the prosthetic group. In contrast to $NAD(P)^+$, FMN and FAD serve as intra-enzymatic redox carriers. The flavin group is strongly bound to the enzyme protein, where it undergoes alternate oxidation and reduction, since the active moiety of the flavins, the isoalloxazine ring, can be reversibly reduced at the nitrogen atoms. Like $NAD(P)^+$, the flavin-based enzymatic reactions are extremely common in biological processes. In quantitative terms, the most important flavoproteins are NADH dehydrogenase, succinate dehydrogenase, dihydrolipoyl dehydrogenase, and the fatty acyl-coenzyme A dehydrogenase.

Other important coenzymes involved in redox reactions are glutathione, lipoic acid, ubiquinone, and cytochromes. Of special interest to the medicinal chemist is the cytochrome

Table 11.2   Examples of enzyme numbers, names, and reactions.

EC number	Systematic name	Trivial name	Reaction catalyzed
1.1.1.27	L-Lactate:NAD$^+$ oxidoreductase	Lactate dehydrogenase	L-Lactate + NAD$^+$ → pyruvate + NADH
1.2.1.3	Aldehyde:NAD$^+$ oxidoreductase	Aldehyde dehydrogenase	Aldehyde + NAD$^+$ + H$_2$O → acid + NADH
1.2.3.2	Xanthine:Oxygen oxidoreductase	Xanthine oxidase	Xanthine + H$_2$O + O$_2$ → uric acid + O$_2^-$
1.3.99.1	Succinate:Acceptor oxidoreductase	Succinate dehydrogenase	Succinate + A(ox) → fumarate + A(red)
1.5.1.3	5,6,7,8-Tetrahydrofolate:NADP$^+$ oxidoreductase	Tetrahydrofolate dehydrogenase	5,6,7,8-Tetrahydrofolate + NADP$^+$ → 7,8-dihydrofolate + NADPH
1.11.1.6	H$_2$O$_2$:H$_2$O$_2$ oxidoreductase	Catalase	H$_2$O$_2$ + H$_2$O$_2$ → O$_2$ + 2H$_2$O
1.13.11.12	Linoleate:O$_2$ oxidoreductase	Lipoxygenase	Linoleate + O$_2$ → 13-HOO-octadecadienoate
1.15.1.1	O$_2^{\bullet-}$:O$_2^{\bullet-}$ oxidoreductase	Superoxide dismutase	O$_2^{\bullet-}$ + O$_2^{\bullet-}$ + 2H$^+$ → O$_2$ + H$_2$O$_2$
2.3.1.6	Acetyl-CoA:choline O-acetyltransferase	Choline acetyltransferase	Acetyl-CoA + choline → CoA + O-acetylcholine
2.4.2.12	Nicotinamidenucleotide: pyrophosphate phosphoribosyl transferase	Nicotinamide phosphoribosyl-transferase	Nicotinamide D-ribonucleotide + pyrophosphate → 5-phospho-α-D-ribose 1-diphosphate + nicotinamide
2.6.1.2	L-Alanine:2-oxoglutarate aminotransferase	Alanine aminotransferase	L-alanine + 2-oxoglutarate → pyruvate + L-glutamate
2.7.1.1	ATP:D-hexose 6-phosphotransferase	Hexokinase	ATP + D-hexose → ADP + D-hexose-6-phosphate
2.8.3.5	Succinyl-CoA:3-oxoacid CoA transferase	3-oxoacid CoA-transferase	Succinyl-CoA + 3-oxoacid → succinate + 3-oxo-acyl-CoA
3.1.1.1	Carboxylic-ester hydrolase	Carboxylesterase	carboxylic ester + H$_2$O → alcohol + carboxylic acid
3.1.3.9	D-Glucose-6-phosphate phosphohydrolase	Glucose-6-phosphatase	D-Glucose-6-phosphate + H$_2$O → D-Glucose + orthophosphate
3.1.4.3	L-3-Glycerophosphocholine glycerophosphohydrolase	Phospholipase C	Phosphatidylcholine + H$_2$O → 1,2-diacylglycerol + choline phosphate

Table 11.2 Continued.

EC number	Systematic name	Trivial name	Reaction catalyzed
3.1.4.17	3':5'-Cyclic nucleotide 5'-nucleotidohydrolase	3':5'-Cyclic nucleotide phosphodiesterase	Nucleoside 3':5'-cyclic phosphate + H_2O → nucleoside 5'-phosphate
3.2.1.1	1,4-α-D-Glucan glucanohydrolase	α-Amylase	Hydrolysis of 1,4-α-D-glucosidic linkages of polysaccharides
3.3.2.3	Epoxide hydrolase	Epoxide hydrolase	Epoxide + H_2O → glycol
3.4.21.4		Trypsin	Unspecific protease
3.4.23.1		Pepsin A	Unspecific protease
3.5.1.5	Urea amido hydrolase	Urease	Urea + H_2O → CO_2 + $2NH_3$
3.5.2.6	Penicillin amido-β-lactamhydrolase	β-Lactamase or Penicillinase	Penicillin + H_2O → Penicillic acid
4.1.1.1	2-Oxoacid carboxy-lyase	Pyruvate decarboxylase	2-oxoacid → aldehyde + CO_2
4.1.3.2	L-Malate glyoxylate-lyase	Malate synthase	L-Malate + CoA → acetyl-CoA + H_2O + glyoxylate
4.2.1.20	L-Serine hydro-lyase	Tryptophan synthase	L-Serine + indoleglycerol phosphate → L-tryptophan + glyceraldehyde phosphate
4.6.1.1	ATP pyrophosphate-lyase	Adenylate cyclase	ATP → 3':5'-cyclic AMP + pyrophosphate
5.1.1.1	Alanine racemase	Alanine racemase	L-Alanine → D-alanine
5.2.1.1	Maleate cis-trans-isomerase	Maleate isomerase	Maleate → fumarate
5.3.1.7	D-Mannose ketol-isomerase	Mannose isomerase	D-Mannose → D-fructose
5.3.99.2	Prostaglandin D-isomerase	Prostaglandin D-isomerase	PGE_2 → PGD_2
6.1.1.22	L-Asparagine:tRNA ligase tRNA ligase	Asparaginyl-tRNA synthetase	ATP + L-asparagine + tRNA → AMP + pyrophosphate + L-asparaginyl-tRNA
6.2.1.1	Acetate:CoA ligase	Acetyl-CoA synthetase	ATP + acetate + CoA → AMP + pyrophosphate + acetyl-CoA
6.5.1.1–3	(DNA repair enzymes)		

P-450 system, which is of great importance to the organism's handling of certain xenobiotics, including drugs. Cytochrome P-450 is a group of microsomal haemoproteins, which is also present in mitochondria of some tissues, e.g. the adrenals. The name of the enzyme originates from the formation of a complex with carbon monoxide, which absorbs light of the wavelength 450 nm. It consists of a group of enzymes of different specificities, but containing the same prosthetic group, haem b. The main function of cytochrome P-450 is to catalyze the oxidation of non-polar compounds in order to facilitate their renal excretion. Oxidation is accomplished by the use of molecular oxygen and NADPH, as shown in equation (2).

$$\overset{|}{\underset{|}{C}}H_2 + NADPH + H^+ + O_2 \longrightarrow \overset{|}{\underset{|}{C}}HOH + NADP^+ + H_2O \qquad (2)$$

Examples of cofactors involved in enzymatic reactions other than redox-processes include those transferring functional groups. Pyridoxal phosphate, a derivative of vitamin B_6, is the prosthetic group of the transaminases, i.e. enzymes catalyzing the transfer of amino groups. Pyridoxal phosphate forms a Schiff's base (–N=CH–) by combination of the aldehyde function with the amino group of the substrate. In this way, an amino group of an amino acid can be transferred to an α-keto acid to form another amino acid in a series of reactions shown in Figure 11.2. Important transaminase reactions are catalyzed by the enzymes alanine transaminase and glutamate transaminase, the latter serving the important role of creating a pool of amino groups in one amino acid, glutamate.

A similarly important coenzyme is coenzyme A, which serve as a prosthetic group of enzymes involved in the transfer of acetyl and fatty acyl groups, which are esterified with the thiol group of the β-aminoethanethiol moiety. The carrier function of coenzyme A is used for the entry of metabolic end-products of carbohydrates, amino acids and fatty acids into the Krebs cycle, and for the oxidation of fatty acids.

11.4 ENZYME KINETICS

A number of conditions determine the rate of an enzyme-catalyzed reaction. The most important are the substrate concentration, pH, and temperature. The effect of the substrate concentration is discussed in the following paragraph.

11.4.1 Effect of the substrate concentration

The theory of the effect on enzyme kinetics has been developed by Michaelis and Menten, using a single substrate reaction model and, although enzyme reactions involving only one substrate are relatively rare, the conclusions that can be reached from the study of one substrate-reactions are in many aspects valid for more complicated systems. The rate of an enzymatic reaction is a function of the substrate concentration in a manner depicted in Figure 11.3. $[S]$ is the substrate concentration, V the reaction velocity, and V_{max} the maximal velocity. The equation of the hyperbola is $(V_{max} - V)[S] = K$, in which K is a constant, and it follows that the reaction is saturable with regard to substrate concentration. In 1913, the saturation phenomenon led Michaelis and Menten to propose a theory for this

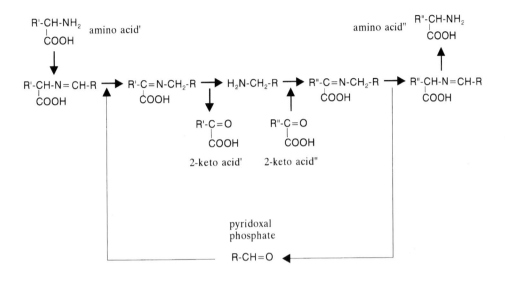

Figure 11.2   The mechanism of amino group transfer catalyzed by transaminases using pyridoxal phosphate as coenzyme.

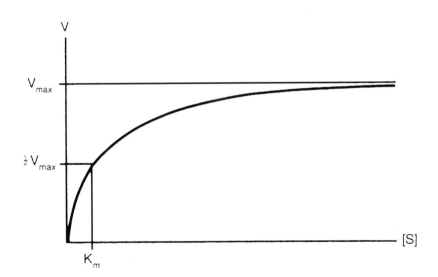

Figure 11.3   The rate, V, of an enzyme-catalyzed reaction as a function of substrate concentration, $[S]$. The value of $[S]$, which gives rise to half-maximal reaction rate, is the Michaelis-Menten constant, K_m.

process, based on the important assumption that the enzyme first forms a complex with the substrate, which subsequently breaks down to liberate the unchanged catalyst (the enzyme) and the product, as shown in equation (3).

$$E + S \underset{k_2}{\overset{k_1}{\rightleftarrows}} ES \overset{k_3}{\rightarrow} E + P \tag{3}$$

In these reactions, the first being essentially reversible, k_1, k_2, and k_3 are the rate constants of the specific reactions as indicated. If $[E]$ is the enzyme concentration, $[ES]$ the concentration of the complex, and the concentration of free enzyme is $[E] - [ES]$, it follows from equation (3) that

$$K_s = \frac{k_2}{k_1} = \frac{([E] - [ES])[S]}{[ES]} \tag{I}$$

in which K_s is the dissociation constant. Rearranging (I) gives

$$[ES]K_s + [ES][S] = [E][S] \tag{II}$$

or:

$$[ES] = \frac{[E][S]}{K_s + [S]} = \frac{[E]}{1 + K_s[S]^{-1}} \tag{III}$$

The rate, V, of the product formation is determined by the breakdown of ES to $E + P$:

$$V = k_3[ES] \tag{IV}$$

and by substituting the expression (III) for $[ES]$, we get

$$V = \frac{k_3[E]}{1 + K_s[S]^{-1}} \tag{V}$$

At high substrate concentrations, $K_s[S]^{-1}$ becomes negligible, and V approaches the maximum velocity, V_{max}, so that

$$V_{max} = k_3[E] \tag{VI}$$

(V) may then be written:

$$V = \frac{V_{max}}{1 + K_s[S]^{-1}} \tag{VII}$$

It follows from equation (VII) that when $[S]$ is equal to K_s, the reaction velocity, V, is $\frac{1}{2}V_{max}$. This particular concentration of S, which can be determined experimentally, is called the Michaelis-Menten constant, K_m (Fig. 11.3). K_m is therefore the substrate concentration, which gives rise to the half-maximal enzymatic reaction rate. Under conditions where equilibrium exists between the concentration of enzyme, substrate, and enzyme-substrate complex, K_s may be replaced by K_m, in which case (VII) gives

$$V = \frac{V_{max}}{1 + K_m[S]^{-1}} \quad \text{(The Michaelis-Menten equation)} \qquad \text{(VIII)}$$

V_{max} and K_m are the two most important constants used to characterize an enzymatic reaction in kinetic terms. By application of various transformations of the equation the determination of these constants from experimental data is facilitated (e.g. "Lineweaver-Burk", "Eadie-Hofstee").

11.5 ENZYME INHIBITION

Whenever an enzymatic reaction is involved in a pathophysiological process, it is obviously of great interest from a pharmacological point of view to apply a drug, which specifically blocks the reaction. A number of factors limits this approach in drug development. Most importantly, relatively few purely "pathophysiological" enzymes have been identified. In many cases, enzymes involved in disease mechanisms are also normally necessary for non-pathological, physiological processes. Inhibition of such enzymes may have therapeutic value, but side-effects related to the removal of important, or even vital, enzymatic products may be intolerable. An example of this limitation is the non-steroidal anti-inflammatory drugs (NSAIDs), which depend on inhibition of prostaglandin synthesis for their activity (see Section 11.6.3.2). Prostaglandins are important mediators of inflammatory disease, but are also natural, gastric mucosal protective agents. Therefore, inhibition of prostaglandin synthesis by administration of NSAIDs inevitably leads to an increased risk of developing gastric ulceration. In other cases, the treatment with enzyme inhibitors is an excellent curative approach. In the case of penicillins, specific bacterial enzymes are inhibited (see Section 11.6.2), which do not play any role in the function of the human organism. Penicillins are therefore devoid of significant side-effects, except in cases when they are recognized as antigens, so that immunological problems preclude their use, or when they upset the normal intestinal bacterial flora, in which case gastrointestinal side-effects may occur.

Enzyme inhibitors may conveniently be classified as belonging to one of two groups: reversible inhibitors and irreversible inhibitors. Irreversible inhibition implies that *de novo* protein synthesis is necessary to regain normal enzyme activity. Well-known examples of irreversible enzyme inhibitors are cyanide, which blocks the enzyme xanthine oxidase (whereas the fatal inhibition by cyanide of cytochrome c oxidase is actually reversible in a noncompetitive manner; see below), nerve poisons like diisopropylphosphofluoridate (DFP), which inhibits acetylcholinesterase, and alkylating agents such as iodoacetamide, which reacts irreversibly with thiol groups essential to the active site of the enzyme. In some cases, irreversible enzyme inhibition may represent a therapeutic advantage. For example, platelets produce thromboxane A_2 from endoperoxides formed by the action of cyclooxygenase on liberated arachidonic acid (see Section 11.6.3.1). Thromboxanes are potentially important mediators of thrombus formation. Very low doses of acetylsalicylic acid (aspirin) inhibit the cyclooxygenase enzyme by irreversible acetylation of the active site. Most tissues quickly regain enzymatic activity by *de novo* protein synthesis, but platelets are anuclei cells, which do not have the capacity for protein synthesis. Therefore, inhibition by aspirin of platelet thromboxane A_2 synthesis lasts for the lifetime of the cell. Since the biological half-life of platelets is more than a week, low-dose aspirin represents a means of thrombosis prophylaxis with a very low frequency of adverse reactions. In fact, low-dose aspirin has been demonstrated to reduce the incidence of stroke and other thrombotic disorders.

11.5.1 Reversible enzyme inhibitors

Reversible inhibitors may be grouped into different classes, depending on the way in which they affect the enzyme kinetics. Those decreasing the substrate affinity (i.e. increasing K_m) are competitive inhibitors. Those decreasing V_{max} are non-competitive inhibitors. Some reversible inhibitors affect both the K_m and the V_{max} values; these are called mixed and incompetitive inhibitors. The latter are not further discussed here.

Competitive inhibitors bind to the active site of the enzyme in a reversible manner, as shown in equation (4).

$$E + I \underset{k_2}{\overset{k_1}{\rightleftharpoons}} EI \tag{4}$$

The dissociation constant of the enzyme-inhibitor complex is

$$K_i = \frac{[E][I]}{[EI]} = \frac{k_1}{k_2} \tag{IX}$$

K_i is called the inhibitor constant. By application of the Lineweaver-Burk plot at different concentrations of the inhibitor, competitive inhibition is recognized as increasing slopes of the straight line with increasing concentrations of the inhibitor (Fig 11.4). The intercept on the V^{-1}-axis (V_{max}^{-1}) is not changed, since a competitive inhibitor does not change V_{max}; by increasing the substrate concentration it is always possible to reach V_{max}, since the substrate competes with the inhibitor for binding to the catalytic site, and the binding of the inhibitor is reversible. However, the intercept of the Lineweaver-Burk plot with the $[S]^{-1}$-axis increases when the inhibitor concentration increases, since the intercept is $-K_m^{-1}$ and a competitive inhibitor increases K_m. The slope of the line is:

$$a = \frac{K_m}{V_{max}} \left(1 + \frac{[I]}{K_i}\right) \tag{X}$$

From this expression, K_i may be calculated:

$$K_i = \frac{K_m[I]}{a \cdot V_{max} - K_m} \tag{XI}$$

when K_m, V_{max}, the inhibitor concentration, and the slope of the inhibited reaction are known from experimental data.

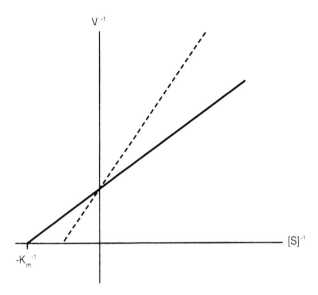

Figure 11.4.   The effect of a competitive inhibitor (broken line) on the Lineweaver-Burk plot.

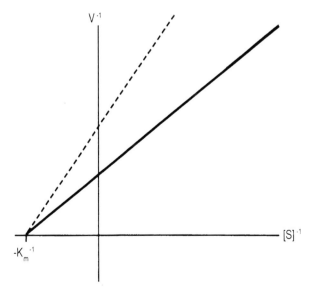

Figure 11.5   The effect of a noncompetitive inhibitor (broken line) on the Lineweaver-Burk plot.

Non-competitive, reversible inhibition cannot be reversed by increasing the substrate concentration, since the inhibition depends on binding of the inhibitor to a site of the enzyme other than the active site. Evidently, the binding still affects the catalytic activity, either by altering the configuration of the active site so as to prevent the proper binding of the substrate, or by interacting with amino acid residues essential to the catalytic activity. Like competitive inhibitors, a noncompetitive inhibitor is recognized by studying the Lineweaver-Burk plot of the enzymatic reaction in the presence of increasing concentrations of the inhibitor (Fig. 11.5). Again, the slope is increased because V_{max} is decreased. However, the intercept on the V^{-1}-axis now increases for the same reason, whereas the intercept on the $[S]^{-1}$-axis $(-K_m^{-1})$ remains constant. The V^{-1}-axis intercept is

$$b = \frac{1}{V_{max}} \left(1 + \frac{[I]}{K_i} \right)$$ (XII)

from which K_i may be calculated as:

$$K_i = \frac{[I]V_{max}}{b \cdot V_{max}^{-1}}$$ (XIII)

A classical example of a competitive inhibitor used in medicine is sulphanilamide, which belongs to the sulphonamide class of antibiotics. These drugs are structural analogues of para-aminobenzoic acid, which serves as a precursor for folic acid. Sulphanilamide blocks the synthesis of folic acid, thereby preventing the formylation of 5-aminoimidazole-4-carboxamide ribonucleotide and, hence, purine nucleotide synthesis in susceptible bacteria. Cyanide is an example of a noncompetitive, reversible inhibitor which forms a stable complex with iron at the catalytic site of cytochrome c oxidase.

11.5.2 Transition state analogues

A special case of reversible inhibition is represented by the transition state analogues. Any chemical reaction passes through a state of higher energy than that of the mixture of the reactants before the products of the reaction are formed. The peak of the energy barrier is called the transition state (Fig. 11.6), and this state of the reactant, R, is usually depicted by the symbol $R‡$. In terms of energy, an enzyme, E, decreases the activation entropy by strongly binding to the substrate, S, in the transition state, $S‡$: $ES‡$. The study of the structure of transition state complexes are important for the understanding of the catalytic mechanism. Obviously, such understanding may help in designing potent and specific enzyme inhibitors.

The concentration of $ES‡$ in any given enzymatic reaction is, however, extremely low, so that direct structural analysis of $ES‡$ is impossible in most cases. An indirect approach is provided by the transition state analogue theory, which was originally described by Pauling. The theory predicts that the enzyme binds the transition state of the substrate much stronger than the substrate, and it follows that a transition state analogue inhibitor will also bind much more tightly to the active site of the enzyme than a simple substrate analogue inhibitor. In other words, the active site of the enzyme is reflected by $S‡$ rather than S, and an analogue of $S‡$ will fit as the key in the lock. Thus, when a hypothetical transition state structure is available it may be possible to design a transition state analogue inhibitor.

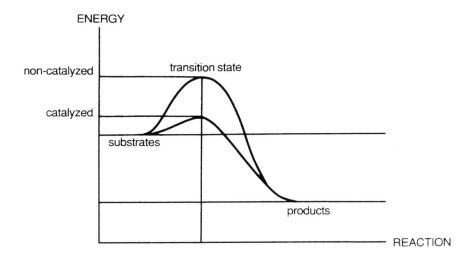

Figure 11.6   Energy diagram of a non-catalyzed and an enzyme-catalyzed reaction.

In practice, a metastable intermediate of high energy represents the analogue replicate. For example, tetrahedral intermediates of the acylation reactions of certain proteases have been postulated, and certain substituted boronic acids, which are known to add OH^- in aqueous solutions, resulting in the formation of negatively charged tetrahedral adducts, are potent inhibitors of protease-catalyzed reactions. Other examples of hypothetical transition states are represented by carbonium ion; X-ray crystallographic analysis indicates that the glycosyl-transfers catalyzed by lysozyme involves the transition state of an alkoxy carbonium ion, and some ∂-lactones are very potent transition state analogue inhibitors of these reactions.

The most convincing examples of transition state analogues are perhaps the enzyme inhibitors produced by plants and animals. The presence of natural transition state analogues is predicted by the principle of natural selection, and their existence strongly supports the transition state theory. Very often, they are species of high molecular weight, and therefore beyond the synthetic possibilities of medicinal chemists. For example, there are polypeptide inhibitors of trypsin having extremely low inhibitor constants (actually in the picomolar range), the bovine pancreatic trypsin inhibitor (BPTI/aprotinin; see Section 11.6.1.3) and the soybean trypsin inhibitor. These inhibitors form a very stable enzyme intermediate, which is close to the transition state of the trypsin-catalyzed reaction. Leupeptin, antipain, and β-lactam antibiotics are other examples of transition state analogue inhibitors.

11.5.3 Irreversible enzyme inhibitors

Reversible enzyme inhibitors are easily distinguished from irreversible inhibitors by simple experiments, such as dialysis, gel-filtration or dilution of the enzyme-inhibitor complex. By such methods, a reversibly inhibited enzyme will restore its normal activity. In contrast to reversible inhibitors, irreversible inhibitors are also time-dependent in their action, because inhibition involves the formation of a covalent bond with the enzyme. Many types of unspecific, irreversible enzyme inhibitors are known, but their lack of specificity do not make them suitable for pharmacological use.

Some irreversible inhibitors show enzyme specificity in the sense that they form a complex with a specific enzyme before they destroy its catalytic site. This may be expressed by equation (5),

$$E + I \underset{k_2}{\overset{k_1}{\rightleftarrows}} EI \overset{k_3}{\rightarrow} E - I \tag{5}$$

in which $E - I$ represents the covalent binding of the inhibitor to the enzyme, and EI the intermediate complex.

Irreversible inhibitors can be divided into two groups, the active site-directed inhibitors and the suicide inhibitors. In both cases, inhibition depends on the irreversible interaction with the active site (destruction of the functional properties), most often by the formation of covalent bonds. Suicide inhibitors, however, differ from the former in that inhibition depends on the enzyme-catalyzed transformation of the compound into an inhibitor product. Thus, the compound itself is not an inhibitor, but in fact an enzyme substrate. The great advantage of such a mechanism is the specificity it provides: inhibition does not occur until a complex has been formed with the target enzyme. Suicide inhibitors have other names, k_{cat} inhibitors and enzyme-activated irreversible inhibitors, but the common term used here gives an adequate and mnemotechnically useful description of the mechanism. The suicide mechanism of inhibitory action has been described for a number of transaminases dependent on pyridoxal phosphate as a cofactor, e.g. GABA-transaminase, aspartate transaminase, ornithine transaminase and alanine transaminase, in which the formation of carbanionic intermediates have been used to design a variety of suicide inhibitors. In particular, the pharmacology of the GABA-transaminase inhibitor, gabaculine (**11.1**), has been studied in detail. As shown in Section 11.6.2.2, suicide inhibitors are used to control bacterial resistance to penicillins.

(**11.1**)

11.6 ENZYME INHIBITORS AS DRUGS

A great number of drugs depend on inhibition of a specific enzyme for their pharmacological activity. The present section deals with some examples of such drugs used to treat cardiovascular disease, infectious disease, and inflammatory disease.

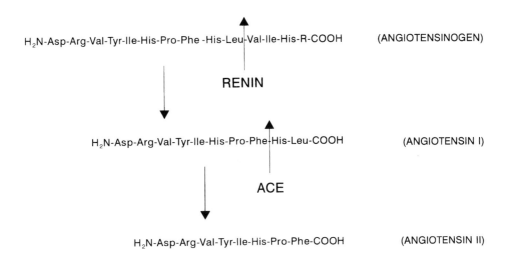

Figure 11.7   The renin-angiotensin system.

11.6.1 Cardiovascular pharmacology

Hypertension is a common disorder predisposing of coronary heart disease, stroke and other serious cardiovascular conditions. It is generally accepted that patients presenting with a diastolic blood pressure above 90–95 mmHg should be treated prophylactically with a blood pressure lowering agent. The most common antihypertensive drugs are the thiazide diuretics, the α- and β-adrenergic receptor antagonists, the centrally acting antihypertensives (e.g. α-methyldopa), the calcium entry blockers, peripheral vasodilators, and angiotensin converting enzyme inhibitors. The latter, as well as a related class of new compounds, the renin inhibitors, are discussed in the following sections. Furthermore, a serine protease inhibitor, aprotinin, a naturally occurring transition state analogue, which can be used to prevent blood loss during open heart surgery, is mentioned in Section 11.6.1.3.

11.6.1.1 Angiotensin converting enzyme inhibitors
Extracts of the kidney contain an enzyme called renin, which was first discovered almost a hundred years ago by Tiegerstedt and Bergman in Sweden. Renin increases the blood pressure when injected intravenously. The mechanism by which the blood pressure is increased has been shown to depend on the catalytic cleavage by renin of angiotensinogen (Fig. 11.7), a hepatically synthesized α-globulin polypeptide circulating in the blood. Angiotensinogen is degraded by renin to release a decapeptide, angiotensin I, which in itself has little pharmacological activity. However, an enzyme present in the blood and, more importantly, on the luminal aspect of vascular endothelial cells, the angiotensin converting enzyme (ACE), cleaves angiotensin I to form the octapeptide, angiotensin II, which has two principal, pharmacological activities: (1) It is one of the most potent vasoconstrictors known, and (2) it stimulates the release of aldosterone from the adrenal cortex. The vasoconstricting

action of angiotensin II primarily involves the arterioles (precapillary vessels), which is the organ determining the vascular tone and, thereby, the blood pressure, since this is the product of the peripheral resistance and the cardiac output. Systemic administration of renin, angiotensin I, or angiotensin II by intravenous injection thus leads to an increase in peripheral vascular resistance. The effect is rapid in onset (<10 sec), and also rapidly declines, since angiotensin II is degraded to inactive peptide fragments by amino and carboxy peptidases in a matter of minutes.

The other important hypertensive mechanism of angiotensin II is the direct stimulation of aldosterone secretion from the adrenal cortex. Aldosterone is a hormone controlling sodium homeostasis by enhancement of renal sodium reabsorption. When the extracellular concentration of sodium increases, the concentration of water also increases by osmotic forces, the net result being an increase in extracellular fluid volume, another determinant of peripheral resistance. In short, by two separate mechanisms, arteriolar smooth muscle contraction and enhancement of sodium reabsorption, angiotensin II increases the blood pressure (Fig. 11.8). It follows from these pharmacological effects of angiotensin II that an approach to the treatment of hypertension is the administration of drugs that prevent the formation of this octapeptide. Although the rationale was originally developed for the subgroup of hypertensive patients characterized by high plasma renin activity it has surprisingly turned out that ACE inhibitors, as they came into clinical use, are effective and well-tolerated antihypertensive agents regardless of the renin activity status of the patients. This seems to indicate that the rate-limiting step in angiotensin II formation is not the plasma renin activity but the endothelial ACE activity.

ACE is a zinc metalloprotein enzyme cleaving dipeptides from the C-terminal end of polypeptides (an exopeptidase). This action, apart from leading to the formation of angiotensin II, inactivates the nonapeptide, bradykinin. Bradykinin is a vasodilator and a diuretic compound, and thus have physiological effects opposite those of angiotensin II. The inactivation of bradykinin may thus theoretically potentiate the hypertensive effect of the action of ACE on angiotensin I; however, the role of bradykinin in the action of ACE is not completely understood. It has been suggested that one of the adverse reactions of ACE inhibitors, coughing, is associated with accumulation of bradykinin in the airways.

The first ACE inhibitors were obtained from snake venoms by Ferreira in 1965. These were polypeptides containing from nine to thirty amino acid residues, and important work by Cushman and Cheung in the 1970s identified the peptide with the most potent antihypertensive effect as Glu-Trp-Pro-Arg-Pro-Glu-Ile-Pro-Pro (SQ 20881). The terminal proline residue is common to all snake venom ACE inhibitors. SQ 20881, the generic name of which is teprotide, is a competitive inhibitor of ACE with a K_i value of 0.10 μM, and shows a duration of antihypertensive activity of up to 16 hrs *in vivo*. Due to the presence in the stomach of a number of unspecific proteases, which rapidly inactivate peptidic drugs, teprotide is only active by parenteral administration, the active dose being 1–4 mg/kg. Although the compound was found to be active in renovascular and malignant hypertensive disease, the lack of oral activity precluded its general use as an antihypertensive compound, and a major goal of the scientists at the Squibb Institute for Medical Research was therefore to develop an orally active ACE inhibitor on the basis of the knowledge of the inhibitory mechanisms of the snake venom polypeptide inhibitors.

The rationales for these drug development projects were established by comparison with earlier mechanistic and structural analyses of a closely related enzyme, carboxypeptidase A.

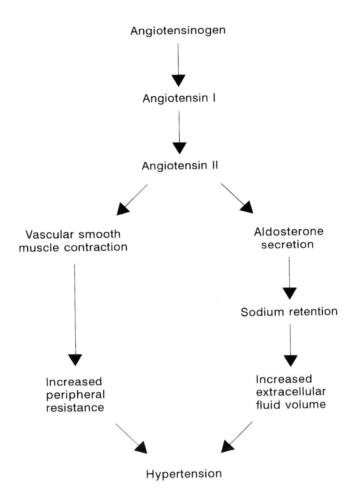

Figure 11.8   Hypertensive mechanisms of angiotensin II.

Carboxypeptidase A is also a zinc metalloprotein, and the exact structure of its active site has been determined by X-ray crystallographic studies. In contrast to ACE, it splits single amino acids from the carboxy-terminal end of peptides. The peptide is held in place by ionic attraction of the terminal carboxyl group to a positively charged arginine residue of the enzyme, and by interactions of the R-group of the terminal amino acid with a hydrophobic surface area of the active site. This positions the >C=O group of the last peptidic bond adjacent to the zinc ion, which subsequently forms a Zn^+-O^--C bond, enhancing the rate of hydrolysis. In much a similar way, ACE is thought to cleave it substrates, although the last peptide bond, which is not hydrolyzed, is thought to be held in place by a hydrogen bond, allowing the second-last peptide bond to be positioned at the zinc ion. These considerations and, in addition, the knowledge from the work with the snake venom inhibitors showing the C-terminal proline to be an important requirement for ACE inhibition, led to the synthesis of succinyl-proline, a relatively weak but specific ACE inhibitor. A number of different substitutions of succinyl-proline established some important structure-activity relationships, but the most significant improvement in inhibitory activity was accomplished, when the putative zinc-binding moiety, $>C=O$, was replaced by a mercapto function. One of these thiols, captopril (**11.2**), showed inhibitory constants in the nanomolar range,

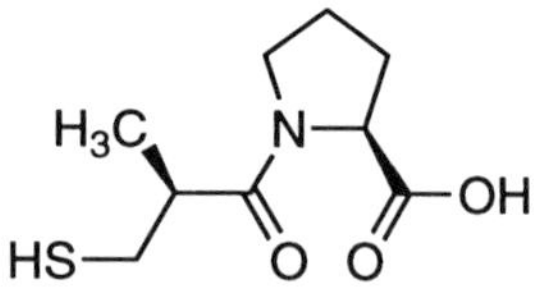

(**11.2**)

and was found to be an orally active antihypertensive compound. Captopril is a relatively safe drug, which does not show acute toxicity at doses required to reach complete inhibition of ACE *in vivo*. A number of adverse reactions, some related to interference with the immune system by the thiol group, have been noted. These effects develop at relatively high doses of captopril, which were commonly used shortly after the introduction of the drug. A daily dose of 50–100 mg is now considered sufficient to achieve blood pressure control, and the reduction in dose has markedly reduced the incidence of side-effects. Like most antihypertensive compounds, captopril shows little effect on blood pressure in normotensive individuals. Approximately half of the hypertensive patient population achieves satisfactory blood pressure control with captopril or similar ACE-inhibitors in monotherapy. This rate is comparable to that of other types of antihypertensive drugs, e.g. diuretics and β-blockers. The advantages of ACE inhibitors over other commonly used blood pressure-lowering drugs are several. They do not cause orthostatic hypotension, as seen with α-adrenergic receptor blockers like prazosin. Patients do not develop tolerance to the drugs, and adequate control of blood pressure is maintained with long-term therapy. There is no rebound effect upon withdrawal, which in the case of the β-adrenergic antagonists may cause severe reactions. Furthermore, the ACE inhibitors seem to cause regression of left ventricular hypertrophy, which is an important complication of untreated hypertension. These, and other benefits demonstrated with the clinical use of captopril, have led to considerable drug development activities, resulting in the introduction of several new ACE-inhibitors. In the newer ACE-inhibitors, the zinc ligand has been replaced by carboxyl (instead of thiol in captopril). A much enhanced rate of absorption from the gastrointestinal tract is often achieved by presenting the compounds in the form of pro-drugs, i.e. esters that are cleaved by esterases to the active ACE-inhibitor during or following passage from the stomach to the blood stream. Thus, enalapril is the ethanol ester of enalaprilate (Fig. 11.9), which is the active, blood pressure lowering agent in this case.

11.6.1.2 Renin inhibitors

The successful introduction of ACE inhibitors as new antihypertensive agents has prompted the search for compounds interfering with the formation of angiotensin II by other

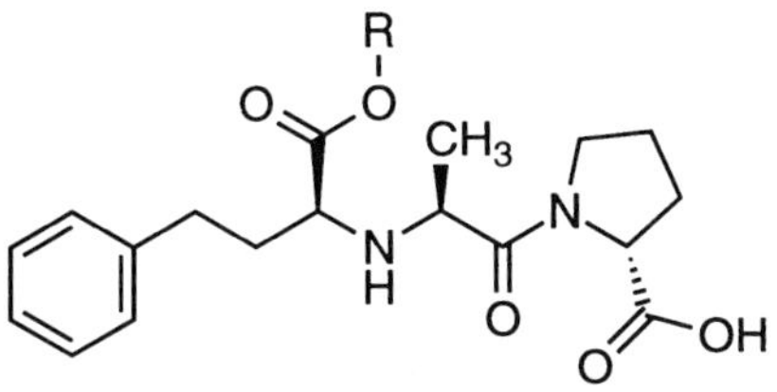

Figure 11.9   Enalapril (R=C$_2$H$_5$) and its active, ACE-inhibiting metabolite, enalaprilate (R=H).

mechanisms. Obviously, inhibition of renin would lead to the same result as inhibition of ACE: a decrease in angiotensin II (see Fig. 11.7). This approach might have some advantages over the ACE inhibitors, since it would not inhibit the degradation of bradykinin, which is hypothesized to be involved in some of the adverse reactions to ACE inhibitors (see Section 11.6.1.1). There is reason to believe that the folding of human renin is similar to that of penicillopepsin, which has been utilized for the modelling of a theoretical structure of the active site. This has recently resulted in the synthesis of a very potent and specific renin inhibitor, KRI-1230 (**11.3**), which contains the unnatural amino acid, norstatine. Another nonpeptidic and orally active renin inhibitor is BW-175 (**11.4**). Both are resistant to proteolytic cleavage; and are orally active in lowering the blood pressure in various experimental models of hypertension. There is thus little doubt that renin inhibitors will be introduced as novel antihypertensive agents in the future.

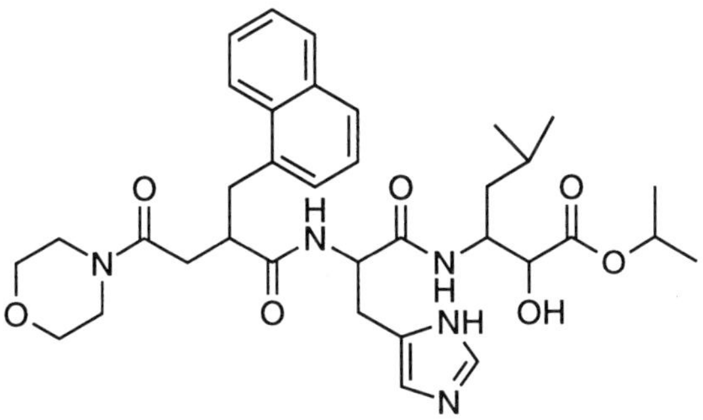

(**11.3**)

(11.4)

11.6.1.3 Aprotinin

SERPINs (serine protease inhibitors) are polypeptides that are able to inhibit proteases with serine residues at their active site. These inhibitors have been grouped into ten families. One important group of SERPINs is the pancreatic trypsin inhibitor (PTI) family, also known as the Kunitz family, named after M. Kunitz who described in 1936 a trypsin inhibitor isolated from bovine pancreas. This inhibitor, which can be isolated in good yields from bovine lung, is known as aprotinin (Trasylol, Bayer), and is becoming an increasingly important drug, primarily due to its effectiveness in prevention of blood loss during open heart surgery. Aprotinin has been cloned and expressed in yeast which provides a convenient production method.

Kunitz inhibitors are relatively small polypeptides (~60 amino acid residues) with a high disulphide content. Aprotinin consists of 58 amino acid residues, has a molecular weight of 6.5 kDa, and is strongly basic (pKa = 10). The molecular structure has been determined by X-ray crystallography, showing a pear-shaped form measuring 29 Å in length and 19 Å in diameter at the widest end. The reactive bond is between Lys-15 and Ala-16. It is a very stable molecule which withstands boiling and TCA treatment, and it is soluble in a wide range of solvents. It is particularly stable at basic pH below its isoelectric point (pH 10.5). By forming stable complexes, aprotinin inhibits a broad spectrum of serine proteases, such as trypsin, chymotrypsin, plasmin and kallikrein. The dissociation constants of the complexes differ, however, from 12 min (bovine chymotrypsin) to 17 weeks (!) (bovine trypsin). The equilibrium constant for the latter interaction is extremely low, 6×10^{-14} M, explaining the extraordinary stability of the aprotinin-trypsin complex. Aprotinin is an example of a naturally occurring transition state analogue inhibitor (see Section 11.5.2).

Aprotinin was used as a drug to treat acute pancreatitis, but more recently the use of aprotinin in shock and conditions of hyperfibrinolytic haemorrhage has been advocated. Plasma proteases/protease inhibitors form a highly regulated network constituting important parts of the clotting, complement, fibrinolytic and kallikrein/kinin systems. Obviously,

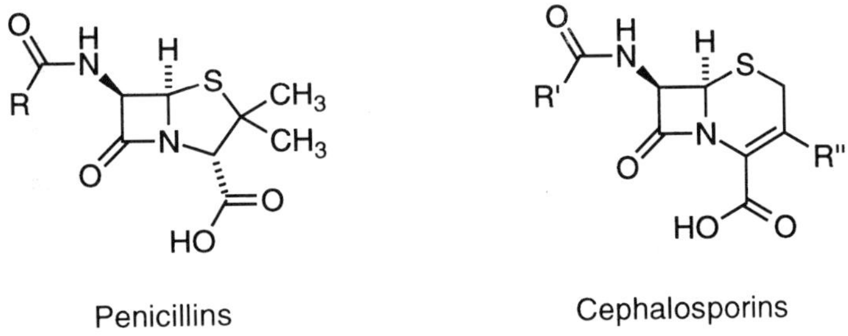

Penicillins   Cephalosporins

Figure 11.10   General structures of β-lactam antibiotics.

a stable serine protease inhibitor with a wide range of target specificity like aprotinin may serve as a pharmacological tool in correcting a pathological imbalance of these systems, as it occurs e.g. in shock and bleeding. Despite good evidence of a beneficial effect of aprotinin in a number of experimental shock models, the therapeutic effect of aprotinin in patients with shock has, however, been difficult to demonstrate.

In 1987, D. Royston demonstrated that a high dose of aprotinin prevented postoperative bleeding after open heart surgery involving extracorporeal circulation, thereby dramatically reducing the need for donor blood transfusions. This new indication for aprotinin is rapidly gaining acceptance and enthusiasm in the clinic, and new interest in the exact mechanism of action by which aprotinin prevents blood loss is emerging, since the elucidation of the mechanism might lead to design of even better drugs. Probably inhibition of plasmin and kallikrein is an important part of the mechanism, but platelet protection by preservation of receptors otherwise destroyed by plasmin or proteases released from leukocytes (such as cathepsin G) has also been suggested to contribute to the beneficial action of aprotinin in open heart surgery.

Aprotinin as a non-human protein carries the risk of some patients becoming sensitized and being at risk of developing a severe anaphylactic reaction should a second course of treatment in a repeat surgical procedure be indicated. Attempts to "humanize" aprotinin by genetic engineering techniques are on-going, as well as the search for a human aprotinin in human tissues.

11.6.2 Antibiotics

The introduction of penicillin and similar β-lactam antibiotics (Fig. 11.10) had a dramatic effect on the mortality rate in consequence of bacterial infection. However, the introduction of penicillin was historically preceded by a different class of antibiotics, the sulfonamides, which were introduced for the treatment of staphylococcal infections in the 1930s.

11.6.2.1 Sulfonamides
Dyes containing an azo-bond were commonly used in the textile industry at the beginning of this century. Some of the dyes were substituted with a sulfonamide group to enhance their

stability, and in 1935 it was discovered by Domagk in Germany that one of these sulfonamide dyes, Prontosil (**11.5**), was able to protect mice from streptococcal infections. It soon became clear that the dye was also an effective antibiotic in humans, and that the activity resided in the sulfanilamide (**11.6**) moiety of the molecule, which is the main metabolite of Prontosil in mammals. A great number of sulfanilamide analogues and prodrugs were subsequently synthesized (e.g. sulfasalazine), partly with the aim of improving the activity, and partly to find a compound that could be patented; sulfanilamide was already an old compound in 1935 and thus beyond commercial protection. Only a few of these compounds are of therapeutic value today.

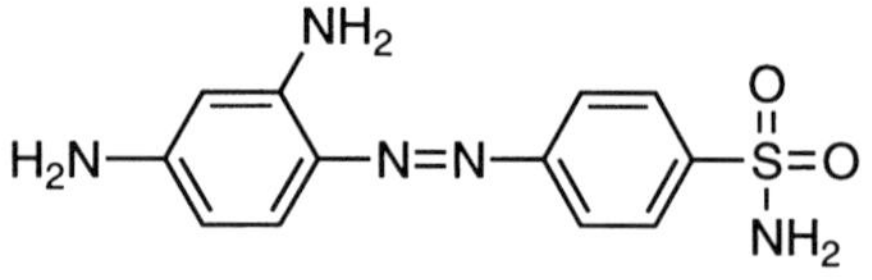

(**11.5**)

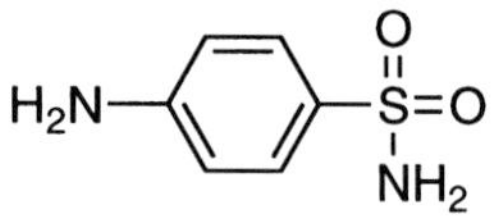

(**11.6**)

Sulfonamides antagonize the microbial growth factor, para-aminobenzoic acid (PABA). PABA is essential in the synthesis of folic acid (Fig. 11.11), which is converted by enzymatic reduction to tetrahydrofolic acid via formation of dihydrofolic acid. The enzyme involved in the terminal reduction is dihydrofolic acid reductase, which catalyses the reaction:

$$\text{NADPH} + \text{H}^+ + \text{dihydrofolic acid} \rightarrow \text{NADP}^+ + \text{tetrahydrofolic acid}$$

Tetrahydrofolic acid is a coenzyme involved in enzymatic one-carbon transfers such as methylation, hydroxymethylation and formylation. Dihydrofolic acid reductase is competitively inhibited by structural analogues of dihydrofolic acid, e.g. methotrexate (**11.7**) and trimethoprim (**11.8**), which are being used in the treatment of hyperproliferative disease and, in combination with sulfamethoxazole, in the treatment of bacterial infections, respectively.

The sulfonamides, on the other hand, are competitive inhibitors of the incorporation of PABA into pteroic acid (Fig. 11.11). Being structural analogues of PABA, the sulfonamides are incorporated instead of PABA, and the result is a non-functional folic acid derivative. Folic acid deficiency in bacteria leads to loss of the ability to synthesize thymidylic acid which is essential to nucleic acid generation. This is the basis for the antibiotic action of the sulfonamides.

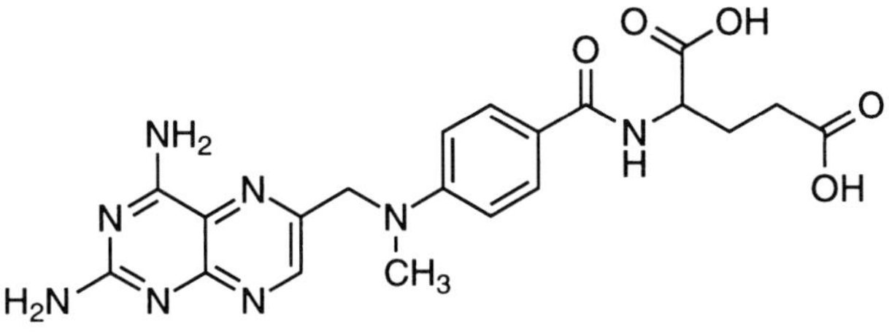

(11.7)

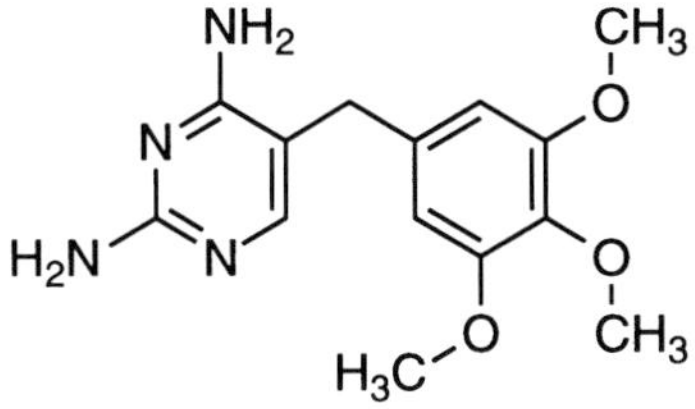

(11.8)

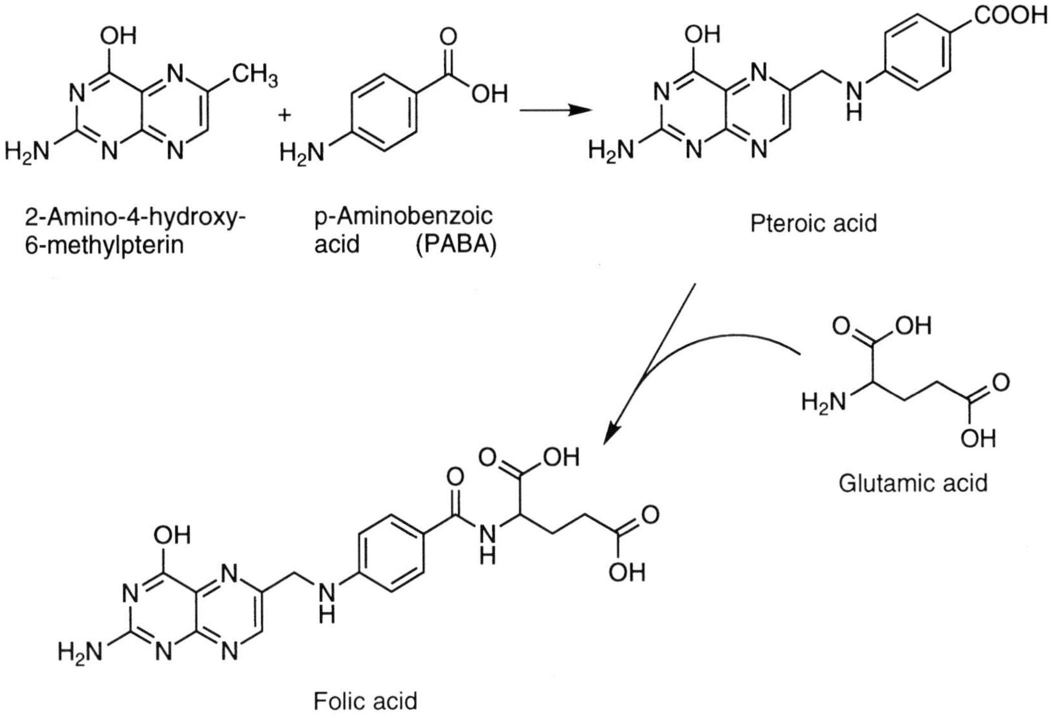

2-Amino-4-hydroxy-
6-methylpterin

p-Aminobenzoic
acid   (PABA)

Pteroic acid

Glutamic acid

Folic acid

Figure 11.11   Pathways in the biosynthesis of folic acid by bacteria. The incorporation of PABA to form pteroic acid is inhibited by the sulfonamides.

Sulfonamides have a broad spectrum of antimicrobial activity and their introduction meant a revolution in the treatment of infectious disease. Unfortunately, the widespread use of these agents resulted in the appearance of numerous sulfonamide resistant strains of bacteria, and they have largely been replaced by penicillins and other β-lactam antibiotics. However, the importance of sulfonamides to the concept of rational drug development must not be underestimated, as these compounds were some of the first examples of drugs to which a molecular mechanism of action could be assigned.

11.6.2.2 β-Lactamase inhibitors

Soon after the introduction of β-lactam antibiotics, bacterial enzymes capable of hydrolyzing the amide bond in the β-lactam ring, the β-lactamases, were recognized. The β-lactamases serve as a bacterial defense mechanism against penicillins and cephalosporins containing a β-lactam ring. Their production is controlled by either chromosomal or plasmid genes, and may be induced by the presence of an antibiotic. The plasmid-mediated β-lactamases are the major determinants of bacterial resistance to β-lactam antibiotics, as plasmid transfer of genetic material is a widespread bacterial phenomenon. Resistance to antibiotics is a growing and serious problem in the clinic, in particular in intensive care units and haematological and urological wards.

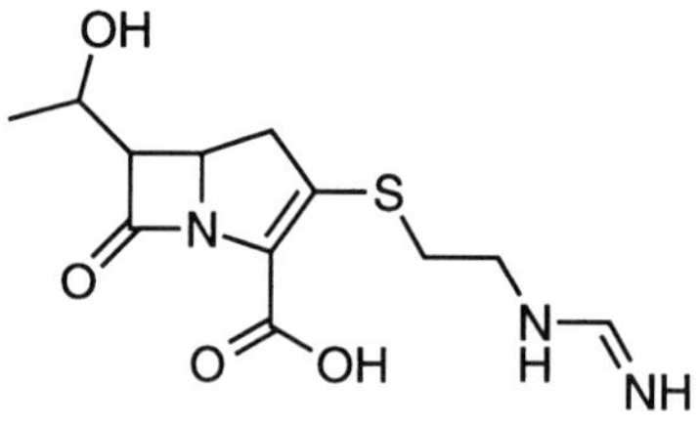

(11.9)

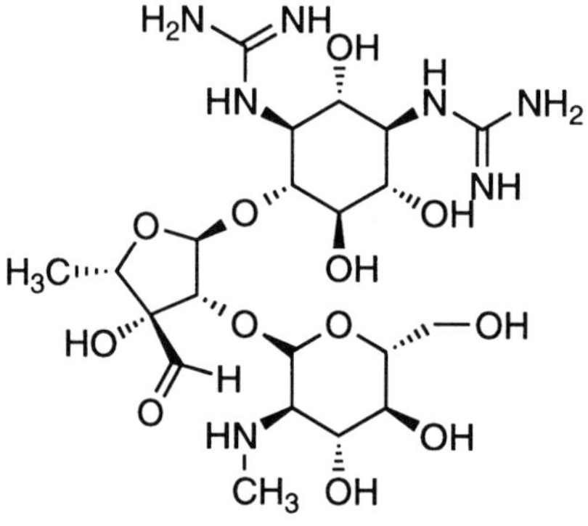

(11.10)

Medicinal chemists have pursued different ways of solving the problems of β-lactamase producing bacteria. One way of circumventing the problem is by introducing enzyme-stable antibiotics, e.g. the carbapenems like imipenem (**11.9**), and the aminoglycosides like streptomycin (**11.10**). A different, promising approach against bacteria in which β-lactamase activity is present is the use of β-lactamase inhibitors in combination with a β-lactam antibiotic. This allows the antibiotic to exert its normal activity without undergoing enzymatic degradation. Several β-lactamase inhibitors have been developed, e.g. clavulanic acid (**11.11**) and sulbactam (**11.12**).

(**11.11**)   (**11.12**)

Clavulanic acid was isolated from Streptomyces clavuligerus in 1976 and represents the first successful attempt to identify an agent capable of protecting susceptible β-lactam antibiotics. A combination of amoxycillin and clavulanate, Augmentin, is now used therapeutically. Clavulanic acid and the other β-lactamase inhibitors are suicide inhibitors that are recognized by the bacterial enzymes as substrates, but the very action of the hydrolytic enzyme leads to the formation of enzyme inhibitors (see Section 11.5.3). The mechanism of inhibitory action has been deduced by Knowles and coworkers at Harvard University, mainly by studies of sulbactam, a compound developed by Pfizer (CP-45,899). When the sulfone is incubated with the β-lactamase enzyme, a hydroxyl group of a serine residue at the active site attacks the β-lactam carbonyl, resulting in the formation of an unstable tetrahedral intermediate, which transforms spontaneously into an acyl-enzyme compound (Fig. 11.12). The acyl-enzyme then undergoes a transimination reaction with a lysine residue of the β-lactamase enzyme, leading to the cross-linkage of two amino acid residues of the active site. This is a true suicide inhibitory mechanism, since the formation of the cross-link requires the normal, hydrolytic cleavage by β-lactamase of the β-lactam ring in the first place.

Careful studies have provided evidence for the inhibitory mechanism outlined above as a general mode of action of the β-lactamase inhibitors *in vitro* using the purified enzyme, as well as in cultures of viable β-lactamase producing bacteria. The elucidation of the mechanism of action of sulbactam and clavulanic acid has made it possible to provide the rationales for development of other β-lactamase inhibitors, and thus represents a significant progress in chemotherapy.

11.6.3 Anti-inflammatory drugs

Inflammation is a natural and beneficial reaction in response to infection and trauma. In some cases, however, the inflammatory reaction fails to subside, and the patient presents with

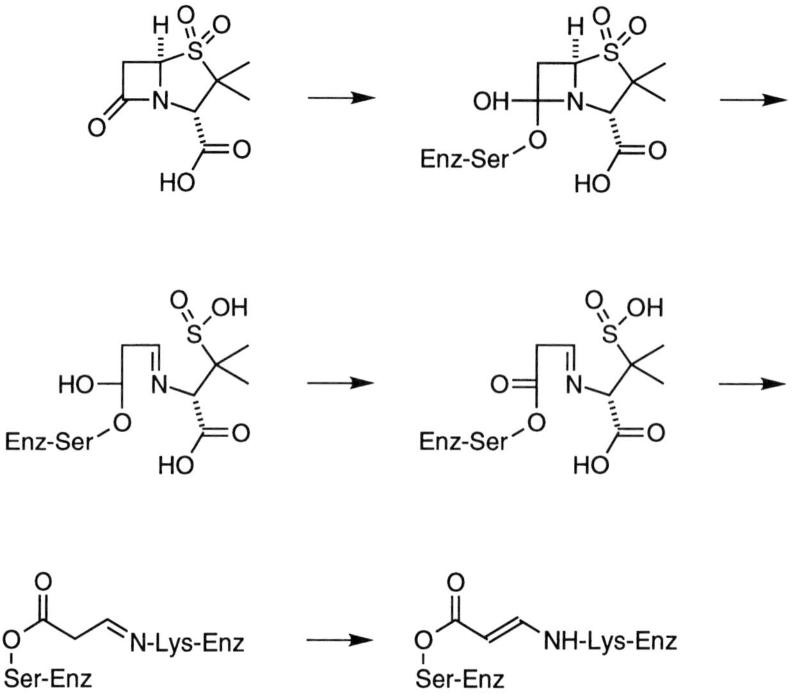

Figure 11.12 Irreversible acylation of the catalytic site of β-lactamase by sulbactam.

chronic inflammation. This condition characterizes a wide range of diseases, notably autoimmune disease (e.g. rheumatoid arthritis), chronic inflammatory bowel disease, psoriasis, and bronchial asthma to mention a few important ones. In recent years, a number of new inflammatory mediators have been identified. The present section focuses on those derived from arachidonic acid, and the drugs which inhibit their formation.

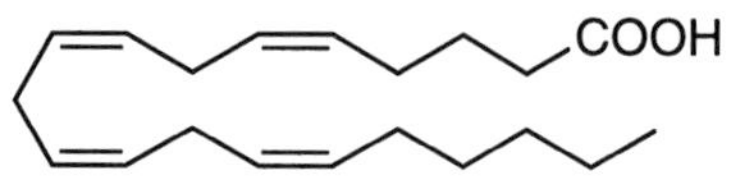

(11.13)

11.6.3.1 Arachidonic acid metabolism

Arachidonic acid (11.13) is a polyunsaturated fatty acid containing 20 carbon atoms. It is ubiquitously present in an esterified form in the phospholipids of all mammalian cell-membranes. It is released by the action of a membrane-bound enzyme, phospholipase A_2, which serves to hydrolyze the carbon-2 ester bond of phospholipids, and to some extent by the concerted action of phospholipase C and diacylglycerol lipase. Arachidonic acid is then oxidized into a number of important autacoids (known as eicosanoids, the name derived from the systematic name for arachidonic acid: eicosatetraenoic acid) by the action of certain lipoxygenases, the most important being cyclooxygenase (COX) and 5-lipoxygenase (5-LO).

COX is present as a constitutive enzyme in most mammalian cells. In addition, an inducible form has recently been described in certain cells (macrophages, endothelial cells and others). COX catalyses the peroxidation of arachidonic acid at carbon-11, leading to the initial formation of 11-hydroperoxyeicosatetraenoic acid, which transforms into the endoperoxides, prostaglandin (PG) G_2 and PGH_2. The endoperoxides are relatively unstable substances, which by the action of other specific enzymes are metabolized to the classical prostaglandins, PGD_2, PGE_2 and $PGF_{2\alpha}$, and to prostacyclin (PGI_2) and thromboxane (TX) A_2. The two latter compounds are unstable, degrading spontaneously to the biologically inactive metabolites, 6-keto-$PGF_{1\alpha}$ and TXB_2, respectively. The subscript of the various prostaglandins and thromboxanes (known under the common name prostanoids) refers to the number of double bonds present in the molecules.

The 5-LO enzyme is present mainly in leukocytes (polymorphonuclear granulocytes, macrophages/monocytes, mast cells, and, possibly, in certain lymphocytes), and is responsible for the formation of some highly active "local" hormones, the leukotrienes (LT), and 5-hydroxyeicosatetraenoic acid (5-HETE). The leukotrienes carry their name because they are produced by *leuko*cytes and contain three conjugated double bonds (*triene*), which provide them with a characteristic UV-absorption spectrum. The first step in leukotriene formation is peroxidation of the carbon-5 atom of arachidonic acid, followed by epoxidation to LTA_4. LTA_4 may either be converted enzymatically to 5,12-dihydroxyeicosatetraenoic acid (LTB_4) or to LTC_4 in a reaction with glutathione. LTC_4 is thus a tripeptide derivative of eicosatetraenoic acid, and by the action of specific enzymes amino acids are successively split from LTC_4 to form LTD_4 and LTE_4, respectively. Although the chemical structure of LTC_4, LTD_4 and LTE_4 was only recently elucidated by Samuelsson's group at the Karolinska Institute in Stockholm (1979), these compounds have collectively been recognized as a physiological principle, the slow-reacting substance of anaphylaxis (SRS-A), for 50 years.

In view of the important role of prostaglandins and leukotrienes in mediating and modulating inflammatory reactions it is not surprising that many inhibitors have been, or are being developed as anti-inflammatory drugs.

11.6.3.2 *Prostaglandins and non-steroidal anti-inflammatory drugs (NSAIDs)*
In the 1930s, von Euler in Sweden identified a lipophilic acid in human semen, which contracted uterine and other tissue-derived smooth muscles. Von Euler named the substance 'prostaglandin', but it was not possible to elucidate the chemical structure until 1962, when it was accomplished by Bergström and Samuelsson, also in Sweden. Prostaglandins are derivatives of prostanoic acid (**11.14**), a 20-carbon fatty acid containing a cyclopentane ring, which is not a naturally occurring compound. In 1964, Bergström and van Dorp showed that the prostaglandins were formed enzymatically when arachidonic acid, and a few other unsaturated fatty acids, were incubated with the microsomal fraction of seminal vesicle homogenates, and the enzyme responsible was named fatty acid cyclooxygenase.

(11.14)

Due to the ubiquitous presence of arachidonic acid and COX, and to the potent biological effects of the prostanoids, these substances have been hypothesized to be implicated as mediator and modulators of a variety of physiological and pathological processes. PGE_2 is a potent bronchodilator, whereas PGD_2, $PGF_{2\alpha}$ and TXA_2 constrict bronchial smooth muscle. The prostanoids are released from the lung in response to antigenic challenge of sensitized lung preparations, and may thus be involved in the increase in bronchial smooth muscle tone characteristic of asthmatics. However, the 5-LO products, the peptido-leukotrienes, are probably more important in this respect (see Section 11.6.3.3). TXA_2 is formed in platelets in response to a variety of stimuli, and seems to be responsible for the second wave of platelet aggregation. In contrast, prostacyclin produced by the arterial wall inhibits platelet aggregation, and the endogenous equilibrium between the level of thromboxane and prostacyclin formation may therefore be of importance to the mechanisms underlying arterial thrombus formation. Furthermore, prostaglandins may be involved in the regulation of renal function and in the physiology of reproduction.

The most interesting role of prostanoids is, however, their involvement in the inflammatory reaction, and in the production of pain and fever. Inflammation is the process elicited in order to protect the organism from injury of tissues by destruction and removal of the agent causing the injury, and by repair of the injured tissue. The five clinical signs of inflammation, pain, heat, redness, swelling, and loss of function, are caused by arteriolar, capillary and venular dilation, followed by an increase in blood flow and vascular permeability leading to plasma exudation, and leukocyte infiltration and activation. When an otherwise normal inflammatory process, initiated to defend the host from invasion by "non-self", fails to turn off after resolution of the injury, or when components of "self" are erroneously recognized as "non-self" by the immune system, as in autoimmune disease, inflammatory disease ensues.

Pharmacological application of prostaglandins may reproduce many of the cardinal signs of inflammation: vasodilation, plasma exudation, and hyperalgesia. Furthermore, prostaglandins are formed in sufficient quantities at inflammatory foci to indicate a pathophysiological function. Thus, two of the three requirements for ascribing a pathological mediator role to an autacoid, as established by H.H. Dale, are valid in the case of the prostanoids in inflammation: (1) By pharmacological application they can reproduce some of the characteristic signs of the disorder, and (2) they are present in the diseased tissues at relevant concentrations. The third condition is that drugs known to specifically inhibit their endogenous synthesis, or antagonize their biological effects, should ameliorate the symptoms of the disease. This condition is amply fulfilled in the case of the prostaglandins, since in 1971 it was reported by Vane in England that a group of drugs known as aspirin-like drugs or non-steroidal anti-inflammatory drugs (NSAIDs) are generally potent inhibitors of COX activity.

NSAIDs constitute a structurally heterogenous group of compounds, which share a number of pharmacological actions and adverse reactions. It is therefore logical to assume that they share a common biochemical activity in spite of their diverse structures, and it is now generally accepted that this is inhibition of prostaglandin biosynthesis. As outlined above, prostaglandins are mediators of inflammation, pain and fever, pathological conditions which are readily controlled by NSAIDs. Although the prostaglandins are not very potent pain-inducing agents *per se*, they substantially increase the pain response to other inflammatory mediators, such as bradykinin. The prostaglandin-induced hyperalgesia seems to be precipitated by the ability of the prostaglandins, in particular those of the E-series, to sensitize pain receptors. The prominent therapeutic actions of the NSAIDs therefore fits with a mechanism of action based on inhibition of COX. Thus, the main pharmacological activities of NSAIDs are the anti-inflammatory, analgesic and antipyretic effects. In fact, the vast majority of NSAIDs have been shown to inhibit prostaglandin synthesis *in vitro* using microsomal seminal vesicle preparations as the enzymatic source and arachidonic acid as the substrate, and *in vivo* after systemic administration of the compounds to human and experimental animals. Furthermore, their potencies in inhibiting prostaglandin synthesis *in vitro* correlate well with their *in vivo* potencies.

Another characteristic feature of the NSAIDs is that they generally share the same side-effects, which to a large extent seem to be action-related. The most common adverse effect of the aspirin-like drugs is gastric ulceration. Since the predominant prostaglandins formed by the gastric mucosa are important gastric mucosal protective agents, which both inhibit gastric acid secretion and promote mucus secretion, a certain incidence of gastric ulceration following administration of prostaglandin synthesis inhibitors is easily rationalized. Furthermore, they prolong the bleeding time by inhibiting the platelet thromboxane synthesis pathway of platelet aggregation, and prolong gestation by inhibition of prostaglandin-mediated induction and progression of labor.

COX inhibition by NSAIDs is most often noncompetitive or "mixed-type". Aspirin (or acetylsalicylic acid) (**11.15**) has a special mode of inhibition, as it acetylates the hydroxyl group of a serine residue of the active site. The implications of this special mechanism for the use of aspirin as a prophylactic agent in thromboembolic disease was discussed in Section 11.5. In the following, the most important classes of NSAIDs are briefly discussed.

Historically, aspirin was the first synthetic NSAID. It was prepared by Hoffman about a hundred years ago in an attempt to provide a substitute for the long known anti-inflammatory agent, salicylic acid, which has been prepared from the bark of willow by a great number of cultures for centuries. Salicylic acid (**11.16**) is the common structural feature of the salicylates, which are widely used as anti-inflammatory and antirheumatic drugs. A more recent salicylate is diflunisal (**11.17**).

Indomethacin (**11.18**) is a very potent inhibitor of COX activity, which was introduced as an antirheumatic drug in 1963. It is a potent NSAID, but its wider use is limited by the toxicological profile. Sulindac (**11.19**) is a closely related substance, which is reduced to the active sulfide metabolite *in vivo*. It is less toxic than indomethacin, but still shows an undesirably high rate of adverse reactions. The pyrazolones constitute another older class of NSAIDs, the most prominent one being phenylbutazone (**11.20**), which was introduced

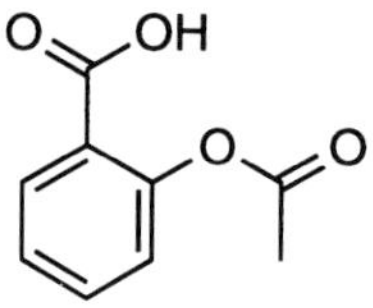

(11.15)

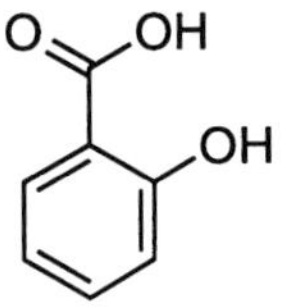

(11.16)

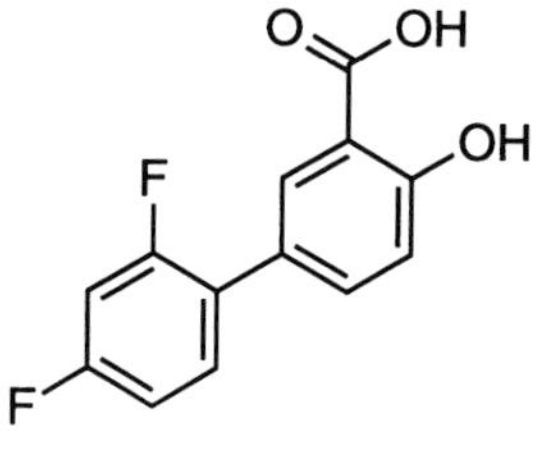

(11.17)

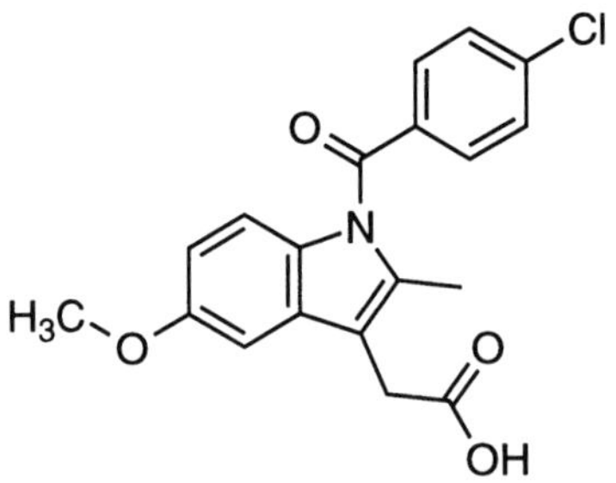

(11.18)

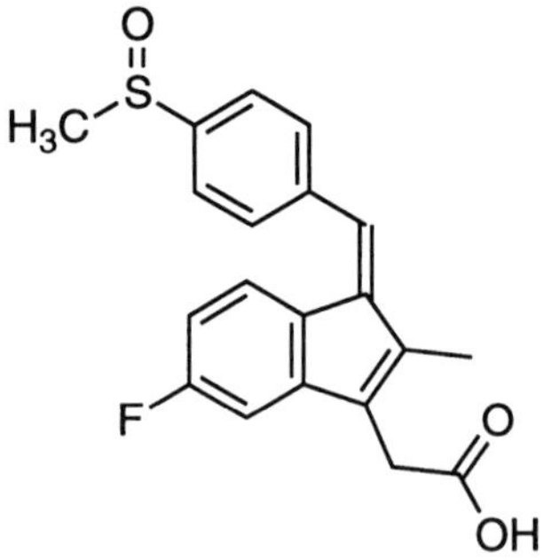

(11.19)

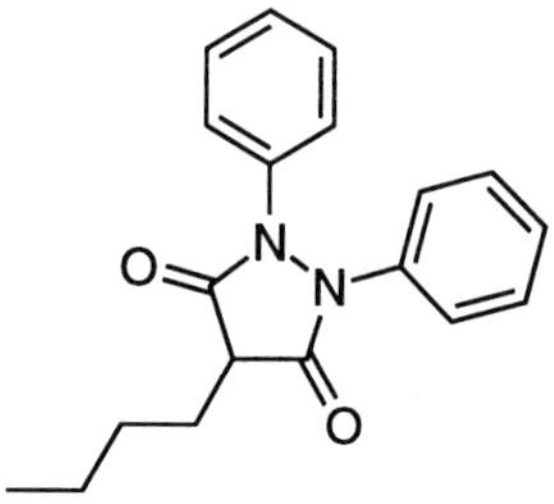

(11.20)

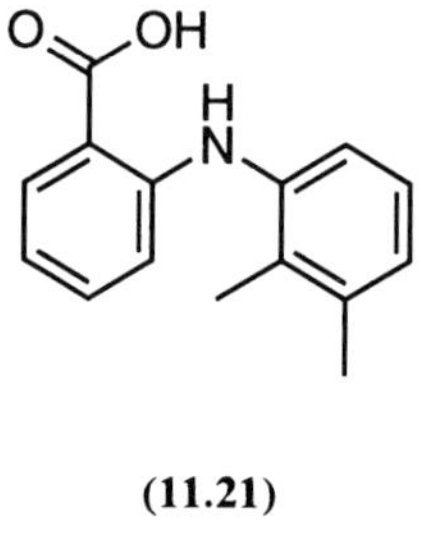

(11.21)

in 1949. As in the case of indomethacin, phenylbutazone has largely been replaced by newer and less toxic NSAIDs, but it is still an important anti-inflammatory drug, especially in veterinary medicine. N-phenyl-substituted anthranilic acid derivatives, the fenamates, comprises a number of important NSAIDs, e.g. mefenamic acid (**11.21**). Naproxen (**11.22**) and ibuprofen (**11.23**) represent the 2-arylpropionic acid derivatives that are widely used as antirheumatic and analgesic drugs. Two more recent NSAIDs are piroxicam (**11.24**) and etodolac (**11.25**).

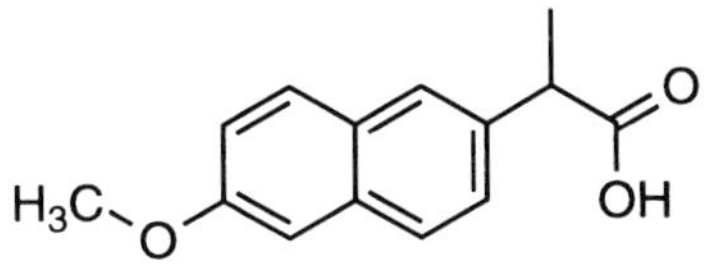

(**11.22**)

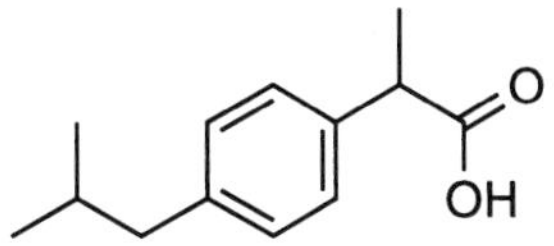

(**11.23**)

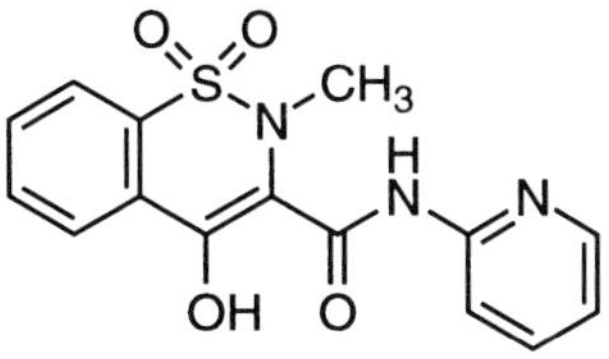

(**11.24**)

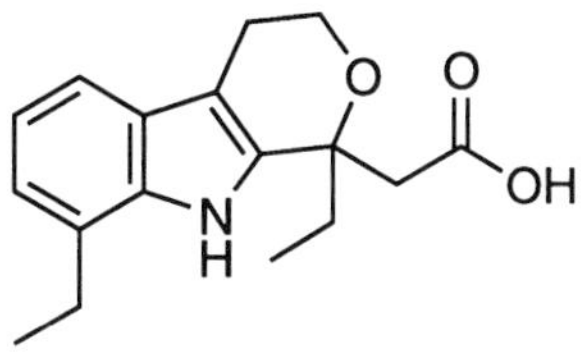

(**11.25**)

The important discovery of the mechanism of action of NSAIDs as inhibition of prostaglandin synthesis made it possible to develop rapid screening methods for the development of better drugs. Although it is impossible to separate the action-related side-effects of these drugs from their beneficial pharmacological effects, and although NSAIDs are drugs giving only symptomatic relief (they do not arrest or alter the course of rheumatic diseases), the summary above of the available major drugs in the market shows that it is possible to develop still better drugs, from the point of view of therapeutic index (ratio between therapeutic and toxic dose), when the enzymatic activity underlying a pathophysiological reaction is known.

As stated above, an inducible form of cyclooxygenase (COX-2) has recently been described in inflammatory cells. This protein is induced by inflammatory stimuli such as bacterial lipopolysaccharides (LPS), and the expression is markedly inhibited by anti-inflammatory glucocorticoids. It is anticipated that new drugs which specifically inhibit COX-2 may show much less toxicity than inhibitors of the constitutive enzyme (COX-1), which is now believed to mainly catalyze the production of cytoprotective prostanoids. Since there is only about 60% homology between COX-1 and COX-2, a new generation of NSAIDs may therefore emerge in the future.

11.6.3.3 Leukotrienes and 5-lipoxygenase inhibitors

LTB_4 is an important activator of polymorphonuclear leukocyte functions (e.g. protease secretion, phagocytosis, superoxide synthesis), and is an extremely potent chemotactic agent for these inflammatory cells. In addition, LTB_4 may have immunomodulating activity, since it has been shown *in vitro* to induce differentiation of T-lymphocytes. The S-cysteinyl substituted leukotrienes, LTC_4, LTD_4 and LTE_4 show smooth muscle contractile actions in ileum, stomach and lung preparations. LTD_4 causes profound bronchoconstriction when inhaled by human volunteers, and the sensitivity is much higher in asthmatics than in healthy subjects. Furthermore, these leukotrienes promote the secretion of airway mucus. The combination of these biological effects suggests that inhibitors of 5-LO, the enzyme responsible for the formation of all leukotrienes, may be of therapeutic value in human bronchial asthma, which is a disease characterized by bronchoconstriction as well as inflammation, and possibly also in a number of other inflammatory disorders.

A great effort has been made since the discovery of the enzyme 5-LO in order to develop specific inhibitors of this enzymatic pathway. In spite of this, it has not yet been possible to introduce such a compound as a new therapeutic agent. One reason is that 5-LO is an enzyme regulated by a great number of co-factors, including Ca^{2+}, ATP and phospholipids. It is therefore very difficult to study the enzyme in a pure form, and in contrast to COX, which is readily available in microsomal preparations of different cells, whole cells must be studied in order to develop 5-LO inhibitors. This approach has limitations, insofar as compounds interfering with normal cell metabolism (e.g. ATP synthesis) may be falsely identified as 5-LO inhibitors. Nevertheless, a number of interesting 5-LO inhibitors have emerged in the course of the last decade: Nordihydroguaiaretic acid (NDGA) (**11.26**), REV 5901 (Revlon) (**11.27**), Zileuton (Abbot) (**11.28**), L 663536 (Merck) (**11.29**), ICI 207968 (I.C.I.) (**11.30**),

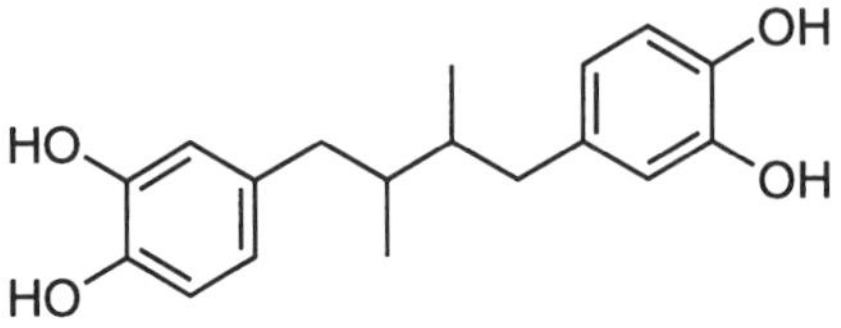

(**11.26**)

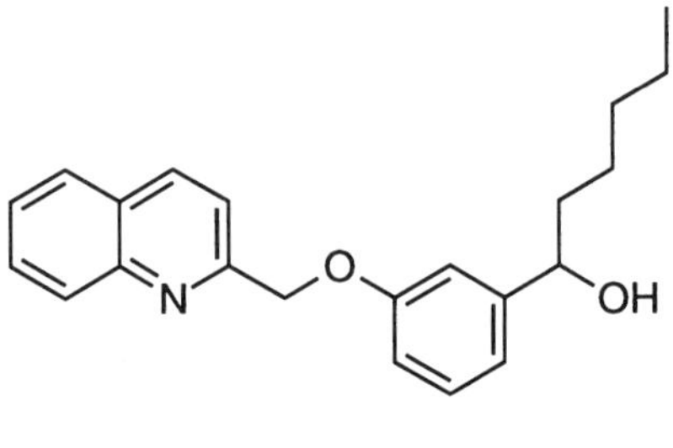

(**11.27**)

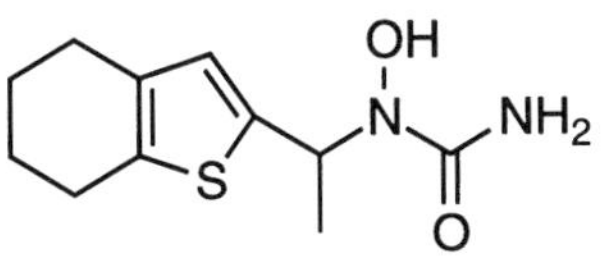

(11.28)

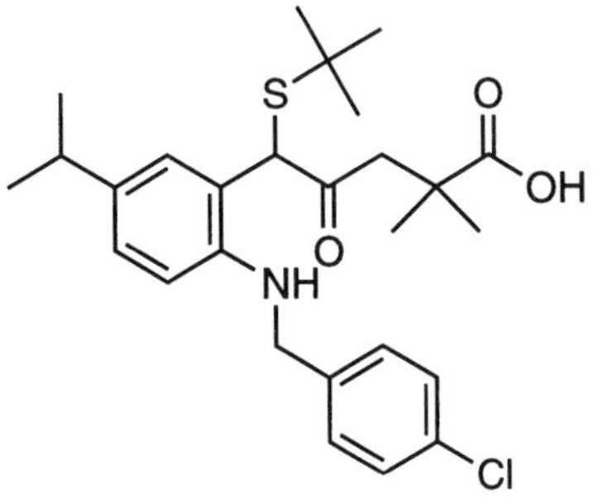

(11.29)

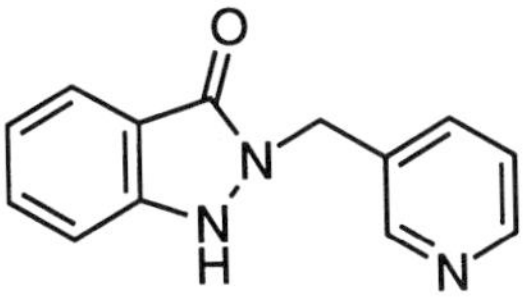

(11.30)

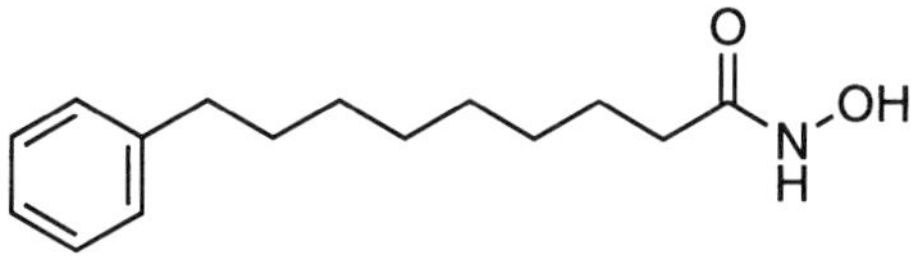

(11.31)

BMY 30094 (Bristol-Myers) (11.31), CGS 8515 (Ciba-Geigy) (11.32), ETH 615 (Leo) (11.33), and others. ETH 615 acts by inhibiting the translocation of the cytosolic 5-LO to its membrane receptor, FLAP (5-LO Activating Protein) which is an obligatory step in the activation of 5-LO. It is still too early to assess the clinical potential of such compounds.

11.6.3.4 Phospholipase A₂ inhibitors

The release of arachidonic acid by the action of phospholipase A$_2$ (PLA$_2$) is the rate-limiting step for the formation of eicosanoids. Anti-inflammatory glucocorticoids (e.g. hydrocortisone) inhibit PLA$_2$ by inducing an inhibitory protein known as lipocortin. Hence, PLA$_2$ is regarded a pro-inflammatory enzyme. Attempts are presently being made in order to design small molecule inhibitors of PLA$_2$; it has recently become clear that at least two main classes of PLA$_2$ exist: The secretory (low-molecular weight enzyme) and the cytosolic (high-molecular weight enzyme) PLA$_2$. It is believed that the secreted enzyme which shows homology with that of PLA$_2$ in snake and bee venom is an important pro-inflammatory enzyme, as it is found in inflammatory exudates such as rheumatoid synovial fluid.

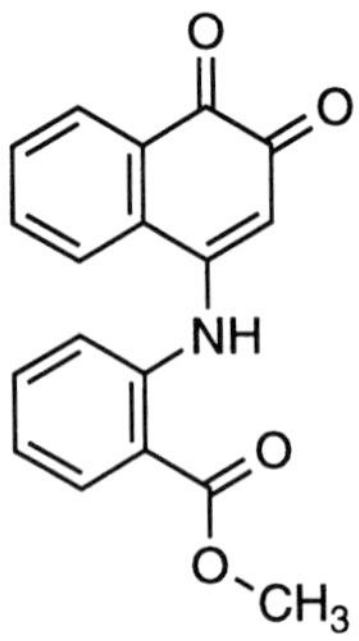

(11.32)

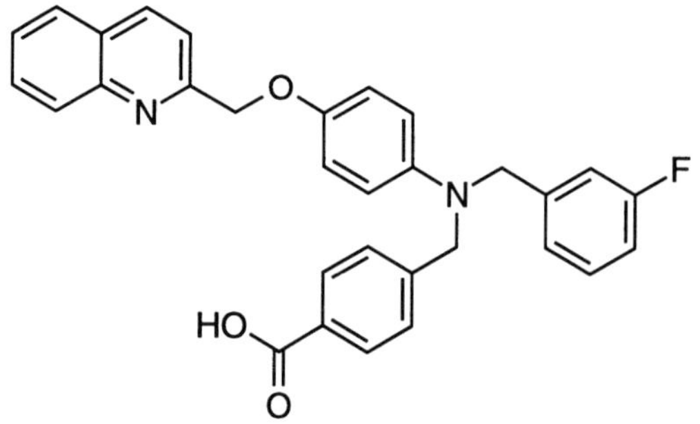

(11.33)

11.7 SUMMARY

The first part of the present chapter deals with the structure, mechanism and inhibition of enzymes. The amino acid sequence determines the three-dimensional conformation of enzyme proteins, including the active, catalytic site, which accommodates substrates and cofactors of the chemical reaction to be catalyzed. The kinetics of enzyme-catalyzed reactions are largely determined by the substrate concentration. A number of different mechanisms exist by which an enzyme may be inhibited. The reversible inhibitors may either be competitive or non-competitive. Competitive inhibitors are often substrate analogues and lower the affinity of the substrate for the active site. Transition state analogues constitute a special case of competitive inhibitors. The noncompetitive inhibitors lower the maximum velocity of the enzymic reaction without interfering with the substrate affinity. Irreversible inhibitors destroy the enzyme's catalytic site, most often by covalent binding to essential amino acid residues.

The involvement of enzymes in disease makes them an obvious target for drugs. All of the inhibitory mechanisms mentioned above are represented in the second part of the chapter. The angiotensin converting enzyme inhibitors, used in the treatment of hypertension, are competitive inhibitors, their development being rationalized from studies of the arrangement of the true substrate, angiotensin I, at the active site. The β-lactam antibiotics and aprotinin are examples of drugs derived from naturally occurring transition state analogues, whereas the β-lactamase inhibitors are a special case of irreversible inhibitors called suicide inhibitors. Most of the non-steroidal anti-inflammatory drugs, on the other hand, are non-competitive or mixed-type inhibitors, with aspirin as a notable exception. Aspirin destroys the catalytic site of its enzyme target by irreversible acylation.

FURTHER READING

Books

Kostis, J.B. and DeFelice, E.A. (eds.) (1987) *Angiotensin Converting Enzyme Inhibitors*. New York: Alan R. Liss, Inc.

Rainsford, K.D. (ed.) (1985) *Anti-inflammatory and anti-rheumatic drugs*. Vol. I, Boca Raton: CRC Press, Inc.

Sandler, M. and Smith, H.J. (eds.) (1989) *Design of Enzyme Inhibitors as Drugs*. Oxford: Oxford University Press.

Kucers, A. and Bennett, N.McK. (eds.) (1987) *The use of antibiotics. A comprehensive review with clinical emphasis*. Fourth edition, London: William Heinemann Medical Books.

Dixon, M. and Webb, E.C. (eds.) (1979) *Enzymes*. Third Edition. London: Longman Group Ltd.

Goodman Gilman, A., Goodman, L.S. and Murad, F. (eds.) (1985) *Goodman and Gilman's The Pharmacological Basis of Therapeutics*. Seventh Edition. New York: MacMillan Publishing Co.

Zollner, H. (ed.) (1993) *Handbook of Enzyme Inhibitors*. Second Edition. Weinheim: VCH Verlagsgesellschaft mbH.

Rokach, J. (ed.) (1989) *Leukotrienes and lipoxygenases. Chemical, biological and clinical aspects*. Amsterdam: Elsevier.

Reynolds, J.E.F. (ed.) (1993) *Martindale. The Extra Pharmacopoeia*. Thirtieth Edition. London. The Pharmaceutical Press.

Barrett, A.J. and Salvesen, G. (eds.) (1986) *Proteinase Inhibitor*. Amsterdam: Elsevier.

Lorand, L. and Mann, K.G. (eds.) (1993) Proteolytic Enzymes in Coagulation, Fibrinolysis and Complement Activation. Part A: Mammalian Blood Coagulation. Factors and Inhibitors. In *Methods in Enzymology*, vol. 222., San Diego: Academic Press, Inc.

Articles

Belz, G.G., Kirch, W. and Kleinbloesem, C.H. (1988) Angiotensin converting enzyme inhibitors. Pharmacodynamics and pharmacokinetics. *Clin. Pharmacokinetics*, **15**, 295–318.

Collen, D. (1987) Molecular mechanisms of fibrinolysis and their application to fibrin-specific thrombolytic therapy. *J. Cell Biochem.*, **33**, 77–94.

Crofford, L.J., Wilder, R.L., Ristimaki, A.P., Sano, H., Remmers, E.F., Epps, H.R. and Hla, T. (1994)

Cyclooxygenase-1 and cyclooxygenase-2 expression in rheumatoid synovial tissues — effects of interleukin-1-beta, phorbol ester, and corticosteroids. *J. Clin. Invest.*, **93**, 1095–1101.

Knowles, J.R. (1985) Penicillin resistance: the chemistry of β-lactamase inhibition. *Acc. Chem. Res.*, **18**, 97–104.

Kostis, J.B. (1988) Angiotensin converting enzyme inhibitors. I. Pharmacology. II. Clinical use. *Am. Heart J.*, **116**, 1580–1605.

Vadas, P., Browning, J., Edelson, J. and Pruzanski, W. (1993) Extracellular phospholipase A_2 expression and inflammation: The relationship with associated disease states. *J. Lipid Med.*, **8**, 1–30.

Williams, J.D. (1988) Importance of β-lactamases and clinical implications of their inhibitors. *Drugs*, **35** (Suppl. 7), 3–11.

12. BIO-INORGANIC CHEMISTRY

OLE JØNS and ERIK SYLVEST JOHANSEN

CONTENTS

12.1 INTRODUCTION

Man needs some 25 elements of the periodic table to have a good, healthy life. More than half of these elements are metals of which most form complexes of crucial importance to the overall metabolism.

Some other metals are imposing toxic hazards to man and they can give rise to acute or chronic diseases.

Since the chemistry of metals is part of inorganic chemistry some topics from this discipline are among the prerequisites of medicinal chemistry. Generally, the reader is referred to a textbook of inorganic or bio-inorganic chemistry for a thorough presentation of these topics. The reader may wish to consult the monographs referred to for more detailed discussion of the topics presented.

12.2 ESSENTIAL AND BENEFICIAL ELEMENTS

The simplest definition of an essential element is that the absence of the element will prevent man from completing the life cycle, reproduction included.

Experimentally, this rigorous criterion cannot always be satisfied and a broader definition is used today. Generally, it is a characteristic of an essential element that insufficient intakes produce an impairment of function, and sufficient intakes prevent or relieve the impairment.

A beneficial element is an element that seems to aid growth or reproduction, but no ill-effects can be ascribed to its absence, perhaps because of the experimental difficulties of proving essentiality of the vanishingly small amounts.

The essential and beneficial elements are concentrated in the upper part of the periodic system (Fig. 12.1).

It can be seen that most metals belong to the first transition series — only molybdenum comes from the second series.

The optimal daily intake can roughly be connected to the total amounts of the elements in a human being (Table 12.1). Effective homeostatic mechanisms are involved in controlling the uptake of most of the essential elements.

As it is seen the units stretch from kilograms to milligrams. The levels can be maintained by daily intakes of amounts smaller in comparison with the total masses, and because of homeostasis, the daily dose can vary within usually rather wide limits. Some trace elements, however, must be supplied within very narrow limits, since too much will have an adverse effect, i.e. the elements become toxic. The optimal daily uptake of an essential element is shown schematically in the dose-response curve (Fig. 12.2).

H													B	C	N	O	F	
Li													B	C	N	O	F	
Na	Mg													Si	P	S	Cl	
K	Ca			V	Cr	Mn	Fe	Co	Ni	Cu	Zn				As	Se		
				Mo													I	

Figure 12.1   Essential elements and the periodic system. Bulk elements in bold typeface and proposed essential elements in italics.

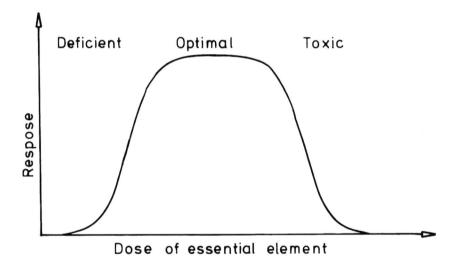

Figure 12.2   Schematical dose — response curve of an essential element.

The figure illustrates that an essential element can be toxic if given in excessive amounts. An example: copper deficiency can lead to anemia, while copper excess is associated with Wilson's disease. Only intakes in the optimal region have no ill-effects.

An especially narrow optimal region is found for selenium, for which the interval corresponds to ca. 50–200 μg per day. Usually the interval allows for much greater variations in daily intake.

Table 12.1   Mass of essential elements in human adult.

Elements	Mass
Main Group Elements	
Sodium	100 g
Potassium	140 g
Magnesium	20–30 g
Calcium	1200 g
Phosphorus	600–800 g
Iodine	10– 20 mg
Selenium	13–20 mg
Transition Series Metals	
Chromium	2 mg
Manganese	10–20 mg
Iron	3–5 g
Cobalt	1–2 mg
Copper	100–150 mg
Zinc	2–4 g

The concentration unit on the horizontal axis in Figure 12.2 is arbitrary, since different elements have very different daily requirements.

12.2.1 The possible role of evolution

The magnitude of reported levels and the distribution in the periodic system reflect to some degree the availability of the elements during the evolution of man. The lighter elements were from the outset much more abundant than the heavier ones, and anomalous large amounts of iron and neighbouring elements from the first transition metal series have facilitated the exploitation of these metals in a great number of metalloproteins and -enzymes.

As a consequence of this selection of essential elements and because evolution did not need to create defensive mechanisms, many heavier metals can have adverse effects on biological systems. The chemistry of toxic metals is similar enough to that of essential metals to compete for binding sites in enzymes and other molecules. But the similarity is limited and the new complexes formed will not function properly.

The modern industrialized society has made these heavy elements available in large quantities and has for a long time not worried about spreading the waste in the environment.

12.2.2 The different roles of essential elements

The most abundant essential elements (Table 12.1) include four metals, sodium, potassium, magnesium, and calcium. These are most often associated with trigger and control mechanisms. The selective distribution of the cations inside and outside the cell is the basis of triggering nerves, muscle contraction, and neurotransmitters. The alkali metals rarely form any complexes. Magnesium and calcium do form coordination compounds with both low and high molecular weight ligands. But a substantial proportion of the dissolved metals are present in the form of naked (hydrated) ions in biological fluids. In the form of complexes, both magnesium and calcium ions stabilize structures such as lipoprotein membranes.

The less abundant transition group metals have a yet greater tendency to form coordination compounds with a specific stereochemistry and accordingly an important role is that of structure promoters. A certain metal ion in a certain oxidation state has the greatest affinity for selected donor atoms according to the principle of hard and soft acids and bases (HSAB), so the possibility exists of controlling the folding of a protein chain in a very specific way and thus bringing important groups together.

Many processes demand some catalysis to proceed at a finite speed. Often acid catalysis is involved, but since most biological fluids have a pH near 7.4 this mechanism cannot be promoted by protons. Lewis acids such as the ions of the first transition series then become important in metalloenzymes, which can act as general acid catalysts. A large number of zinc-containing enzymes is found in this group, i.e. carbonic anhydrase, alcohol dehydrogenase, and alkaline phosphatase.

The last role of the transition metals to mention is that of redox mediators, since they can have several oxidation states. In metalloenzymes they are important in the controlled metabolic degradation of food and drugs, and they also act as transporters of electrons. Iron in several cytochromes and molybdenum in xanthine oxidase are examples of this role.

12.2.3 Toxic elements

As already mentioned, essential elements in excessive amounts are toxic to the healthy organism. Even supplements in the agreed optimal region can be toxic to non-healthy persons. A well-known example is Wilson's disease (an impaired copper metabolism caused by an inherited genetic defect).

Another recent example is the harm caused by zinc supplements to Alzheimer's patients. Indeed it seems that zinc could play a crucial role in the formation of amyloid plaques found in the brains of Alzheimer's patients.

Toxic metals often, but not invariably, have enough resemblance to essential elements to expel the latter from enzymes and the like. Since the chemistry will differ in some respects, the coordination compound formed often has a changed symmetry or a different folding of protein chains as a consequence of the enhanced affinity for soft donor atoms like sulphur. The principle of HSAB is indeed a good guide for the prediction of such interactions in a sensible way.

The classical examples of toxic elements are mercury and arsenic. They are both classified as soft elements by HSAB, and it does seem that softness and toxicity are related to each other. The toxic elements have been spread into the environment by careless handling of waste, leading of petrol, and so on. Since metals, in contrast to most organic molecules, cannot be destroyed, the toxic elements will continue to present a rather unpleasant problem for many years to come.

When considering the toxicity of mercury it is necessary to specify the oxidation state and the ligands. Metallic mercury for example is quite nontoxic and only prolonged exposure to the vapour will give rise to any harm. In contrast, Hg^{2+} ions are acutely toxic and CH_3-Hg^+ which is easily formed by biomethylation is especially nasty because its ambivalent lipophilic/hydrophilic character makes it possible for the ion to traverse even the blood-brain barrier.

Table 12.2   Nutritional aspects of essential trace elements.

Element	Recommended daily dietary allowance*	Functions	Deficiency
Iron	10–15 mg	Heme respiratory carrier system. Immune system. Enzymes.	Tiredness. Anemia. Reduced resistance.
Zinc	12–15 mg	Many metabolic enzymes. Nucleic acid and protein synthesis. Immune system and wound healing.	Skin lesions. Growth weakness. Delayed appetite and sexual maturation.
Copper	1.5–3 mg	Enzymes in blood and skeletal synthesis. Immune system. Protein metabolism.	Rare for healthy humans. Anemia. Neurological defects.
Manganese	2.0–5 mg	Enzymes in protein and energy metabolism. Antioxidant.	Rarely known. Growth failure.
Fluorine	1.5–4 mg	Structural component of bones and teeth.	Carries in teeth.
Molybdenum	75–250 μg	Enzymes in metabolism of xanthine and sulfites.	Reduced metabolism of xanthine.
Chromium	50–200 μg	Maintenance of normal glucose tolerance.	Disturbance in glucose and lipid metabolism.
Selenium	55–70 μg	Antioxidant against free radicals. Heavy metal protection.	Keshan disease. Muscle weakness.
Iodine	150 μg	Thyroid hormones.	Goiter.
Cobalt	2 μg vitamin B_{12}	Erythropoisis.	Only as vitamin B_{12}.
Nickel	—	Nucleic acid. Lipid metabolism.	Unknown.
Silicon	—	Structural components in nails and hair.	Unknown.
Vanadium	—	Lipid metabolism. Regulation of cholesterol synthesis.	Unknown.

*Adults. Recommended Dietary Allowances, 10th Edition 1989, National Academy Press, Washington D.C.

12.3 NUTRITIONAL ASPECTS OF THE ESSENTIAL TRACE ELEMENTS

There has been a great increase in the general interest in knowledge of the biology of essential trace metals, as witnessed by the number of publications in the scientific world and by the ever increasing supply of nutritional supplements offered to people through pharmacies and druggists. Some nutritional and metabolic aspects of essential trace elements are shown in Table 12.2.

Because of the economic importance the deficiency and toxicological aspects of the trace elements has been known in agriculture for a long time. Problems in practical agriculture with farm animals have caused much more attention on supplements of trace elements to food products. Pig food-stuff has thus for many years been supplemented with selenium.

In human nutrition, however, the situation is somewhat different. The need for iron in connection with anemia and iodine in connection with goiter were recognized many years ago. The recognition of deficiencies of zinc, copper and selenium in different parts of the world has been made in the last thirty years.

From the years after World War Two the advertising sentence for oatmeal: "contains calcium, iron, phosphorus and vitamin B" is well known. The U.S. National Academy of Science has set up recommended daily dietary allowances (RDA) figures for some trace elements based on the requirements for growth and maintenance, excretion and absorption. Cobalt is required only in the form of vitamin B_{12}. The figures are based on the usual intake from a Western-type diet by a healthy adult person assumed to be obtaining sufficient quantities of the trace elements. The authorities only recommend supplementary trace elements to certain risk groups. Iron deficiency is a problem for 1–2 years old children and for some menstruating women. Iodine deficiency is a problem in some areas and is commonly remedied by the supplementation with salt. Selenium is discussed intensely in these years. In some parts of the world, e.g. Finland the selenium level in soil is low and supplement could be necessary.

Deficiencies of chromium, copper, molybdenum, selenium, and zinc have been reported in patients receiving long-term total parenteral nutrition unsupplemented with trace elements. Genetic defects in the trace element metabolism may result in deficiency syndromes e.g. for copper in the Menke's Steely Hair Syndrome. An optimal level of all trace elements in the body is dependent on both sufficient and balanced supplementation of the trace elements. Numerous synergistic or antagonistic effects have been observed involving two essential metals or an essential element and a toxic metal. The absorption of zinc is impaired by iron(II) and a high zinc intake influences the absorption of copper. In the human body zinc and cadmium presumably are competitors for the protein binding sites (on metallothionein) and a sufficiently high zinc level is likely to mitigate the effect of cadmium accumulation in the tissues. In Greenland, the local population has a high level of mercury in the blood in comparison with other Danish people, but they also have a much higher level of selenium. Both elements stem from the food coming primarily from the sea. Selenium might be a natural antidote protecting against mercury poisoning.

In order to recommend figures for dietary intake one must know the bioavailability of the element in the food. Iron is known to be absorbed to different extents from different types of food. The bioavailability of iron depends mainly on the form in which it is present. Diets containing compounds such as sugar and vitamin C may enhance its bioavailability, whereas others like phytate and tannic acid may reduce iron absorption. Several iron preparations are found in the pharmacy and chemist's store. Simple iron salts such as sulphate will cause gastric irritation and iron in a chelated form is therefore usually applied. Preparations with iron(II)fumarate, iron(II)gluconate, and iron(II)glycinate are commonly used. Iron(III) in soluble form will not give a better absorption, and only a fraction of the total iron will be absorbed.

The bioavailability of other essential trace elements is also markedly affected by the composition of the diet. Cereals and other plant foods contain e.g. phytate which can bind zinc strongly, thus making it unavailable for absorption. In human milk the availability of zinc is much higher than it is in cow milk and infant formulas. This might be due to the presence in human milk of a specific enhancing zinc-binding ligand, picolinic acid.

Also the form in which the element is present will influence its metabolism. Toxicologists know that the chemical form or valence state of an element can affect its metabolic behaviour in the body. Arsenic(V) is relatively harmless but in the trivalent state arsenium is a highly toxic substance. Nevertheless, it has been found that arsenobetain $((CH_3)_3As^+CH_2COO^-)$, which can be found in fish and other sea food fortunately is relatively nontoxic. Much research in the field of speciation has been going on in recent years. In supplemental products containing selenium it is found that those products with yeast-selenium or selenomethionin will cause the selenium level in the blood to rise more quickly than products containing inorganic selenium at the same concentration.

Research in the field of nutritional aspects continues. Deficiencies will be found in new geographic areas and as a function of changes in the environment, new food habits and improvements of our food products. Therefore an understanding of the mode of action of an element and its metabolism in the body is important.

12.4 THERAPEUTIC CHELATING AGENTS

Toxicity of metal ions is generally based on formation of metal chelates with naturally occurring ligands. Metal ions are toxic because they can bind to enzymes and other ligands in biological systems and so prevent these molecules from functioning in a normal manner. A therapeutic chelating agent is a compound to be used as an antidote for metal ion poisoning. The mode of action of such compounds is based on competition with metal ions for binding sites on the molecules in biological systems. The goal of chelate therapy is a complexation with the toxic metal ion and facilitation of its excretion.

The use of therapeutic chelating agents goes back to the Second World War in connection with the use of the organoarsenic toxic gas, Lewisite (**12.1**) acting on lungs and skin. Peters and co-workers found that the action of Lewisite on pyruvate oxidase could be reversed by a thiol-containing compound. The result of their research was the selection of 2,3-dimercaptopropanol-1 or BAL (British Anti-Lewisite) (**12.2**) as the first chelating agent which clearly demonstrated the successful chelation therapy in humans.

$$CI-CH=CH-As\begin{cases} CI \\ CI \end{cases}$$

$$\begin{array}{c} CH_2OH \\ | \\ CHSH \\ | \\ CH_2SH \end{array}$$

12.1   **12.2**

In chelation therapy it is desirable to use selective agents which bind the target metal ion very strongly while not interfering with the metabolism of vulnerable essential elements. An ideal agent should be capable of penetrating into the body compartment where the toxic meal ion is to be found. And the drug must be non-toxic, resistant to metabolic degradation, cheap and, if possible, useful for oral administration.

12.4.1 Properties of chelating agents

12.4.1.1 Coordination chemistry
Chelation therapy is the formation of complexes with polydentate ligands with the aim of removing a metal ion from a biomolecular site where it is producing a "biochemical lesion".

In chemistry terms, the agent acts as a ligand binding the central metal ion in a coordination compound. The formation of one or more five- or six-membered chelate rings makes a significant contribution to the stability of the complex. The ability of a chelating agents or a ligand to bind metal ions may be expressed quantitatively as the equilibrium constant of the reaction. Charges are omitted for the sake of clarity.

We distinguish between formation constants and stability constants. If more than one ligand is added to the metal ion in the complex we get $K_1, K_2, \ldots, K_N$, the stepwise formation constants.

$$M + L = ML; \quad K_1 = \frac{[ML]}{[M][L]}$$

$$ML + L = ML_2; \quad K_2 = \frac{[ML_2]}{[ML][L]}$$

Another way to express the equilibrium relations give $\beta_1, \beta_2, \ldots, \beta_N$, the stepwise stability constants.

$$M + L = ML; \quad \beta_1 = \frac{[ML]}{[M][L]}$$

$$M + 2L = ML_2; \quad \beta_2 = \frac{[ML_2]}{[M][L]^2}$$

This means that $K_1 = \beta_1$, $K_1 \cdot K_2 = \beta_2$ etc. Often the complexes found are simple ML and ML_2 complexes, but protonated species like MHL and hydroxy complexes, for example $ML(OH)$ will also be found in many cases. In the literature many stability constants can be found. They are often practical constants and not thermodynamic constants valid only at zero ionic strength. They are determined under controlled circumstances e.g. at a given temperature and constant ionic strength (potassium nitrate, sodium chloride or sodium perchlorate).

The *in vivo* concentration of a metal chelate is not only a function of the stability constant but is also affected by the other components in the solution. This means that we have to use the conditional constant which takes into consideration those side reactions.

12.4.1.2 *Selectivity*

Some compounds like ethylenediaminetetraacetic acid (EDTA) will form stable complexes with nearly all the metal ions, i.e. it is not a selective agent and there is a great danger that the side-effects caused by interference with the essential metal ions may limit the usefulness. The chemical basis for selecting selective chelating agents is established by the concept of HSAB (Table 12.3).

The general rule is that "soft" metal ions such as Ag(I), Hg(II), Cd(II), Au(I) and Cu(I) will prefer interaction with a "soft" donor atom such as sulfur. In contrast, "hard" metal ions like Ca(II), Mg(II), Fe(III) will form complexes preferably with species containing "hard" oxygen donor atoms. The "intermediate" metal ions such as Cu(II), Fe(II), Zn(II) and Ni(II) will preferably bind to nitrogen donors but most often to a mixture of both "hard" and "soft" donor atoms.

Table 12.3   Some hard and soft acids and bases.

Hard Acids:
  alkali metals
  alkaline earth metals
  La^{3+}, Ce^{4+}, Th^{4+}, UO^{2+}, Ti^{4+}, Zr^{4+}, Cr^{3+}, Mn^{2+}, Fe^{3+}, Co^{3+}, Au^{3+}, Sn^{4+}

Border Line:
  Fe^{2+}, Co^{2+}, Ni^{2+}, Cu^{2+}, Zn^{2+}, $Sb(III)$, Bi^{3+}, Sn^{2+}, Pb^{2+}

Soft Acids:
  Cu^+, Ag^+, Cd^{2+}, Hg_2^{2+}, Hg^{2+}, Tl^+

Hard Bases:
  NH_3, H_2O, OH^-, O^{2-}, CO_3^{2-}, NO_3^-, PO_4^{3-}, SO_4^{2-}, ClO_4^-, $-COO^-$, F^-, $EDTA$, Cl^-

Border Line:
  N_3^-, NO_2^-, SO_3^{2-}, Br^-

Soft Bases:
  CN^-, SNC^-, $S_2O_3^{2-}$, S^{2-}, I^-

12.4.1.3 Kinetics

The rate of an exchange reaction for a complex with a given ligand is also important in relation to the use of chelating agents as drugs. Those complexes for which substitution reactions are rapid are called labile, whereas those for which substitution reactions proceed slowly are called inert.

Most metal ion complexes are normally labile, with the notable exceptions of Cr(III), Co(III) and sometimes Fe(II) which have slow kinetics because of inert complexes. The vitamin B_{12} is an example of a cobalt(III) complex being stabilized as an inert complex.

If a toxic metal ion is bound deeply within a big protein molecule one can imagine how slow the substitution reactions might be. A mobilization of the metal ions is generally necessary. The essential metal ions are unevenly distributed between body compartments and, furthermore, ions will be found either in labile form, i.e. aquated ions, low molecular weight complexes with e.g. amino acids or in protein molecules or in more inert form firmly bound or precipitated in bones or other tissues. For instance, iron is bound in ferritin from which iron is mobilized only by metabolic processes and not directly by a concurrent complexing agent.

12.4.1.4 Lipophilicity

It applies to the chelating agents as well as to other drugs that the lipophilicity of the agents is of great importance for the absorption into the body and to their ability to pass the biological membranes. Nonpolar and electrically neutral agents and complexes have the highest lipophilicity, while compounds which exist as charged species cannot diffuse through biological membranes. Cisplatin (**12.12**) is an example where the absorption and action is a function of the concentration of chloride ions in the gastrointestinal tract and in the cells.

Also, the composition of the metal complex is important for the excretion of the metal or the activity of the drug used. In the classical Albert study the bacteriostatic activity of 8-hydroxyquinoline is due to the passive diffusion of the neutral 1:3 iron(III) complex through the bacterial cell membrane. When inside the cell the complex dissociates to 1:2 and 1:1 complexes being responsible for the bactericidal effect.

12.4.1.5 Other properties

A chelating agent should of course be of low inherent toxicity for clinical use and the complexes formed should also possess low toxicity. Metabolic stability of the agent is also of importance. Some otherwise excellent ligands like citrate are metabolized too rapidly to be useful. In the case of EDTA, no metabolism is found and the metal ions will be excreted from the body in complexed form.

These strict requirements for an ideal chelating agent cannot at all be fulfilled by any single compound. In the following discussion of individual chelating agents advantages and disadvantages are mentioned. The only chelating agents commercially available in Denmark are BAL, D-penicillamine, calcium-EDTA and desferrioxamine.

12.4.2 Computer simulations

In a discussion of the therapeutic chelating agents computer simulations based on models with several equilibria are useful. A blood plasma model is based on known concentrations of the essential metal ions like Ca, Mg, Zn, Cu and of amino acids, peptides, inorganic anions and other ligands found in blood plasma. In the model, these concentrations are combined with the dissociation and stability constants found in the literature. With this plasma model, it is possible to calculate a given concentration of a complex or species, for example the concentration of the copper(II)histidine 1:1 complex or the concentration of free, hydrated calcium ions. This equilibrium model is vizualized with e.g. the Plasma Mobilizing Index (PMI), of May and Williams.

The PMI function is defined as:

$$PMI = \frac{\text{Concentration of low-molecular-weight species in blood plasma in the presence of exogenous ligand drug}}{\text{Concentration of low-molecular-weight species in normal blood plasma}}$$

Figure 12.3 shows log (PMI) curves for ethambutol (EMB) and a metabolite of ethambutol, 2,2′-(ethylenediamino)dibutyric acid (EDBA) together with various other ligands. Ethambutol will have no effect on the level of low-molecular-weight complexes in plasma or on the distribution of copper(II) and zinc(II). The concentration of EMB needed to raise the PMI value would be unrealistically high. In contrast, EDBA causes a moderate increase in the concentration of low-molecular-weight zinc(II) and copper(II) fractions, but the effect is smaller that the one given by DTPA at the same molar concentration. The conclusion is that any disturbance of the metal ion metabolism caused by the use of ethambutol for treatment over a long period of time cannot be explained by ethambutol itself. The recognized effect is believed to be chelation by the metabolite, EDBA.

This computer model has its limitations mainly related to the simplification introduced by the use of only stability constants as a basis for the calculations. Other computer models are under development which include rate constants for the various processes involved in the mobilization, transport and excretion of a toxic metal ion in the presence of

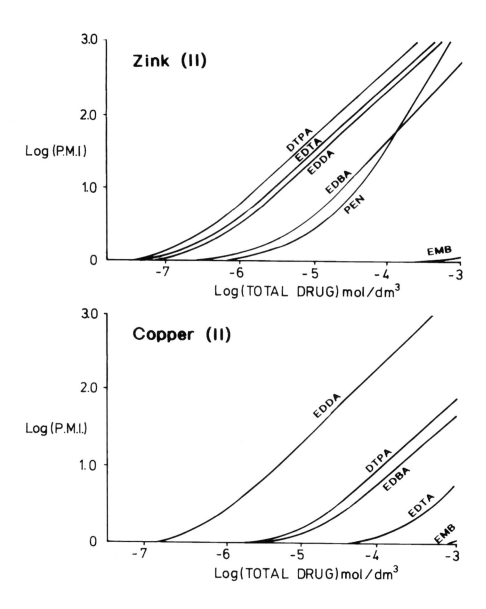

Figure 12.3 Log (PMI) curves for various ligands including EDBA and ethambutol. EMB = ethambutol; PEN = D-penicillamine; EDBA = 2,2'-(ethylenediamine)dibutyric acid; EDDA = ethylenediaminediacetic acid; EDTA = ethylenediaminetetraacetic acid; DTPA = diethylenetriaminepentaacetic acid.

Source: Reprinted by permission from A. Cole, P.M. May and D.R. Williams; *Agents and Actions*, **11** (1981) 296.

a chelating agent. Such a compartment distribution model is analogous to those used in clinical pharmacokinetic studies.

12.4.3 Synergistic chelation therapy

In practical chelation therapy two compounds with different mode of action are often used. One agent will remove the metal ion from the tissue into the bloodstream as a neutral lipophilic complex. Then the second agent takes over and forms a charged complex which can pass through the kidneys. In the treatment of lead toxification penicillamine is used to remove the lead from the tissue and EDTA takes over the lead as a charged complex ready for excretion with urine. EDTA and its complexes are highly charged and are not able to penetrate lipophilic membranes. Another example is the increase in the excretion of iron when desferrioxamine (**12.8**) treatment is combined with the use of ascorbic acid.

12.4.4 Selected chelating agents

12.4.4.1 BAL and other dithiols

BAL
Although BAL (**12.2**) was the first chelating agent used clinically (see previous section), it is still in use even though more efficient and less toxic agents are available. With two "soft" thiol groups, it will complex most heavy metals which also form stable sulfides. It is the best choice for arsenic, gold and inorganic mercury detoxification. Usually it is recommended exclusively for the treatment of gold poisoning due to overload in gold drug treatment. BAL is a yellow liquid which has only limited solubility in water.

There are several disadvantages connected with this compound. It is decomposed through oxidation and it smells very badly with a strong garlic-like odour. The inherent toxicity is high and it is metabolized rather quickly. The advantage of BAL is its lipophilic capacity, making it able to penetrate into the tissues where the toxic metal is accumulated. The complex formed is electrically neutral and is also able to penetrate membranes. This can, on the other hand, also be a disadvantage. If used in the treatment of mercury poisoning the complex is sufficiently lipophilic to increase the accumulation of mercury, including methyl mercury, in the brain.

UNITHIOL (SODIUM 2,3-DIMERCAPTOPROPANE-1-SULFONATE)
This agent also has two neighbouring thiol groups which chelate readily to the same series of heavy metals as BAL. Unithiol (**12.3**) is water-soluble and the complexes formed are stable and water-soluble too as a result of the charged sulfonate group.

$$CH_2SH$$
$$CHSH$$
$$CH_2SO_3Na$$

12.3

In contrast to BAL, it cannot lead to an increased concentration of the metal in the brain, but it reduces the body concentration of metal acting primarily in the extracellular fluids. Unithiol is reported to be useful in the treatment of acute inorganic mercury and cadmium poisoning and is also shown to be efficient in the removal of methylmercury, copper, nickel, lead and others. Most of the literature describing its applications comes from Russia, where it is widely used. Only now it is on its way to the Western market. It has a much lower inherent toxicity than BAL and the complexes too have low toxicity. It can be administrated orally or by injection of aqueous solutions.

2,3-DIMERCAPTOSUCCINIC ACID (DMSA)

2,3-dimercaptosuccinic acid (DMSA) (**12.4**) is another dithiol compound investigated as a probable chelating agent. The two pK_a-values for the carboxyl groups are 2.45 and 3.50. Like Unithiol, it is water-soluble and forms stable, water-soluble complexes. Its inherent toxicity is very low (LD_{50} value for mice is 5 g/kg when given orally). In application it covers the same series of metals as BAL and Unithiol.

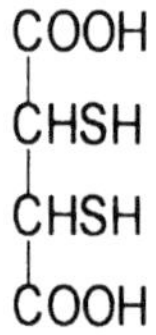

$$
\begin{array}{c}
COOH \\
| \\
CHSH \\
| \\
CHSH \\
| \\
COOH
\end{array}
$$

12.4

DMSA has been used in the case of lead, mercury and methylmercury poisoning. In the case of lead poisoning it is reported to be as efficient as calcium-EDTA. PMI calculations show that low-molecular-weight cadmium complexes will account for more that 95% with DMSA, Unithiol and BAL. The antimony complex of DMSA has been used in the treatment of schistosomiasis with fewer side effects than the potassium antimonyl tartrate commonly used.

12.4.4.2 D-penicillamine

D-penicillamine (PEN) (**12.5**) is a degradation product of penicillin. The structure with three different types of donor groups: $-COOH$, $-NH_2$ and $-SH$ gives a universal chelating agent for metal ions preferring S as well as N and O donors. However, the compound is a cysteine derivative and the organism possesses an enzymatic system for the metabolism. D-cysteine itself would be a fairly good metal binding compound, but it is metabolized too quickly.

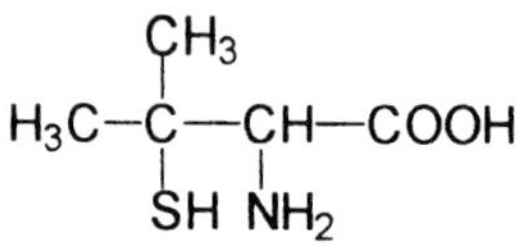

$$
\begin{array}{c}
CH_3 \\
| \\
H_3C-C-CH-COOH \\
| \quad\ | \\
SH\ \ NH_2
\end{array}
$$

12.5

PEN is water-soluble and stable and can be administrated orally. The inherent toxicity is low. The L-isomer is a vitamin B_6 antagonist with a correspondingly higher toxicity. PEN has achieved a wide application area and several preparations are on the market. It is used as a chelating agent and is the one which can replace BAL in most of its applications. It is used in treatment of lead poisoning in combination with EDTA and finds some use against mercury and gold poisoning too. A special application is in the treatment of Wilson's disease. A genetic defect leads to an excessive accumulation of copper in the kidney, liver and brain, which untreated causes malfunctions of the kidney, liver failure and neurological disturbances. Treatment with PEN will enhance the copper excretion in urine up to 20 times.

The compound is further found to be efficient in the control of rheumatoid arthritis. The basis for this application can be understood when one realizes that PEN acts as a copper mobilizing agent. The copper bound in an inert form in liver and kidney proteins, such as metallothionein, is mobilized by PEN which brings the copper into a low-molecular-weight labile form. The copper is then accessible to other important molecules in the organism such as the copper-enzymes superoxide dismutase and lysozyme oxidase — enzymes related to the inflammatoric reactions in rheumatoid arthritis. D-penicillamine has been called a "wonder drug". It shows only few side effects, but some patients develop hypersensitivity reactions to the drug. A realistic alternative for the treatment of Wilson's disease is the compound triethylenetetraamine, TRIEN, which shows almost the same properties and stability of complexes.

12.4.4.3 Polyaminocarboxylic acids

The polyaminocarboxylic acids, EDTA (**12.6**) and analogues, are less selective as chelating agents than the compounds with S and N donor atoms mentioned earlier. Their broad field of use as chelating agent is well known from analytical chemistry.

$$\begin{array}{ccc} HOOCCH_2 & & CH_2COOH \\ & N-CH_2-CH_2-N & \\ HOOCCH_2 & & CH_2COOH \end{array}$$

12.6

The complexes formed when both N and O are bound to the same metal ion involve five-membered rings. Often two or more chelate rings are formed (a phenomenon known as the "chelate effect") resulting in complexes of high stability. The application area is the "hard" and intermediate metal ions. Although the stability of the Hg^{2+} complex is high it is not stable enough to compete with the biological "soft" molecules found in tissue.

EDTA is not metabolized and has a biological half-life of one hour. Both Na_2H_2EDTA and $Na_2CaEDTA$ are water-soluble, but are poorly absorbed from the gastrointestinal tract. The administration of EDTA is therefore done in the form of intravenous injections of Na_2H_2EDTA or $Na_2CaEDTA$. Used as a chelating agent for lead poisoning, $Na_2CaEDTA$ is recommended. Na_2H_2EDTA has a tendency to lower the serum calcium concentration resulting in muscle cramps if calcium depletion is carried too far.

In the United States, Na_2H_2EDTA is commonly used in the treatment of artheriosclerosis. These treatments have been going on since the 1950s with the intent of lowering the plasma calcium level and consequently reduce metastatic calcium deposits. This chelating treatment is an alternative to ordinary operations. The rationale is unclear since the artheriosclerotic deposits are not just calcium salts.

EDTA forms complexes with many of the essential metal ions and it is usually necessary to supplement the diet with minerals.

$$HOOCCH_2\diagdown \\ \qquad\qquad N-CH_2-CH_2-N-CH_2-CH_2-N \\ HOOCCH_2\diagup \qquad\qquad\qquad\; |\qquad\qquad\qquad\qquad \diagup\diagdown \\ \qquad\qquad\qquad\qquad\qquad CH_2COOH$$

CH$_2$COOH ... CH$_2$COOH ... CH$_2$COOH

12.7

Diethylenetriaminepentaacetic acid (DTPA) (**12.7**) forms complexes with the same type of metal ions as EDTA but the stability constants are higher with DTPA. DTPA was found to be the most efficient chelating agent known for the removal of internally deposited transuranium elements, such as plutonium, in humans. In clinical use, the zinc complex, $Na_3ZnDTPA$ is preferred because of its low toxicity, which is even lower than that of the calcium complex.

12.4.4.4 Desferrioxamine
From the bacteria *Actinomycetes* the quite selective iron(III) chelators, desferrioxamines (DFOAs), can be isolated. The structure of one commercially available DFOA (**12.8**) is:

$$H_2N-(CH_2)_5-\underset{\underset{OH}{|}}{N}-\overset{\overset{O}{\|}}{C}-(CH_2)_2-\overset{\overset{O}{\|}}{C}-NH-(CH_2)_5-\underset{\underset{OH}{|}}{N}-\overset{\overset{O}{\|}}{C}-(CH_2)_2-\overset{\overset{O}{\|}}{C}-NH-(CH_2)_5-\underset{\underset{OH}{|}}{N}-\overset{\overset{O}{\|}}{C}-CH_3$$

12.8

It contains a series of "hard" oxygen donor atoms ready to complex with iron(III). The stability constant for the formation of a 1:1 complex is determined to be 10^{31} mol l^{-1}. This value is many orders of magnitude larger than that for other essential elements, making this compound especially iron selective.

DFOA is used as the water-soluble methanesulfonate salt. Only about 15% of the compound is absorbed from the gastrointestinal tract and parenteral administration is usually required. The metabolic destruction and the excretion is rather quick.

DFOA is used as an antidote for acute iron intoxications and in the treatment of Cooley's anemia where the iron contents of the liver and the heart continually increase. The compound enhances the excretion of iron in the urine. The coordination chemistry of aluminium and plutonium is similar to that of iron(III), and DFOA has been used in treatments of overloads of those two elements. Aluminium intoxification is seen as a result of the aluminium treatment of patients with renal failure.

12.5 DRUG INTERACTIONS WITH METAL IONS

Many drugs have excellent chelating abilities and consequently interact with metal ions in plasma, tissue and the intestinal tract. The interaction is often unwanted, since it counteracts the absorption of the drug, but it can also be crucial to the uptake, transport and effect of the drug. The topic is complicated and involves considerations of the selectivity of complex formation (since many low-molecular-weight ligands compete) and the charge of the complex (which determines the ability to cross lipophilic membranes).

Combining the HSAB principle with knowledge of concentrations of the metals in labile complexes in the biological phase will give some guidance. Only a few examples of interactions will be given below.

12.5.1 Unsuitable interactions

A classical example of unwanted interaction with supplied metals is the hindered uptake of tetracyclines by calcium, zinc, iron and/or aluminium from diet, antacid or mineral supplementation formulations.

12.9

The formula for tetracycline (**12.9**) shows that the drug has several donor atoms belonging to the group of hard bases, indicating that some interaction with hard acids can be expected. The above mentioned incompatible metals are characteristic hard acids in agreement with the principle. Indeed, the antibacterial activity of the drug seems to be connected with its ability to chelate magnesium.

12.5.2 Suitable interactions

The complex formation between copper ions and some drugs are examples of wanted interactions.

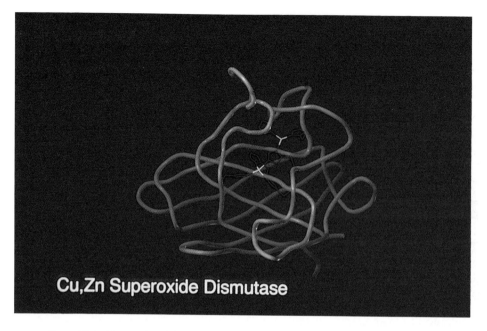

Figure 12.4   Structural model of superoxide dismutase displaying the zinc and copper centers.
(See Color Plate V.)

Copper is involved in many metalloenzymes:

Cytochrome c oxidase

Superoxide dismutase (SOD) (Fig. 12.4)

Tyrosinase

Dopamine hydroxylase

Lysyl oxidase

Amine oxidases.

An increase in the amount of copper-containing species (low- and high-molecular-weight) is observed as a general response to infections, arthritis and cancers.

The anti-inflammatory effect of salicylic acid and other ligand drugs has been examined and it has been demonstrated that copper complexes of the drugs were active in tissue repair and ulcer prevention.

In this connection, the activation of lysyl oxidase and SOD has been suggested as the chemical mechanism for the anti-inflammatory activity. Lysyl oxidase is required to catalyze the cross-linking of connective tissue and SOD is required to prevent the accumulation of superoxide in the cellular fluid matrix. Reduced SOD activity has been suggested as the cause of inflammatory disease.

The anticancer drug, bleomycin, which is thought to cleave DNA as an iron(II) complex *via* oxygen activation, is discussed in Chapter 17.

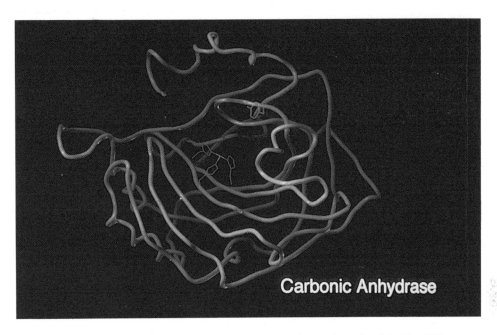

Figure 12.5   Structural model of the zinc enzyme, carbonic anhydrase. (See Color Plate VI.)

Another example with rather complicated gross mechanism is the effect of some drugs on the zinc enzyme, carbonic anhydrase (Fig. 12.5), in the treatment of epilepsy. Zinc has the function of a Lewis acid at the active site of the enzyme catalyzing among others the process

$$CO_2 + H_2O = HCO_3^- + H^+$$

in the kidneys. Acetazolamide will coordinate directly to zinc at the active site and thus block the catalyst. The result is probably that an increase in CO_2 concentration will lower the pH in the brain and it has been suggested that this will influence the GABA concentration either by enhancing GABA synthesis or by slowing down its metabolism (see also Chapter 10).

12.6 METAL IONS AND CHELATES IN THERAPY

Metal ions and their chelates have been used in the treatment of diseases since more than 2000 years BC. Metallo-organic compounds with arsenic and mercury were developed at the beginning of this century. A wide range of arsenicals were used for the treatment of syphilis and other parasitic infections. In the same way, mercurials were used as bacteriostatic antiseptics. A few years ago the use of mercury compounds in ophthalmic liniments and ointments was still common. However, the current use of inorganic compounds as drugs and diagnostic agents shows that many of the elements in the periodic system are involved.

12.6.1 Lithium

Lithium is an efficient sedative used in the treatment of the manic phase of manic-depressive patients. Relatively little is known about the mechanism of action of lithium, but the effect is well documented.

The lithium ion is able to pass through all biomembranes and thus has access to many important control sites. The chemistry of lithium indicates that lithium may interfere with aspects of the sodium, potassium, magnesium or calcium metabolisms. The diagonal rule (from inorganic chemistry) suggests a competition between lithium and magnesium on the magnesium sites to be the most probable. A comparison of the stability constants suggests that lithium is unable to compete with any other cations. But the other cations may be bound firmly by ligands such as ATP and the free lithium ion could compete for other biologically important ligands containing hard donor atoms. In connections with magnesium complexes, elevated lithium concentration can lead to lithium occupation of about 25% of the binding sites.

A theory for the lithium action suggests that it acts as an inhibitor of the enzyme adenylate cyclase which is a hormone-stimulated enzyme catalyzing the formation of cyclic AMP from ATP. Lithium has also been proposed to have an antiviral effect on herpes viruses based on a replacement of magnesium as the viral enzymatic co-factor (see also Chapter 6).

12.6.2 Gold

Gold(I) chelates are used in the treatment of difficult cases of rheumatoid arthritis. The mechanism of action of these drugs is largely unknown.

Gold with oxidation number +1, Au(I), is unstable and will disproportionate into Au(0) and Au(III) if not stabilized with a suitable ligand. Currently, a number of such complexes are used as drugs and only two of them are shown here, aurothiomalate ("Myocrisin") (**12.10**) and (2,3,4,6-tetrakis-*O*-acetyl-1-thiol-β-D-glucopyranosido)-gold(I)triethylphosphin, ("Auranofin") (**12.11**).

12.10   **12.11**

The water-soluble aurothiomalate has to be injected intramuscularly, whereas the lipophilic "Auranofin" can be given orally with equally good results.

12.6.3 Platinum complexes

In the group of cytostatica currently in use, one is remarkable in being a heavy metal complex — cisplatin, *cis*-diamminedichloroplatinum(II) (*cis*-DDP). In the early 1960s, Rosenberg studied the growth of *E. coli* bacteria under the influence of an electric field. The bacteria failed to divide, but continued to grow now forming long filaments. These unexpected effects were finally attributed to the formation of platinum complexes in trace amounts as a result of electrolytic oxidation of the platinum electrode used in ammonium chloride medium. The platinum complexes found to be active were shown to be the *cis*-isomers $Pt(NH_3)_2Cl_2$ ("cisplatin") (**12.12**) and *cis*-diamminetetrachloroplatinum(IV) (**12.13**).

12.12   **12.13**

Intense investigations have lead to the use of cisplatin as a leading anticancer drug for the treatment of ovarian and testicular tumors with promising results (see also Chapter 17).

How is the mode of action of these compounds? Two possible explanations for the observation of the active compounds to possess a *cis* geometry have been proposed. One is the influence of the ligands *trans* to labile groups (known as the "trans-effect"), and the other is a stereospecific interaction between the platinum compound and some cellular components.

The *trans* effect (from inorganic chemistry) has its origin in the ability of a given ligand to labilize the metal-ligand bond *trans* to it.

The chloro groups in *cis*-DDP are more labile than the ammonia groups. In blood plasma the high concentration of chloride ions (>0.1 mol l^{-1}) will result in a very slow replacement of chloride by other ligands. During transport through membranes, *cis*-DDP will thus probably remain unchanged. Inside cells the chloride concentration is $4 \cdot 10^{-3}$ mol l^{-1}, and the substitution will take place with the result that the *cis* complex binds strongly to biological ligands. The platinum complexes react with DNA in the tumour cells and the DNA replication is inhibited. The transcription (RNA synthesis) and other metabolic processes are maintained at small concentrations of the active drug. At higher concentrations, the cells die. Especially the studies that make use of NMR techniques have contributed to a better understanding of the manner in which DNA fragments react with the platinum complex. The binding of *cis*-DDP to DNA is presumed to start with the loss of both chloride ions. The theory, now accepted, is that the platinum complex $Pt(NH_3)_2^{2+}$ binds intrastrand crosslink to two N7 donor atoms on adjacent guanosine bases on a single strand. Other anticancer agents, the alkylating agents, also react preferentially at the guanosine moiety of DNA. The *trans*-form of $Pt(NH_3)_2Cl_2$ (**12.14**) has been found to be toxic and inactive. *Trans*-$Pt(NH_3)_2^{2+}$ can also chelate to DNA sequences through two guanine N7 atoms. The distorsion of DNA after such *trans*-binding is likely to be very pronounced. The hypothesis has been put forward that repair enzymes recognize and remove the *trans* compound more easily than the *cis* compound.

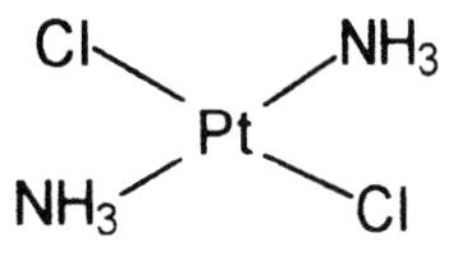

12.14

The discovery of the anitumour activity of cisplatin has generated considerable interest in the pharmacology of metal complexes both in order to minimize the toxic side-effects and to find a broader treatment area. The basic rule in the design of an active platinum complex is to make a neutral *cis* diammine complex with two labile ligands coordinated. Many platinum complexes have been synthesized, but other metal complexes as well have been investigated; two examples are shown below, (**12.15**) and (**12.16**).

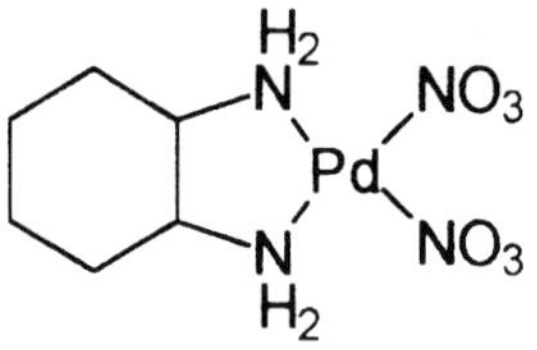

12.15

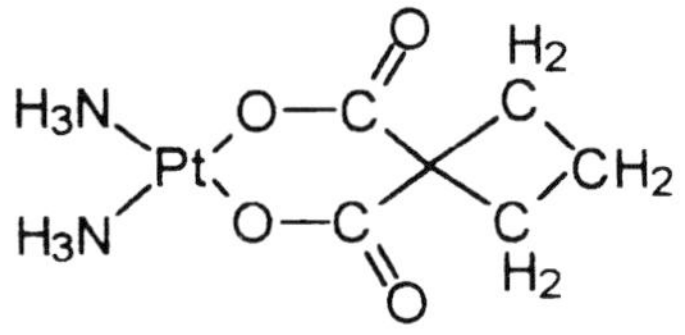

12.16

12.6.4 Sodium nitroprusside

Sodium nitroprusside, $Na_2[Fe(NO)(CN)_5] \cdot 2H_2O$, known from qualitative inorganic analysis as a reagent for the sulfide ion, is used in surgery for the control of blood pressure. The hypotensive action of the drug is dependent on the NO ligand in the complex. Indeed, the small molecule, NO, has recently been demonstrated to be a neurotransmitter with functions in the synaptic transmission between neurones and relevant to the effects of this drug on the control of blood pressure by relaxing muscles in the blood vessels. The small NO molecule has an uneven number of electrons and is consequently a reactive radical with a short lifetime in the organism ($\sim$10 sec). Its biosynthesis from arginine is controlled by nitric oxide synthase.

12.6.5 Contrast agents in medicinal diagnosis

In medicinal diagnosis, contrast agents are used in X-ray Imaging, Magnetic Resonance Imaging (MRI), and Nuclear Medicine. The radiographic contrast agents increase the absorption of X-rays when they pass through the different organs of the body. In MRI the contrast agents enhance the images resulting from the absorption of energy by atomic nuclei.

The insolubility of barium sulphate ($BaSO_4$) allows its safe use as a contrast agent for X-ray imaging of the gastrointestinal tract. Other often used contrast agents for X-ray imaging are iodinated ionic or non-ionic organic compounds. The radiodensity of these agents depends on their iodine content. Ionic compounds in high concentrations will result in hypertonic solutions, and this has led to the development of non-ionic iodinated contrast agents. An example of a non-ionic, monomeric X-ray contrast agent for intrathecal and parenteral use is iopamidol (**12.17**).

12.17

Contrast agents for NMR imaging or MRI (the term used by the medical community for NMR) are chemically very different from iodinated compounds. The main contrast parameters in MRI are tissue proton densities and the relaxation times in tissue. Paramagnetic ions mainly reduce the relaxation time of the surrounding protons resulting in increased MR signal intensity. An effective paramagnetic metal ion is gadolinium(III), Gd(III), which has seven unpaired 4f electrons. Ordinary salts of Gd(III) are too toxic for use in humans but chelated complexes with e.g. DTPA (**12.7**), $[Gd(III)DTPA]^{2-}$, are rapidly excreted through the kidneys and can be injected safely in gram quantities. A local $[Gd^{3+}]$ level of at least 50 μM is needed in order to observe MR contrast in organs. Complexes of manganese(II) (high-spin $3d^5$) have also been investigated for their ability to give an effective MRI contrast. Several MRI contrast agents are now commercially available. These include low molecular weight hydrophilic chelates with extracellular biodistribution and renal elimination, for use in brain, spine and other organ systems, lipophilic chelates for liver imaging, macromolecular compounds for blood pool studies and particle/liposomes for diagnosis in the reticuloendothelial organs.

Radiopharmaceutical agents are used in medicine for diagnostic purposes and as sources of radiation for therapy. The most commonly used radionuclei is the technetium isotope, ^{99m}Tc, with a half-life of 6 hours. The decay of ^{99m}Tc (m for metastable) releases γ-rays with a favourable energy. The radioisotopes are used in inorganic form, e.g. ^{131}I-iodide, but most often complex compounds which are able to target specific macromolecules found in biological systems, are used. The hexakis-(2-methoxy-2-methylpropylisocyanide) complex of technetium(I), $[Tc(RNC)_6]^+$, (**12.18**) is an example of a radiopharmaceutical agent used for the investigation of cardiac perfusion.

12.18

FURTHER READING

Bulman, R.A. (1989) The Chemistry of Chelating Agents in Medicinal Sciences. *Structure and Bonding*, **67**, 91–141.

Cotton, F.A. and Wilkinson, G. (1984) *Advanced Inorganic Chemistry* (4th ed.) Interscience Publishers, New York.

Frausto Da Silva, J.J.R. and Williams, R.J.P. (1991) *The Biological Chemistry of the Elements: The Inorganic Chemistry of Life*, Oxford University Press.

Frieden, E. (ed.) (1984) *Biochemistry of the Essential Ultratrace Elements*, Plenum Press, New York.

Jones, M.M., Wilson, D.J., Topping, R.F. and Laurie, S.H. (1988) The Role of Rate Determining Steps in the Decorporation of Toxic Metal Ions. *Inorg. Chim. Acta*, **152**, 159–170.

Kaim, W. and Schwederski, B. (1994) *Bioinorganic Chemistry. Inorganic Elements in the Chemistry of Life.* John Wiley & Sons, Chichester.

Sadler, J.P. (1991) Inorganic Chemistry and Drug Design. *Advances in Inorganic Chemistry*, **36**, 1–48.

Sigel, H. (ed.) Vol. 1 — (1973) *Metal Ions in Biological Systems*. Marcel Dekker Inc., New York. (Comprehensive series covering all aspects of bioinorganic chemistry).

Sorenson, J.R.J., Kishore, V., Pezeshk, A., Oberley, L., Leuthauser, S.W.C. and Oberley, T.D. (1984) Copper Complexes: A Physiological Approach to the Treatment of 'Inflammatory Diseases'. *Inorg. Chim. Acta*, **91**, 285–294.

13. DESIGN AND APPLICATION OF PRODRUGS

GITTE JUEL FRIIS and HANS BUNDGAARD[†]

CONTENTS

[†] Deceased.

13.1 DEFINITION OF THE PRODRUG CONCEPT

During the past 25 years it has become more obvious that the commonly used processes of delivering therapeutic agents to the sites of their action within the body are generally inefficient and unreliable. Optimization of the drug delivery and consequently improvement in drug efficacy implies an efficient and selective delivery and transport of a drug substance to its site of action. Recognition of the importance of drug delivery for the therapeutic indices of many types of drugs has been followed by a large increase in research activities in this area, and much attention has been focused on approaches which aim at enhancing the efficacy and reducing the toxicity and unwanted effects of drugs controlling their absorption, blood levels, metabolism, distribution and cellular uptake.

Prodrug design comprises an area of drug research, which is concerned with the optimization of drug delivery. A prodrug is a pharmacologically inactive derivative of a parent drug molecule, which requires spontaneous, i.e. non-enzymatic, or enzymatic transformation within the body in order to release the active drug. A prodrug has improved delivery properties over the parent drug molecule.

A molecule with optimal structural configuration and physico-chemical properties for eliciting the desired therapeutic response at its target site does not necessarily possess the best molecular form and properties for its delivery to its site of ultimate action. Usually, only a minor fraction of doses administered reaches the target area and since most agents interact with non-target sites as well, an inefficient delivery may result in undesirable side-effects. This fact of differences in transport and *in situ* effect characteristics for many drug molecules is the basic reason why bioreversible chemical derivatization of drugs, i.e. prodrug formation, is a means by which a substantial improvement in the overall efficacy of drugs can often be achieved.

Prodrugs are designed to overcome pharmaceutically and/or pharmacokinetically based problems associated with the parent drug molecule, which otherwise would be of limited clinical use. The prodrug approach can be illustrated as shown in Figure 13.1. The usefulness of a drug molecule can be limited by its suboptimal physico-chemical properties, e.g. if it shows poor biomembrane permeability. By attachment of a pro-moiety to the molecule or by otherwise modifying the compound, a prodrug is formed, which overcomes the barrier for the usefulness of the drug. Once past the barrier, the prodrug is ideally reverted quantitatively to the parent compound by a post-barrier enzymatic or non-enzymatic process. Prodrug formation can thus be considered as conferring a transient chemical cover to alter or eliminate undesirable properties of the parent drug molecule.

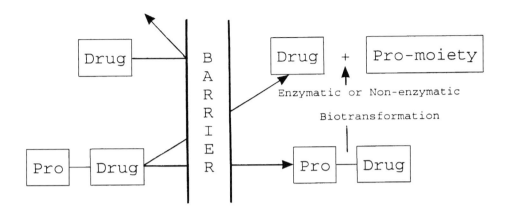

Figure 13.1   Schematic illustration of the prodrug concept.

A number of barriers may limit the clinical usefulness of a drug. In the *pharmaceutical phase*, i.e. the incorporation of a potential drug entity into a practically useful drug delivery system or dosage form, the barriers may be represented by formulation problems due to physico-chemical properties of the drug, such as poor water solubility, and by aesthetic properties of the drug, such as taste and tissue irritation.

In the *pharmacokinetic phase*, i.e the absorption, distribution, metabolism and excretion of the drug, major barriers which may limit the usefulness of a drug are:

1. Incomplete absorption of the drug across biological membranes such as the gastrointestinal mucosa or the blood-brain barrier.
2. Incomplete systemic bioavailability of a drug due to presystemic metabolism (first-pass metabolism).
3. Too rapid absorption or excretion of the drug when a longer duration of action is desired.
4. Toxicity problems related to local irritation or distribution into tissues other than the desired target organ.
5. Poor site-specificity of the drug.

The design of prodrugs in a rational manner requires that the underlying cause, which necessitate or stimulate the use of the prodrug approach is defined and clearly understood. It may then be possible to identify the means by which the difficulties can be overcome. *The rational design of prodrugs* can thus be divided into three basic steps:

1. Identification of the drug delivery problem.
2. Identification of the physico-chemical properties required for maximum efficacy or delivery.
3. Selection of a prodrug derivative, which has the proper physico-chemical properties and which can be cleaved in the desired biological compartment.

Several criteria should be considered in the design of a prodrug:

1. Which functional groups on the parent molecule are amenable to chemical derivatization?
2. What mechanisms and systems are available in the organism for the required bioactivation of the prodrug derivative?
3. Synthesis and purification of the prodrug should be relatively simple.
4. The prodrug should be chemically stable in bulk form and compatible with ingredients in the dosage form formulation.
5. The parent drug molecule must be regenerated (ideally quantitatively) from the prodrug *in vivo*, i.e the prodrug must be bioreversible.
6. Toxicity of the pro-moiety attached to the drug molecule as well as the toxicity of the prodrug *per se* must be considered.

13.2 PRODRUGS OF VARIOUS FUNCTIONAL GROUPS

13.2.1 Introduction

A basal requisite for the prodrug approach to be useful in solving drug delivery problems, is the ready availability of chemical derivative types satisfying the prodrug requirements, the most prominent of these being reconversion of the prodrug to the parent drug *in vivo*. This prodrug to drug conversion may take place before absorption (e.g. in the gastrointestinal tract), during absorption, after absorption or at the specific site of drug action in the body, all dependent upon the specific goal for which the prodrug is designed. Ideally, the prodrug should be converted to the drug as soon as the goal is reached. The prodrug *per se* is an inactive species and therefore, once its job is completed, intact prodrug represents unavailable drug. For example, prodrugs designed to overcome solubility problems in formulating intravenous injection solutions should preferably be converted immediately to the drug following injection so that the concentration of circulating prodrug would rapidly become insignificant in relation to that of the active drug. Conversely, if the objective of the prodrug is to produce a sustained drug action through rate-limiting prodrug conversion, the rate of the conversion should not be too high.

The necessary conversion or activation of prodrugs to the parent drug molecules in the body can take place by a variety of reactions. The most common prodrugs are those requiring a hydrolytic cleavage mediated by enzymatic catalysis. Active drug species containing hydroxy or carboxyl groups can often be converted to prodrug esters from which the active forms are regenerated by esterases within the body, e.g. in the blood or liver. In other cases, active drug substances are regenerated from their prodrugs by biochemical reductive or oxidative processes. Besides usage of the various enzyme systems of the body to carry out the necessary activation of prodrugs, the buffered and relatively constant value of the physiological pH (pH 7.4) may be useful in triggering the release of a drug from the prodrug. In these cases, the prodrugs are characterized by a high degree of chemical lability at pH 7.4 while preferably exhibiting a higher stability at for example pH 3–4. As will be discussed below examples of such prodrugs are *N*-Mannich bases. A serious drawback of prodrugs requiring chemical (non-enzymatic) release of the active drug is the inherent lability of the compounds, raising some stability-formulation problems at least in the cases of solution preparations. As will be shown later such problems have, in particular cases, been overcome by using a more sophisticated approach involving pro-prodrugs or double prodrugs where use is made of an enzymatic release mechanism prior to the spontaneous reaction.

In recent years several types of bioreversible derivatives have been exploited for utilization in the design of prodrugs. An outline of some commonly used prodrugs is given below.

13.2.2 Esters as prodrugs for compounds containing carboxyl or hydroxy groups

The popularity of using esters as a prodrug type of drugs containing carboxyl or hydroxy functions (or thiol groups) primarily stems from the fact that the organism is rich in enzymes capable of hydrolysing esters. The distribution of esterases is ubiquitous and several types can be found in the blood, liver and other organs or tissues. In addition, by appropriate esterification it is possible to obtain derivatives with almost any desirable hydro- or lipophilicity as well as in vivo lability, the latter being dictated by electronic and steric factors. Accordingly, a great number of drugs with hydroxy or carboxylic acid groups have been modified for a multitude of reasons using the ester prodrug approach as will be described in Section 13.3 of this chapter.

While the chemical reactivity of esters is readily predictable on the basis of the steric and electronic properties of the substituents in both the acyl and alcohol moieties, this does not apply for the enzymatic hydrolysis. Steric effects generally alter non-enzymatic and enzymatic ester hydrolysis rates in the same directions, but exceptions do exist. For enzymatic ester hydrolysis the hydrophilic properties and charge of the ester may play a major role and non-enzymatic hydrolysis cannot be used as a reliable guide to predict enzyme-catalysed reactions. The best way to get an early impression of the rate of hydrolysis of an ester prodrug in vivo may be measurement of the rate of ester hydrolysis in vitro in the presence of an appropriate enzyme source such as plasma or a homogenate from liver, intestine, skin or cornea, dependent on the intended route of administration of the prodrug. In this respect, it can be noted that large differences in the ease of enzymatic ester hydrolysis exist between different species. Thus, esters are usually hydrolysed markedly faster in rat plasma than in human plasma whereas dog plasma often is less efficient than human plasma.

To illustrate the influence of chemical structure on the chemical and enzymatic lability, the data obtained for various esters of the same acid (benzoic acid) can be considered (examples are given in Table 13.1). The hydroxide ion-catalysed hydrolysis of these esters is primarily determined by the polar effects exhibited by the alcohol portions of the esters, because the steric proportions can be considered to be almost constant (there is a methylene group connected to the oxygen in all compounds). With few exceptions, e.g. compound 6, where intramolecular catalysis by the carboxylate group occurs, the rates of hydrolysis of these esters, and other esters of the same compound not mentioned here, are correlated by the following equation:

$$\log k_{OH} = 0.54\sigma^* + 0.74 \quad (n = 16; r = 0.962) \tag{13.1}$$

where the Taft polar substituent parameter σ^* refers to R in RCH_2OH for the alcohols. Thus, the variation of the rates of hydrolysis can be accounted for in terms of the different polarity of the leaving alcohol group.

Table 13.1 Rate data for the alkaline and enzymatic hydrolysis of various benzoic acid esters at 37 °C.

| $C_6H_5-COOCH_2-R$ | | | k_{OH} | 80% human plasma | |
Compound	R	σ^* for R	$(M^{-1} min^{-1})$	k (min^{-1})	$t_{1/2}$ (min)
1	H	0.49	13.6	6.4×10^{-3}	108
2	CH_3	0.00	6.6	3.3×10^{-3}	210
3	C_2H_5	−0.10	5.5	1.5×10^{-2}	46
4	C_4H_9	−0.25	5.3	2.9×10^{-2}	24
5	C_6H_5	0.75	13.0	3.7×10^{-2}	19
6	COO^-	−1.06	6.3	$<10^{-4}$	>100 h
7	$COOCH_3$	2.00	70.1	2.0×10^{-1}	3.5
8	$CONH_2$	1.68	69.9	1.7×10^{-2}	40
9	$CON(CH_3)_2$	1.94	19.2	>5.0	<8 sec
10	$CH_2N(CH_3)_2$	0.49	9.8	>8.0	<5 sec
11	$CH_2N(CH_3)_3^+$	1.90	95.1	>8.0	<5 sec

However, the plasma-catalysed hydrolysis of the esters cannot be correlated in the same way. By increasing the chain length in the alkyl esters, it can be seen that the enzymatic reactivity increases except when going from methyl to ethyl. The N,N-dimethylglycolamide ester 9 is seen to be cleaved extremely fast in human plasma although being highly stable chemically. The rapid rate of hydrolysis of ester 9 has been attributed to pseudo-cholinesterase present in plasma. The protonated esters 10 and 11 are also cleaved very rapidly by plasma enzymes in contrast to the benzoylglycolic acid (compound 6). The high resistance of compound 6 towards enzymatic hydrolysis is due to its negative charge at physiological pH like various other esters with an ionized carboxylate group such as hemisuccinate esters which are also known to be poor substrates for hydrolytic plasma enzymes (see Section 13.3.5).

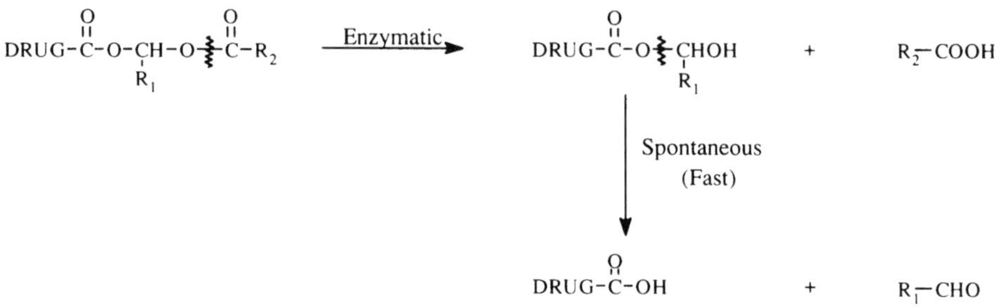

Scheme 13.1

Not only the charge and steric effects within the alcohol portion have influence on the enzymatic hydrolysis of esters. The enzymatic hydrolysis is also highly sensitive to the steric effects within the acyl portion. In penicillins, for example, the environment around the carboxyl group is highly sterically hindered, and simple aliphatic or aromatic esters are not sufficiently labile *in vivo* to function as prodrugs. This shortcoming can be overcome by preparing a double ester type, (acyloxy)alkyl or [(alkoxycarbonyl)-oxy]alkyl esters in which the terminal ester grouping is less sterically hindered. The first step in the hydrolysis of such an ester is enzymatic cleavage of the terminal ester bond with formation of a highly unstable α-hydroxyalkyl ester which rapidly dissociates to the parent acidic drug and an aldehyde (Scheme 13.1). For examples of this approach see Section 13.3.1.2.

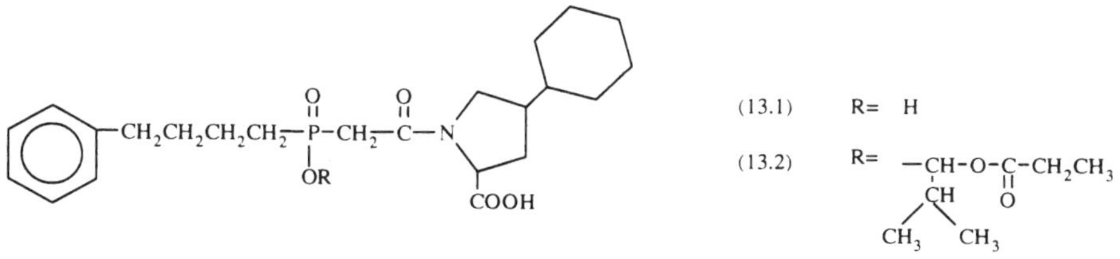

Scheme 13.2

The applicability of α-acyloxyalkyl esters as biologically reversible transport forms has also been extended to include the phosphate group, phosphonic acids and phosphinic acids. An example is compound (**13.1**), an angiotensin converting enzyme (ACE) inhibitor, where the phosphinic acid group has been α-*O*-acyloxyalkylated to provide fosenopril (**13.2**) which is better absorbed orally than the parent active drug due to its greater lipophilicity (Scheme 13.2).

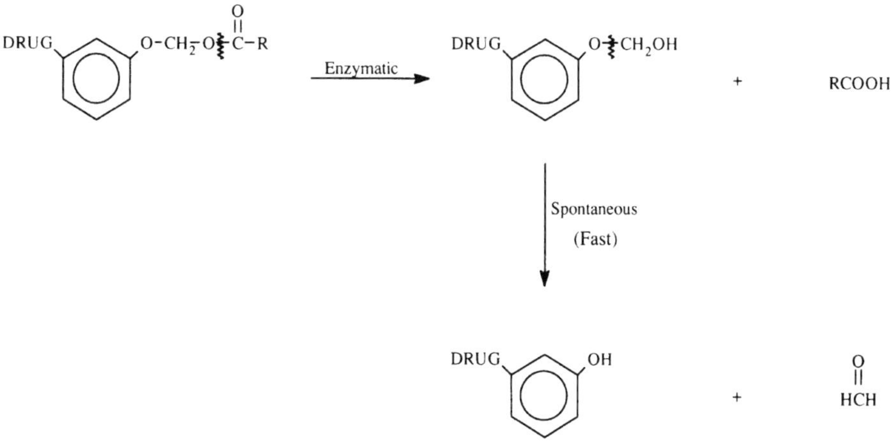

Scheme 13.3

O-α-Acyloxyalkyl ethers may be a useful prodrug type for compounds containing a phenol group. Such derivatives are hydrolysed by a sequential reaction involving the formation of an unstable hemiacetal intermediate (Scheme 13.3), and they are as susceptible as normal phenol esters to undergo enzymatic hydrolysis by e.g. human plasma enzymes. The O-α-acyloxyalkyl ethers are, however, more stable against chemical (hydroxide ion-catalyzed) hydrolysis than phenolate esters and this may make them more favourable in prodrug design. Analogously, S-α-acyloxyalkyl ethers have been described as prodrug derivatives of drugs containing an aliphatic or aromatic thiol group. For information about different ester types introduced to improve the water-solubility of drugs containing a hydroxy group (Drug-OH) see Section 13.3.5.

13.2.3 Prodrugs for amides, imides and other NH-acidic compounds

13.2.3.1 N-Mannich bases

N-Mannich bases can function as prodrug candidates for NH-acidic compounds such as various amides, imides, carbamates, hydantoins and urea derivatives as well as for aliphatic and aromatic amines (see Section 13.2.4.3). They are generally formed by reacting an NH-acidic compound with formaldehyde, or in very rare cases, other aldehydes and a primary or secondary aliphatic or aromatic amine. The process can be considered a N-aminomethylation (in the case of the NH-acidic component being an amide) (Scheme 13.4).

$$R\text{–}CONH_2 + CH_2O + R_1R_2NH \rightleftharpoons R\text{–}CONH\text{–}CH_2\text{–}NR_1R_2 + H_2O$$

Scheme 13.4

N-Mannich bases are readily hydrolysed in aqueous solution. The rate of hydrolysis usually increases with increasing pH, resulting in a sigmoidal (S-shaped) pH-rate profile obtained when log k_{obs} (the degradation rate) is plotted against pH. The pH-rate profile can be accounted for by assuming spontaneous decomposition of the free Mannich base (B) and the protonated form (BH^+). The expression for the pseudo-first-order rate constant (k_{obs}) is:

$$k_{obs} = k_1 f_B + k_2 f_{BH^+} = \frac{k_1 K_a}{a_H + K_a} + \frac{k_2 a_H}{a_H + K_a} \tag{13.2}$$

where f_B and f_{BH^+} is the fraction of the N-Mannich species on basic or acidic form, respectively, K_a is the apparent ionization constant of the protonated N-Mannich bases, a_H is the hydrogen ion activity, and k_1 and k_2 are the apparent first-order rate constants for the spontaneous degradation of B and BH^+, respectively.

The reaction mechanism proposed for the decomposition involves as rate-determining step a unimolecular N–C bond cleavage with the formation of an amide (or imide) anion and an imminium cation. In subsequent fast steps, a solvent molecule transfers a proton to the anion and a hydroxide ion to the immonium ion, giving hydroxymethylamine which rapidly dissociates to formaldehyde and amine (Scheme 13.5).

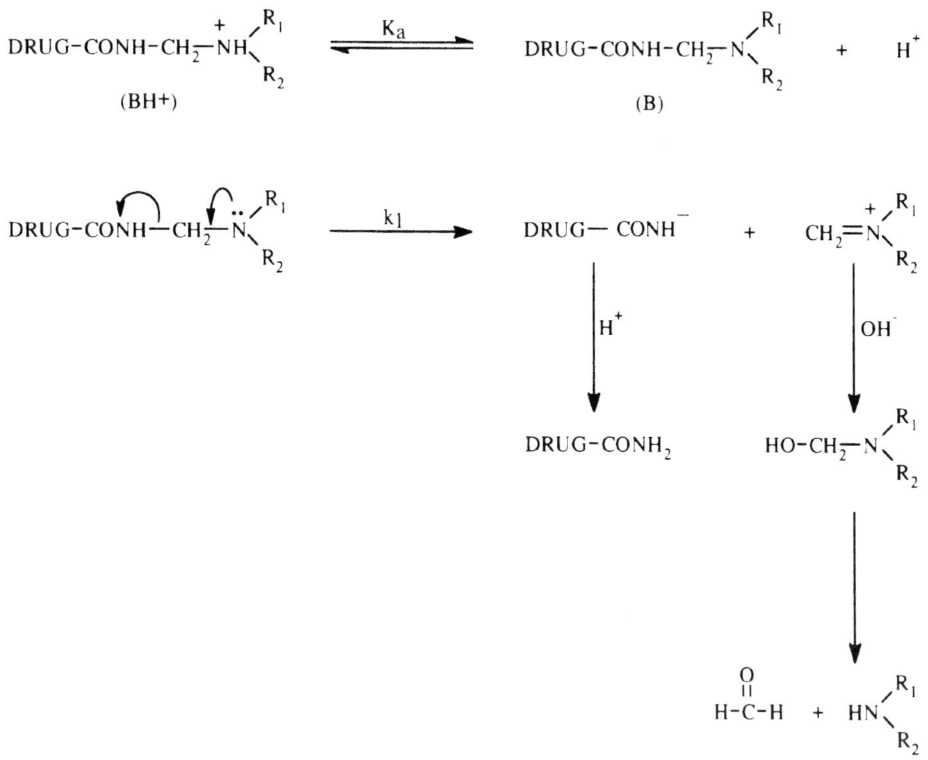

Scheme 13.5

The structural effects on the decomposition rate of the N-Mannich bases derived from carboxamides, thioamides, sulphonamides or imides and aliphatic or aromatic amines involve steric effects and basicity of the amine component and acidity of the amide-type component. These factors are most pronounced with respect to the rate constant k_1 and, accordingly, to the decomposition rate in weakly acidic to basic solutions. The rates of the hydrolysis of unprotonated Mannich bases are accelerated strongly by (a) increasing steric effects within the amine substituent, (b) increasing basicity of the amine component and (c) increasing acidity of the parent amide-type compound.

By appropriate selection of the amine component, it should be feasible to obtain prodrugs of a given amide type-drug with varying degrees of *in vivo* lability, and also to vary the physico-chemical properties of the parent compound such as aqueous solubility, dissolution rate and lipophilicity. Transformation of an amide into an N-Mannich base introduces a readily ionizable amino moiety which may allow the preparation of derivatives with increased water-solubility at slightly acidic pH values where the stability at the same time may be quite high.

The concept of N-Mannich base formation of NH-acidic compounds to yield more soluble prodrugs has been used in the case of rolitetracycline (**13.4**). This highly water-soluble N-Mannich base of tetracycline and pyrrolidine, which is used clinically, is decomposed quantitatively to tetracycline (**13.3**). The half-life is 40 min at pH 7.40 and 37 °C (Scheme 13.6). Since the breakdown of this prodrug (**13.4**) and other N-Mannich bases does not rely on enzymatic catalysis, similar rates of hydrolysis are seen in buffer solution and plasma.

$$(13.3) \quad R = \quad H$$

$$(13.4) \quad R = \quad -CH_2-N$$

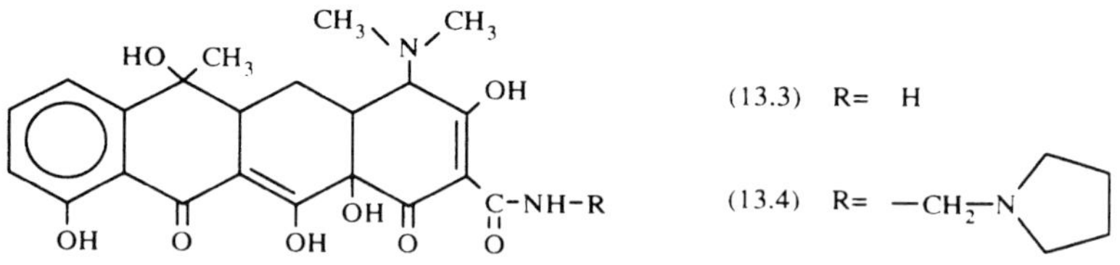

Scheme 13.6

In addition, the concept may be useful for improving the dissolution behaviour of poorly soluble drugs in an effort to improve the oral bioavailability. Thus, it has been shown that N-Mannich base formation of various NH-acidic drugs (e.g phenytoin, acetazolamide and allupurinol) increases the intrinsic dissolution rates in 0.1 M HCl in comparison with the parent compounds.

13.2.3.2 N-Hydroxymethyl derivatives
When an acidic compound is allowed to react with formaldehyde in absence of a primary or secondary amine, N-hydroxymethylation occurs (Scheme 13.7):

$$R\text{–}CONH_2 + CH_2O \leftrightharpoons R\text{–}CONH\text{–}CH_2OH$$

Scheme 13.7

The rate of decomposition of N-hydroxymethyl derivatives in aqueous solution increases with increasing pH and increasing acidity of the parent compound. The following linear correlation has been found between log half-life ($t_{1/2}$) (hydrolysis at pH 7.4 and 37 °C) and the pK_a of the parent NH-acidic compound:

$$\log t_{1/2} = 0.77\text{p}K_a - 8.34 (t_{1/2} \text{ in min, } 37\,°C) \tag{13.3}$$

This relationship allows one to predict the reactivity of an N-hydroxymethyl derivative solely from the knowledge of the pK_a of the parent compound. Thus, it can be predicted that the requirement for a half-life of the decomposition reaction of less than 1 h at pH 7.4 and 37 °C is that the NH-acidic compound possesses a pK_a value of less than 13.1, or that a pK_a value of less than 10.8 is required for a half-life of less than 1 min.

The mechanism for the decomposition of N-hydroxymethyl derivatives involves a stepwise pathway with an N-hydroxymethyl anion as an intermediate undergoing rate-determining N–C bond cleavage as illustrated in Scheme 13.8. The degradation of the N-hydroxymethyl derivative is a spontaneous reaction, i.e. a non-enzymatic degradation. The half-life seen in a buffer solution and plasma is therefore similar.

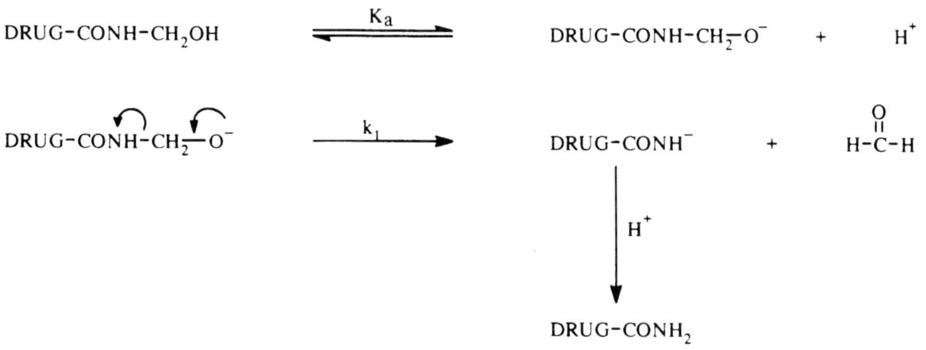

DRUG-CONH-CH$_2$OH $\xrightleftharpoons{\text{K}_a}$ DRUG-CONH-CH$_2$-O$^-$ + H$^+$

DRUG-CONH-CH$_2$-O$^-$ $\xrightarrow{\text{k}_1}$ DRUG-CONH$^-$ + H-C-H (O)

$\downarrow$ H$^+$

DRUG-CONH$_2$

Scheme 13.8

The N-hydroxymethyl derivatives of amide- or imide-type compounds are more water-soluble than the parent compounds thus suggesting a potential use of the prodrug type for nitrogenous molecules, e.g. for increasing dissolution rates and hence oral bioavailability. By replacing a hydrogen bound to a nitrogen atom by a hydroxymethyl group, intra- or intermolecular hydrogen bonding in such molecules may be decreased, leading to a corresponding decrease in melting point and increase in water solubility.

From the structure-reactivity data given above, it is readily evident that N-hydroxymethyl-ation is not a universally applicable approach to bioreversible derivatization of NH-acidic compounds. This approach is limited to compounds possessing a pK$_a$ value of less than about 10.5–11 in order to provide a sufficient rate of drug regeneration at physiological pH. For example, N-hydroxymethyl derivatives of carboxamides (pK$_a$ 14–15) are relatively stable, the half-life for decomposition of e.g. benzamide and nicotinamide being 183 and 37 h, respectively, at pH 7.4 and 37 °C. Derivatives obtained from other aldehydes than formaldehyde possess, however, a greater lability (e.g. N-α-hydroxybenzyl benzamide, prepared by condensation of benzamide with benzaldehyde, has a half-life of only 6.5 min at pH 7.4 and 37 °C).

It should be pointed out that although N-hydroxymethyl derivatives may be useful as prodrug forms, the most important aspect of N-hydroxymethylation resides in the fact that the hydroxy group introduced by this process is readily amenable to bioreversible derivatization, e.g. by esterification to produce water-soluble or lipophilic N-acyloxymethyl derivatives.

13.2.3.3 N-α-Acyloxyalkyl derivatives

In recent years N-α-acyloxyalkylation has become a commonly used approach to obtain pro-drugs of various secondary amides, imides, hydantoins, uracils, tertiary or N-heterocyclic amines and other NH-acidic compounds. By varying the acyl portion of such derivatives it is possible to control the rate of regeneration of the parent drug and to obtain prodrugs with varying physico-chemical properties such as water-solubility and lipophilicity. Whereas the derivatives, similar to other esters, show good stability in aqueous solution *in vitro*, they are in general rapidly cleaved *in vivo* by virtue of enzyme-mediated hydrolysis. The regeneration of the parent NH-acidic drug takes place via a two-step reaction (Scheme 13.9). Enzymatic cleavage of the ester results in the formation of an N-α-hydroxyalkyl derivative, which subsequently decomposes spontaneously to the corresponding aldehyde and the NH-acidic drug as described above. Thus, the rate of drug formation is solely dependent on the rate of the initial ester cleavage, which can be controlled by steric and electronic factors.

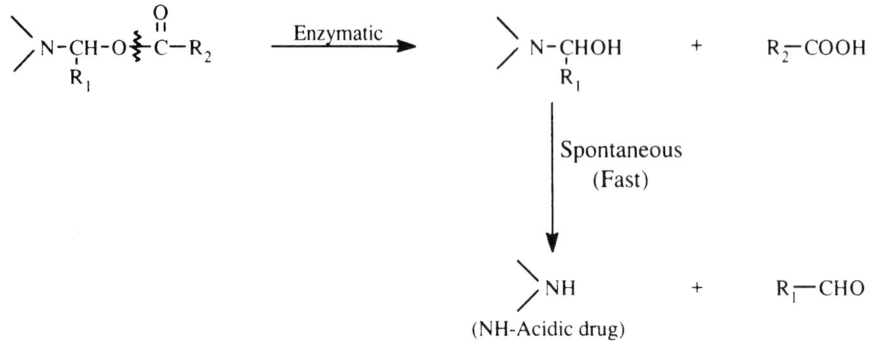

Scheme 13.9

The most commonly used α-acyloxyalkyl derivatives are acyloxymethyl compounds, i.e. derivatives from which formaldehyde is released from the N-hydroxymethyl intermediate. As discussed above the N-acyloxymethylation approach is limited to NH-acidic compounds possessing a pK_a value lower than about 10.5–11. When this is fulfilled the intermediate N-hydroxymethyl derivative will only have transitory existence in the overall process of the drug release as outlined in Scheme 13.9. However, by using other aldehydes than formaldehyde for the derivatization, the N-α-hydroxyalkyl intermediate formed will be more unstable than the N-hydroxymethyl analogue as discussed above, hence expanding the usefulness of N-α-acyloxyalkylation as a means of obtaining prodrug forms of weakly NH-acidic drugs.

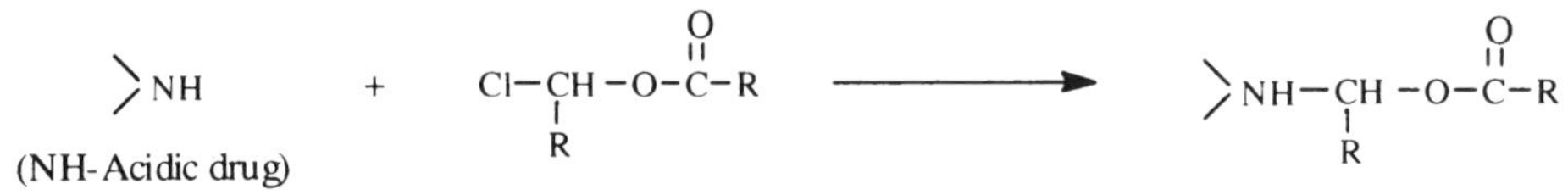

Scheme 13.10

Although the synthetic availability of N-α-hydroxyalkyl derivatives other than those derived from formaldehyde is very limited, this does not restrict a broad utility of N-α-acyloxyalkyl derivatives as prodrug forms. The reason for this is that besides being obtainable by esterification of the intermediate N-α-hydroxyalkyl derivative, such derivatives are readily, and most often, obtained by reacting the NH-acidic drug substance with an α-acyloxyalkyl chloride (Scheme 13.10). The latter compounds are easily available from the reaction of an acid chloride with a variety of aldehydes including for instance acetaldehyde or benzaldehyde as well as formaldehyde.

It should be pointed out that N-α-hydroxyalkylation of NH-acidic compounds like primary amides, carbamates and sulphonamides is not a feasible method to obtain *in vitro* stable prodrug derivatives. Such derivatives are extremely unstable in aqueous solution. In contrast, N-α-acyloxyalkyl derivatives of most secondary amides or imide-type structures behave as normal esters with respect to hydrolysis and stability. It should also be added that N-α-acyloxyalkylation of primary and secondary amines, which can be regarded as very weakly NH-acidic compounds, likewise are not useful because of the extreme lability of such derivatives.

By introduction of an amino group (see Section 13.3.1.3) or a phosphate group in the acyl moiety, derivatives with a high water-solubility can be obtained. Besides being influenced by the hydrophilic or hydrophobic properties of the acyl moiety, the water-solubility or lipophilicity of N-α-acyloxyalkyl derivatives can be affected by the fact that the N-α-acyloxyalkylation may lead to decreased intermolecular hydrogen bonding in the crystal lattice.

13.2.3.4 N-Acyl derivatives

N-Acylation of amide- or imide-type compounds may be a useful prodrug approach in some cases because of plasma-catalyzed hydrolysis of the N-acyl derivatives. Thus N_3-acetyl-5-fluorouracil (**13.5**) and N_1-ethoxycarbonyl-5-fluorouracil (**13.6**) hydrolyse with half-lives of 40 and 550 min, respectively, at pH 7.4 and 37 °C, whereas the half-lives in the presence of 80% human plasma are only 2–4 min. As a result of their changed physico-chemical properties and easy bioconversion, these prodrug derivatives of 5-fluorouracil have shown improved ocular and rectal absorption compared to the parent drug (Scheme 13.11). Further examples are given in Section 13.3.1.5.

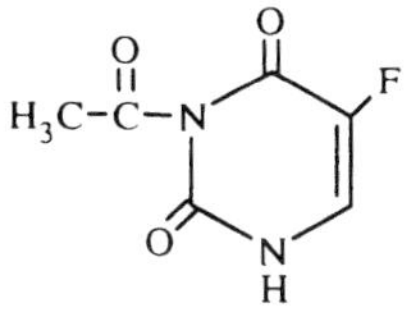

(13.5) 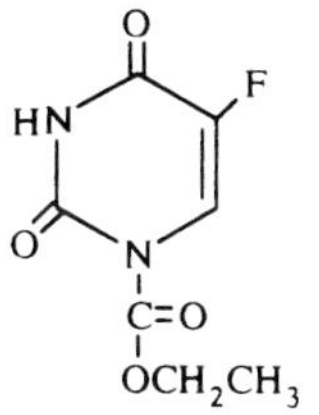   (13.6)

Scheme 13.11

13.2.4 Prodrugs for amines

13.2.4.1 Amides

N-Acylation of amines to give amide prodrugs has been used only to a limited extent due to the relatively high stability of amides *in vivo*. However, certain activated amides are sufficiently chemically labile and likewise certain amides are formed with amino acids susceptible to enzymatic cleavage *in vivo*.

Thus, γ-glutamyl derivatives of sulphamethoxazole (**13.53**) are readily hydrolysed by γ-glutamyl transpeptidase *in vivo* and, as described in Section 13.3.2.2, have been promoted as kidney-specific prodrugs because of their preferential bioconversion in the kidney. Other examples of enzymatically labile amides or peptides include the *N*-L-isoleucyl derivative of dopamine and the *N*-glycyl derivative midodrin (**13.8**), the latter being an orally absorbable prodrug of compound (**13.7**) (Scheme 13.12). The latter is cleaved readily by aminoacylarylamidase, an enzyme which is particularly abundant in renal tissue.

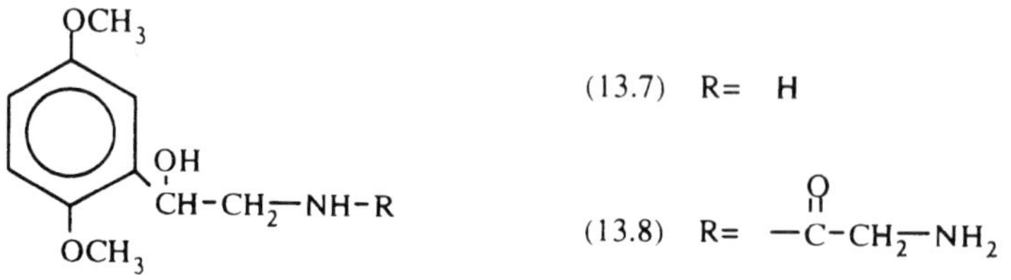

(13.7)   R= H

(13.8)   R= $-\overset{\overset{O}{\|}}{C}-CH_2-NH_2$

Scheme 13.12

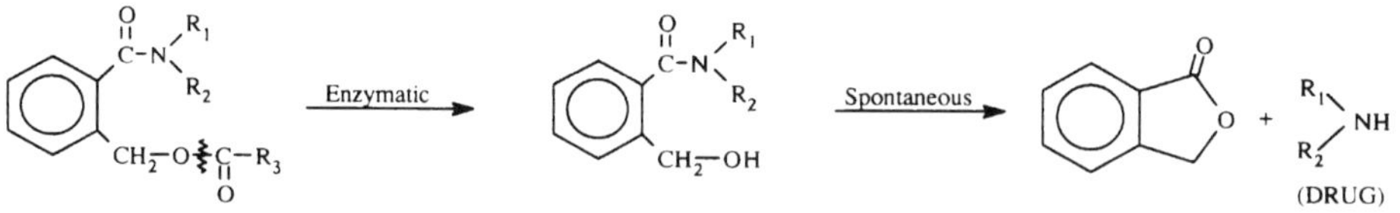

Scheme 13.13

A promising approach to obtain an amide prodrug capable of releasing the parent amine drug at physiological pH and temperature is to make use of intramolecular chemical assistance of the amide hydrolysis. Thus, 2-(hydroxymethyl)benzamides undergo a relatively rapid cyclization in aqueous solution to give phthalide and free amine. By masking the hydroxy function in these derivatives by esterification, chemically stable 2-(acyloxymethyl)benzamides are obtained and a double prodrug is produced. This way the lactonization is blocked and must be preceded by hydrolysis of the ester group, i.e. by the action of esterases *in vivo* (Scheme 13.13).

13.2.4.2 N-(Acyloxyalkoxycarbonyl) derivatives

The utility of carbamates as prodrug derivatives for amines (–NH–(C=O)–OR) is limited due to the general resistance of carbamates to undergo enzymatic cleavage *in vivo*. By introduction of an enzymatically hydrolysable ester function in the carbamate structure it is, however, possible to circumvent this problem. Thus, *N*-(acyloxyalkoxycarbonyl) derivatives of primary or secondary amines may be readily transformed to the parent amine *in vivo*. Enzymatic hydrolysis of the ester moiety in such derivatives lead to a (hydroxyalkoxy)carbonyl derivative, which spontaneously decomposes into the parent amine via an unstable carbamic acid (Scheme 13.14). Such (acyloxy)alkyl carbamates may be promising biolabile prodrugs for amino functional drugs since they are neutral compounds and combine a high stability in aqueous solution with a high susceptibility to undergo enzymatic regeneration of the parent amine by ester hydrolysis. For primary amines, however, an intramolecular acyl transfer reaction leading to the formation of a stable N-acylated parent amine may compete with the reaction sequence in Scheme 13.14 at physiological pH and thus diminish the yield of amine regenerated. Such intramolecular N-acylation is structurally impossible in the derivatives of secondary amines. Therefore, the utility of acyloxyalkoxycarbonyl derivatives as prodrugs of primary amines relies on a high rate of enzymatic ester hydrolysis to compete with the undesired intramolecular reaction.

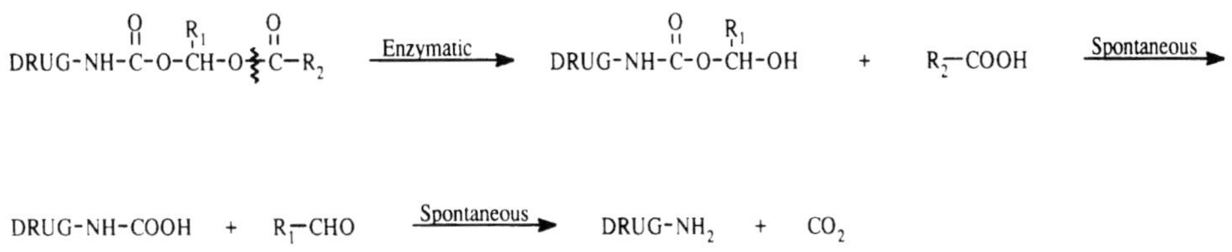

$$DRUG-NH-\overset{O}{\overset{\|}{C}}-O-\overset{R_1}{\overset{|}{C}}H-O\overset{O}{\overset{\|}{C}}-R_2 \xrightarrow{\text{Enzymatic}} DRUG-NH-\overset{O}{\overset{\|}{C}}-O-\overset{R_1}{\overset{|}{C}}H-OH + R_2-COOH \xrightarrow{\text{Spontaneous}}$$

$$DRUG-NH-COOH + R_1-CHO \xrightarrow{\text{Spontaneous}} DRUG-NH_2 + CO_2$$

Scheme 13.14

13.2.4.3 N-Mannich bases

Preparation of N-Mannich bases is a useful prodrug approach for amide-type compounds (see Section 13.2.3.1) and the method is used similarly for prodrugs of primary and secondary amines, in which case the amide-type component acts as a pro-group. N-Mannich base formation lowers the pK_a values of the conjugate acids of amines by about 3 units. Therefore, a potentially useful purpose for transforming amino compounds into N-Mannich prodrugs is to increase the lipophilicity of the parent amines at physiological pH. This leads to depression of protonation, resulting in enhanced biomembrane-passage properties. The selection of biologically acceptable amide-type transport groups affording an appropriate cleavage rate of a Mannich base of a given amine at pH 7.4 is restricted. In a search for useful candidates, it has been found that N-Mannich bases of salicylamide (**13.9**) and different aliphatic amines including amino acids show an unexpectedly high cleavage rate at neutral pH, thus suggesting the utility of salicylamide (Scheme 13.15).

Although the salicylamide N-Mannich bases are more stable in weakly acidic solutions (pH 2–5) than at pH 7.4, a drawback of this prodrug type, requiring chemical (non-enzymatic) release of the parent amine drug, is still the limited *in vitro* stability. This raises some stability-formulation problems, but a method for improving the stability may be further derivatization of the salicylamide Mannich bases in such a manner that an enzymatic release mechanism is required prior to the spontaneous decomposition of the Mannich bases. Since the hydroxy group in the salicylamide Mannich base is responsible for the great reactivity of these derivatives, possibly by intramolecular catalysis, protection of this group may afford derivatives with enhanced stability. By O-acyloxymethylation it is possible to increase the stability *in vitro* and still obtain a rapid rate of amine release under conditions similar to those encountered *in vivo* due to the enzymatic lability of the *O*-acyloxymethyl group introduced. The *O*-acyloxymethyl derivative (**13.10**) is considerably more stable than the *N*-Mannich base (**13.9**) at pH 2–8. In the presence of human plasma the ester group is rapidly hydrolysed by virtue of enzymatic catalysis and (**13.11**) is formed, which spontaneously degrades to (**13.9**). In addition to providing an *in vitro* stabilizing effect, the concept of *O*-acyloxymethylation makes it possible to obtain prodrug derivatives of a given amine drug with varying physico-chemical properties of importance for drug delivery, such as lipophilicity and water solubility. This can simply be effected by the selection of an appropriate acyloxymethyl group (varying the R_3 group).

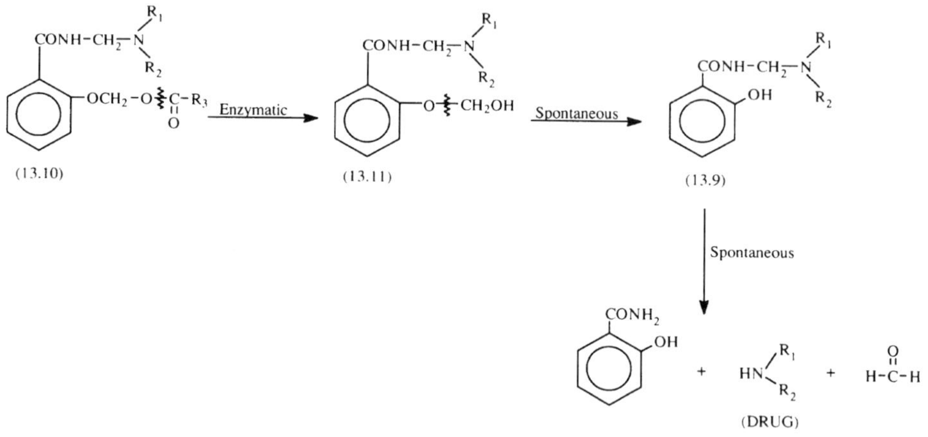

Scheme 13.15

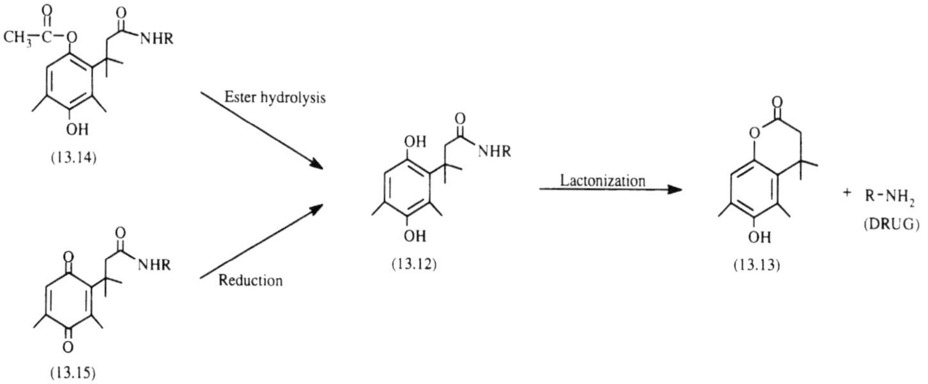

Scheme 13.16

13.2.4.4 Redox and esterase sensitive prodrugs, which utilize hydroxy amide lactonization
The highly chemically reactive phenolic amide derivative (**13.12**) can function as a prodrug
of an amine drug. The lactonization, affording the parent amine drug and the lactone (**13.13**),
proceeds with a half-life of approximately 1 min at physiological pH and temperature. The
reactivity of this compound is attributed to the presence of the "trimethyl lock" (methyl
groups at positions 3, 3 and 6′). The half-life of 1 min is, however, too short to give a
useful prodrug system for amines. In order to transform (**13.12**) into a chemically stable
and yet enzymatically labile prodrug the double prodrugs (**13.14**) and (**13.15**) have been
developed. The parent amine is regenerated via a two-step process. The initially enzymatic
step may be catalyzed by esterases or reductive mechanisms, the ester portion in (**13.14**)
and the quinone portion in (**13.15**) being transformed to (**13.12**), respectively, followed by
the non-enzymatic lactonization (Scheme 13.16).

13.3 APPLICATIONS OF THE PRODRUG APPROACH

Different prodrug types of various functional groups have been discussed above and
illustrated with a few examples on specific drugs. The prodrug approach has, however,
been successfully applied to a wide variety of drugs. Most of the applications have
involved (a) enhancement of bioavailability and passage through various biological
barriers, (b) increased duration of pharmacological effects, (c) increased site-specificity,
(d) decreased toxicity and adverse reactions, (e) improvement of organoleptic properties
and (f) improvement of stability and solubility properties. These aspects will be further
illustrated in the following.

13.3.1 Bioavailability and biomembrane passage

13.3.1.1 Transport theory
It has been shown that the rate of transport by passive diffusion across a biological membrane
will increase exponentially with increasing lipophilicity of a given compound until a certain
level of lipophilicity. For compounds of high lipophilicity the rate of transport levels off and
reaches a constant level and may decrease, due to dissolution problems in the aqueous layers
connected to the biomembrane. This behaviour is explained by the frequently inversely
proportional relation between aqueous solubility and lipophilicity. The lipophilicity for a
given compound has traditionally been expressed by the *n*-octanol-water system partition
coefficients (P). The optimal values for solubility and log P to ensure good absorption
depend on the nature of the biomembrane and the volume of the aqueous phase adjacent
to the membrane. If dissolution phenomena are not rate-limiting, a log P value of about 2
appears to be optimal for gastrointestinal absorption.

Thus, it is clear that both aqueous solubility and lipophilicity are most important factors in
drug absorption, which usually takes place by passive diffusion. Drugs, which are too polar
or hydrophilic often exhibit poor transport properties, whereas those that are too non-polar
or lipophilic frequently have low bioavailability because of their poor aqueous solubility
and dissolution characteristics.

Since many drugs are either weak acids or bases or salts of these, dissociation must
be regarded as an important factor in determining absorbability. It is generally accepted

that the unionized (most lipophilic) form of an acidic or basic drug is absorbed far more efficiently than the ionic species. Although the latter is more water-soluble, the increase in the partition coefficient gained by going from a salt to free acid (or free base) usually exceeds the corresponding decrease in solubility by several orders of magnitude.

Since the partition coefficient of the ionic species is usually negligible, the partition coefficient of a weak acid at a given pH value can be expressed as:

$$P_{pH} = P_{HA} f_{HA} \tag{13.4}$$

where P_{HA} is the intrinsic partition coefficient of a weak acid and f_{HA} is the fraction of the undissociated species at the particular pH values. Equation 13.4 can also be written as:

$$\log P_{pH} = \log P_{HA} - \log(1 + 10^{(pH-pKa)}) \tag{13.5}$$

where K_a is the ionization constant of the acid.

The analogous expression for a basic drug is:

$$\log P_{pH} = \log P_B - \log(1 + 10^{(pKa-pH)}) \tag{13.6}$$

where P_B is the intrinsic partition coefficient of a weak base.

Since biomembrane passage of a drug depends primarily on its physico-chemical properties (water-solubility and lipophilicity), and the prodrug principle involves transient modification of these properties, it is readily evident that this principle is perfectly suitable to improve drug absorption through epithelial tissue. A number of examples are given in the following, the examples being classified according to the route of administration.

13.3.1.2 Oral absorption

Poor bioavailability of an orally administered drug may be due to too low lipophilicity, too low water-solubility, low acid-stability or extensive first-pass metabolism of the drug in intestine or liver.

Some of the best examples of increasing the lipophilicity of agents in order to enhance absorption of a polar drug by prodrug modification are seen with various ampicillin derivatives. Being zwitterionic in the pH range in the gastrointestinal tract, ampicillin (**13.16**) possesses a low lipophilicity and only about 30–40% is absorbed following oral administration. Altering the polarity of the penicillin by esterifying the free carboxyl group to form the prodrugs pivampicillin (pivaloylmethyl ester) (**13.17**), bacampicillin (ethoxycarbonylethyl ester) (**13.18**) or talampicillin (phthalidyl ester) (**13.19**) has proven successful, resulting in essentially complete absorption of ampicillin (Scheme 13.17). During or after absorption these clinically used prodrug derivatives are rapidly cleaved by enzymatic hydrolysis to yield free ampicillin. A discussion of the mechanism of cleavage of these double esters is given in Section 13.2.2.

In recent years, simple ethyl esters of various peptidic ACE inhibitors have been exploited for improvement of the oral bioavailability of the parent drugs by increasing the lipophilicity. Enalapril (**13.21**) and pentopril (**13.23**) are such ethyl ester prodrugs of their parent active acids (**13.20**) and (**13.22**), respectively. Although the esters are much better absorbed than the very polar active agents, they are only rather slowly cleaved in the organism

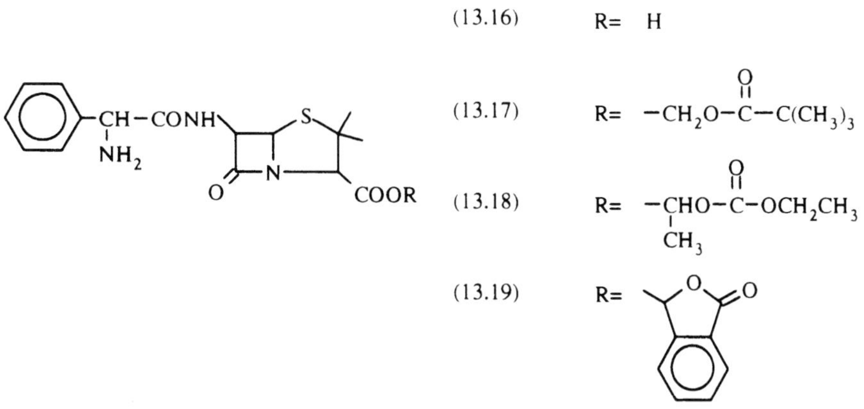

| | (13.16) | R= | H |

(13.17) R= $-CH_2O-\overset{\overset{O}{\|}}{C}-C(CH_3)_3$

(13.18) R= $-\underset{\underset{CH_3}{|}}{CH}O-\overset{\overset{O}{\|}}{C}-OCH_2CH_3$

(13.19) R=

Scheme 13.17

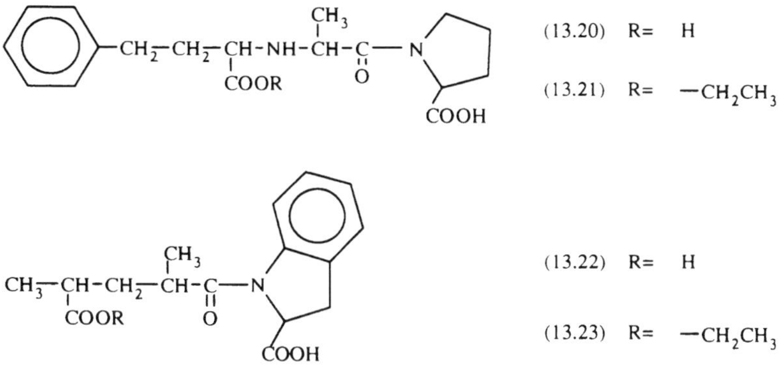

(13.20) R= H

(13.21) R= $-CH_2CH_3$

(13.22) R= H

(13.23) R= $-CH_2CH_3$

Scheme 13.18

(by liver esterases) and especially in the case of pentopril appreciable quantities of intact and biologically inactive prodrug are excreted in the urine. It is of interest to note that these ACE-inhibitors have been marketed only in their prodrug forms, thus indicating the increasing awareness of the utility of the prodrug approach at an early stage of new drug development (Scheme 13.18).

Several drugs show poor and variable oral absorption characteristics as a result of insufficient aqueous solubility ($<0.1\%$) and absorption becomes dissolution rate-limited. An example of a prodrug used to increase the aqueous solubility and dissolution behaviour is the water-soluble dipotassium salt of clorazepate (**13.24**). It is marketed as a prodrug of the slightly soluble desmethyldiazepam (**13.25**). In acidic solution clorazepate spontaneously decarboxylates to the parent drug, which is the form absorbed (Scheme 13.19).

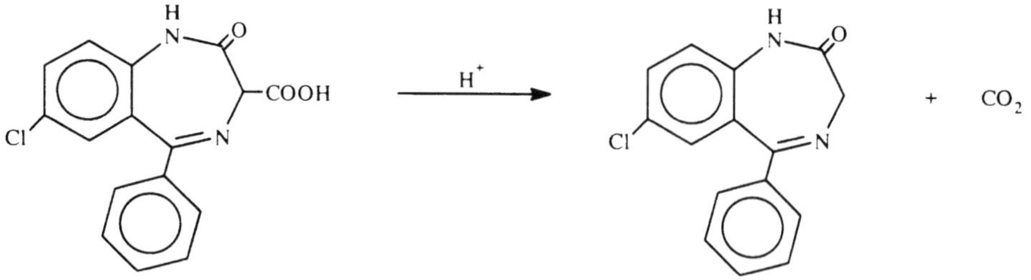

(13.24)   (13.25)

Scheme 13.19

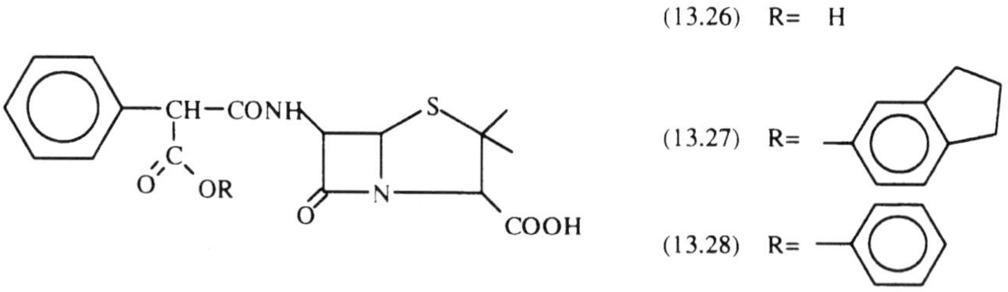

(13.26)   R=   H

(13.27)   R=

(13.28)   R=

Scheme 13.20

The poor gastrointestinal absorption of carbenicillin (**13.26**) is due to acid-catalysed destruction of the drug in the stomach as well as to its strongly polar character. By bioreversible esterification of the side-chain carboxyl group the more acid-stable (by a factor of 6 at pH 2) and lipophilic derivatives (**13.27**) (carindacillin) and (**13.28**) (carfecillin) are obtained (Scheme 13.20). Upon absorption carbenicillin is released in the blood by enzymatic hydrolysis from these clinically used prodrugs.

13.3.1.3 Rectal absorption
Drug absorption from the rectum does not differ significantly from that taking place in other parts of the gastrointestinal tract. Passive diffusion is the main mechanism and therefore, the solubility and lipophilicity of the drug or prodrug are of great importance. Because only little fluid (about 10 ml) is present in the rectum, a greater water-solubility is required for rectal absorption than for oral absorption.

Because of its low water and lipid solubility allupurinol (**13.29**) is only very poorly (<5%) absorbed following rectal administration. In addition, allupurinol shows strong intermolecular hydrogen bonding and therefore has a strong crystal lattice energy resulting in a high melting point. The rectal absorption of allupurinol has been improved by various N-acyloxymethyl prodrug derivatives containing a sligthly basic amino function

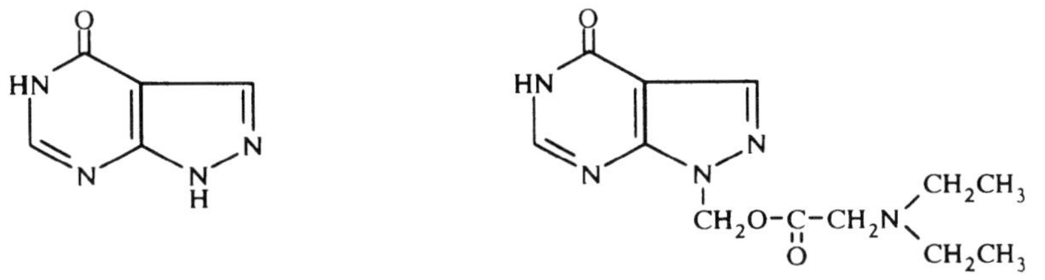

(13.29)

(13.30)

Scheme 13.21

in the ester moiety. These derivatives combine good aqueous solubility with an adequate lipophilicity at pH values corresponding to those in the rectum (pH 7.5–8). Thus, 1-(N,N-diethylglycyloxymethyl)allupurinol (**13.30**) possesses a pK_a value of 7.0, a log P value of 0.20 in octanol/aqueous buffer pH 8.0 and a water-solubility of 4.5 mg ml^{-1} as free base which is about 10 times greater than that observed for allupurinol (Scheme 13.21). The log P value of allupurinol is –0.55. Thus it can be seen that derivative (**13.30**) is both more water-soluble and lipophilic than the parent drug. Likewise, by blocking the NH-acidic group by N-acyloxymethylation, the intermolecular hydrogen bonding is decreased as reflected by a decreased melting point. Thus, the water and lipid solubility is increased and the increase is dependent on the nature of the acyl group. Following rectal administration to man the prodrug (**13.30**) affords an absolute bioavailability of allupurinol of about 40%. The mechanism of cleavage and other properties of the N-acyloxymethyl derivatives have previously been discussed in Section 13.2.3.3.

13.3.1.4 Ocular drug delivery

A major problem in ocular therapeutics is the attainment of an optimal drug concentration at the site of action within the eye. The difficulty is largely due to precorneal factors (e.g. solution drainage, tear turnover and conjunctival absorption) that rapidly remove the drug from the conjunctival sac, where it is applied, and to the mismatch of the physico-chemical properties of the drug with those of the cornea. The net result is that less than 10%, typically 1% or less, of the instilled dose is ocularly absorbed.

The cornea is a trilaminate structure consisting of a hydrophilic stromal layer sandwiched between a very lipophilic epithelial layer and a much less lipophilic endothelial layer. Consequently, drugs with extremes in partition coefficient penetrates the cornea poorly. The optimal log P (octanol/buffer pH 7.4) for transcellular corneal drug penetration has been reported to be 2–3. This forms the basis for the chemical modification of hydrophilic ophthalmic drugs to yield lipophilic prodrugs, which, following corneal absorption, are converted back either chemically or enzymatically to the parent drugs in the eye.

Epinephrine (**13.31**) has long been used for the treatment of glaucoma although its corneal absorption is poor because of its high polarity and rapid, metabolic destruction. The development of the prodrug, dipivefrin (**13.32**), has led to a markedly improved ocular delivery of epinephrine (Scheme 13.22). This dipivalate ester prodrug is much more lipophilic than epinephrine and the esterification of the metabolically susceptible phenolic

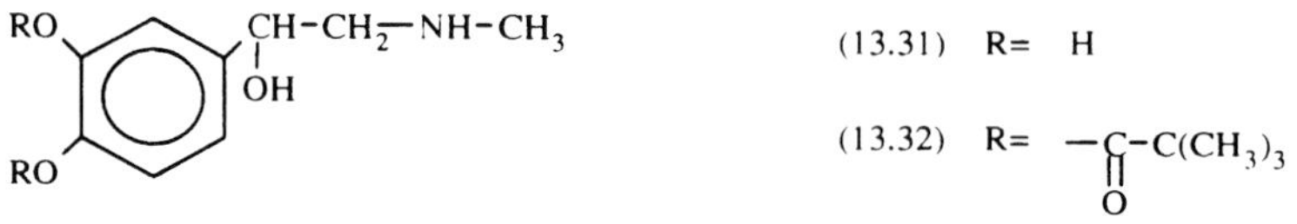

RO—⬡(CH—CH₂—NH—CH₃ / OH)—RO

(13.31) R= H

(13.32) R= $-\overset{O}{\underset{\|}{C}}-C(CH_3)_3$

Scheme 13.22

hydroxyl groups affords a delay in metabolic destruction. These properties coupled with a sufficiently high susceptibility to undergo enzymatic hydrolysis in the eye during and after absorption are responsible for the approximately 20 times greater antiglaucoma activity of the prodrug in comparison with the parent drug upon local administration in humans. In addition, untoward cardiac side-effects due to epinephrine absorption from the tear duct overflow are diminished because lower doses of the prodrug can be used. Dipivefrin also has a longer duration of action than epinephrine, because the metabolism of the latter, which involves a methylation of the phenolic OH-groups, is prevented until the prodrug has undergone conversion to epinephrine.

Similarly, the corneal absorption of other hydrophilic agents such as pilocarpine, phenylephrine and timolol has been improved by the prodrug approach. Timolol (**13.33**) is a β-adrenergic receptor blocker widely used in the treatment of glaucoma. A major problem in its use in glaucoma therapy is, however, its relatively high incidence of cardiovascular and respiratory side-effects. These effects arise as a result of absorption of the topically applied drug into the systemic circulation and are essentially the same as those seen with oral timolol.

Timolol contains a secondary amino group with a pK_a of 9.2 and since this group is highly protonated at pH 7.4, the compound shows a low lipophilicity at physiological pH ($\log P = -0.04$), which in turn is unfavourable for corneal penetration. The corneal absorption characteristics of timolol has recently been improved by esterification of the hydroxy group in the molecule to yield more lipophilic compounds (**13.34** and **13.35**) (Scheme 13.23). These esters have been shown to penetrate the cornea more rapidly than timolol as a result of their higher lipophilicities, and to be converted by enzymatic hydrolysis to the parent timolol within the eye. Most important, the increase in corneal penetration achieved with the esters was not paralleled to the same magnitude in penetration of the conjunctival and nasal biomembranes giving rise to systemic absorption and thus side-effects.

The O-butanoyl timolol (**13.34**) has a log P of 2.08 which leads to a four- to sixfold increase in the corneal absorption of timolol following topical administration in rabbits and the systemic absorption of timolol is unaffected or even slightly reduced compared to timolol. Besides this improved topical/systemic bioavailability ratio, this prodrug also shows a greatly extended duration of action in comparison with the parent timolol in an experimental animal model. The greater lipophilicity of the ester probably results in enhanced reposit of the prodrug in ocular tissues serving as a depot from which the active parent drug is slowly released. Just as favourable findings have been obtained with some other timolol esters such as the 1-methylcyclopropanecarboxylate ester (**13.35**).

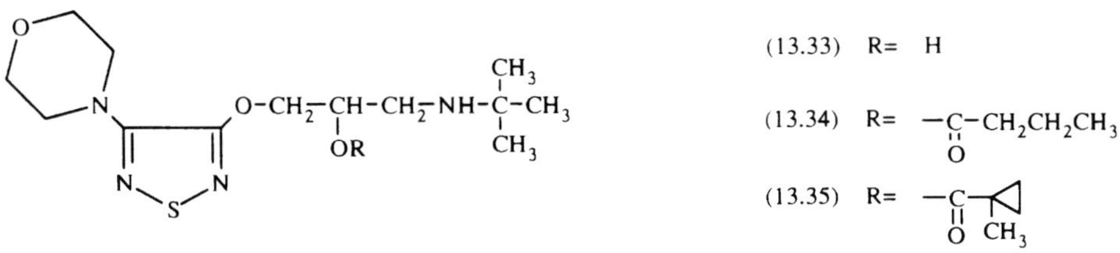

(13.33) R= H

(13.34) R= $-\overset{O}{\underset{||}{C}}-CH_2CH_2CH_3$

(13.35) R= $-\overset{O}{\underset{||}{C}}-\overset{CH_3}{\triangleleft}$

Scheme 13.23

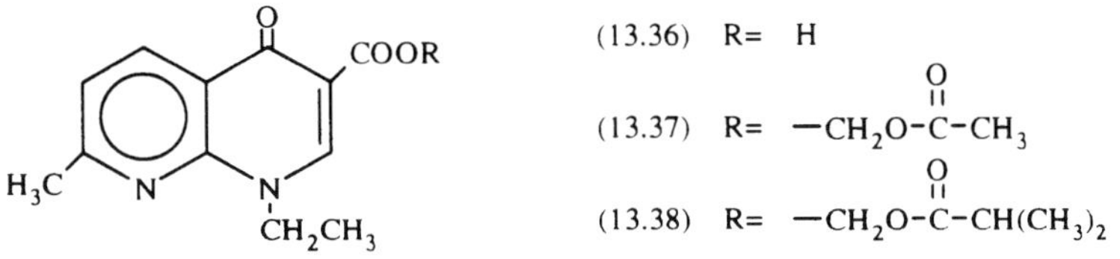

(13.36) R= H

(13.37) R= $-CH_2O-\overset{O}{\overset{||}{C}}-CH_3$

(13.38) R= $-CH_2O-\overset{O}{\overset{||}{C}}-CH(CH_3)_2$

Scheme 13.24

13.3.1.5 *Dermal drug delivery*

Most drugs diffuse poorly through the skin, in particular through the stratum corneum, because of unfavourable physico-chemical properties (water and lipid solubility). Several studies have demonstrated a biphasic solubility profile for absorption through the skin, i.e. in order to diffuse readily through the skin a compound should possess adequate water as well as lipid solubility. This can often be achieved by the prodrug approach and, in fact, the dermal delivery of several drug molecules such as steroids, antiviral and antipsoriasis agents have in recent years been improved by this approach.

Nalidixic acid (**13.36**) is a promising agent for treatment of psoriasis, but its physico-chemical properties are suboptimal for an efficient topical absorption. By esterification of the carboxylic acid group by *O*-acyloxymethylation, the prodrug derivatives (**13.37** and **13.38**), both being more lipid and water-soluble, have been obtained (Scheme 13.24). Diffusion studies *in vitro* using human skin have shown that the derivatives enhance the delivery of nalidixic acid from polar and apolar vehicles. The double esters are enzymatically hydrolysed to nalidixic acid during the transport through the skin.

Thyrotropin-releasing hormone (TRH, pGlu-L-His-L-Pro-NH$_2$) (**13.39**) is the hypothalamic peptide that regulates the synthesis and secretion of thyrotropin from the anterior pituitary gland. TRH has been proposed as a potential drug in the management of various neurologic and neuropsychiatric disorders. The clinical utilization of TRH is, however, greatly hampered due to its rapid metabolism and clearance as well as by its very hydrophilic nature and poor access to the central nervous system. By modification of the imidazole ring in histidine various *N*-alkoxycarbonyl prodrugs have been prepared. Application of

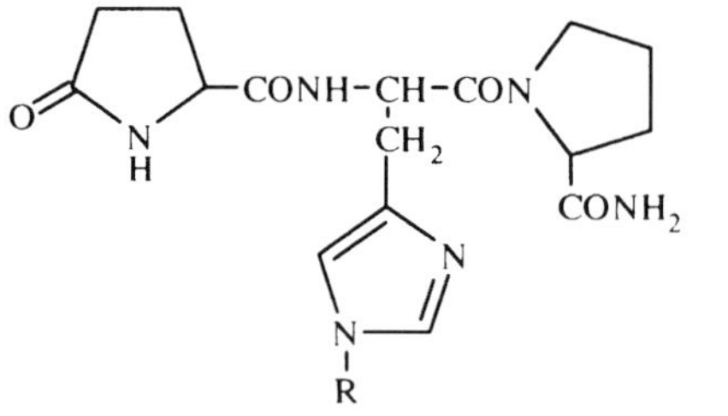

(13.39) R= H

$$O$$
$$\|$$
(13.40) R= $-C-OC_8H_{17}$

Scheme 13.25

the N-octyloxycarbonyl-TRH derivative (**13.40**) (Scheme 13.25) showed a very efficient delivery of TRH in a human skin diffusion model. Essentially, all of the prodrug applied was converted to the parent TRH during diffusion through the skin samples.

13.3.1.6 Prevention of first-pass metabolism

Several drugs are efficiently absorbed from the gastrointestinal tract, but show limited systemic bioavailability due to presystemic (or first-pass) metabolism or inactivation before reaching the systemic circulation. This metabolism can occur in the intestinal lumen, at the brush border of the intestinal cells, in the mucosal cells lining the gastrointestinal tract or in the liver. In addition to decreasing the percentage of dose reaching its intended site of action, extensive first-pass metabolism often results in significant variability in bioavailability. First-pass metabolism can be avoided by other routes of administration such as sublingual, inhalation and partly by the rectal route. The oral route is, however, generally preferred.

A major class of drugs undergoing extensive first-pass metabolism are those containing phenolic hydroxyl groups. The rapid inactivation of these drugs (e.g. salicylamide, morphine, isoprenaline, dopamine and β-oestradiol) is mainly due to sulphation, glucuronidation and methylation of the phenolic moieties, the conjugation action being catalyzed by enzymes present in the gut and liver.

The prodrug approach can sometimes be very useful to reduce first-pass metabolism. Most attempts performed in the past have been concerned with phenolic drugs. The traditional approach has been to mask the metabolizable moiety, i.e. to derivatize the phenolic group with e.g. an acid to yield an ester prodrug. This approach will only be useful if the prodrug to drug conversion occurs mainly in an organ other than the intestine or liver. If the demasking of the protective group already occurs in the intestinal wall or liver, the active parent drug will subsequently be metabolized within the same organ. One should also be aware that ester derivatives of a given compound sometimes can increase the extent of first-pass metabolism. Apparently, the lipophilic prodrug ester is entering the lipoidal microsomal media in the liver to a higher extent than the parent drug, and is subsequently hydrolysed and conjugated.

Nevertheless, a number of recent examples show the potential usefulness of protecting the metabolizable phenolic moiety into a bioreversible derivative. Thus, anthranilate and acetylsalicylate (or salicylate) esters of naltrexone (**13.41**), nalbuphine and β-oestradiol have been found to result in greatly increased systemic bioavailability of the parent drugs following oral administration in dogs due to depressed first-pass metabolism.

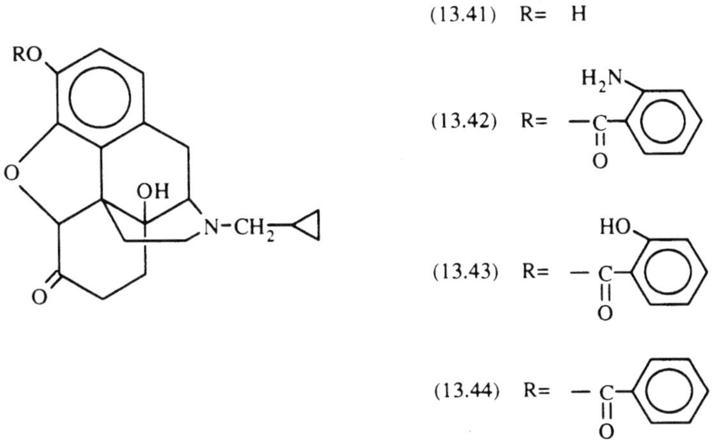

(13.41)   R=   H

(13.42)   R=   [structure: anthranilate ester with H₂N]

(13.43)   R=   [structure: salicylate ester with HO]

(13.44)   R=   [structure: benzoate ester]

Scheme 13.26

For example, the anthranilate ester (**13.42**) and the salicylate ester (**13.43**) of naltrexone (**13.41**) resulted in a bioavailability of the parent drug of 49 and 31%, respectively. Naltrexone itself gave only a bioavailability of 1% whereas the benzoate ester (**13.44**) did not improve the bioavailability (Scheme 13.26). Hydrolysis data indicated that ester (**13.42**) and (**13.43**) are more stable toward enzymatic degradation than the benzoate ester, which indicate that these esters are able to survive presystematic hydrolysis to a greater extent.

Another way to protect a phenolic moiety against presystemic metabolism is to prepare an ester with a built-in esterase inhibiting function, so that the prodrug can slow down its own rate of hydrolysis, and thereby pass intact through the gut wall and liver. A nice example of this strategy is the bronchodilator prodrug bambuterol (**13.45**), which is the bis-*N*,*N*-dimethylcarbamate of terbutaline (**13.48**). *N*,*N*-disubstituted carbamate esters are generally very stable against both chemical and enzymatic hydrolysis and have, in addition, esterase-inhibiting properties. Bambuterol has been found to possess these properties, being a potent inhibitor of pseudocholinesterase. Upon oral administration, the compound is readily absorbed and passes unmetabolized through the gut wall so that most of the dose reaches the liver and the systemic circulation unchanged. The generation of the active terbutaline from the prodrug takes place by a multi-step reaction involving an initial enzyme-mediated oxidation at the methyl groups in the carbamate moiety to give *N*-hydroxymethyl carbamates (**13.46**), which are subsequently decomposed spontaneously to formaldehyde and monomethyl carbamates (**13.47**). The latter are then enzymatically hydrolysed by virtue of pseudo-cholinesterase (Scheme 13.27). This enzyme is selectively inhibited by bambuterol, i.e. the prodrug inhibits its own hydrolysis, and the result is a slow formation of the parent drug and a sustained action. In addition to these desirable gains in bioavailability and duration of action, bambuterol has been shown to afford enhanced delivery of the parent drug to its site of action, the lungs, with concomitant reduction of

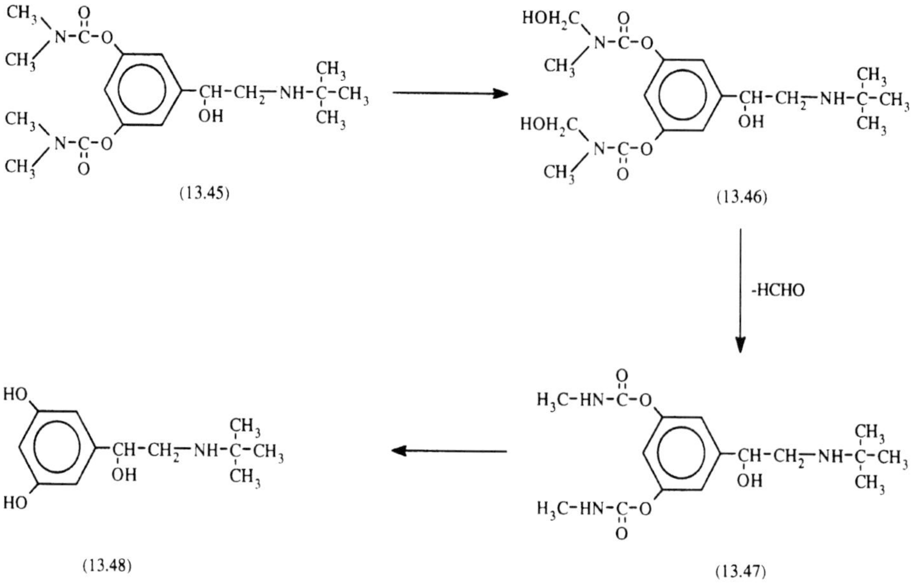

(13.45)

(13.46)

-HCHO

(13.48)

(13.47)

Scheme 13.27

side-effects such as muscle tremor due to the lower plasma levels of terbutaline. Apparently, bambuterol and its hydroxylated metabolites have greater affinity for lung tissue than terbutaline and are somewhat retained in this tissue. Following lung uptake, terbutaline is regenerated from the prodrug and its primary metabolites.

A third approach to depress presystemic metabolism is to derivatize the susceptible drug molecule at some other position in the molecule so that the prodrug obtained is no longer a substrate for the presystemic metabolizing enzyme, even though the functional group originally attacked is not directly masked. An example illustrating this approach is propranolol (13.49), which is undergoing extensive first-pass metabolism in the liver, in particular through cytochrome P 450-mediated oxidation. By esterification of the hydroxy group, which is attacked only to a minor extent during first-pass metabolism, to the acetate (13.50) or hemisuccinate (13.51), derivatives of (13.49) with a significant protection against first-pass metabolism has been obtained (Scheme 13.28).

13.3.2 Site-specific drug delivery

Two approaches to the design of site-specific drug delivery of drugs via the prodrug concept can be visualized. First, one can aim at designing a bioreversible derivative (prodrug), which affords an increased or selective transport of the parent drug to the site of action (*site-directed drug delivery*). The site-directed drug delivery can further be divided into *localized site-directed drug delivery* and *systemic site-directed drug delivery*. Second, the

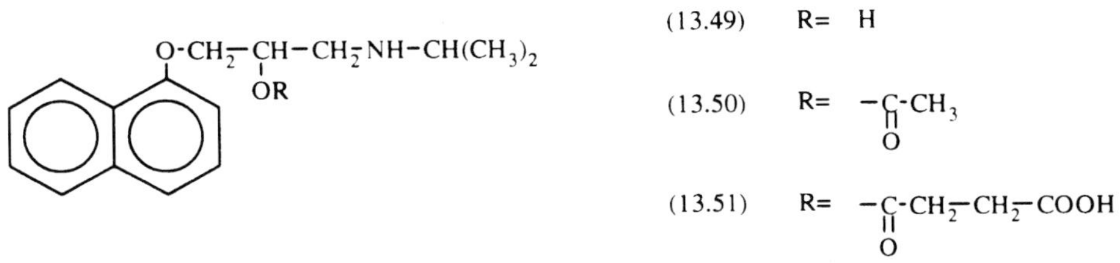

O·CH$_2$-CH-CH$_2$-NH-CH(CH$_3$)$_2$
OR

(13.49)   R=   H

(13.50)   R= $-\underset{\underset{O}{\|}}{C}$-CH$_3$

(13.51)   R= $-\underset{\underset{O}{\|}}{C}$-CH$_2$-CH$_2$-COOH

Scheme 13.28

objective can be accomplished by designing a derivative that goes everywhere, but which undergoes bioactivation only at the desired target (*site-specific bioactivation or site-specific drug release*). In the following, examples will be given to illustrate the possible utilization of these principles to achieve site-directed drug delivery or targeting of drug molecules, i.e. site-specific bioactivation. In several cases site-specific drug delivery has been obtained by a combination of site-directed drug delivery and site-specific bioactivation.

13.3.2.1 Site-directed drug delivery
Until now, most successes in achieving site-directed drug delivery via prodrugs have been through localized site-directed drug delivery, i.e. where the drug input is applied directly to the target organ such as the skin or eye. The therapeutic success achieved stems primarily from increased absorption or transport of the prodrug across the biological membrane to which it is applied. Thus, as described above, improved localized site-directed drug delivery of the antiglaucoma agents epinephrine (**13.31**) or timolol (**13.33**) has been achieved with prodrugs possessing improved corneal permeability characteristics. This, in turn, leads to decreased concentrations of the parent drug at sites where it is unwanted such as the systemic circulation. The net result obtained is a reduction of the dose necessary for eliciting the pharmacological effect and hence a reduction in side-effects.

Systemic site-directed drug delivery, i.e. delivery to a specific internal site or organ, through a selective drug transport is more difficult to achieve than localized site-directed drug delivery, since the drug must be transported in the blood to the desired organ or tissue, passing various complex barriers on the way. Despite the difficult goal some successful examples have appeared.

An example is a method for systemic site-directed drug delivery of drugs to the brain. The drug (D), which is aimed to be delivered to the brain, is coupled to a quaternary carrier (e.g. *N*-methylnicotinic acid) (QC)$^+$ and the obtained (D-QC)$^+$ is reduced chemically to the neutral, lipophilic dihydro form (dihydrotrigonelline) (D-DHC) (Scheme 13.29). After administration of this compound, it is distributed quickly throughout the body, including the brain. The lipophilic form is then enzymatically oxidized back to the original quaternary salt (D-QC)$^+$, which, because of its ionic, hydrophilic character prevents it from passing through the blood-brain barrier and thus, it has been trapped in the brain. Slow enzymatic cleavage of (D-QC)$^+$ in the brain will then result in a steady release of the parent drug there. Because of the facile elimination of (D-QC)$^+$ from the general circulation,

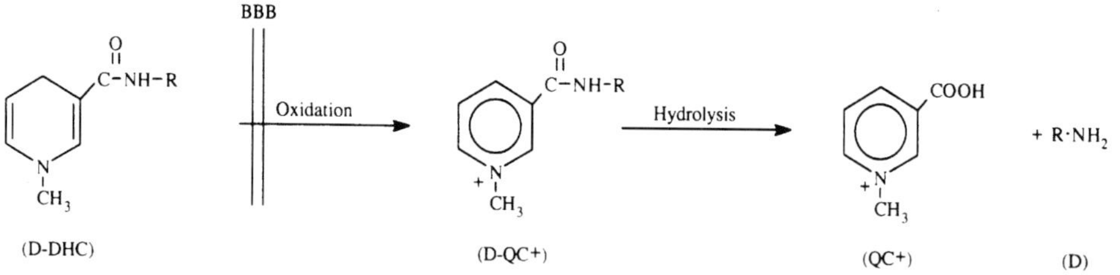

Scheme 13.29

only small amounts of the free drug are released in the blood and the overall result is a fairly high concentration of the drug at its site of action within the brain. This system has been applied successfully to several drugs, e.g. dopamine, phenytoin or penicillins, in order to achieve brain-specific or brain-enhanced delivery. The chemical linkage connecting the drug with $(QC)^+$ can be an amide or ester bond if the drug contains an amino or hydroxy group, respectively. For a carboxylic acid drug acyloxymethyl derivatives have been used.

13.3.2.2 Site-specific bioactivation

Site-specific drug delivery through a site-specific prodrug bioactivation may be accomplished by the utilization of a specific property at the target site, such as changed pH or high activity of certain enzymes relative to non-target tissues, affording conversion of prodrug to drug.

It has been shown that the kidney is highly active in the uptake and metabolism of γ-glutamyl derivatives of amino acids and peptides. This property is due to the high concentration of γ-glutamyl transpeptidase in the kidney, an enzyme capable of cleaving γ-glutamyl derivatives of amino acids and other compounds containing an amino function. Another example of an enzyme present in high concentrations in the kidney is N-acylamino acid acylase. N-Acetyl-γ-glutamylsulphamethoxazole (**13.52**) is a prodrug requiring the action of both enzymes in order to release the parent compound. Besides being dependent on γ-glutamyl transpeptidase, the release of sulphamethoxazole (**13.53**) from this derivative requires the initial action of N-acylamino acid deacylase (Scheme 13.30). This way it is possible to obtain a kidney-selective accumulation of sulfamethoxazole. Thus, this example and other examples of kidney specific γ-glutamyl derivatives indicate that γ-glutamyl or N-acyl-γ-glutamyl prodrug derivatives of a variety of drugs may be of general use when it is desired to obtain a drug action in the kidney and/or the urinary tract. A prerequisite for the applicability of this concept is, however, that the γ-glutamyl derivative of a given drug substance can function as a substrate for γ-glutamyl transpeptidase.

The anti-ulcer agent omeprazole (**13.54**) is an excellent example of a prodrug showing a high degree of site-specific bioactivation resulting in site-specific drug delivery. The drug is an effective inhibitor of gastric acid secretion by inhibiting the gastric H^+, K^+-ATPase. This enzyme is responsible for the gastric acid production, and is located in the secretory membranes of parietal cells. Omeprazole itself is not an active inhibitor of this enzyme,

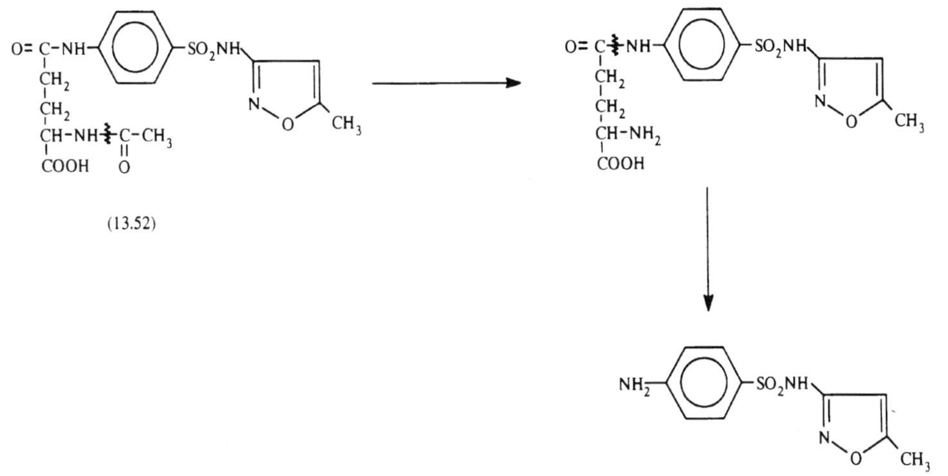

O= C-NH—⟨benzene⟩—SO₂NH—(isoxazole)—CH₃
| CH₂
| CH₂
| CH-NH—C-CH₃
| COOH   O

(13.52)

⟶

O= C⧧NH—⟨benzene⟩—SO₂NH—(isoxazole)—CH₃
| CH₂
| CH₂
| CH-NH₂
| COOH

↓

NH₂—⟨benzene⟩—SO₂NH—(isoxazole)—CH₃

(13.53)

Scheme 13.30

but is transformed within the acid compartments of the parietal cells into the active inhibitor, a cyclic sulphonamide (**13.55**). This reacts with the thiol groups in the enzyme and forms a disulphide complex (**13.56**), thus inactivating the H^+, K^+-ATPase (Scheme 13.31). The high specificity in the action of omeprazole is due to a combination of factors:

1. Omeprazole is a weak base (pK_a of the pyridine nitrogen is 4.0) and therefore concentrates in acidic compartments, i.e. in parietal cells, which have the lowest pH of the cells in the body.
2. The low pH value of the parietal cells causes the conversion of omeprazole into the active inhibitor close to the target enzyme.
3. The active inhibitor (**13.55**) is a permanent cation with limited possibilities to penetrate the membranes of the parietal and other cells, and thus will be retained at its site of action.
4. In the neutral part of the body omeprazole has good stability and only slight conversion to the active species occurs.

Another example of site-specific bioactivation is two colon specific prodrugs of 5-aminosalicylic acid (mesalazine) (**13.59**), namely sulphasalazine (**13.57**) and olsalazine (**13.58**) (Scheme 13.32). Both are azo-linked prodrugs, which release the parent drug by the action of azo-reductases produced by anaerobic colonic bacteria. Whereas sulphasalazine suffers from the fact that the released sulphapyridine, formed upon degradation of the prodrug, is absorbed from the colon and contributes to the side-effects of the prodrug, olsalazine is cleaved to give two molecules of the parent drug (a twin prodrug). The benefits by site-specific drug delivery of these 5-aminosalicylic acid prodrugs, which are commonly used for the treatment of ulcerative colitis, are not only due to the site-specific bioactivation,

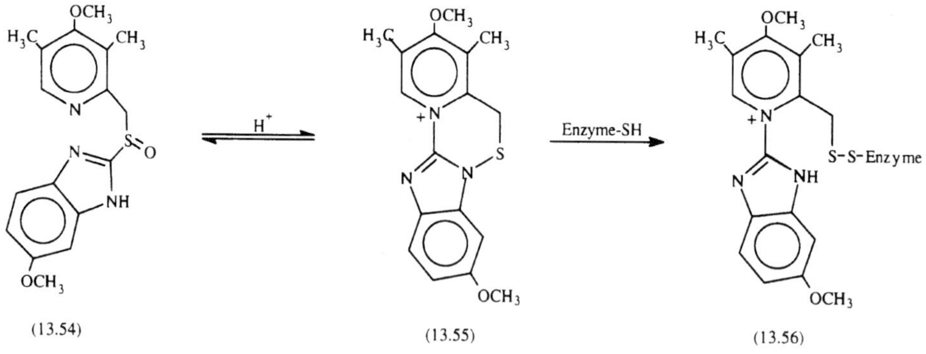

(13.54)   (13.55)   (13.56)

Scheme 13.31

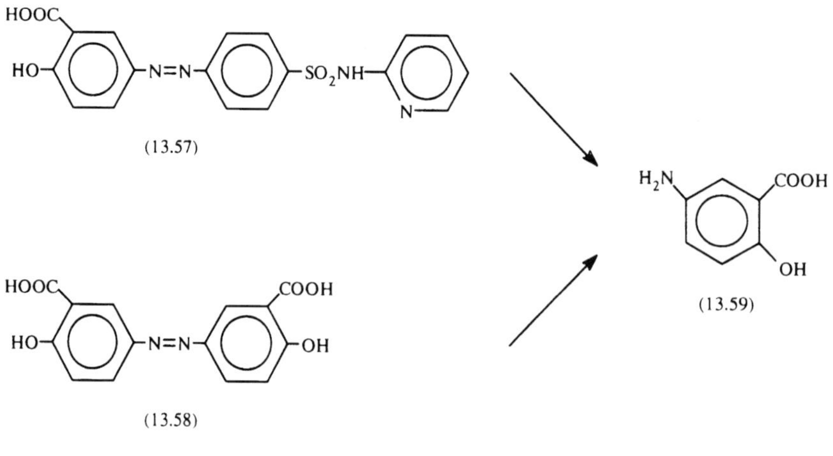

(13.57)

(13.58)

(13.59)

Scheme 13.32

but also to the fact that these very polar prodrugs are not significantly absorbed from the small intestines.

The examples cited above in this section and Section 13.3.2.1 are examples of utilization of the prodrug concept to achieve site-specific drug delivery. For the design of prodrugs directed selectively to their site of action, the following basal criteria must be taken into consideration:

- the prodrug should be able to reach the site of action
- the prodrug should be converted efficiently to the drug at the site of action
- the parent active drug should be somewhat retained or trapped at the target site for a sufficient period of time to exert its effect.

The reason why attempts to promote site-specific drug delivery via prodrugs have failed in many past cases, is that not all these criteria have been met. Thus, although a prodrug will release the parent drug at its target site in a highly selective manner due to a target-specific cleavage mechanism, it will not be successful if the prodrug is not able to reach the target tissue. Both conditions should be fulfilled at the same time. Likewise it is desirable that the prodrug is retained at the site of action and followed by conversion to the parent drug as described above for the brain-directed delivery system (Scheme 13.29).

13.3.3 Reduction of side-effects

As described above increased site-specific delivery of drugs usually results in diminishing the toxicity or unwanted side-effects. As exemplified with epinephrine and timolol improved drug absorption can also afford a reduction of side-effects due to the reduction in dose needed because of the improved bioavailability (see Section 13.3.1.4). Prolongation of drug delivery may also minimize toxic effects through a decrease of plasma peak concentrations. In addition, side-effects such as gastric irritation and pain at an injection site can be overcome or reduced by the prodrug approach.

The induction of gastric or intestinal ulceration, bleeding or irritation is a recognized problem in patients treated with most non-steroidal anti-inflammatory drugs. The gastrointestinal lesions produced by these drugs are generally believed to be caused by two different mechanisms: a direct contact mechanism on the gastrointestinal mucosa and a generalized systemic action appearing after absorption, which can be demonstrated following parenteral dosing. The relative importance of these mechanisms may vary from drug to drug. Since the locally mediated ulcerogenic effect is unrelated to the anti-inflammatory activity, it should be feasible to reduce the former by the prodrug approach in such a manner that the prodrug passes intact through the stomach and, following absorption, is converted back to the parent drug by e.g. plasma esterases. Decreased gastrointestinal irritation with retainment of the desired anti-inflammatory activity has, in fact, been demonstrated for various prodrugs of non-steroidal anti-inflammatory agents. Thus, various prodrug esters and amides of these carboxylic acid agents have been shown to possess such properties, e.g. the guiacol ester (**13.61**) of ibuprofen (**13.60**) (Scheme 13.33). Following absorption, these derivatives are hydrolysed to give the parent acids. The exposure of the gastrointestinal mucosa to the active substances is reduced by giving them as prodrug derivatives resulting in low gastrointestinal irritation.

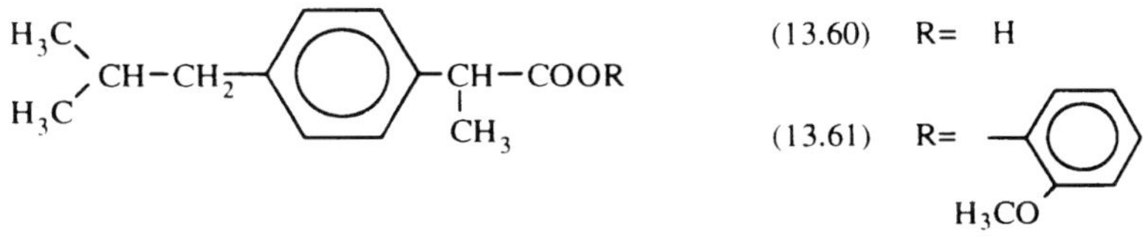

Scheme 13.33

Another type of local toxicity is tissue irritation and pain sometimes produced upon intramuscular administration of injection preparations of poorly water-soluble drugs. These problems may be overcome by transforming the drugs into water-soluble prodrugs, which can revert to the parent drug once in the body. There are many examples showing the use of this approach as discussed in Section 13.3.5.

13.3.4 Prolonged duration of action

Prolonging the duration of action of a drug can, in principle, be done in two ways:

1. Through sustained delivery of the prodrug form to the systemic circulation; or
2. Through design of prodrugs possessing a slow conversion rate to the parent drug in the organism.

The use of the first method to prolong the duration of action has been very extensive, especially in the area of hormonal steroids and neuroleptics. Virtually all long-acting steroids and neuroleptics are prodrugs given in an oil vehicle by the intramuscular route. These prodrugs are generally highly lipophilic esters, which are dissolved in an oil vehicle (e.g. sesame oil) and exhibit a sustained-release profile due to their high oil/water partition coefficients and a subsequent slow release from the injection site. After entry into the bloodstream the prodrug ester is in general rapidly hydrolysed. Thus, the selection of a combination of a lipophilic prodrug and an oil vehicle enables one to control the duration of action. By increasing the lipophilicity and hence the oil/water partition coefficients of the prodrug the rate of release from the vehicle to the bloodstream is decreased, resulting in increased duration of action. This can be illustrated with fluphenazine (**13.62**). After intramuscular injection in a sesame oil vehicle the duration of action of this neuroleptic is 6–8 h, whereas the more lipophilic enanthate prodrug ester (**13.63**) and decanoate ester (**13.64**) show a duration of action of 1–2 and 3–4 weeks, respectively (Scheme 13.34). Clinically, depot neuroleptics possess several advantages over the short-acting oral forms, such as enhanced patient compliance, reduced relapse and rehospitalization rate and reduced and more efficient daily dosage.

The second method involving slow conversion of a prodrug to the parent drug to obtain sustained drug action has already been exemplified earlier with the prodrugs bambuterol (**13.45**) and dipivefrin (**13.32**).

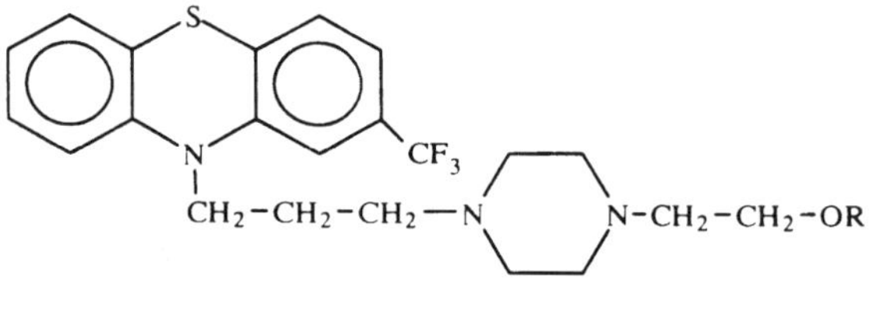

(13.62) R= H

(13.63) R= $-\overset{O}{\underset{\|}{C}}-C_6H_{13}$

(13.64) R= $-\overset{O}{\underset{\|}{C}}-C_9H_{19}$

Scheme 13.34

13.3.5 Improvement of drug formulation

The prodrug approach can be used to solve organoleptic problems. By preparing derivatives with greatly depressed aqueous solubility the bitter taste of several drugs can be masked. In the gastrointestinal tract or following absorption the derivatives are cleaved with the formation of the parent drug. Examples are the palmitate ester of chloramphenicol and metronidazole, both formulated in oral mixtures. *In vitro* stabilization has also been achieved in some cases. Methenamine (hexamethylentetramine), for instance, is a crystalline derivative which is hydrolysed to formaldehyde and ammonia in the urinary tract. It is frequently used as a formaldehyde prodrug for the purpose of disinfection.

The greatest utility of the prodrug approach in solving pharmaceutical formulation problems is probably to increase the aqueous solubility of drugs so that a convenient solution dosage form for intravenous or ophthalmic usage can be obtained.

Ester formation has long been recognized as an effective way to increase the aqueous solubility of drugs containing a hydroxy group (Drug-OH) with the aim of developing prodrug preparations suitable for parenteral administration. Two physico-chemical strategies can be employed to increase aqueous solubility: (1) introduction of an ionic or ionizable group by the pro-moiety and (2) derivatization in such a manner that the prodrug shows a decreased melting point. The most commonly used esters for increasing the aqueous solubility of hydroxy-containing agents are dicarboxylic acid hemiesters (notably hemisuccinates), sulphate esters, phosphate esters, α-amino or related short-chained aliphatic amino acid esters. However, the use of some of the ester types listed above are not without problems considering the ideal properties of such prodrugs. They should possess a high water-solubility at the pH of optimum stability, sufficient stability in aqueous solution to allow long-term storage (>2 years) of a ready to use solution and yet they should be converted quantitatively and rapidly *in vivo* to the parent drug.

Hemisuccinate esters have limited solution stability and, in addition, they show a slow and incomplete conversion *in vivo* to the parent drug. This has been reported for esters of various corticosteroids, chloramphenicol and metronidazole. Sulphate esters are, in contrast, rather stable in solution, but their deficiency is a high resistance to enzymatic hydrolysis *in vivo*. Phosphate esters as sodium salts are freely water-soluble, generally readily hydrolysed *in vivo* and more stable, allowing, in some cases, the formulation of solutions with practical shelf-lives. Vidarabine-5'-phosphate (**13.66**) as a sodium salt has thus a predicted shelf-life ($t_{10\%}$) of more than 10 years in aqueous solution at pH 6.8 and is used as a water-soluble prodrug of vidarabine (**13.65**) (Scheme 13.35). α-Amino or related short-chained aliphatic amino acid esters are in general readily hydrolysed by plasma enzymes but exhibit a poor stability in aqueous solution as exemplified with esters of metronidazole, corticosteroids and paracetamol. Thus, N,N-dimethylglycine esters of these drugs have a shelf-life of only a few days in aqueous solution at pH 3–5, and can therefore only be used in formulations to be reconstituted as solution prior to use (Table 13.2).

The major reason for the high instability of α-amino and short-chained aliphatic amino acid esters in aqueous solution at pH values affording their favourable water-solubility (i.e. pH 3–5) is the strongly electron-withdrawing effect of the protonated amino group. This protonation activates the ester linkage toward hydroxide ion attack, especially by intramolecular catalysis or assistance as a neighbouring group of ester hydrolysis. An effective and simple method of blocking the hydrolysis facilitating effect of the amino group

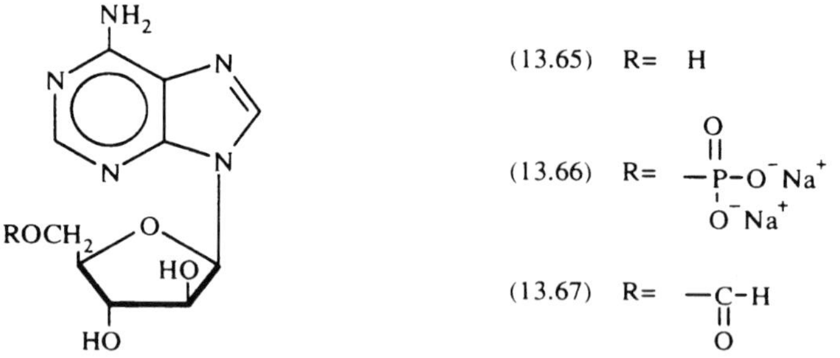

(13.65)   R=   H

(13.66)   R= $-\overset{\overset{\displaystyle O}{\|}}{\underset{\underset{\displaystyle O^-Na^+}{|}}{P}}-O^-Na^+$

(13.67)   R= $-\overset{}{\underset{\underset{\displaystyle O}{\|}}{C}}-H$

Scheme 13.35

and yet retain a rapid rate of enzymatic ester hydrolysis is to incorporate a phenyl group between the ester moiety and the amino group. By doing so the intramolecular catalytic reactions of the amino group are no longer possible for sterical reasons. Because of the requirement of a pK_a value greater than 5–6 for the amino group and for solubility reasons, the group is not directly attached to the phenyl nucleus but separated from this by an alkyl group, most often a methylene group. Such N-substituted 3- or 4-aminomethylbenzoate esters have been found to be readily soluble in water at weakly acidic pH values and to possess a very high stability in such solutions combined with a high susceptibility to undergo enzymatic hydrolysis in the presence of plasma (Table 13.2).

For drugs containing an NH-acidic group (e.g. amides, hydantoins, imides and imida-zoles) N-α-acyloxymethylation can be used to obtain prodrug derivatives. As described in Section 13.2.3.3, the regeneration of the parent drug from these derivatives occurs via a two-step reaction, enzymatic cleavage of the ester group followed by a spontaneous decomposition of the N-α-hydroxymethyl intermediate. By incorporation of an ionizable acyl group such as those described above, derivatives with increased water-solubility have been obtained as exemplified with the allupurinol prodrug (**13.29**).

A high crystal lattice energy of a crystalline compound as manifested in a high melting point results in poor solubility (in all solvents). Therefore, an approach to reduce this energy may result in improved solubility. An example of the usefulness of this approach in prodrug design concerns vidarabine (**13.65**), which has a low water-solubility (0.5 mg ml^{-1}). This is primarily due to the occurrence of intermolecular hydrogen bonding in the crystalline state as reflected by its melting point ($260\,^\circ$C). By esterification of the $5'$-hydroxy group this possibility to form hydrogen bonds is reduced, and further more, by choosing a polar acyl group like formyl, a vidarabine ester with greatly increased solubility (30 mg ml^{-1}) has been obtained. The $5'$-formate ester (**13.67**) is rapidly hydrolysed in human blood with a half-life of about 6–8 min, and it appears to be a useful parenteral delivery form of vidarabine, although the solution stability of this prodrug is rather limited (Scheme 13.35). Other examples of using this approach to increase solubilities of drugs is given in other sections of this chapter, e.g. the allupurinol prodrug (**13.30**) described in Section 13.3.1.3.

Table 13.2 Examples of water-soluble prodrug derivatives of drugs containing a hydroxyl group (Drug-OH) and their chemical and enzymatic reactivity.

Prodrug derivatives		Stability in solution	Enzymatic lability
Hemisuccinates	Drug–O–C(=O)–CH$_2$–CH$_2$–COO$^-$	Limited	Limited
Sulphates	Drug–O–SO$_3^-$	High	Poor
Phosphates	Drug–O–PO$_3^{--}$	High	High/Limited
α-Amino acid esters	Drug–O–C(=O)–CH–NH$_3^+$ | R	Limited	High
Dialkylaminoacetates	Drug–O–C(=O)–CH$_2$ –$\overset{+}{\underset{\text{R}}{\text{NH}}}$– R	Limited	High
Aminomethyl benzoate esters*	Drug–O–C(=O)–⟨benzene⟩–CH$_2$ –$\overset{+}{\underset{\text{R}}{\text{NH}}}$– R	High	High

*3 or 4 position.

FURTHER READING

Bundgaard, H. (Ed.) (1985) *Design of Prodrugs*. Amsterdam: Elsevier.

Bundgaard, H. (1989) The double prodrug concept and its application. *Adv. Drug Delivery Rev.*, **3**, 39–65.

Bundgaard, H. (1992) Means to enhance penetration. Prodrugs as a means to improve the delivery of peptide drugs. *Adv. Drug Delivery Rev.*, **8**, 1–38.

Oliyai, R. and Stella, V.J. (1993) Prodrugs of peptides and proteins for improved formulation and delivery. *Annu. Rev. Pharmacol. Toxicol.*, **32**, 521–544.

Roche, E.B. (Ed.) (1987) *Bioreversible Carriers in Drug Design. Theory and Application*. New York: Pergamon Press.

Sinkula, A.A. and Yalkowsky, S.H. (1975) Rationale for design of biologically reversible drug derivatives: Prodrugs. *J. Pharm. Sci.*, **64**, 181–210.

Sloan, K.B. (Ed.) (1992) *Prodrugs, Topical and Ocular Drug Delivery*. New York: Marcel Dekker Inc.

Stella, V.J., Mikkelsen, T.J. and Pipkin, J.D. (1980) Prodrugs: the control of drug delivery via bioreversible chemical modifications. In *Drug Delivery Systems. Characteristics and Biomedical Applications*, edited by R.L. Juliano, pp. 112–176. New York: Oxford University Press.

Stella, V.J., Charman, W.N.A. and Naringkar. V.H. (1985) Prodrugs. Do they have advantages in clinical practice? *Drugs*, **29**, 455–473.

Yalkowski, S.H. and Morozowich, W. (1980) A physical chemical basis for the design of orally active prodrugs. In *Drug Design, Vol IX*, edited by E.J. Ariëns, pp. 121–185. New York: Academic Press.

14. PEPTIDES AND PEPTIDOMIMETICS

KRISTINA LUTHMAN and ULI HACKSELL

CONTENTS

14.1 INTRODUCTION

A large number of endogenous peptides have been isolated and characterized (Table 14.1). These peptides are involved in a wide range of important physiological processes both

Table 14.1 Some important endogenous peptides.

Peptide	Amino acid sequence
Adrenocorticotropic hormone (ACTH)	SYSMEHFRWGKPVGKKRRPVKVYPNGAEDESAEAFPLEF
Angiotensin I (Ang I)	DRVYIHPFHL
Angiotensin II (Ang II)	DRVYIHPF
Bradykinin	RPPGFSPFR
Calcitonin (CT)	CGNLSTCMLGTYTQDFNKFHTFPQTAIGVGAP-amide
Calcitonin-gene-related-peptide (α-CGRP)	ACNTATCVTHRLAGLLSRSGGMVKSNFVPTNVGSKAF-amide
Cholecystokinin (CCK-33)	KAPSGRVSMIKNLQSLDPSHRISDRDY (SO$_3$H)MGWMDF-amide
Dynorphin B	YGGFLRRIRPKLKWDNQ
β-Endorphin	YGGFMTSEKSQTPLVTLFKNAIIKNAYKKGQ
Endothelins (ET-1)	CSCSSLMDKECVYFCHLDIIW
(Leu)Enkephalin	YGGFL
(Met)Enkephalin	YGGFM
Galanin	GWTLNSAGYLLGPHAIDNHRSFHDKYGLA-amide
Gastrin	pEGPWLEEEEEAY(SO$_3$H)GYGWMDF-amide
Gastrin-releasing peptide (GRP)	APVSVGGGTVLAKMYPRGNHWAVGHLM-amide
Growth hormone-releasing factor (GH-RF)	YADAIFTNSYRKVLGQLSARKLLQDIMSRQQGESNQERGARARL -amide
Gonadotropin-releasing hormone (Gn-RH)	pEHWSYGLRPG-amide
Neurokinin A (NKA)	HKTDSFVGLM-amide
Neurokinin B (NKB)	DMHDFFVGLM-amide
Neuropeptide Y (NPY)	YPSKPDNPGEDAPAEDMARYYSALRHYINLITRQRY-amide
Neurotensin (NT)	pELYQNKPRRPYIL
Oxytocin	CYIQNCPLG-amide
Somatostatin	AGCKNFFWKTFTSC
Substance P (SP)	RPKPQQFFGLM-amide
Thyrotropin-releasing hormone (TRH)	pEHP-amide
Vasoactive intestinal peptide (VIP)	HSDAVFTDNYTRLRKQMAVKKYLNSILN-amide
Vasopressin (AVP)	CYFQNCPRG-amide

centrally and peripherally and medicinal chemists have used them as interesting starting points in drug discovery efforts.

14.1.1 Peptide structure

Already in 1902 Hofmeister and Fischer independently reported that peptides consist of amino acids (Table 14.2) linked via amide bonds (peptide bonds). A peptide is defined as having a chain length between 2–50 amino acids whereas proteins include more than 50 amino acids. The different properties of the individual amino acids together with the

Table 14.2   The chemical name of the 21 common amino acids together with their 3 and 1 letter codes.

Alanine	Ala	A	Lysine	Lys	K
Arginine	Arg	R	Methionine	Met	M
Asparagine	Asn	N	Phenylalanine	Phe	F
Aspartic acid	Asp	D	Proline	Pro	P
Cystein	Cys	C	Serine	Ser	S
Glutamic acid	Glu	E	Threonine	Thr	T
Glutamine	Gln	Q	Tryptophan	Trp	W
Glycine	Gly	G	Tyrosine	Tyr	Y
Histidine	His	H	Valine	Val	V
Leucine	Leu	L			

Figure 14.1   Structures of L- and D-amino acids.

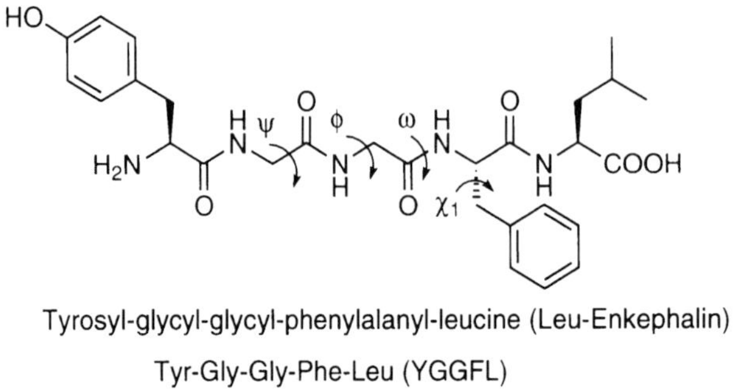

Tyrosyl-glycyl-glycyl-phenylalanyl-leucine (Leu-Enkephalin)

Tyr-Gly-Gly-Phe-Leu (YGGFL)

Figure 14.2   Structures of Leu-enkephalin. Also shown are the ψ, ϕ, ω and the χ torsion angles.

amino acid sequence (the primary structure) determine the physico-chemical properties of the peptides. All amino acids except glycine are chiral (Fig. 14.1). In Nature, the L-configuration is predominating but peptides from microorganisms and some opioid peptides isolated from the skin of amphibians also contain D-amino acids.

Peptides are very flexible and frequently adopt a large number of conformations in solution. This flexibility is caused by the rotation about single bonds within each amino acid. The torsions in the backbone of particular interest for peptide over-all conformations are the ψ, ϕ and ω angles (Fig. 14.2). Many combinations of ψ and ϕ angles are disallowed because of unfavourable steric interactions. The relationship between ψ, ϕ and

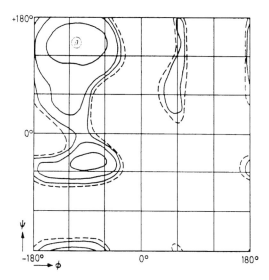

Figure 14.3   Ramachandran map (ϕ,ψ map) from Ramachandran *et al.*, *Biophys. J.*, 1966, **6**, 849–872.

energy is often visualized in Ramachandran maps (Fig. 14.3) in which the approximate areas of allowed ψ/ϕ angles can be identified. Short peptides exist in a multitude of conformations in solution whereas longer peptides may adopt stable secondary structures such as α-helices, β-sheets, or turns.

14.1.2 Solid phase peptide synthesis

A major milestone in peptide chemistry was achieved in 1953 with the isolation, charac-terization and synthesis of the peptide hormones oxytocin and vasopressin (*J. Am. Chem. Soc.*, 1953, 75, 4879 and 4880). Another major step in the synthesis of biologically active peptides and peptide analogues was the introduction of the solid phase synthetic method by Merrifield in 1963 (*J. Am. Chem. Soc.*, 1963, 85, 2149). In this method, the peptide is synthesized from the *C*-terminal to the *N*-terminal end. The *C*-terminal amino acid is linked to an insoluble polystyrene based polymer and the peptide is then conveniently synthesized by sequential coupling of properly protected amino acids. The most commonly used *N*-terminal protecting groups are the acid labile *tert*-butoxycarbonyl (Boc) and the base labile 9-fluorenylmethoxycarbonyl (Fmoc) moieties. The carboxylic acid function has to be activated before coupling. Protecting groups and coupling reagents are improved continuously.

The synthesized peptide is cleaved from the polymer resin and fully deprotected by HF- or TFA-treatment. The synthesis may be performed either by using single amino acid couplings or the fragment condensation technique. The latter strategy is mainly used in the synthesis of longer peptides and small proteins, but also in the synthesis of modified peptides using nonpeptidic building blocks.

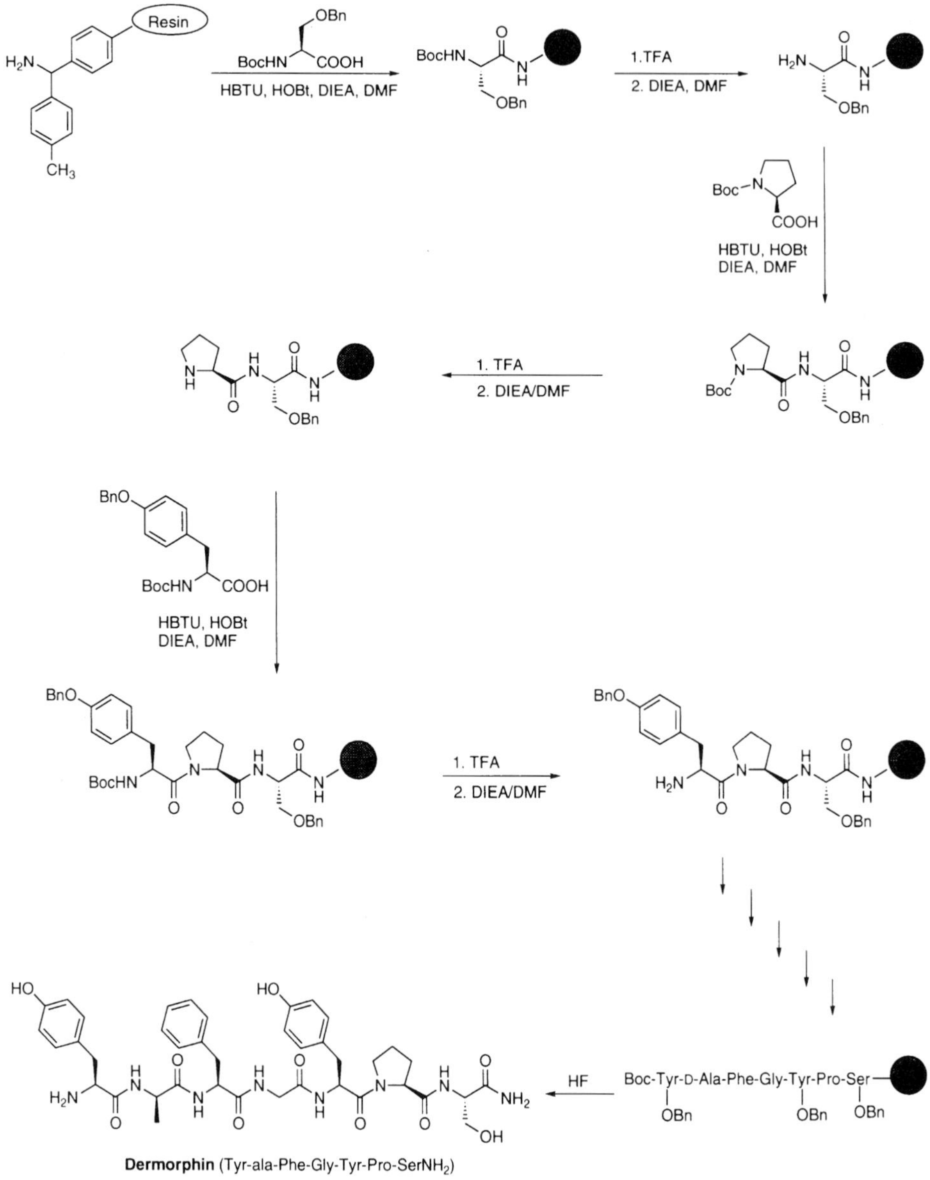

Figure 14.4   Solid phase synthesis of the amphibian heptapeptide dermorphin. HBTU: 2-(1H-benzotriazol-1-yl)-1,1,3,3-tetramethyluronium hexafluorophosphate; HOBt: 1-hydroxybenzotriazole; DIEA: diisopropylethylamine; DMF: dimethylformamide; TFA: trifluoroacetic acid; ●: polystyrene resin with a specific spacer for synthesis of C-terminal amidated peptides.

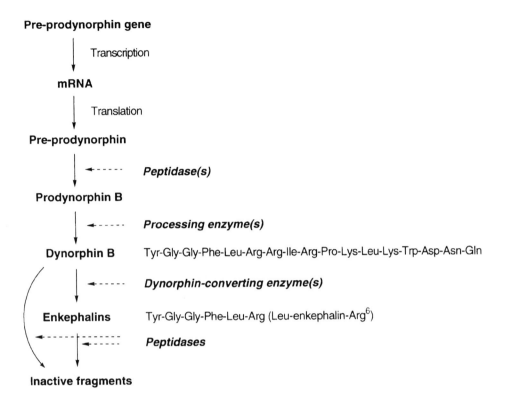

Pre-prodynorphin gene

  | Transcription

mRNA

  | Translation

Pre-prodynorphin

  | ← - - - - - *Peptidase(s)*

Prodynorphin B

  | ← - - - - - *Processing enzyme(s)*

Dynorphin B   Tyr-Gly-Gly-Phe-Leu-Arg-Arg-Ile-Arg-Pro-Lys-Leu-Lys-Trp-Asp-Asn-Gln

  | ← - - - - - *Dynorphin-converting enzyme(s)*

Enkephalins   Tyr-Gly-Gly-Phe-Leu-Arg (Leu-enkephalin-Arg^6)

  ← - - - - - ← - - - - - *Peptidases*

Inactive fragments

Figure 14.5   Flowchart showing the biosynthesis of dynorphin B and its breakdown.

The peptide synthesis of today has been automated. However, manual solid phase synthesis of shorter peptides can easily be performed in plastic syringes. Although the synthesis of a peptide is rather trivial a considerable amount of time has to be spent on its purification, usually using reversed phase HPLC or electrophoresis techniques. Synthesized peptides are characterized by amino acid analysis, mass spectrometry, and NMR-spectroscopy. Sequence analyses can be performed by Edman degradation and mass spectrometry (FAB-MS and MS-MS). Production of endogeneous peptides and proteins may also be achieved using genetic engineering techniques.

14.1.3 Biosynthesis of peptides

Peptide precursors are biosynthesized on the ribosome as higher molecular forms (pre-propeptides) (Fig. 14.5). During the transport through the endoplasmatic reticulum to the Golgi apparatus, an *N*-terminal signal peptide of 20–30 amino acids is cleaved off to generate a propeptide. This cleavage is catalyzed by specific peptidases. The propeptides are further processed to their active forms and structural modifications like acetylation,

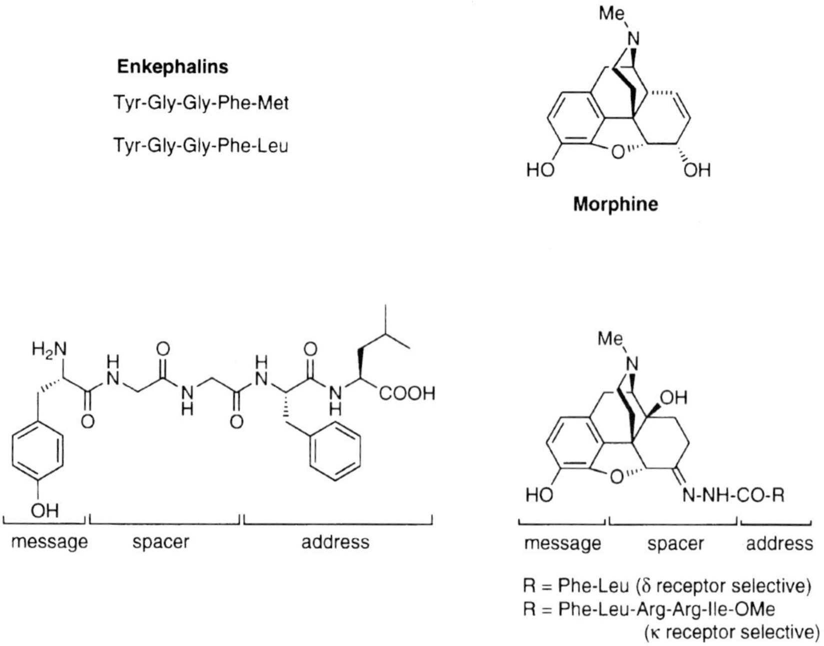

Figure 14.6 Structural relationship between the enkephalins and the peptidomimetic morphine. Also illustrated is the concept of message and address parts of peptides.

glycosylation, sulphation, phosphorylation, or *C*-terminal amidation may occur. The peptides are stored in synaptic vesicles and are released into the environment by appropriate stimuli. The transportation to the site of action is diffusion controlled. The peptides act mainly as neurotransmitters, neuromodulators, and hormones, thus influencing a series of vital functions such as metabolism, immune defense, digestion, respiration, sensitivity to pain, reproduction, behavior, and electrolyte levels. The breakdown of a peptide *in vivo* is frequently less specific than that of small molecule transmitters since it involves peptidases of low specificity. The peptide fragments formed on peptide degradation may be inactive or display biological activity; e.g. dynorphin B produces the potent hexapeptide Leu-enkephalin-Arg^6 on degradation.

14.1.4 Peptide-receptor interactions

Frequently, peptide receptors belong to the G-protein coupled receptor super family. In many peptides only a small number of amino acids (4–8) are responsible for the recognition and activation of the receptor (the "message" part). These important amino acids can be identified by amino acid substitutions which should lead to pronounced changes in the biological response. The part of the peptide not directly involved in the binding of the ligand to the receptor (the "address" part) serves to fix the important amino acids in a proper spatial arrangement and confers additional affinity and selectivity for the receptor. The concept of address and message parts in enkephalin is illustrated in Figure 14.6.

14.2 STRATEGIES FOR THE DEVELOPMENT OF PEPTIDOMIMETICS

The peptide receptors and the enzymes involved in the biosynthesis and degradation of peptides have become attractive targets in drug discovery research. Most biologically active peptides display receptor affinities (K_D) in the nM – pM range ($10^{-9} - 10^{-12}$ M). However, peptides are in themselves not suitable as drugs due to their (i) low oral bioavailability, (ii) rapid degradation by endogenous peptidases, (iii) rapid excretion through liver and kidneys, and (iv) side effects due to their interaction with several different receptors (lack of selectivity). Hence, current research in the field mainly deals with the challenging task of circumventing these limitations; Orally effective and metabolically stable analogs of peptidic hormones, neurotransmitters, and neuromulators are needed and could lead to drugs with useful pharmacological/therapeutical profiles. These compounds are often referred to as "peptide mimetics" or "peptidomimetics".

According to Morgan and Gainor, peptidomimetics can be defined as *"structures which serve as appropriate substitutes for peptides in interactions with receptors and enzymes. The mimics must possess not only affinity, but also efficacy or substrate function."* The most well-known peptidomimetic is probably morphine which is an agonist on opiate receptors (Fig. 14.6). The research on peptidomimetics deals with peptides and proteins as lead compounds for the discovery of other classes of compounds through a variety of research strategies. Since peptide-receptor antagonists do not interact with receptors in the same way as the endogenous peptide they should not be regarded as peptidomimetics. However, all ligands for peptide receptors or peptide degrading enzymes are termed peptidomimetics in the current literature.

In general, a successfully designed peptidomimetic should be metabolically stable, have good (preferably oral) bioavailability, have high receptor affinity and selectivity, and have minimal side effects. However, today it is not known how to rationally convert (*de novo*) a peptide into a nonpeptide while maintaining the biological activity. There is no strategy which guarantees the discovery of ligands with high affinity, efficacy, and specificity. In general, the discovery of novel ligands for peptide receptors has not been based on a thorough understanding of the key-intermolecular interactions. Instead, receptor-based random screening has been the most rewarding method. Below follows an outline of different strategies used in the development of peptidomimetics.

14.2.1 Development of peptidomimetics by design

A design process which is based on the primary structure of a peptide and insight into its biological activity may be used for the development of peptidomimetics. Such a process requires a close collaboration between specialists from the areas of chemistry, NMR-spectroscopy, crystallography, molecular modelling, and biology. In 1980, Farmer described how to convert a peptide into a peptidomimetic. He defined a set of rules (The Farmer's rules) for this process:

(a) *"The design of nonpeptidic analogs of a bioactive peptide should start from the simplest conceivable structure that might possibly have specific peptidomimetic activity."* Large parts of the peptides can be removed without loss of activity and determination of the smallest active fragment can be performed by a stepwise cleavage of amino acids from both the *N*- and the *C*-terminal ends of the natural ligand. Hydrophobic residues are usually important for receptor binding but polar residues are likely to be essential for intrinsic activity.

(b) *"A nonpeptidic analog of a bioactive peptide should not occupy space outside that believed to be occupied by the peptide itself."* In addition, the functional groups should be maintained during the first stages of the conversion of a peptide into a nonpeptide.

(c) *"Conformational flexibility should be maximized until lead activity is discovered in a nonpeptidic structure."* At least some conformational flexibility should be retained in the first set of mimetic compounds. Potency and selectivity may then be improved by introduction of conformational constraints.

(d) *"The design of nonpeptidic peptidomimetics should not rely heavily on mimicking the topology of backbone peptide bonds, especially where there are regular secondary structures."* Analogs of secondary structures such as α-helices or β-sheets are unlikely to exhibit selectivity. Analogs mimicking tertiary structures should be more useful.

Experimental studies of designed drugs should be performed continuously during the design process and should involve biological activity, absorption, first-pass metabolism, CNS-penetration (if important), and water solubility. In addition, structure-activity relationships should be deduced. Several examples are available in the literature which demonstrate that Farmer's rules can be successfully employed.

14.2.1.1 Amino acid manipulations

Following the identification of the smallest active fragment of a peptide the role of each amino acid should be determined. Initially, a systematic replacement of the side chains with methyl groups, i.e., exchange of one amino acid at the time for alanine (Ala-scan), can be performed. This should allow the identification of side chains of importance either for the receptor interaction or for folding of the peptide into its bioactive conformation. A systematic replacement of L-amino acids with D-amino acids may be informative in the initial exploration of structural requirements for receptor recognition and binding. A more elaborate strategy may also involve the systematic introduction of conformational constraints by, e.g., *N*- or α-methylations (the conformational flexibility of the modified peptide could change dramatically due to the limited rotation around the ψ/ϕ bonds). Several unnatural amino acids which differ in physico-chemical parameters compared to the natural amino acids have been designed and synthesized. Some examples are shown in Figure 14.7. The common feature of these structures is the conformationally constrained side chains. The amino acids **Tic** and **Aib** are frequently used as replacements for Phe and Ala, respectively.

14.2.1.2 Peptide backbone modifications

In large peptides the backbone serves as a structural matrix and its conformation positions the side chains in defined spatial positions which allow optimal interactions with the enzyme or receptor protein. The amide bonds themselves may also be of importance for binding

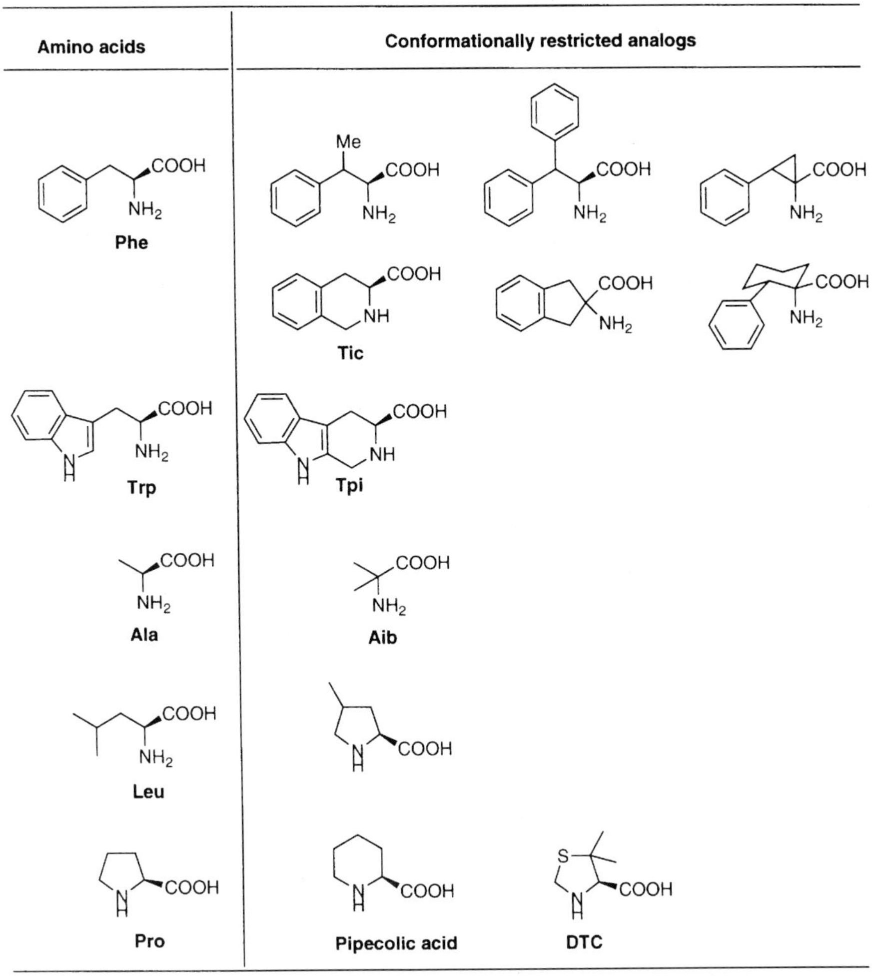

Figure 14.7   Some unnatural amino acids which impose conformational constraints when introduced in peptides.

to enzymes or receptors. Several amide bond isosteres have been designed, synthesized, and introduced into peptide analogs. These fragments are mainly used to enhance the stability towards protease degradation but may also be useful tools in studies of structural mimicry. An appropriate amide bond replacement should, e.g., exhibit similar geometrical, conformational, electrostatical, and hydrogen bonding properties as the amide bond itself. Although a large number of amide isosteres are known "*a convincing imitation of the amide bond in the ground state has not yet been achieved*" according to Giannis and Kolter. Some examples of amide isosteres are shown in Figure 14.8.

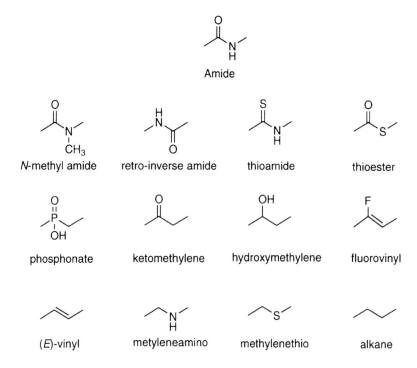

Figure 14.8   Some amide isosteres.

Retro-inverse isosteres not only reverse the direction of the peptide but also have the L-amino acids exchanged for D-amino acids. Incorporation of a retro-inverse isostere results in a pseudopeptide with a similar topology as the native peptide, however, it is no longer sensitive to protease degradation.

14.2.1.3 Di(oligo)peptidomimetics

Replacement of larger structural moieties with di- or tripeptidomimetic structures are of interest since these modified peptides bridge the gap between peptide analogues and nonpeptidic structures. Several lactams have been synthesized as bridging elements to stabilize certain backbone conformations. These mimetic structures are based on side chain to side chain, or side chain to backbone cyclizations (Fig. 14.9). Mimetic moieties involving the peptide bond, such as azole-derived mimetics, have also been successfully used as dipeptide replacements. It should be noted, however, that the incorporation of a specific di(oligo)peptidomimetic moiety into different peptides may affect the biological activity differently.

14.2.1.4 Local or global conformational constraints

The bioactive conformation of a peptide is the conformation recognized by and/or interacting with the binding domain(s) of a receptor or enzyme. Unfortunately, the bioactive conformation of a peptide may be poorly populated in the absence of the

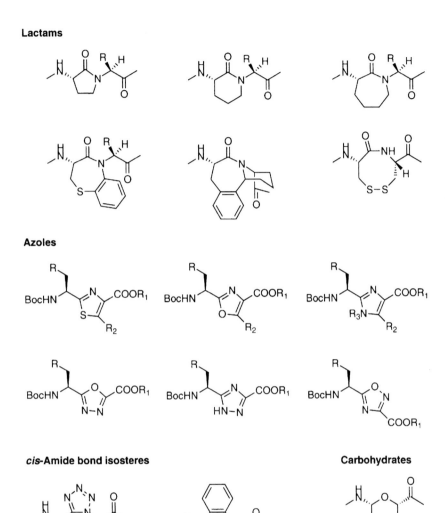

Figure 14.9 Some dipeptidomimetics.

receptor and, consequently, it may be quite different from conformations observed by e.g. NMR-spectroscopy or X-ray crystallography. Molecular mechanics calculations and molecular dynamic studies of isolated peptides have also been performed in attempts to deduce bioactive conformations of peptides but, in general, these studies are noninformative. Recently, computational studies have been performed in which the peptide has been allowed to interact with the receptor structure. However, bioactive conformations are probably best deduced by use of conformationally restricted mimetics.

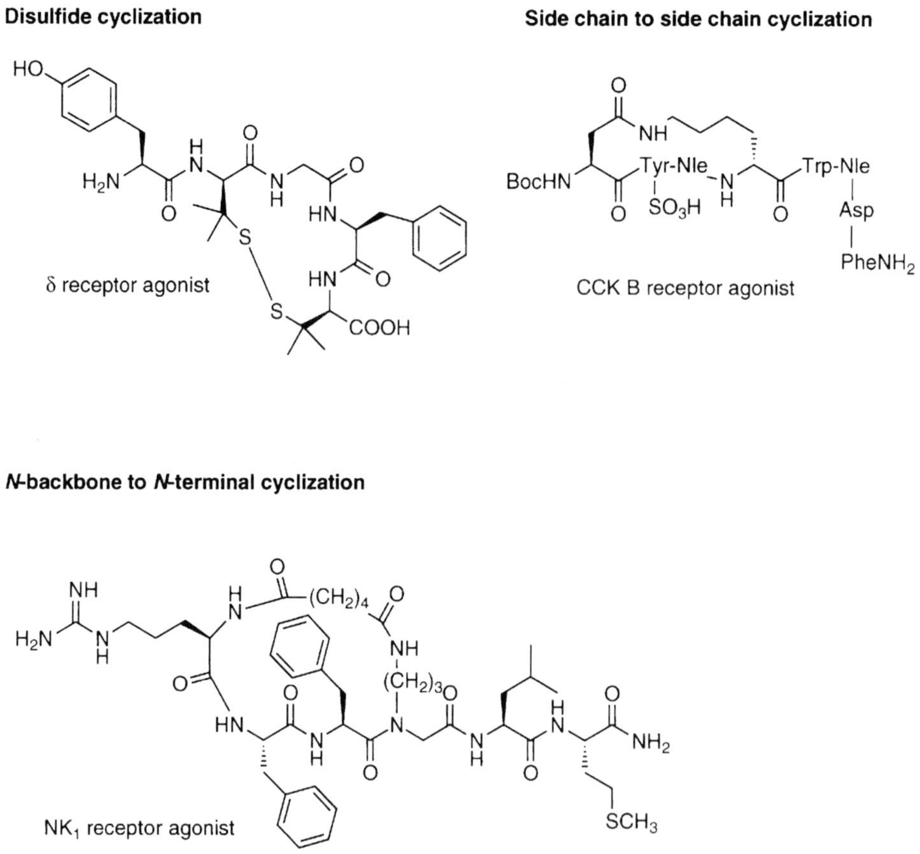

Disulfide cyclization   **Side chain to side chain cyclization**

δ receptor agonist   CCK B receptor agonist

N-backbone to N-terminal cyclization

NK$_1$ receptor agonist

Figure 14.10   Some peptides which have been cyclized to restrict global conformational mobility.

Introduction of conformational constraints aims to produce either local or global conformational effects. Local conformational constraints could include the replacement of the amide moiety by isosteres (methylamino, ketomethylene, inverse amide, etc) and introduction of amino acid residues/mimics which restrict the conformational flexibility. A disadvantage with these approaches is that the introduction of local constraints may have unpredictable effects on the over-all conformational equilibrium. Global constraints may involve cyclic disulfide bridges. Alternatively, side chains not involved in the receptor recognition/interaction could be connected by cyclization. Backbone to backbone cyclizations provide another type of global conformational constraints (Fig. 14.10).

14.2.1.5 Mimics of peptide secondary structures

There are three classes of secondary structure elements of a peptide: α-helices, β-sheets, and turns or loops. A secondary structure mimetic is a structural moiety that, when incorporated into a peptide, forces the peptide to adopt a specific conformation.

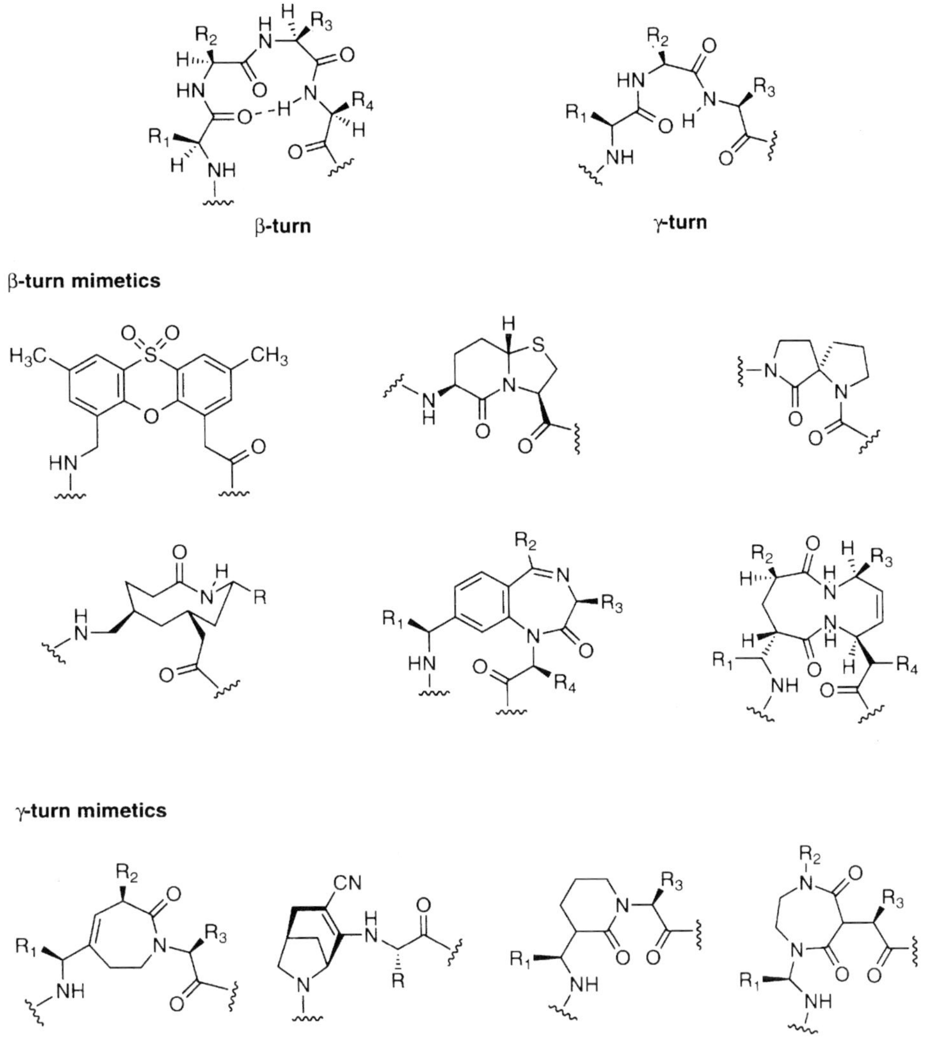

Figure 14.11 The structures of β- and γ-turns (top). Also shown are some β- and γ-turn mimetics.

14.2.1.6 β- and γ-turn mimetics

Turns and loops are important conformational characteristics of peptides and proteins. A β-turn is formed from four amino acids and is stabilized by a hydrogen bond between the first and the fourth amino acid. A γ-turn is formed in a similar way from three amino acids (Fig. 14.11). Large numbers of turn mimetics have been designed and synthesized but most have resulted in inactivity when incorporated into peptides. A selection of turn mimetics are shown in Figure 14.11.

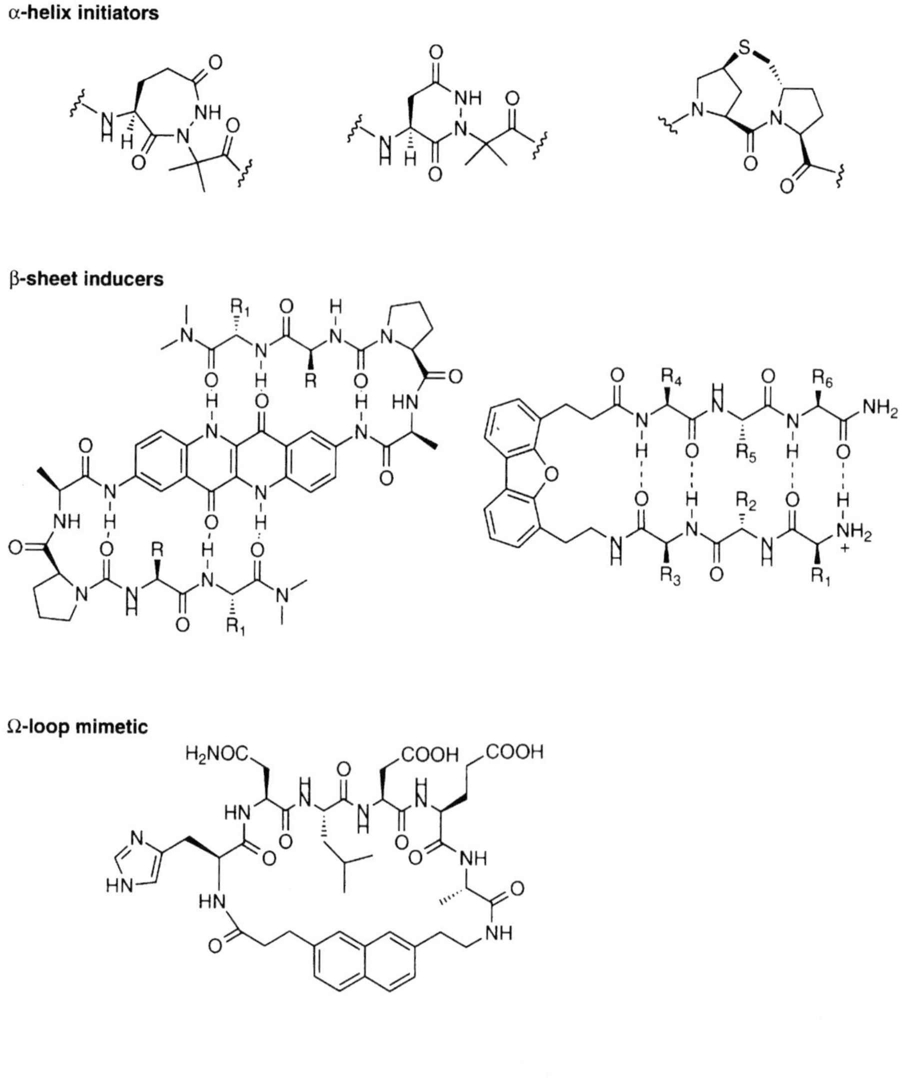

α-helix initiators

β-sheet inducers

Ω-loop mimetic

Figure 14.12   Structures mimicking various aspects of peptide secondary structure.

14.2.1.7 α-helix, β-sheet, and Ω-loop mimetics

α-Helix and β-sheet motifs are well characterized structural features of peptides and proteins. Some examples of α-helix initiators and β-sheet inducers are shown in Figure 14.12. Recently, an Ω-loop mimetic was described (Fig. 14.12). Ω-loops are large, conformationally stabilized curves in peptides involving 6–16 amino acid residues, and are believed to play an important role in biological recognition.

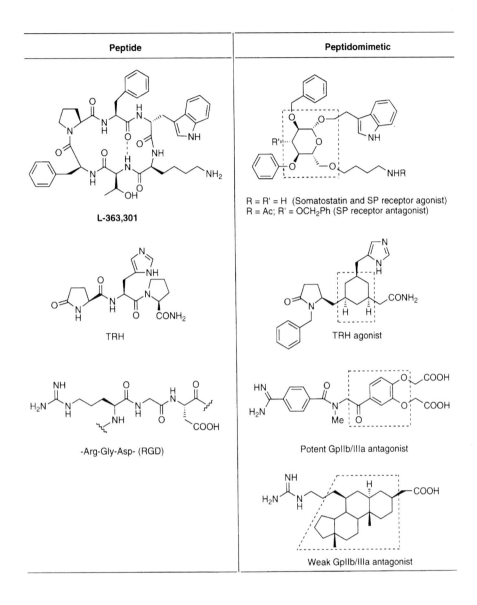

Figure 14.13 Some examples of scaffold-based peptidomimetics.

14.2.1.8 Scaffold mimetics

Topological constraints may also provide information about the bioactive conformation; important amino acid side chains are positioned in proper relative positions onto a molecular template (scaffold), that is, in agreement with the bioactive topology. The optimal molecular scaffold appears to be a highly fuctionalized small (5–7-membered) ring of defined stereochemistry. In Figure 14.13 some interesting scaffold mimetics are shown.

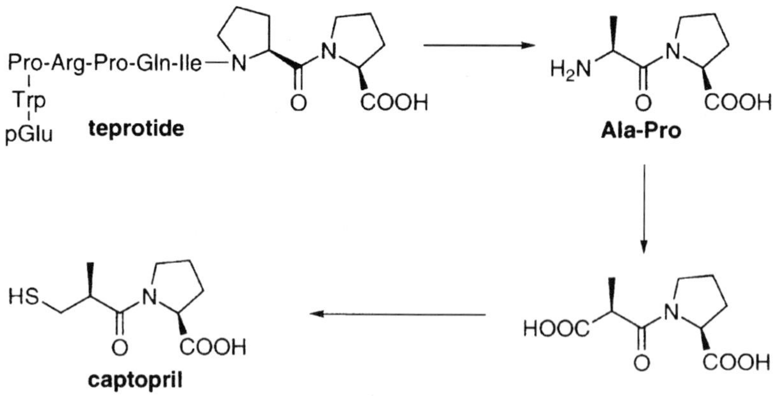

Figure 14.14   The process leading to the discovery of captopril.

The strategies described above are empirical and time consuming. Novel combinatorial chemistry techniques that permit the controlled synthesis of peptide libraries in which various mimetic moieties are introduced should lead to a more efficient research process.

14.3 SOME EXAMPLES OF DRUG DISCOVERY

14.3.1 Angiotensin converting enzyme (ACE) inhibitors

Access to the detailed structure of the binding site of a peptide receptor or an enzyme active site would make it possible to use structure-based design technology in attempts to generate efficient agonists/substrates or antagonists/inhibitors. Unfortunately, our knowledge about the structure of ligand binding sites on receptors is very limited. However, structures of several active sites of enzymes have been obtained. In addition, their mechanisms of action have been deduced and this information can also be used in the design process as examplified by the discovery of the angiotensin converting enzyme (ACE) inhibitors (Fig. 14.14).

The ACE-inhibitors were discovered using the nonapeptide teprotide, that was isolated from snake venom, as the molecular lead. The design started from the weak inhibitor Ala-Pro, a modified C-terminal fragment of teprotide. ACE is known to be a metalloprotease with a Zn^{2+} ion in the active site and a carboxylic acid group was introduced to increase the coordination of the inhibitor to the enzyme. The successful result of this modification led to the replacement of the carboxylic acid group by a thiol function which coordinates even stronger to Zn. The resulting compound, captopril, has been used as an orally active antihypertensive drug for several years.

14.3.2 Peptide receptor ligands from receptor based screening

Extensive efforts have been put into peptide-receptor based screening of small molecules, natural products, or microbial broths. Although identified leads may show quite weak

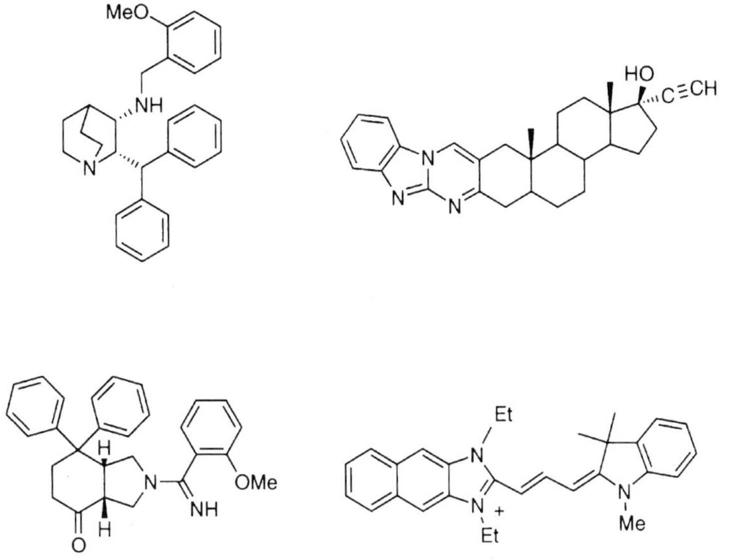

Figure 14.15 Structures of some substance P (NK1)-receptor antagonists.

Asp-Tyr(SO$_3$H)-Met-Gly-Trp-Met-Asp-Phe-NH$_2$ (CCK-8)

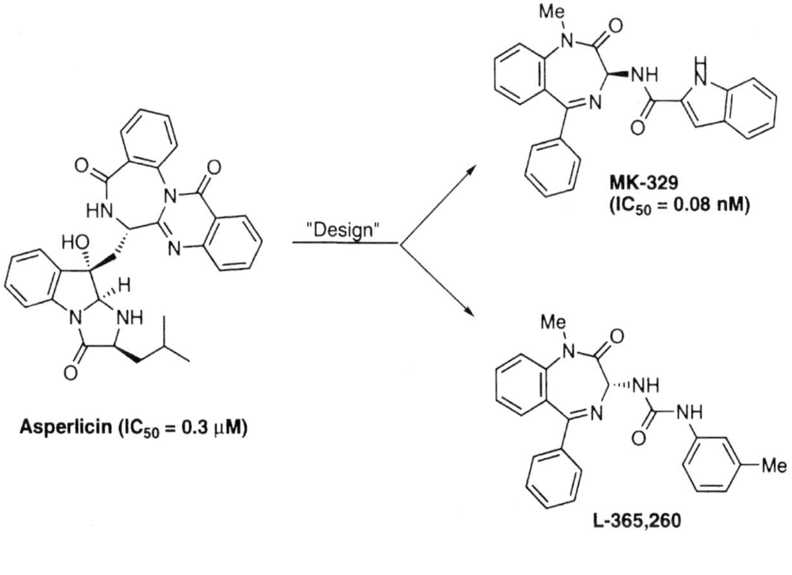

MK-329
(IC$_{50}$ = 0.08 nM)

"Design"

Asperlicin (IC$_{50}$ = 0.3 μM)

L-365,260

Figure 14.16 Peptide-receptor ligands from receptor-based random screening. Two CCK receptor antagonists have been developed from asperlicin.

Asp-Arg-Val-Tyr-Ile-His-Pro-Phe (Ang II)

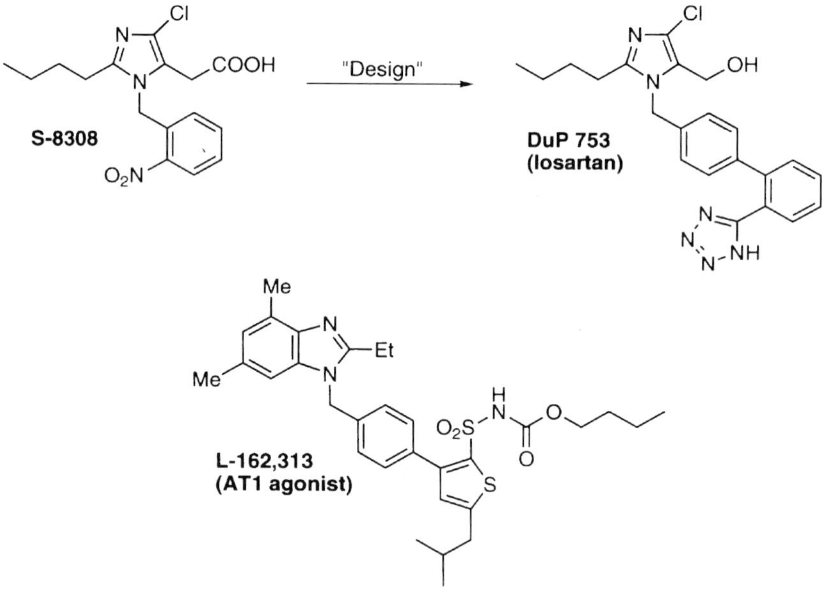

Figure 14.17   The AT$_1$-antagonist DuP753 was developed from S-8308. Recently a structurally related nonpeptidic agonist was also discovered.

affinity structural optimization may improve both affinity and selectivity. Most frequently, receptor antagonists have been discovered using this approach. Antagonists for a particular receptor may exhibit a large structural diversity as exemplified by the substance P (NK$_1$)-receptor antagonists (Fig. 14.15).

An example of discovery of nonpeptidic peptide-receptor ligands by receptor based screening followed by design is provided by the CCK antagonists MK-329 and L-365,260 (Fig. 14.16) that were developed from Asperlicin (cf. Chapter 1). These antagonists contain the benzodiazepine structure. The benzodiazepine moiety is also present in other nonpeptidic peptide-receptor ligands, e.g., trifluadom, which is a κ receptor agonist with effective analgesic activity but without side effects like respiratory depression or addictive potential. The benzodiazepine moiety has been termed a "priviledged structure" for peptide receptor affinity.

The angiotensin II receptor (AT1) antagonist DuP753 (Losartan, Fig. 14.17) was developed from S-8308 and is based on an imidazole moiety. The design was carried out using computer modelling and it has been suggested that the side chains of amino acids Tyr, Ile, and Phe in AngII are mimicked correctly by DuP753. Recently, also an AT1 receptor agonist, L-162,313 was discovered (Fig. 14.17).

REFERENCES

Adang, A.E.P., Hermkens, P.H.H., Linders, J.T.M., Ottenheijm, H.C.J. and van Staveren, C.J. (1994) Case histories of peptidomimetics: progression from peptide to drugs. *Recl. Trav. Chim. Pays-Bas*, **113**, 63–78.

Benz, H. (1994) The role of solid-phase fragment condensation (SPFC) in peptide synthesis. *Synthesis*, 337–358.

Borg, S., Estenne-Bouhtou, G., Luthman, K., Csöregh, I., Hesselink, W. and Hacksell, U. (1995) Synthesis of 1,2,4-oxadiazole, 1,3,4-oxadiazole, and 1,2,4-triazole-derived dipeptidomimetics. *J. Org. Chem.*, **60**, 3112–3120.

Boyle, S., Guard, S., Higginobottom, M., Horwell, D.C., Howson, W., McKnight, A.T, Martin, K., Pritchard, M.C., O'Toole, J., Raphy, J., Rees, D.C., Roberts, E., Watling, K.J., Woodruff, G.N. and Hughes, J. (1994) Rational design of high affinity tachykinin NK₁ receptor antagonists. *Bioorg. Med. Chem.*, **2**, 357–370.

Chorev, M. and Goodman, M. (1993) A dozen years of retro-inverso peptidomimetics. *Acc. Chem. Res.*, **26**, 266–273.

Duncia, J.V., Carini, D.J., Chiu, A.T., Johnson, A.L., Price, W.A., Wong, P.C., Wexler, R.R. and Timmermans, P.B.M.W.M. (1992) The discovery of DuP753, a potent, orally active nonpeptide angiotensin II receptor antagonist. *Med. Res. Rev.*, **12**, 149–191.

Evans, B.E., Bock, M.G., Rittle, K.E., DiPardo, R.M., Whitter, W.L., Veber, D.F., Anderson, P.S. and Freidinger, R.M. (1986) Design of potent, orally effective, nonpeptidal antagonists of the peptide hormone cholecystokinin. *Proc. Natl. Acad. Sci. USA*, **83**, 4918–4922.

Farmer, P.S. (1980) Bridging the gap between bioactive peptides and nonpeptides: some perspectives in design. *Drug Design*, Vol X, pp. 119–143.

Gallop, M.A., Barrett, R.W., Dower, W.J., Fodor, S.P.A. and Gordon, E.M. (1994) Applications of combinatorial technologies to drug discovery. 1. Background and peptide combinatorial libraries. *J. Med. Chem.*, **37**, 1233–1251.

Gante, J. (1994) Peptidomimetics — tailored enzyme inhibitors. *Angew. Chem. Int. Ed. Engl.*, **33**, 1699–1720.

Giannis, A. and Kolter, T. (1993) Peptidomimetics for receptor ligands — Discovery, development, and medical perspectives. *Angew. Chem. Int. Ed. Engl.*, **32**, 1244–1267.

Gilon, C., Halle, D., Chorev, M., Selinger, Z. and Byk, G. (1991) Backbone cyclization: a new method for conferring conformational constraint on peptides. *Biopolymers*, **31**, 745–750.

Golic Grdadolnik, S., Mierke, D.F., Byk, G., Zeltser, I., Gilon, C. and Kessler, H. (1994) Comparison of the conformation of active and nonactive backbone cyclic analogs of substance P as a tool to elucidate features of the bioactive conformation: NMR and molecular dynamics in DMSO and water. *J. Med Chem.*, **37**, 2145–2152.

Gordon, E.M., Barrett, R.W., Dower, W.J., Fodor, S.P.A. and Gallop, M.A. (1994) Applications of combinatorial technologies to drug discovery. 2. Combinatorial organic synthesis, library screening strategies, and future directions. *J. Med. Chem.*, **37** 1385–1401.

Graf von Roedern, E. and Kessler, H. (1994) A sugar amino acid as a novel peptidomimetic. *Angew. Chem. Int. Ed. Engl.*, **33**, 687–689.

Hirschmann, R. (1991) Medicinal chemistry in the golden age of biology: Lessons from steroid and peptide research. *Angew. Chem. Int. Ed. Engl.*, **30**, 1278–1301.

Hirschmann, R., Nicolaou, K.C., Pietranico, S., Leahy, E.M., Salvino, J., Arison, B., Cichy, M.A., Spoors, P.G., Shakespeare, W.C., Sprengler, P.A., Hamley, P., Smith III, A.B., Reisine, T., Raynor, K., Maechler, L., Donaldson, C., Vale, W., Freidinger, R.M., Cascieri, M.R. and Strader, C.D. (1993) *De novo* design and synthesis of somatostatin non-peptide peptidomimetics utilizing β-D-glucose as a novel scaffolding. *J. Am. Chem. Soc.*, **115**, 12550–12568.

Houghten, R.A. (1985) General method for the rapid solid-phase synthesis of large numbers of peptides: Specificity of antigen-antibody interaction at the level of individual amino acids. *Proc. Natl. Acad. Sci. USA*, **82**, 5131–5135.

Houghten, R.A., Pinilla, C., Blondelle, S.E., Appel, J.R., Dooley, C.T. and Cuervo, J.H. (1991) Generation and use of synthetic peptide combinatorial libraries for basic research and drug discovery. *Nature*, **354**, 84–86.

Howson, W. (1995) Rational design of tachykinin receptor antagonists. *Drug News Perspect.*, **8**, 97–103.

Hruby, V.J. (1982) Conformational restrictions of biologically active peptides via amino acid side chain groups. *Life Sci.*, **31**, 189–199.

Hruby, V.J., Al-Obeidi, F. and Kazmierski, W. (1990) Emerging approaches in the molecular design of receptor-selective peptide ligands: conformational, topographical and dynamic considerations. *Biochem. J.*, **268**, 249–262.

Hruby, V.J. (1993) Conformational and topographical considerations in the design of biologically active peptides. *Biopolymers*, **33**, 1073–1082.

Höllt, V. (1986) Opioid peptide processing and receptor selectivity. *Ann. Rev. Pharmacol. Toxicol.*, **26**, 59–77.

Hölzemann, G. (1991) Peptide conformation mimetics part 1 and 2. *Kontakte (Darmstadt)*, 3–12 and 55–63.

Kahn, M. (1993), Peptide secondary structure mimetics: recent advances and future challenges. *Synlett*, 821–826.

Kessler, H. (1982) Conformation and biological activity of cyclic peptides. *Angew. Chem. Int. Ed. Engl.*, **21**, 512–523.

Kivlighn, S.D., Huckle, W.R., Zingaro, G.J., Rivero, R.A., Lotti, V.J., Chang, R.S.L., Schorn, T.W., Kevin, N., Johnson Jr, R.G., Greenlee, W.J. and Siegl, P.K.S (1995) Discovery of L-162,313: a nonpeptide that mimics the biological actions of angiotensin II. *Am. J. Physiol.*, R820–823.

Kreil, G. (1994) Peptides containing a *D*-amino acid from frogs and molluscs. *J. Biol. Chem.*, **269**, 10967–10970.

Liskamp, R.M.J. (1994) Conformationally restricted amino acids and dipeptides, (non)peptidomimetics and secondary structure mimetics. *Recl. Trav. Chim. Pays-Bas*, **113**, 1–19.

Morgan, B.A. and Gainor, J.A. (1989) Approaches to the discovery of non-peptide ligands for peptide receptors and peptidases. *Ann. Rep. Med. Chem.*, **24**, 243–252.

Olson, G.L., Bolin, D.R., Bonner, M.P., Bös, M., Cook, C.M., Fry, D.C., Graves, B.J., Hatada, M., Hill, D.E., Kahn, M., Madison, V.S., Rusiecki, V.K., Sarabu, R., Sepinwall, J., Vincent, G.P. and Voss,'M.E. (1993) Concepts and progress in the development of peptide mimetics. *J. Med. Chem.*, **36**, 3039–3049.

Ostresh, J.M., Husar, G.M., Blondelle, S.E., Dörner, B., Weber, P.A. and Houghten, R.A. (1994) "Libraries from libraries": Chemical transformation of combinatorial libraries to extend the range and repertoire of chemical diversity. *Proc. Natl. Acad. Sci. USA*, **91**, 11138–11142.

Ramachandran, G.N. and Sasisekharan, V. (1968) Conformation of polypeptides and proteins. *Adv. Prot. Chem.*, **23**, 283–437.

Saulitis, J., Mierke, D.F.‡Byk, G., Gilon, C. and Kessler, H. (1992) Conformation of cyclic analogues of substance P: NMR and molecular dynamics in dimethyl sulfoxide. *J. Am. Chem. Soc.*, **114**, 4818–4827.

Schulz, G.E. and Schirmer, R.H. (1979) Principles of Protein Structure. Springer Verlag, New York.

Spatola, A.F. (1983) Peptide backbone modifications: a structure-activity analysis of peptides containing amide bond surrogates, conformational constraints, and related backbone replacements. *Chemistry and Biochemistry of Amino Acids, Peptides, and Proteins. Vol VII*, (Ed: Weinstein, B.), Marcel Dekker, New York, pp. 267–357.

Toniolo, C. (1990) Conformationally restricted peptides through short-range cyclizations. *Int. J. Peptide Protein Res.*, **35**, 287–300.

Wiley, R.A. and Rich, D.H. (1993) Peptidomimetics derived from natural products. *Med. Res. Rev.*, **13**, 327–384.

15. BIOACTIVE ETHER-LINKED PHOSPHOLIPIDS: PLATELET-ACTIVATING FACTOR (PAF) AND ANALOGS

FRED SNYDER

CONTENTS

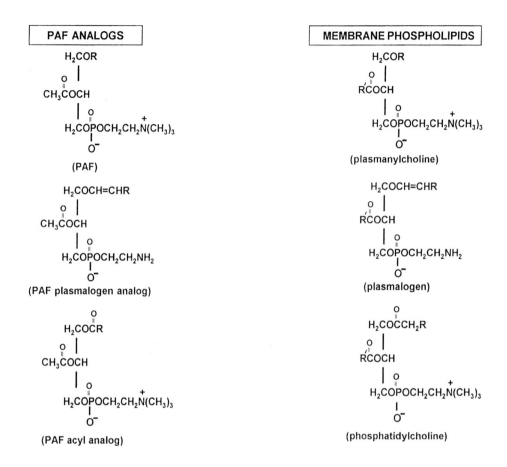

Figure 15.1   Comparison of chemical structures of PAF and its analogs with related phospholipids found in mammalian membranes.

15.1 INTRODUCTION

The ether bond in lipids exists as either an O-alkyl or O-alk-1-enyl moiety linked to the *sn*-1 carbon of a glycerol moiety (Fig. 15.1); glycerolipids containing the O-alk-1-enyl moiety are called plasmalogens. Usually, the *sn*-2 carbon contains esterified fatty acids (acyl group) and the *sn*-3 position an esterified fatty acid, phosphate, or phosphobase (P-choline or P-ethanolamine) moiety. A group of Japanese investigators initially reported the presence of alkyl lipids in several different fish oils some seventy years ago. Although the general properties of plasmalogens were initially described in the late 1920s by a German group, the complete chemical structure was not elucidated until 1957. Except for liver, both types of ether lipids are prominent components of most mammalian cells.

Perhaps the greatest impact in the ether lipid field occurred in 1979 when the chemical structure of platelet-activating factor (PAF) was identified as 1-alkyl-2-acetyl-*sn*-glycero-3-phosphocholine (Fig. 15.1), one of the most potent cellular mediators yet discovered. It is surprising that the relatively simple chemical structure of PAF could express such diverse and profound biological activities (see Section 15.5); moreover, the variety of responses elicited by this molecule in different cell types points out the inadequacy of its name, which was originally based on the ability of PAF to aggregate platelets. In most cells, the O-alkyl moiety of PAF contains 16 carbon atoms (hexadecyl species), although alkyl species possessing other chain lengths do exist.

A neutral glycerolipid precursor of PAF (1-alkyl-2-acetyl-*sn*-glycerol) also possesses biological properties similar to PAF and many of its actions, but not all, are thought to be due to the conversion of the alkylacetylglycerols to PAF. Other derivatives of PAF (acyl, plasmalogen, and ethanolamine analogs) (Fig. 15.1) also appear to participate as modulators of cellular functions, but they have not been as extensively studied as PAF.

It is well established that PAF is a contributing factor to most inflammatory and allergic reactions, but PAF is also thought to be an important physiological mediator of cellular functions involved in reproduction, fetal development, and blood pressure control. However, most research efforts in the PAF field have focused on its pathological ramifications and the role of PAF in a variety of diseases that include asthma, hypertension, acute allergic reactions, anaphylaxis, psoriasis, thrombocytopenic purpura, systemic lupus erythematosus, kidney disorders, pulmonary hypertension and edema, ischemic bowel necrosis, and endotoxin shock.

A large number of anti-PAF drugs (PAF receptor antagonists) have been developed and are now in clinical trials for the treatment of inflammatory diseases. Despite the therapeutic potential of these receptor antagonists, the magic bullet for blocking hypersensitivity reactions would appear to be a drug that possesses multiple receptor antagonistic properties since cellular responses leading to inflammation are caused by many different types of mediators that include PAF, eicosanoid and phosphatidylinositol metabolites, histamine, peptides, etc. Therefore, a challenge to medicinal chemists in PAF research is to successfully design and synthesize new classes of anti-inflammatory antagonists that can interact with more than a single type of agonist receptor, but at the same time not interfere with essential physiological processes of PAF or other mediators.

Except for the availability of PAF receptor antagonists, little attention has been devoted to developing other types of therapeutic agents of possibly even greater usefulness. For example, some synthetic analogs of PAF have been described that are more pronounced in their hypotensive action than in their ability to affect platelet and neutrophil aggregation (see Ohno *et al.* reference). Thus, it is likely that novel antihypertensive drugs related to the chemical structure of PAF could be synthesized that do not possess the undesirable actions of PAF; unfortunately research efforts along these lines are still lagging. Also, very little progress has been made in the development of selective inhibitors for specific enzymes that produce PAF in inflammatory processes without affecting those enzymes that maintain the required normal physiological levels of PAF in tissues and blood. The design of appropriate enzyme inhibitors would permit the highest degree of selectivity for pharmacological intervention in preventing the deleterious effects of PAF from occurring since the anti-PAF receptor antagonists have the disadvantage of blocking both the pathological- and physiologically-induced responses of PAF. One other area of considerable interest from

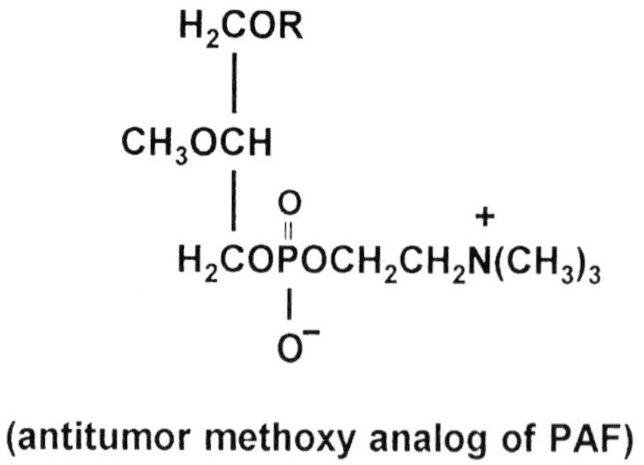

$$\text{H}_2\text{COR}$$
$$|$$
$$\text{CH}_3\text{OCH}$$

$$
\begin{array}{c}
| \quad \overset{\text{O}}{\underset{\|}{}} \qquad\quad + \\
\text{H}_2\text{COPOCH}_2\text{CH}_2\text{N(CH}_3)_3 \\
| \\
\text{O}^-
\end{array}
$$

(antitumor methoxy analog of PAF)

Figure 15.2   An example of an ether-linked phospholipid possessing selective antitumor properties; such lipids appear to be membrane-targeted.

a medicinal chemistry viewpoint concerns a group of synthetic unnatural analogs of PAF (Fig. 15.2) that possess highly selective cytotoxic activities towards a number of different types of cancer cells.

In view of the vast amount of information available about PAF, this chapter can only provide a limited introductory coverage of some of the chemical, biochemical, pharmacological, and biological aspects of PAF and its structurally-related biologically active lipid molecules. In addition, the close metabolic relationship of these phospholipid mediators to the generation of other bioactive molecules (e.g., eicosanoid metabolites) is also emphasized when pertinent.

15.2 CHEMICAL REACTIVITY AND CHROMATOGRAPHY

The ether-linkage at the *sn*-1 position imparts a great deal of chemical and metabolic stability to glycerolipids. Nevertheless, both the O-alkyl and O-alk-1-enyl moieties can be cleaved chemically and enzymatically. The chemical reactivity of the ether linkage will be discussed in this section along with some useful derivatives for identification purposes (Figs. 15.3 and 15.4).

15.2.1 Chemical cleavage of ether-linked moieties

Although both the O-alkyl and O-alk-1-enyl groups attached to the glycerol moiety of lipids are sensitive to strong acid hydrolysis, the alkyl linkage is much more resistant. The alkyl ether bond can be cleaved by nucleophilic attack of a strong acid with the formation of an alkyl halide. Hydriodic acid is much more effective in this cleavage than hydrobromic acid or hydrochloric acid. The alkyl iodide product formed in the reaction with hydriodic acid has been used to characterize the ether-linked aliphatic chain by gas-liquid chromatographic analysis. However, other types of derivatives, as mentioned later in this section, are more advantageous to use because the HI reaction can also form interfering side products (e.g., secondary alkyl iodides produced from olefinic compounds).

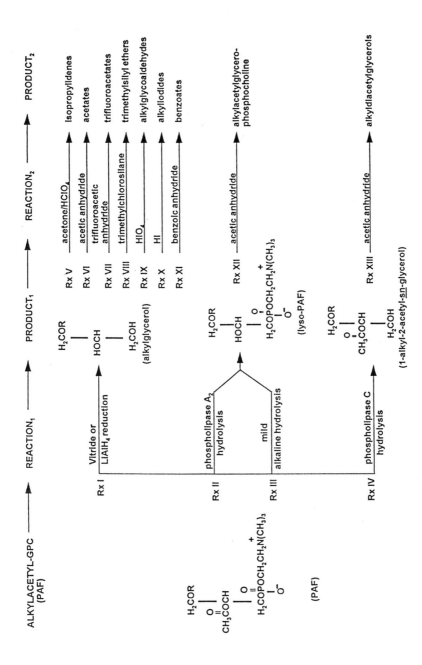

Figure 15.3 Chemical reactions (Rx) and derivatives used in the identification of PAF and other types of O-alkylglycerolipids.

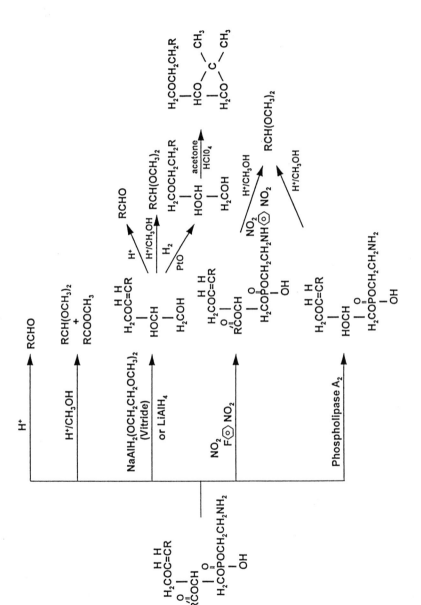

Figure 15.4   Chemical reactions and derivatives used in the identification of plasmalogens (O-alk-1-enyl-linked glycerolipids).

The O-alk-1-enyl group in plasmalogens is readily hydrolyzed to fatty aldehydes by any strong acid. If acid hydrolysis of plasmalogens is carried out in the presence of methanol, dimethylacetals are formed, which are relatively stable and can be readily characterized by gas-liquid chromatography.

15.2.2 Derivatives of ether-linked glycerolipids and their chromatographic behavior

There are many useful chemical derivatives for identifying specific subclasses or molecular species of ether lipids. The first step always requires the separation of the main classes of lipids in total lipid extracts by adsorption chromatography (thin-layer chromatography or high performance liquid chromatography) before carrying out the appropriate resolution of subclasses and the subsequent chemical reactions to produce useful derivatives for chromatographic analyses. Neutral lipid subclasses can be easily separated into alk-1-enyl-, alkyl-, and acyl-types directly from total lipid extracts, whereas the diacyl-, alkylacyl- and alk-1-enylacyl subclasses of phospholipids are not easily resolved by adsorption chromatography. Therefore, with phospholipids it is usually essential to first remove the phosphobase moiety by using phospholipase C; the products of this enzymatic reaction are diacyl-, alkylacyl-, and alk-1-enylacyl-glycerols. Although these diradylglycerols can be separated from one another by adsorption chromatography, it is generally best to prepare sn-3 benzoate, acetate, etc. derivatives, so that migration of the acyl group at the sn-2 position is minimized or prevented. Derivatives such as benzoates are especially useful since they can be readily resolved by chromatography and subsequently quantitated on the basis of their UV absorbing properties.

Another approach for establishing the chain length and degree of unsaturation of ether-linked glycerolipids is to remove the esters at either the sn-2 and/or sn-3 positions. For example, Vitride [$NaAlH_2(OCH_2CH_2OCH_2)_2$] and $LiAlH_4$ are excellent reducing agents since they remove all esterified substituents (acyl and phosphobase moieties) without altering the chemical character of the alkyl or the alk-1-enyl ether groupings at the sn-1 position of the glycerol moiety. The reduced products, alkylglycerols and alk-1-enylglycerols, can then be characterized as isopropylidene, acetate, or benzoate derivatives by chromatographic analyses. Acyl groups are reduced to fatty alcohols by chemical reduction.

Phospholipase A_2 or mild alkaline (monomethylamine) hydrolysis are generally used to selectively hydrolyze the sn-2 acyl moiety of phospholipids. The lyso-phospholipid products or their benzoate or acetate derivatives can be subsequently identified via adsorption chromatography and the fatty acids analyzed by chromatographic methods.

General schemes that illustrate key reactions used to analyze the alkyl and plasmalogen (alk-1-enyl) types of ether-linked lipids and the resulting derivatives formed (e.g., isopropylidenes, benzoates, acetates) are depicted in Figures 15.3 and 15.4. Earlier reviews and/or books on ether lipids (see Further Reading) should be consulted for more specific details of the original literature that describe these methodologies.

15.3 NATURAL OCCURRENCE

Ether-linked glycerolipids are found in most mammalian cells but only to a limited extent in some bacteria, plants, and other lower forms of life. Reviews by Horrocks and by Sugiura

Table 15.1 Ether lipid subclasses in choline and ethanolamine phosphoglycerides of mammalian tissues and cells.

Tissue	percentage of subclass			
	P-choline	P-choline	P-ethanolamine	P-ethanolamine
Brain	1.0–5.6	tr–4.4	1.1–8.0	50.0–68.1
Erythrocytes	1.9–3.9	0–0.6	2.1–11.5	20.5–59.7
Heart (rat)	0.6–1.4	1.7–3.8	3.2–5.9	12.4–15.1
(species other than rat)	1.6–5.2	33–52	5.8–9.4	42.0–64.1
Kidney	tr–6.2	0–3.7	0–8.8	9.6–33.8
Liver	0–2.4	0–0.14	0–2.0	0–3.7
Lung	2.1–5.9	tr–2.5	4.3–8.7	33.5–50.0
Lymphocytes	10.2–23.2	2.2–3.2	3.9–9.7	40.7–49.9
Macrophages	13.5–35.2	2.3–5.6	0.8–11.4	41.2–61.2
Plasma	0.9–5.5	0–0.2	4.6–20.7	13.8–30.8
Platelets	4.5–18.0	1.4–8.8	1.7–29.1	27.0–57.6
Polymorphonuclear leukocytes	16.4–50.2	tr–9.4	3.0–23.9	32.7–65.5
Spermatozoa	17.1–54.9	23.2–62.8	27.0–49.2	40.0–54.0
Testes	5.6–9.8	0.4–2.6	8.3–16.2	25.5–36.9

Values represent a range for the subclasses of ether-linked phospholipids for tissues and cells from different species (unless indicated otherwise) and experiments. These data are based on calculations from a detailed review by Sugiura and Waku. Trace quantities are indicated by tr.

and Waku have compiled data from the literature for both the quantity and composition of ether-linked glycerolipids in a wide variety of tissues from numerous animal species. Some typical cells and tissues of mammals that contain relatively high proportions of alkyl and/or alk-1-enyl types of phospholipids are listed in Table 15.1.

It is especially noteworthy that the naturally occurring ether-linked aliphatic chains have a simple composition in comparison to their acyl counterparts. Only saturated or monoenoic ether-linked hydrocarbon chains are found in mammals with 16:0:, 18:0, and 18:1 moieties (number of carbon atoms:number of double bonds) predominating. Other types of O-alkyl chains have been reported in studies of the molecular species of PAF, but these are of very minor occurrence and their biological significance questionable. On the other hand it is possible to modify both the quantity and chain length/unsaturation composition of the ether-linked moieties by feeding appropriate precursors (e.g., fatty alcohols or alkylglycerols) to animals or cultured cells.

15.4 PHYSICAL PROPERTIES

The presence of the ether bonds in lipids can influence the physical properties of biological membranes, especially when the proportion of ether lipids is relatively high. Studies of pure preparations of ether-linked lipids conducted with artificial model membranes (monolayer and liposomal preparations) have shown the replacement of ester bonds with ether bonds affects primarily hydrophobic-hydrophilic interactions. The closer linear packing arrangements possible with ether-linked chains can also influence the polar head group region of these molecules. In addition, the unique location ($\Delta 1$) of the double bond adjacent to the ether bond in plasmalogens can alter the configuration of lipid arrangements in membranes.

Model membranes of ether lipids exhibit lower ion permeability, surface potential, and phase transition temperatures than their diacyl counterparts. Nevertheless, it is difficult to make general statements about the influence of ether linkages of lipids on membrane functions since it is known the dialkyl analog of phosphatidylcholine deviates from its expected behavior by having a higher phase transition temperature than the corresponding alkylacyl analog. Also, the interpretation of physical effects of ether lipids on the properties of native biological membranes is further complicated by their secondary effects on cholesterol and protein components which influence membrane packing arrangements.

15.5 BIOLOGICAL FUNCTION: PHYSIOLOGICAL AND PATHOLOGICAL ASPECTS

Ether-linked glycerolipids serve as both structural components of cell membranes and as cellular mediators. The determinant factor in this dualistic function appears to be the chain length of the acyl chain at the sn-2 position of phospholipids and the base group at the sn-3 position. Those ether-linked phospholipids with long chain sn-2 acyl groups ($>12:0$) are the structural analogs of phosphatidylcholine and phosphatidylethanolamine and, therefore, they have a comparable role as constituents of cell membranes, albeit differences do exist in the physical and metabolic properties of ether- vs. ester-linked glycerolipids. In contrast, those ether-linked glycerolipids possessing short chain sn-2 acyl moieties ($<6:0$) exhibit biological activities associated with lipids classified under the generic term of PAF. Needless to say, the precise physiological functions of ether lipids as membrane components and cell mediators are not fully understood but it is clear that their prominence in most mammalian cells emphasizes their importance.

The diverse nature of the biological properties of PAF can be seen from the list of biological responses induced by PAF (Table 15.2). Stimulation of PAF production via the remodeling pathway of biosynthesis (see Section 15.7 on Metabolism) is a contributing factor to most inflammatory and allergic reactions associated with a wide variety of diseases (see following paragraph). On the other hand PAF is also thought to be an important physiological mediator of cellular functions, especially those involved in reproduction, fetal development, and blood pressure control. For example, PAF appears to be required for the successful implantation of the fertilized egg in the uterus. The treatment of human pre-embryos with PAF causes an increase in the pregnancy rate, which strongly suggests PAF plays a significant role in embryonic development. In addition, other convincing evidence supports the involvement of PAF in normal fetal development and parturition. These findings coupled with the implication of PAF as a possible renal factor in blood pressure control indicates that PAF has an essential physiological role, a fact that has often been overlooked because of the considerable emphasis placed on specific inflammatory reactions and diseases involving PAF. A book edited by Barnes, Page and Henson and a review by Braquet, Touqui, Shen, and Vargaftig are excellent sources of information about the role of PAF in human disease.

Table 15.2   *In vivo*, tissue, and cellular responses or conditions induced by PAF.

In Vivo	Tissues/Organs	Cellular
Anaphylaxis	↑ Hepatic glycogenolysis	Aggregation (N, P)
Systemic hypotension	Constricts ileum and lung strips	Degranulation (N, P)
Pulmonary hypertension and edema	↑ Vascular permeability	Shape changes (P)
↓ Dynamic lung compliance		↑ Ca^{2+} uptake (P)
↑ Pulmonary resistance		↑ Chemotaxis and chemokinesis (N)
Neutropenia		↑ Respiratory burst and superoxide production (N)
Thrombocytopenia		↑ Protein phosphorylation (P)
Intestinal necrosis		↑ Arachidonate turnover (N, P)
Broncoconstriction		↑ Phosphoinositide turnover (P)

The letters N and P in parenthesis designate neutrophils and platelets, respectively.

15.6 CHEMICAL STRUCTURE AND BIOLOGICAL ACTIVITY RELATIONSHIPS OF ETHER LIPIDS

Very few modifications can be made in the chemical structure of PAF without a loss in the potency of its biological activity. Replacement of the ether group at the *sn*-1 position for an ester group greatly diminishes or abolishes the bioactivity of PAF. Also, the potency of PAF in eliciting cellular responses is proportionately reduced as the *sn*-2 acyl group increases in length beyond three carbon atoms, e.g., PAF analogs with long chain esters at the *sn*-2 position are totally devoid of bioactivity. The same general loss of PAF activity is seen when the choline moiety is altered by the removal of its methyl groups. Dimethyl- and monomethyl-ethanolamine analogs of PAF exhibit moderate PAF activity, whereas 1-alkyl-2-acetyl-*sn*-glycero-3-phosphoethanolamine exhibits no activity. Molecules closely related to the structure of PAF, e.g., alkylacetylglycerols, alk-1-enylacylglycerophosphoethanolamines (plasmalogen analogs of PAF), acylacetyl-glycerophosphocholines, and alkylglycerols are also produced in cells that synthesize PAF but little is known about the structure/functional relationships and biological significance of these lipids. Results obtained with nonhydrolyzable substituents (ethoxy or methylcar-bamoyl groups) indicate such analogs have PAF-like activity, albeit considerably less than the parent structure; these data suggest the hydrolysis of the *sn*-2 acetate moiety of PAF is not required for its biological activity to be expressed. However, the acetate moiety of PAF can be transferred to other lipids by a PAF transacetylase.

The possibility that different mechanisms (e.g., different receptor sites) are involved in the hypotensive versus inflammatory properties of PAF has been implicated in studies by Ohno and co-workers in Japan who synthesized a novel PAF agonist, (*S*)-1-methyl PAF. This small change in chemical structure resulted in an analog that was 2500 times more potent in its hypotensive response than PAF itself; yet it was much weaker in its ability to aggregate platelets or neutrophils. These interesting findings support the notion that beneficial properties of PAF, such as its hypotensive action, might be harnessed through the creation of specific types of PAF analogs useful as antihypertensive drugs.

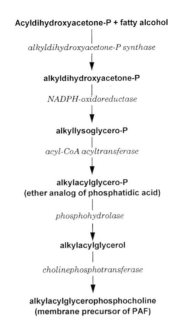

Figure 15.5 Enzymatic reactions involved in the formation of the O-alkyl bond in glycerolipids and the sequence of reactions responsible for the biosynthesis of the membrane ether-linked phospholipid (alkylacylglycerophosphocholine) that serves as a precursor of PAF in the remodeling pathway of PAF biosynthesis.

15.7 METABOLISM

15.7.1 Biosynthesis

15.7.1.1 Formation of ether-linked lipids

The O-alkyl ether bond in glycerolipids is formed in a unique reaction catalyzed by alkyldihydroxyacetone-P synthase, an enzyme that is capable of substituting long-chain fatty alcohols for the acyl moiety of acyldihydroxyacetone-P to produce alkyldihydroxyacetone-P, the first detectable lipid intermediate that contains an ether linkage (Fig. 15.5). The fatty alcohol precursor in this initial reaction is derived from the reduction of fatty acids catalyzed by an acyl-CoA reductase, whereas the other precursor, acyldihydroxyacetone, is generated by an acyl-CoA acyltransferase that utilizes dihydroxyacetone-P (produced from *sn*-glycero-3-P) as a substrate.

Alkyldihydroxyacetone-P can be converted to phospholipids that serve as constituents of biological membranes through a series of enzymatic steps involving an NADPH-dependent oxidoreductase, acyl-CoA acyltransferases, phosphatidate phosphohydrolase, and choline- or ethanolamine-phosphotransferases as illustrated for the biosynthesis of plasmanylcholine in Figure 15.5. The biosynthesis of PAF and its analogs can occur by either remodeling of membrane phospholipids (Fig. 15.6) or by the *de novo* sequence of reactions depicted in Figure 15.7. The remodeling enzymes are thought to be primarily responsible for producing the excessively high levels of PAF in inflammatory responses; whereas the *de novo* enzymes are believed to maintain essential physiological levels of PAF for normal cell functions.

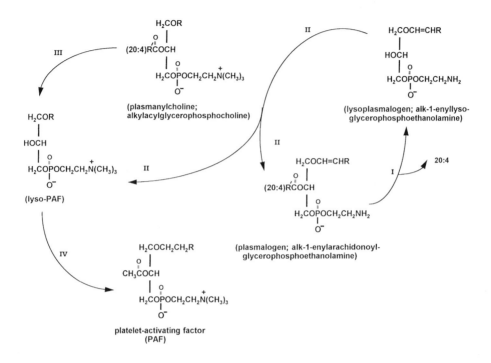

Figure 15.6   Biosynthesis of PAF by the remodeling of a membrane phospholipid (alkylacylglycerophospho-
cholines). The remodeling sequence to form lyso-PAF can occur via the indirect (Reactions I and II) or direct
action (Reaction III) of a phospholipase A$_2$. As shown, the indirect action of a phospholipase A$_2$ (Reaction I) is
coupled to a CoA-independent transacylase (Reaction II) to form lyso-PAF. Lyso-PAF is then acetylated by an
acetyl-CoA-dependent acetyltransferase (Reaction IV).

15.7.1.2 PAF remodeling pathway

Cell stimuli of various sorts (e.g., calcium ionophore, formylmethionylleucylphosphorylala-
nine peptide, zymosan, thrombin, etc.) can trigger the biosynthesis of PAF via the remodeling pathway in a reaction sequence involving (a) the hydrolysis of the *sn*-2 acyl moiety of
a membrane phospholipid precursor of PAF (1-alkyl-2-acyl-*sn*-glycero-3-phosphocholine)
to form lyso-PAF and (b) the acetylation of the lyso-PAF intermediate to produce PAF
(Fig. 15.6). Until recently little was known about the precise mechanism in the initial step
involving acyl group hydrolysis in the remodeling pathway of PAF biosynthesis, although it
has been apparent for some time that membrane alkylarachidonoylglycerophosphocholine
species are selectively utilized as the precursor for the production of the lyso-PAF
intermediate. In the past the hydrolytic reaction was always presumed to be catalyzed
by a putative phospholipase A$_2$ (PLA$_2$); however, at the present time there is still no
direct evidence for the expression of a specific PLA$_2$ activity when PAF formation is
elevated following cell stimulation with calcium ionophore A23187 or various physiological
agonists.

On the other hand, several independent investigations of the remodeling pathway of
PAF biosynthesis have revealed that the lyso-PAF intermediate can be produced from

alkylarachidonoylglycerophosphocholines through reactions involving a CoA-independent transacylase activity, an enzyme thought to possess both intrinsic PLA_2 and acyltransferase activities. The transacylation reaction results in the transfer of arachidonate from alkylarachidonoylglycerophosphocholines to a lyso-phospholipid acceptor which produces lyso-PAF; no release of free arachidonic acid occurs in this step. Considerable evidence indicates the lyso-phospholipid acceptor molecule required as a substrate for the transacylase is thought to be generated *in situ* from ethanolamine plasmalogens (alk-1-enylacyl type) by a PLA_2. Acyl and alkyl species of either choline- or ethanolamine-containing species of lyso-glycerophosphatides also can serve as acyl acceptor molecules for the transacylase. In contrast, other lyso-phospholipids containing serine/inositol, neutral lipids with free hydroxy groups, or cholesterol are not acyl acceptors for the CoA-independent transacylase. The coupled transacylase/A_2 and the PLA_2 reactions also appear to be responsible for generating other lyso-phospholipid acceptor molecules (acyl and alk-1-enyl forms) that contribute to the formation of the acyl and plasmalogen analogs of PAF following agonist stimulation. Plasmalogen and acyl analogs of PAF can also be produced via transfer of the acetate from PAF to their corresponding lyso analogs in a reaction catalyzed by a CoA-independent transacetylase.

Of primary importance is the fact that the lyso-PAF generated by the CoA-independent transacylase has been shown to be directly linked to the synthesis of PAF via the acetyl-CoA:lyso-PAF acetyltransferase. Thus, PAF production can be significantly increased simply by adding the ethanolamine lysoplasmalogen acyl acceptor for the transacylase to enzymatic membrane preparations containing acetyl-CoA. The overall reaction sequence for PAF formation through the combined reactions catalyzed by a PLA_2, a transacylase/A_2, and the acetyltransferase is illustrated in Figure 15.6. Whereas the transacylase-induced formation of lyso-PAF introduces a new concept for how PAF can be biosynthesized in the remodeling pathway, the reader is cautioned that at least at the present time these findings do not completely rule out the existence of a single, direct PLA_2 activity being responsible for the formation of lyso-PAF. Certainly complex regulatory controls of a PLA_2 activity by activation/inactivation mechanisms (e.g., phosphorylation/dephosphorylation) not yet understood could account for the current lack of experimental proof for the sole involvement of the direct action of a PLA_2 in PAF biosynthesis via the remodeling route.

15.7.1.3 PAF de novo pathway

1-Alkyl-2-lyso-*sn*-glycero-3-P (Fig. 15.5) is at a key intermediary metabolic branch point in that it can serve either as the initial precursor in the synthesis of membrane phospholipids or as the starting point for the subsequent committed reaction steps necessary for the *de novo* synthesis of PAF (Fig. 15.7). All or at least some of the enzymes required for the *de novo* synthesis of PAF appear to be present in most mammalian cells. The *de novo* steps consist of (1) the acetylation of alkyllysoglycero-P to form alkylacetylglycero-P by an acetyltransferase, (2) the dephosphorylation of alkylacetylglycero-P to produce alkylacetylglycerols, and (3) the transfer of the choline-P moiety of cytidinediphosphate (CDP)-choline to the alkylacetylglycerols to form PAF by a dithiothreitol (DTT)-insensitive choline phosphotransferase. The enzyme activities in the *de novo* route appear to be novel in that their properties differ from other enzyme activities in ether lipid metabolism involving long-chain acyl groups at the *sn*-2 position.

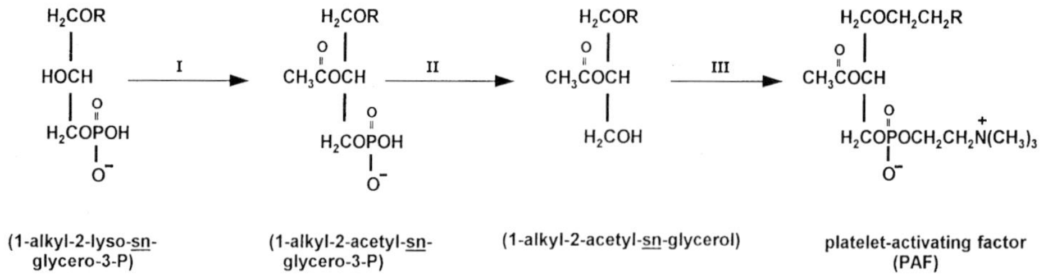

Figure 15.7 Biosynthesis of PAF via the *de novo* pathway. Alkyllysoglycero-P, a branch-point metabolic intermediate, is produced by the reduction of alkyldihydroxyacetone-P as depicted in the pathway outlined in Figure 15.5. The *de novo* sequence of reactions are catalyzed by an acetyl-CoA acetyltransferase (Reaction I), a phosphohydrolase (Reaction II), and a cholinephosphotransferase (Reaction III).

A significant difference between the remodeling and *de novo* routes of PAF biosynthesis is that the *de novo* route is not affected by inflammatory stimuli and glycerolipids containing arachidonate or other polyunsaturated acids are not involved as precursors. Although calcium and other factors are known to influence specific enzymes in the production of PAF, little information is currently available about the regulatory controls responsible for the *in vivo* regulation of PAF biosynthesis.

15.7.2 PAF catabolism

The enzyme of greatest importance in PAF catabolism is PAF acetylhydrolase in that it inactivates PAF (via deacetylation) to form lyso-PAF (Fig. 15.8) and its activity appears to be ubiquitously distributed among mammalian tissues. The lyso-PAF intermediate can then be either converted to a membrane lipid component (alkylacylglycerophosphocholine) or catabolized further to other metabolites (Fig. 15.8) by a lyso-phospholipase D, a phosphohydrolase and/or an alkyl cleavage enzyme (a tetrahydropteridine-dependent monooxygenase). Other enzymes such as phospholipase C and D or other lipases/esterases appear to play a minimal role in the metabolism of PAF and its metabolic products.

15.7.3 Enzyme inhibitors

Very little progress has been made in the design of selective inhibitors for enzymes involved in the metabolism of ether-linked glycerolipids. Moreover, the inhibitors that have been described are not very specific and/or require relatively high concentrations to be effective.

Various isomers of monopalmitoyl-1,2,3-trihydroxyeicosane-1-P have been reported to be inhibitors of alkyldihydroxyacetone-P synthase. Thus, these analogs, at concentrations in the range of 1.3×10^{-4} M, can inhibit the initial step in the formation of the ether linkage in glycerolipids. However, with intact cell systems these inhibitors would probably not block ether lipid biosynthesis since the free phosphate moiety of such analogs would presumably prevent them from crossing the plasma membranes of cells.

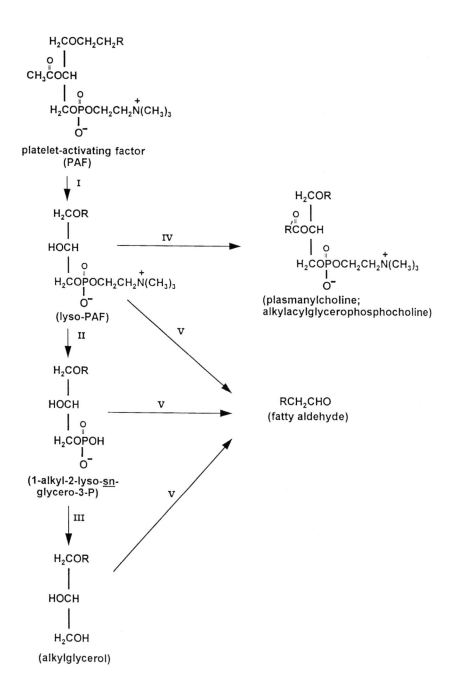

Figure 15.8   Primary enzymatic reactions involved in the catabolism of PAF and its metabolites. The Roman numerals indicate the reactions catalyzed by PAF acetylhydrolase (I), lysophospholipase D (II), a phosphohydrolase (III), a CoA-independent transacylase (IV), and the O-alkyl cleavage enzyme, a tetrahydropteridine-dependent monooxygenase (V).

Investigators at Merck, Sharp and Dohme Research Laboratories reported that 2-(N-palmitoyl-amino)propylphosphocholine and 3-(N-palmitoylamino)propylphosphocholine were able to inhibit the acetyltransferase activities in the remodeling pathway. Both of these synthetic lipids inhibit the acetyltransferase activity in rat spleen microsomes, with an IC_{50} value of 5 μM; they have also been shown to inhibit the synthesis of PAF by intact mouse peritoneal leukocytes stimulated with calcium ionophore A23187. However, it is possible this inhibition of PAF biosynthesis in intact cells by such amino-containing lipids could be explained on the basis of inhibiting a PLA_2 in the remodeling pathway, since it is known that a similar analog, (N-palmitoylamino)ethylphosphocholine, inhibits both acetyltransferase and PLA_2 activities.

Clearly, a fruitful area of research in medicinal chemistry would be the development of specific inhibitors of PAF related enzymes for use in mechanistic studies designed to better understand the cellular role of ether-linked lipids. Moreover, highly selective enzyme inhibitors of the CoA-independent transacylase, acetyltransferase, or PLA_2 in the remodeling pathway of PAF biosynthesis could lead to exciting new drugs, independent of PAF receptors, for the treatment of inflammatory diseases involving PAF.

15.8 PAF RECEPTORS AND RECEPTOR ANTAGONISTS

The PAF receptor from a number of different cell types has been cloned. Each of these studies have revealed that the PAF receptor possesses the typical amino acid composition of other known G-protein coupled receptors such as rhodopsin, β_1 and β_2 adrenergic, D_2-dopamine, and M1–M5 muscarinic receptors. Therefore, it is thought many, if not most, of the actions of PAF must occur through the activation of the cellular signal transduction system involving G-proteins. However, intracellular binding sites for PAF have been described which raises the issue of whether some PAF-induced responses are initiated at sites other than the plasma membrane.

Receptors highly specific for PAF have been characterized on the surface membranes of platelets, neutrophils, differentiated HL-60 cells (granulocytic form induced by dimethyl-sulfoxide), smooth muscle cells, and a cell culture line of murine macrophages ($P388D_1$). Evidence for these high affinity PAF binding sites is based on results obtained with [^{3}H]PAF binding and competition experiments with receptor antagonists and structural analogs of PAF or known PAF antagonists. The number of specific PAF receptors per cell is extremely low for platelets (estimates of 150–400 per cell in rabbits and 250 in humans) in contrast to human neutrophils ($\sim$1100 per cell) and differentiated HL-60 cells (neutrophil form) ($\sim$5200 per cell).

Major pharmaceutical firms have developed a large number of synthetic and natural PAF receptor antagonists. The large number of PAF antagonists available have been discussed in reviews by T.Y. Shen and coworkers and by Pierre Braquet and collaborators (see Further Reading). Examples of the chemical structures of some natural and synthetic PAF receptor antagonists are illustrated in Figure 15.9. Antagonists such as CV-3988 closely resemble the chemical structure of PAF, whereas others such as kadsurenone, L-652,731, and BN 52021 appear structurally different. All of these PAF receptor antagonists have been shown to effectively block cellular responses induced by PAF.

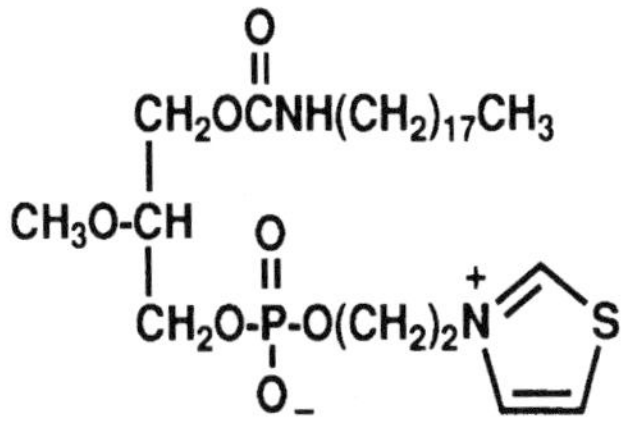

CV-3988

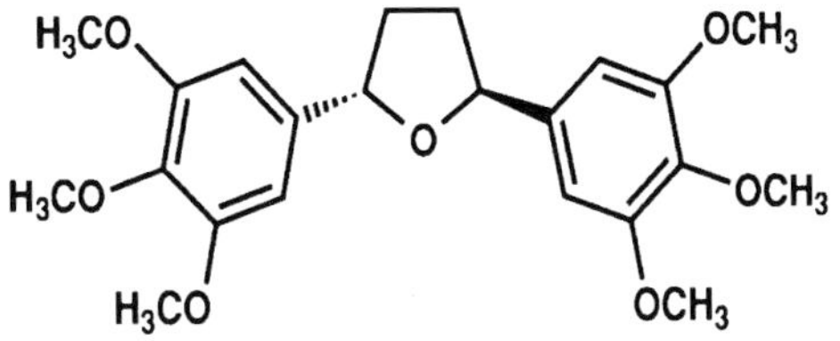

L-652,731

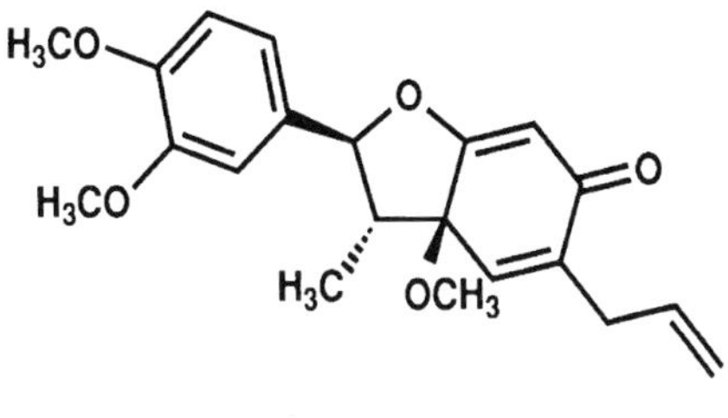

Kadsurenone

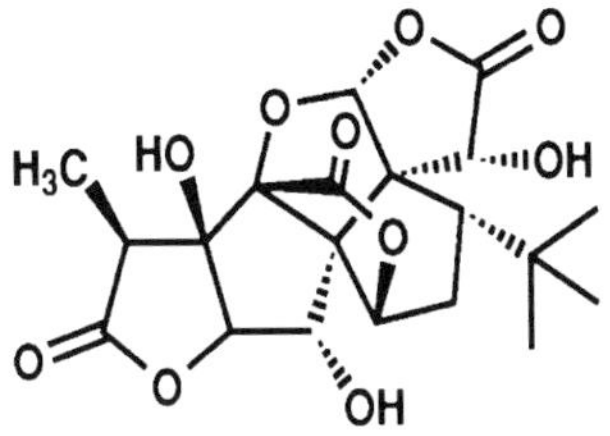

Ginkgolide B
(BN 52021)

Figure 15.9 Examples of synthetic (CV-3988 and L-652,731) and naturally-occurring (Kadsurenone and Ginkgolide B) receptor antagonists of PAF.

15.9 ANTITUMOR ANALOGS OF PAF

A variety of studies have shown that a number of O-alkyl ether-linked phospholipids possess highly selective antineoplastic activities towards certain sensitive cancer cells (see reviews by Berdel and co-workers and Bittman and Lohmeyer). The most extensively investigated lipid of this type is 1-alkyl-2-methoxy-*sn*-glycero-3-phosphocholine (Fig. 15.2), a structural analog of PAF that has a nonhydrolyzable ether-linked methyl group substituted for the acetate group at the *sn*-2 position of PAF. This methoxy analog of PAF is also known as ET-18-OCH_3 (ET-18-O-methyl) or by the commercial drug name, edelfosine. PAF analogs of this type exhibit a direct antiproliferative and cytotoxic activity towards certain tumor cells, whereas normal healthy cells such as human polymorphonuclear cells are highly resistant; however, it should be noted that various resistant lines of cancer cells also exist. Some clinical trials suggest these membrane-targeted ether-linked phospholipid drugs may be useful in cancer therapy. Recently, a related ether lipid, alkylphosphocholine, which does not contain the glycerol moiety, was introduced in Germany under the drug name of miltefosine for topical use in treating cutaneous breast cancer.

Unlike conventional chemotherapeutic cancer drugs that act on the cell nucleus, the cytotoxic ether-linked phospholipid agents are plasma membrane-targeted. Both protein kinase C and Na$^+$, K$^+$-ATPase in HL-60 cells are inhibited by the methoxy analog of PAF as well as its metabolite, alkylmethoxyglycerol. However, the inhibition of protein kinase C does not appear to be directly correlated with the antineoplastic activity of this drug. Different types of transport systems involving lipid precursors, amino acids, and carbohydrates are also inhibited in the sensitive HL-60 cells by the methoxy analog, a finding that suggests nutrient starvation plays an important role in the cytotoxic response of cancer cells to the methoxy analog of PAF. Despite the progress made in accruing a large amount of descriptive knowledge about the biochemical behavior of these unique antitumor lipids, the crucial component(s) of the plasma membrane and the mechanism responsible for the selective cellular responses elicited in certain tumor cells by the methoxy analog remain to be identified.

FURTHER READING

Barnes, P.J., Page, C.P., and Henson, P.M. (eds.) (1989) *Frontiers in Pharmacology & Therapeutics: Platelet Activating Factor and Human Disease*. Oxford, England: Blackwell Scientific Publications.

Blank, M.L. and Snyder, F. (1994) Chromatographic analysis of ether-linked glycerolipids, including platelet-activating factor and related cell mediators. In *Lipid Chromatographic Analysis*, edited by T. Shibamoto, pp. 291–316. New York, NY: Marcel Dekker, Inc.

Braquet, P., Touqui, L., Shen, T.Y., and Vargaftig, B.B. (1987) Perspectives in platelet-activating factor research. *Pharmacol. Rev.*, **39**, 97–145.

Chao, W. and Olson, M.S. (1993) Platelet-activating factor: receptors and signal transduction. *Biochem. J.*, **292**, 617–629.

Horrocks, L.A. (1992) Content, composition, and metabolism of mammalian and avian lipids that contain ether groups. In *Ether Lipids: Chemistry and Biology*, edited by F. Snyder, pp. 177–272. New York, NY: Academic Press.

Horrocks, L.A. and Sharma, M. (1982) Plasmalogens and O-alkyl glycerophospholipids. In *Phospholipids*, edited by J.N. Hawthorne and G.B. Ansell, pp. 51–93. Amsterdam, The Netherlands: Elsevier Biomedical Press.

Lee, T.-c. and Snyder, F. (1985) Function, metabolism, and regulation of platelet activating factor and related ether lipids. In *Phospholipids and Cellular Regulation*, edited by J.F. Kuo, pp. 1–39. Boca Raton, FL: CRC Press.

Muirhead, E.E. (1980) Antihypertensive functions of the kidney: Arthur C. Corcoran memorial lecture. *Hypertension*, **2**, 444–464.

Ohno, M., Fujita, K., Shiraiwa, M., Izumi, A., Kobayashi, S., Yoshiwara, H., Kudo, I., Inoue, K. and Nojima, S. (1986) Molecular design toward biologically significant compounds based on platelet activating factor: a highly selective agent as a potential antihypertensive agent. *J. Med. Chem.*, **29**, 1812–1814.

Paltauf, F. (1983) Ether lipids in biological and model membranes. In *Ether Lipids: Biochemical and Biomedical Aspects*, edited by H.K. Mangold and F. Paltauf, pp. 309–353. New York, NY: Academic Press.

Snyder, F. (1989) Biochemistry of platelet-activating factor: A unique class of biologically active phospholipids. *Proc. Soc. Exp. Biol. Med.*, **190**, 125–135.

Snyder, F. (ed.) (1987) *Platelet-Activating Factor and Related Lipid Mediators*, pp. 1–471. New York, NY: Plenum Press.

Snyder, F. (1995) Platelet-activating factor: the biosynthetic and catabolic enzymes. *Biochem. J.*, **305**, 689–705.

Snyder, F. (1995) Platelet-activating factor and its analogs: metabolic pathways and related intracellular processes. *Biochim. Biophys. Acta*, **1254**, 231–249.

Snyder, F., Lee, T.-c. and Wykle, R.L. (1985) Ether-linked glycerolipids and their bioactive species: enzymes and metabolic regulation. In *The Enzymes of Biological Membranes*, edited by A.N. Martonosi, Vol. 2, pp. 1–58. New York, NY: Plenum Press.

Sugiura, T. and Waku, K. (1987) Composition of alkyl ether-linked phospholipids in mammalian tissues. In *Platelet Activating Factor and Related Lipid Mediators*, edited by F. Snyder, pp. 55–85. New York, NY: Plenum Press.

16. CLASSICAL ANTIVIRAL AGENTS AND DESIGN OF NEW ANTIVIRAL AGENTS

P. HERDEWIJN and E. DE CLERCQ

CONTENTS

16.1 CLASSICAL ANTIVIRAL AGENTS

16.1.1 Introduction

Thirty-five years have elapsed since the discovery of the first antiviral agent: 5-iodo-2'-deoxyuridine. In contrast to the evolution in other fields, the antiviral chemotherapy has evolved very slowly. The reasons therefore are multiple:

- close association between the replicative cycle of the virus and the metabolism of the cell;
- the intracellular location of the virus;
- viruses possess considerable fewer virus-associated or -encoded enzymes than bacteria;
- effective vaccines have been developed for the prevention of some severe viral infections;
- antiviral research is a high risk research for industry.

However, the interest in antiviral chemotherapy has raised considerably since the discovery, now more than 10 years ago, of HIV (human immunodeficiency virus) as the causative agent of the acquired immunodeficiency syndrome.

Viral infections can vary from mild and transient to severe and irreversible, and occasionally lead to death. Viral infections can cause chronic degenerative disease and are also implicated in various forms of cancer in man. Many viral infections, even if not life-threatening, have an important socio-economic impact.

The antiviral agents that are, at present, used in the clinic have all evolved from random screening and serendipity. With few exceptions these compounds are nucleosides, and their antiviral activity depends on interactions with virus-encoded enzymes. Also this situation will change. As progress in the molecular biology of viral-host interaction will uncover new targets for antiviral chemotherapy, the development of selective antiviral drugs will keep pace with the molecular biological advances. In the first part of this chapter an overview is given of classical antiviral agents. In the second part recent developments in antiviral drug design are summarized.

5-Iodo-2′-deoxyuridine (IdUrd) (**16.1**) has a structure that is very similar to that of the natural nucleoside thymidine (**16.2**). The van der Waals radius of an iodo group is somewhat greater than that of a methyl group, and the pKa of 5-iodouracil is about 1.5 units lower than that of thymine. This results from the inductive effect of the iodo group in the 5-position. These slight differences are apparently sufficient for IdUrd to become a rather selective antiviral agent. IdUrd was synthesized first by W.H. Prusoff in 1959 by iodination of 2′-deoxyuridine with iodine/nitric acid. IdUrd is active against the multiplication of *Herpes simplex* virus type 1 (HSV-1), herpes simplex virus type 2 (HSV-2) and vaccinia virus (VV) *in vitro* and has proven efficacious in the treatment of herpes eye infections (i.e. herpetic keratitis). Its toxicity, however, does not allow systemic use.

(**16.1**)   (**16.2**)   (**16.3**)

Also there is a great resemblance in the structures of thymidine and 3′-azido-3′-deoxythymidine (AZT) (**16.3**). Here, the 3′-position is substituted with an azido group. This compound was the first to be approved by the Food and Drug Administration (FDA) for the treatment of AIDS patients. It was synthesized first by J.P. Horwitz in 1964 starting from thymidine. Also, the modes of action of IdUrd and AZT are quite similar. They have to be metabolized intracellularly to their 5′-triphosphate derivatives and these triphosphates then interact with DNA synthesis.

These two nucleoside analogues, which resemble very well their natural counterpart, have had a tremendous impact on antiviral research. IdUrd has long been a model compound for the design of new and more selective anti-herpes agents. The advent of AIDS, the identification of a retrovirus as the causative agent of the disease and the observation that its replication can be blocked by simple nucleosides, gave an important incentive to the search for new antiviral agents.

In this chapter we will see how selectivity can be obtained by interference with virus-specific targets. The identification of virus-encoded enzymes has proved the key step in the design of new antiviral compounds.

In the design of new nucleoside analogues, targeted at viral DNA synthesis, the discovery of HPMPC [(*S*)-1-(3-hydroxy-2-phosphonylmethoxypropyl)cytosine] (**16.4**) and PMEA [9-(2-phosphonylmethoxyethyl)adenine] (**16.5**) as potent inhibitors of HSV and HIV, respectively, could be considered as important progress. Although the mode of action of these compounds has not yet been completely elucidated, their antiviral activity clearly indicates that mimicking nucleoside metabolites, e.g. monophosphate, can overcome at least the first step of intracellular phosphorylation. It also proves that such phosphonate analogues can be taken up by the cell sufficiently well to exhibit their antiviral action. This brings us one step nearer to the target (viral DNA) site.

(**16.4**)   (**16.5**)

Nucleosides are natural occurring molecules which play a crucial role in cell multiplication and function. As a consequence, cells contain a whole battery of enzymes for the anabolism and catabolism of nucleosides. All these enzymes are potential targets for the action of the modified nucleosides, and this can lead to premature death of the cell.

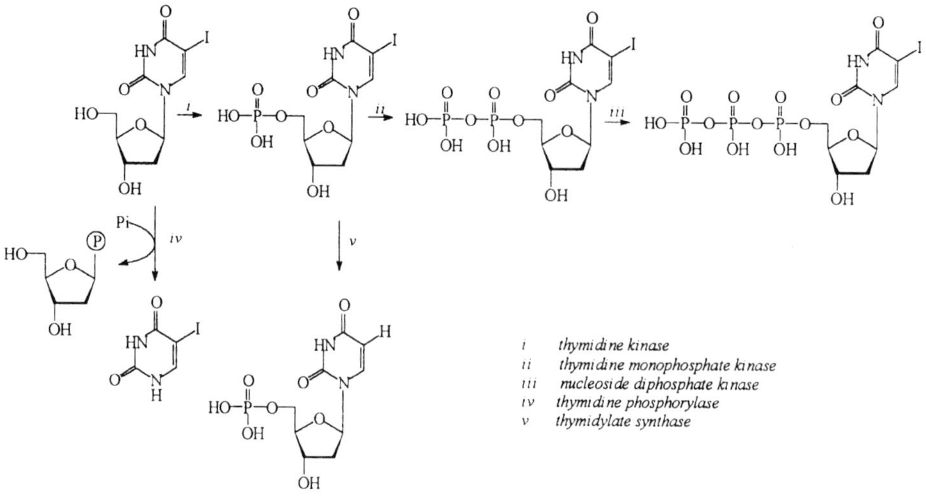

Scheme 16.1

Especially the interaction of the inhibitor with normal cellular DNA may be hazardous in that it could lead to mutagenicity, carcinogenicity or teratogenicity. Moreover, good *in vitro* antiviral activity not necessarily predicts equivalent *in vivo* activity. These considerations make the design of new nucleoside antivirals both a difficult and challenging task.

16.1.2 Base-modified pyrimidine nucleosides as antiherpes agents

The intracellular metabolism and mode of action of IdUrd (**16.1**) can be presented as follows (Scheme 16.1):

IdUrd can be phosphorylated by both cellular and virus-encoded thymidine kinase (*i*). However, IdUrd is phosphorylated more efficiently by the HSV-encoded thymidine kinase than by the cellular thymidine kinase, which explains its (modest) selectivity as an anti-herpes agent. IdUrd 5′-monophosphate is then phosphorylated to the diphosphate (*ii*) and triphosphate (*iii*). IdUrd can be incorporated in both cellular and viral DNA. This incorporation impairs the subsequent transcription and replication processes and is believed to be the major reason for the activity and toxicity of IdUrd. As also evident from the above reaction scheme (Scheme 16.1), IdUrd is a substrate for thymidine phosphorylase (*iv*) and for thymidylate synthase (*v*). Both processes lead to deactivation. Together with the feedback inhibition of the phosphorylated products on the regulatory enzymes of nucleotide biosynthesis, the general biochemical reaction scheme as depicted for IdUrd also holds for most other pyrimidine nucleoside analogues, and could explain their antiviral activity and toxicity.

A crucial enzyme in the anabolism of pyrimidine 2′-deoxynucleosides is the thymidine kinase which phosphorylates the nucleoside to its 5′-monophosphate derivative. Some herpes viruses (i.e. HSV-1, HSV-2) and also *Varicella-zoster* virus (VZV) encode for their own thymidine kinase. Introduction of a substituent in the 5-position has led to compounds with higher affinity for the virus-encoded enzyme than for the cellular enzyme, and thus greater selectivity as antiviral agents. Pertinent examples of this "second" generation of antiviral compounds are 5-ethyl-2′-deoxyuridine (EtdUrd) (**16.6**) and, even more so, 5-(*E*)-bromovinyl-2′-deoxyuridine (BVdUrd) (**16.7**).

(16.6)   (16.7)

There is a marked difference in the phosphorylation capacity of the thymidine kinases of different herpes viruses. While the HSV-1-encoded thymidine kinase is capable of converting BVdUrd to its 5′-monophosphate and further onto its 5′-diphosphate, the HSV-2-encoded thymidine kinase is unable to further phosphorylate BVdUrd monophosphate onto its diphosphate. This differential behavior in phosphorylation may explain the differences found in the activity of BVdUrd against HSV-1 and HSV-2.

BVdUrd and EtdUrd can also be incorporated into DNA. Because of the specific phosphorylation of EtdUrd and BVdUrd by the virus-infected cells, only the virus-infected cells that have allowed phosphorylation of the compounds will be sensitive to their eventual antiviral action (following incorporation into DNA).

The first, but unpractical, synthesis of BVdUrd was carried out by condensing bis(trimethyl)silylated 5-(*E*)-bromovinyluracil with 1-chloro-2-deoxy-3,5-di-(*O*)-p-toluoyl-α-D-*erythro*-pentofuranose followed by separation of the α/β-anomers (Scheme 16.2). A more practical route to BVdUrd has been worked out starting from 2′-deoxyuridine *via* the 5-chloromercuri nucleoside. This procedure has been modified for industrial application with IdUrd (**16.1**) as the starting material: BVdUrd can be synthesized in three steps from IdUrd without the need of chromatographic purifications.

EtdUrd could be considered for the topical treatment of mucocutaneous HSV-1 and HSV-2 infections. BVdUrd is superior to any other anti-herpes agent in the topical treatment of herpetic (HSV-1) eye infections. It has also proven efficacious, and should be seriously considered, for the treatment of VZV infections, as it is 1000-fold more active *in vitro* against VZV than the drug (acyclovir) which is currently used for the treatment of VZV infections. Also, BVdUrd is markedly active against Epstein Barr virus (EBV), but not cytomegalovirus (CMV). A close analogue of BVdUrd, BVaraU, while less active against

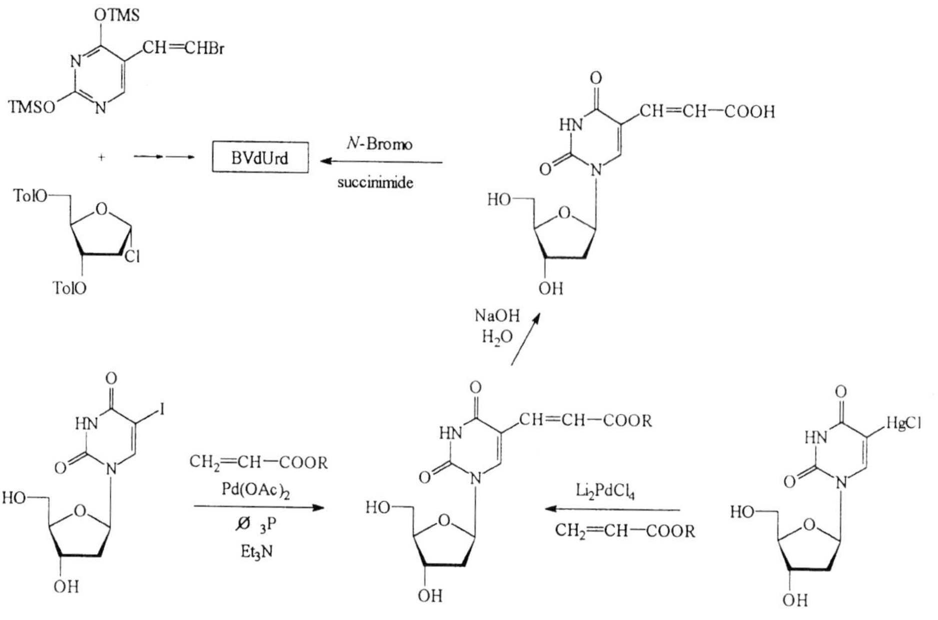

Scheme 16.2

HSV-1, is as potent and selective as BVdUrd against VZV and has been pursued for the treatment of VZV infections. In contrast with BVdUrd, BVaraU is less susceptible or even resistant to phosphorolytic cleavage by mammalian thymidine phosphorylase. However, it appears to be readily cleaved by the bacterial phosphorylases of the gut.

IdUrd monophosphate can be dehalogenated by thymidylate synthase to give dUrd mono-phosphate (Scheme 16.1), which is the natural substrate for the enzyme. Thymidylate synthase is responsible for the conversion of dUrd monophosphate to dThd monophosphate using N^5,N^{10}-methylenetetrahydrofolic acid as methyl donor. This is the key enzyme in the *de novo* biosynthesis of the dThd metabolites (Scheme 16.3).

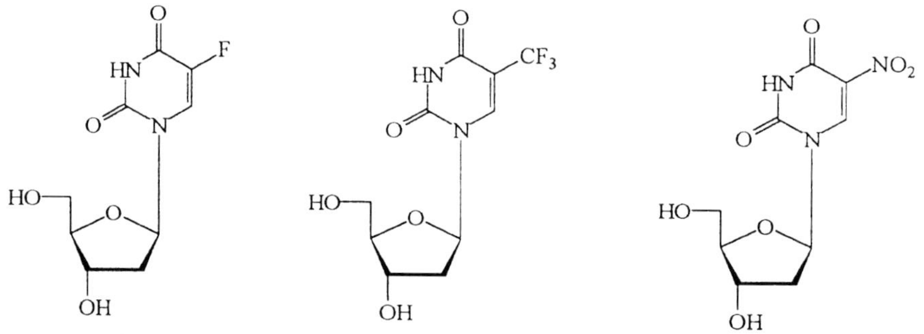

(16.8)   (16.9)   (16.10)

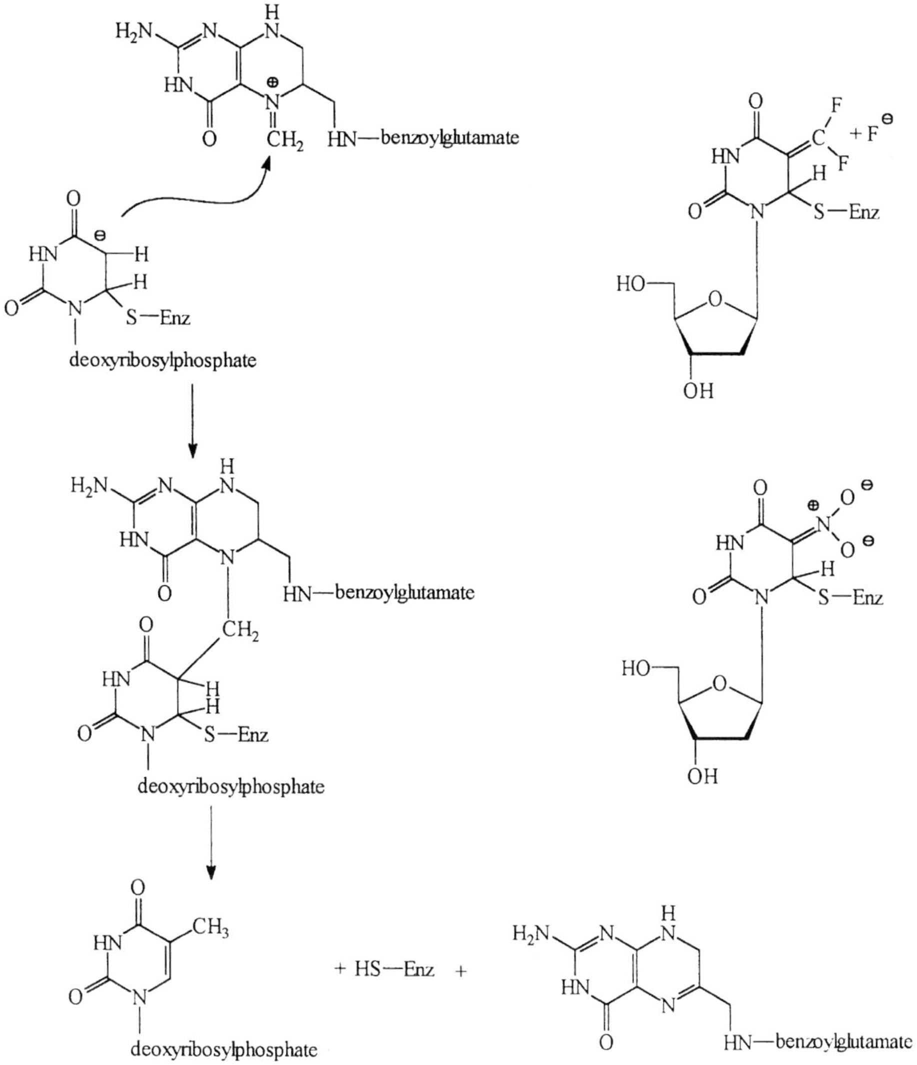

Scheme 16.3

When the iodo group of IdUrd (**16.1**) is replaced by a strong electron withdrawing substituent (X) which forms a stable C-X bond, the compound could inhibit thymidylate synthase without functioning as a substrate. This is the case for 5-fluoro-2′-deoxyuridine (**16.8**), 5-trifluoromethyl-2′-deoxyuridine (**16.9**) and 5-nitro-2′-deoxyuridine (**16.10**).

The pKa of 5-fluorouracil is 8.04, as compared to 7.35 for 5-trifluoromethyluracil and 9.94 for thymine.

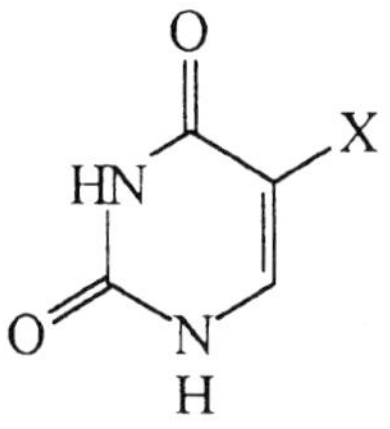

X	pKa
CH_3	9.94
H	9.38
I	8.25
F	8.04
CF_3	7.35
NO_2	5.56

While 5-fluorouracil is used only in cancer chemotherapy, 5-trifluoromethyl-2′-deoxyuridine (F₃dThd, TFT) (**16.9**) is used for the topical treatment of herpetic keratitis. 5-Nitro-2′-deoxyuridine (**16.10**) is of no practical use. 5-Trifluoromethyl-2′-deoxyuridine was first synthesized by C. Heidelberger starting from 5-trifluoromethyluracil and thymidine using an enzymatic transglycosylation reaction.

F₃dThd (**16.9**) is phosphorylated by viral and cellular kinases to the monophosphate and further to the di- and triphosphate. Here again, phosphorylation is more efficient in HSV-infected than uninfected cells. Incorporation into DNA occurs and could contribute to the antiviral activity of F₃dThd. However, F₃dThd owes its antiviral activity mainly to the inhibition of thymidylate synthase. The mode of action of F₃dThd can be explained by assuming a nucleophilic attack of the enzyme at the 6-position of the heterocyclic base which leads to the generation of a reactive difluoromethylene at the 5-position (Scheme 16.3). This enzyme is an interesting target for those viruses which do not encode for a functional thymidine kinase. These viruses must rely on the *de novo* biosynthesis of dThd monophosphate starting from *N*-carbamoylaspartate to form the necessary quantities of dThd triphosphate that are needed for their own DNA synthesis.

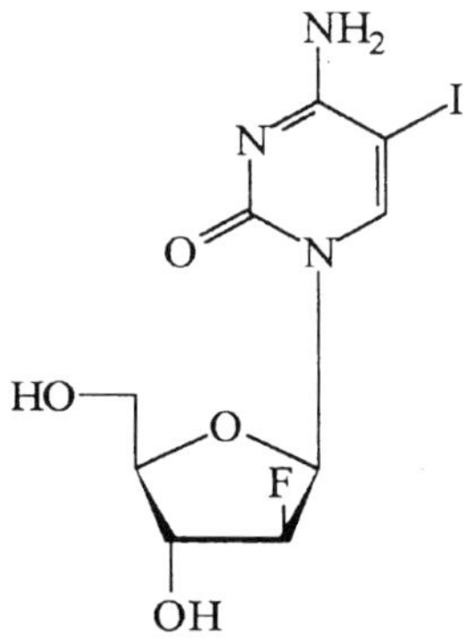

(16.11)

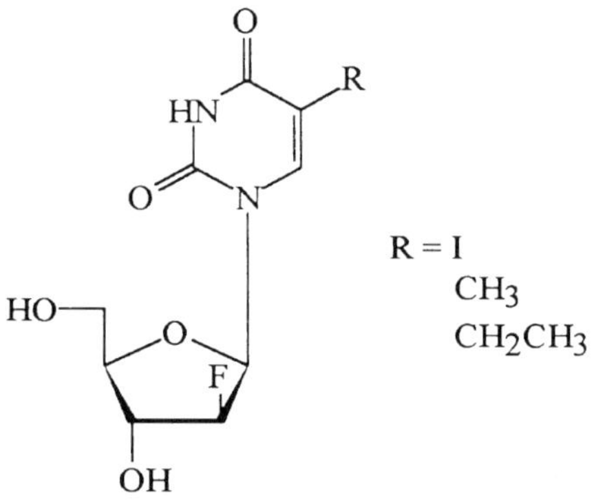

R = I
CH₃
CH₂CH₃

(16.12)

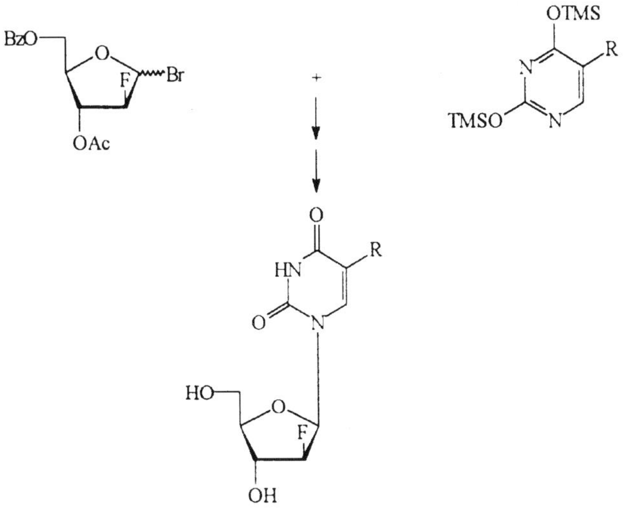

Scheme 16.4

Most antiviral nucleosides are modified in either the base or the carbohydrate moiety. Double-modified nucleosides have seldom proved to be good antivirals. An apparent exception is 5-iodo-1-(2-deoxy-2-fluoro-β-D-arabinofuranosyl)cytosine (FIAC) (**16.11**). This compound is markedly active against HSV-1, HSV-2, VZV, CMV and EBV. The corresponding uracil, thymine (5-methyluracil) and 5-ethyluracil analogues, FIAU (**16.12**, R = I), FMAU (**16.12**, R = CH$_3$), FEAU (**16.12**, R = CH$_2$CH$_3$) have the same activity spectrum as FIAC. In addition, the latter analogues have also proved to be active against hepatitis B virus (HBV).

This group of compounds was synthesized by J.J. Fox's group through condensation of the silylated heterocyclic base with 1-bromo-3-O-acetyl-5-O-benzoyl-2-deoxy-2-fluoro-D-arabinofuranose (Scheme 16.4). FIAU (**16.12**) has been pursued for the treatment of HBV infections, and, while effective in reducing the viral parameters of HBV infections, it led to unacceptable delayed toxicity and even deaths.

The mechanism of action of FIAC, FIAU, FMAU and FEAU is similar to that of BVdUrd (**16.7**). The DNA polymerase is the target enzyme for the antiviral action of these compounds. As FIAC is rapidly metabolized by deiodination and deamination (Scheme 16.5), it is not very clear which metabolite represents the active form of FIAC. However, the deaths of hepatitis B patients following treatment with FIAU has put the whole class of 1-(2-deoxy-2-fluoro-1-β-D-arabinofuranosyl)pyrimidines in an unfavourable light.

16.1.3 Sugar-modified purine nucleosides

9-(β-D-Arabinofuranosyl)adenine (**16.13**) is a naturally occurring nucleoside which was synthesized, 8 years before its isolation, from 3',5'-di-O-protected 9-(β-D-xylofuranosyl)-adenine (Scheme 16.6).

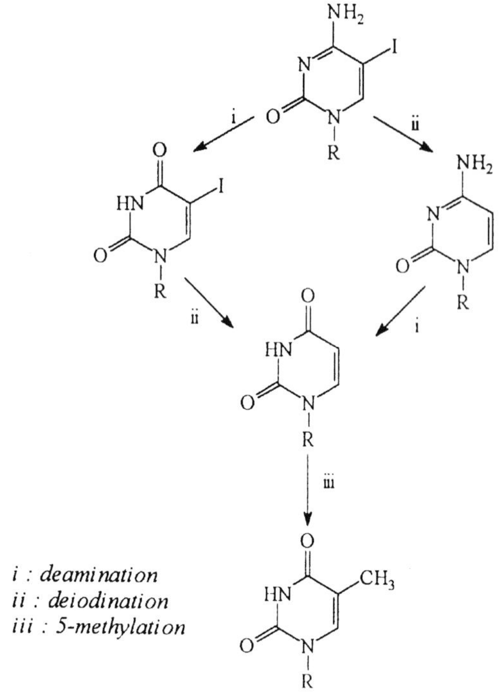

i : deamination
ii : deiodination
iii : 5-methylation

Scheme 16.5

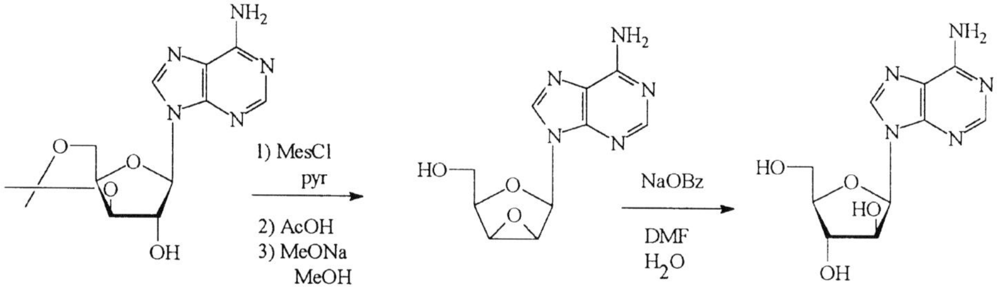

(**16.13**)

Scheme 16.6

Ara-A (**16.13**) is an antiviral agent with a multiple mode of action. Theoretically, drugs that have multiple modes of action are most likely to avoid drug-virus resistance but, they may also have the highest risk for toxic side effects. The relative role of the different actions in the overall antiviral activity of ara-A is not well known. Ara-A is phosphorylated to its monophosphate and further to its di- and triphosphate. This triphosphate inhibits DNA polymerases, which could explain the activity of ara-A against DNA viruses. Ara-A can also be incorporated into both host cell DNA and viral DNA. Ara-A also inhibits methyltransferase reactions presumably through inhibition of S-adenosylhomocysteine hydrolase and accumulation of S-adenosylhomocysteine. The latter acts as a product inhibitor of transmethylation reactions such as those involved in the maturation of viral mRNA. Ara-A has been used for the treatment of HSV-1 encephalitis and *Herpes zoster* in immunocompromised patients, but is now surpassed by acyclovir for this purpose. A major disadvantage of ara-A is that it is promptly deaminated *in vivo* by adenosine deaminase. The resulting hypoxanthine analogue has a markedly reduced antiviral activity as compared to ara-A.

The search for inhibitors of the adenosine deamination reaction has led to the discovery by the Wellcome Research Laboratories of 9-(2-hydroxyethoxymethyl)guanine (acyclovir) (**16.14**) as an antiviral agent. This compound, whose action is surprisingly similar to that of the aforementioned pyrimidine nucleoside analogues, has oriented research in the direction of the acyclic nucleoside analogues. This research has yielded a number of active congeners, i.e. 9-(1,3-dihydroxy-2-propoxymethyl)guanine (DHPG, ganciclovir) (**16.15**) and 9-(4-hydroxy-3-hydroxymethylbut-1-yl)guanine (penciclovir) (**16.16**).

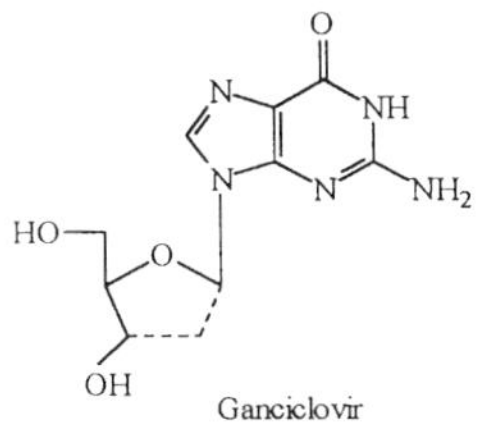

Ganciclovir

(16.15)

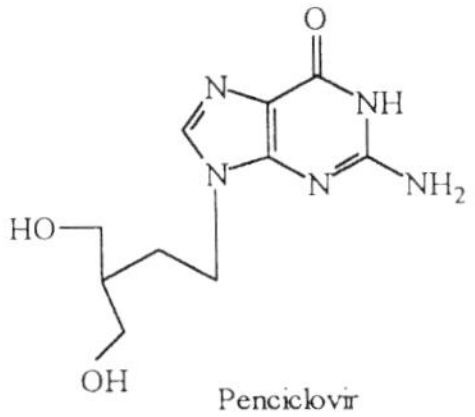

Penciclovir

(16.16)

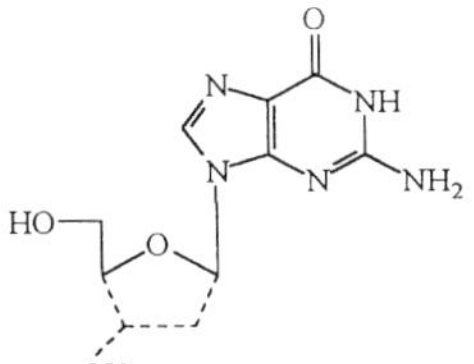

Acyclovir

(16.14)

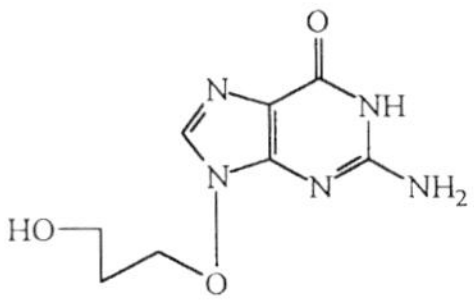

(16.17)

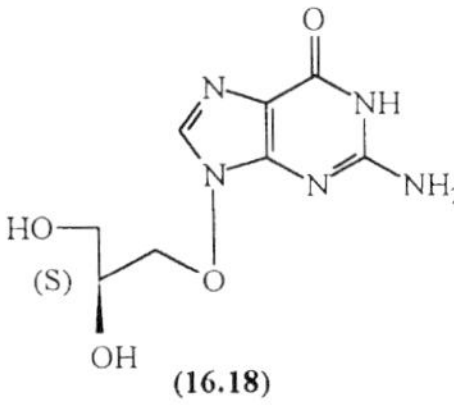

(16.18)

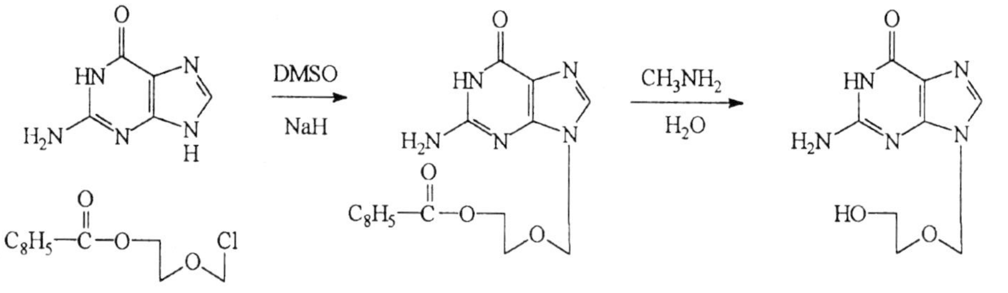

Scheme 16.7

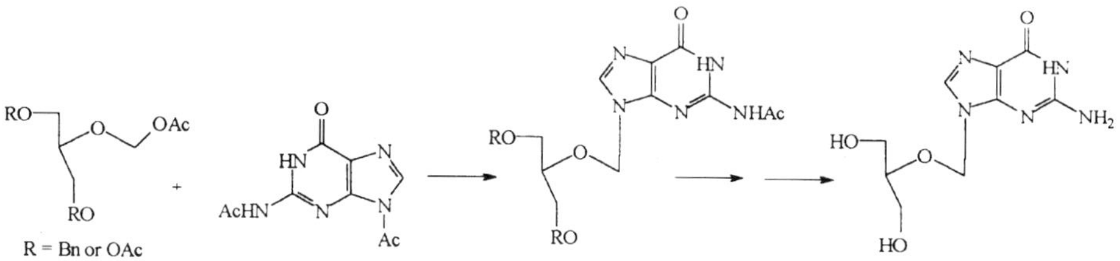

Scheme 16.8

All these compounds can be considered as analogues of $2'$-deoxyguanosine or carbocyclic $2'$-deoxyguanosine (*vide infra*) from which the $2'$-carbon (ganciclovir, penciclovir) or both the $2'$- and $3'$-carbons (acyclovir) have been deleted. The antiviral activity of acyclovir was discovered by accident, whereas DHPG (**16.15**) was the result of logical design starting from acyclovir as model compound. From a structural viewpoint, DHPG is more closely related to $2'$-deoxyguanosine than is acyclovir.

Acyclovir (**16.14**) was first synthesized by reaction of 2,6-dichloropurine with 2-benzoyloxyethylchloromethyl ether in the presence of triethylamine followed by conversion of the dichloropurine to the guanine base. The synthesis was later improved by direct reaction of the sodium salt of guanine, in the presence of sodium hydride in dimethylsulfoxide, with the same ether followed by removal of the blocking group of the acyclic side chain with aqueous methylamine (Scheme 16.7).

For the synthesis of ganciclovir (**16.15**), di-acetylated guanine was reacted with 1,3-di-O-protected 2-O-acetoxymethylglycerol in the presence of a sulphonic acid followed by deprotection of the base and the aliphatic side chain (Scheme 16.8).

The reaction of silylated N^2-acetylguanine with 1,3-di-O-benzyl-2-O-chloromethyl-glycerol has also been used.

The antiviral activity of acyclovir (**16.14**) can be explained by the same biochemical re-action scheme as presented for IdUrd (Scheme 16.1). There are, however, subtle differences that explain the broader activity spectrum and greater selectivity of acyclovir. Acyclovir is phosphorylated to its monophosphate by a virus-specific thymidine/deoxycytidine kinase, which actually recognizes acyclovir as a deoxycytidine analogue. Viruses which encode for such an enzyme (HSV-1, HSV-2, VZV, but not CMV) are susceptible to the antiviral action of acyclovir. Although the natural substrates for this enzyme are pyrimidine nucleosides, it apparently accepts purine derivatives as substrates. In uninfected cells, phosphorylation occurs to a limited extent. The monophosphate of acyclovir is phosphorylated to the diphosphate by GMP kinase and further to its triphosphate by various cellular enzymes. The triphosphate of acyclovir is a competitive inhibitor of dGTP for the viral DNA polymerase and can also function as a substrate resulting in the incorporation of acyclovir into DNA and chain termination. Acyclovir is given orally or intravenously in the treatment of HSV and VZV infections, and topically in the treatment of HSV infections (i.e. herpetic keratitis and *Herpes labialis*).

As compared to acyclovir, ganciclovir (**16.15**) is more easily phosphorylated in CMV-infected cells and its triphosphate has a 5-fold greater affinity than ACV triphosphate for CMV DNA polymerase. Ganciclovir can be incorporated both internally and at the 3'-terminal end of DNA. Ganciclovir is active against HSV-1, HSV-2, VZV, CMV and EBV. It is fairly toxic for the bone marrow (neutropenia). Its clinical use is restricted to the treatment of CMV infections in immuno-compromised patients.

Penciclovir (**16.16**) possess the same antiviral spectrum as acyclovir. As compared to acyclovir, penciclovir leads to higher triphosphate concentrations in virus-infected cells and its antiviral activity persists for a longer time after removal of the compound. In fact, after removal of acyclovir, antiviral activity rapidly disappears. Not only penciclovir, but also BVdUrd (**16.7**), FIAC (**16.11**) and ganciclovir (**16.15**) show persistent antiviral activity after the drugs have been removed from the medium. This is due to the greater stability of their triphosphates as compared to that of acyclovir triphosphate.

An acyclovir (**16.14**) isomer, 9-(3-hydroxypropoxy)guanine (**16.17**), has the N^9 of guanine linked to an oxygen (instead of a carbon) and would be more active than its alkoxymethyl counterpart (acyclovir) against HSV-1, HSV-2, VZV and EBV. A similar increase in activity was noted for (S)-9-(2,3-dihydroxypropoxy)guanine (**16.18**) relatively to its 9-(2,3-dihydroxybutyl)guanine counterpart.

16.1.4 Ribavirin

In contrast with the preceding compounds, ribavirin (Virazole®) (**16.19**) has a broad spectrum activity against RNA and DNA viruses both *in vitro* and *in vivo*. Ribavirin (1-β-D-ribofuranosyl-1,2,4-triazole-3-carboxamide) was first synthesized by R.K. Robins' group.

This synthesis was based upon the acid-catalyzed fusion reaction between methyl 1,2,4-triazole-3-carboxylate and 1,2,3,5-tetra-O-acetyl-β-D-ribofuranose or the glycosylation reaction of the same trimethylsilylated heterocycle with 2,3,5-tri-O-acetyl-D-ribofuranosyl bromide (Scheme 16.9). The carbomethoxy group was then converted to a carboxamide group with ammonia in methanol. The fusion method gave predominantly the 1-glycosyl-3-substituted 1,2,4-triazole. The glycosylation method gave a 1/1 mixture of this compound with the 1-glycosyl-5-substituted-1,2,4-triazole.

The structural requirements for the broad-spectrum antiviral activity of ribavirin are very stringent. The compound shows its greatest potency against myxo (influenza) and paramyxo (respiratory syncytial) virus infections. Ribavirin also shows activity against some

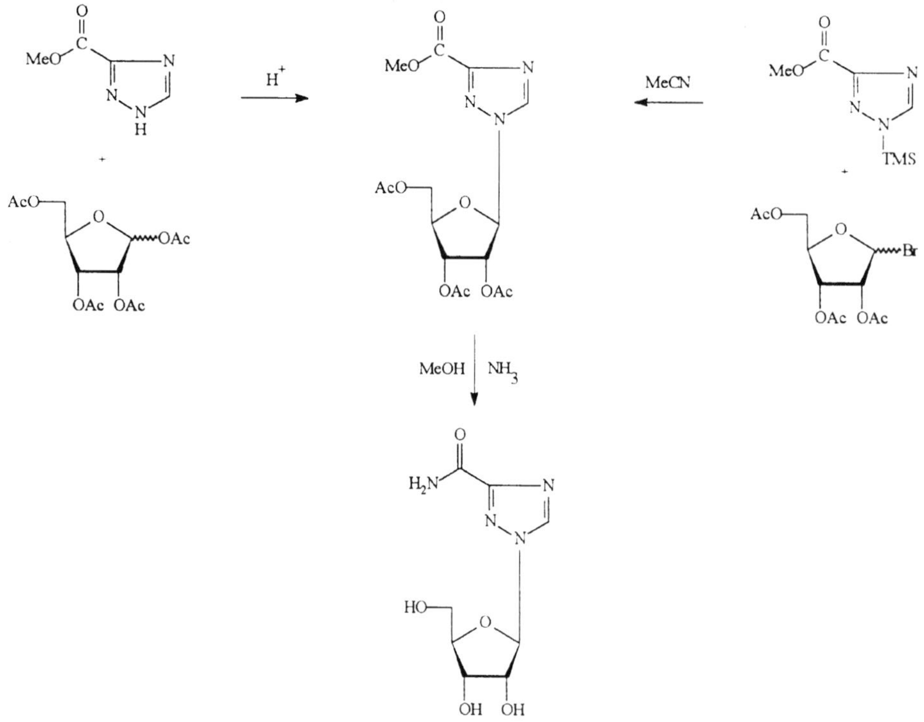

MeO–C=O ... N, N, N–H

H$^+$ →

MeO–C=O ... N, N, N

← MeCN

MeO–C=O ... N, N, N–TMS

AcO ... O ... OAc, OAc OAc

+

AcO ... O ... OAc OAc

AcO ... O ... Br, OAc OAc

MeOH | NH$_3$

H$_2$N–C=O ... N, N, N

HO ... O ... OH OH

(16.19)

Scheme 16.9

hemorrhagic fever viruses such as Lassa, Machupo, Pichinde, Rift Valley and Hantaviruses. Therapeutic efficacy has been demonstrated with ribavirin, given as a small-particle aerosol, in infants suffering from respiratory syncytial virus (RSV) infection. The compound has been approved for the treatment of this disease.

The mode of action of ribavirin (**16.19**) is multi-pronged and may also vary from one virus to another. Ribavirin can be considered as an analogue of AICAR (Scheme 16.10) which is the precursor of both AMP and GMP.

As has been elucidated by X-ray crystallography studies, there is a good resemblance between ribavirin and guanosine; by rotating the amide group, also good resemblance is found between ribavirin and adenosine (Scheme 16.10). The possible target enzymes for ribavirin are presented in Scheme 16.11.

Because of its resemblance to purine nucleosides, ribavirin (**16.19**) can be phos-phorylated by cellular purine nucleoside kinases to its monophosphate and by other cellular enzymes to its triphosphate. In its monophosphate form, ribavirin inhibits

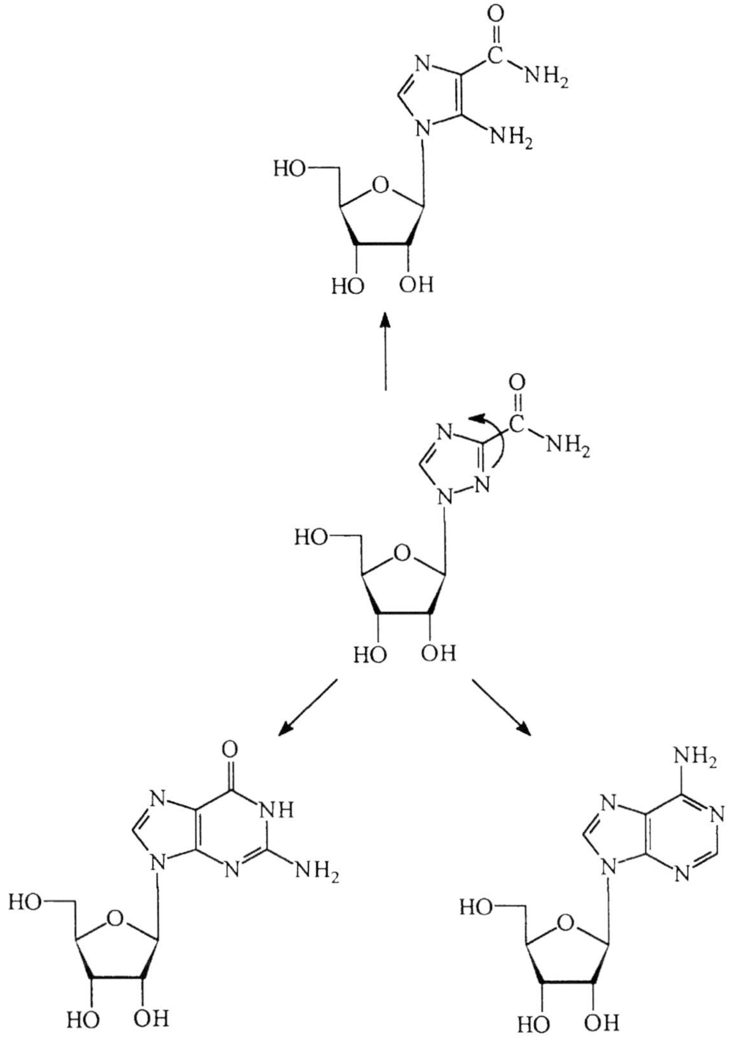

Scheme 16.10

inosine monophosphate (IMP) dehydrogenase and in this way prevents the formation of GMP. In its triphosphate form, ribavirin inhibits 5'-terminal guanylylation of un-capped mRNA and N^7-methylation of the terminal guanine residue. Also, ribavirin monophosphate could replace GMP in the cap. Ribavirin 5'-triphosphate has been shown to inhibit RNA polymerase (i.e. of influenza virus) in competition with GTP and ATP.

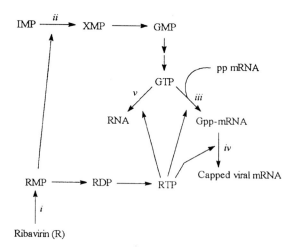

i   : adenosine kinase
ii : inosine monophosphate dehydrogenase
iii : guanylyl transferase
iv : mRNA-guanine-N^7-methyl transferase
v   : RNA polymerase

Scheme 16.11

16.1.5 Compounds which inhibit the replication of the human immunodeficiency virus (HIV)

HIV is a retrovirus, which means that, once it has infected the cell, its genomic RNA is transcribed to proviral DNA by a virus-specific enzyme: reverse transcriptase. This enzyme has a broader substrate specificity than cellular DNA polymerases, and has since long been recognized as a target for antiviral chemotherapy. Here the task of design specific antiviral agents is somewhat more difficult than for herpes viruses since HIV does not code for a virus-specific kinase which could confine the metabolism of the nucleoside analogues to the virus-infected cells.

The first drug which was approved for the treatment of AIDS patients was azidothymidine (zidovudine, AZT), (16.3). Approval then followed for 2′,3′-dideoxyinosine (didanosine, DDI) (16.20), 2′,3′-dideoxycytidine (zalcitabine, DDC) (16.21) and 2′,3′-didehydro-2′,3′-dideoxythymidine (stavudine) (16.22).

Azidothymidine is phosphorylated by the cellular thymidine kinase to its 5′-monophosphate (Scheme 16.12). This 5′-monophosphate is then phosphorylated to the di- and triphosphate by thymidylate kinase and, presumably, nucleoside-5′-diphosphate kinase, respectively. As the efficiency of conversion of azidothymidine-5′-monophosphate to its diphosphate by thymidylate kinase is much lower than the efficiency of phosphorylation of the natural substrate, azidothymidine-5′-monophosphate accumulates in the cells.

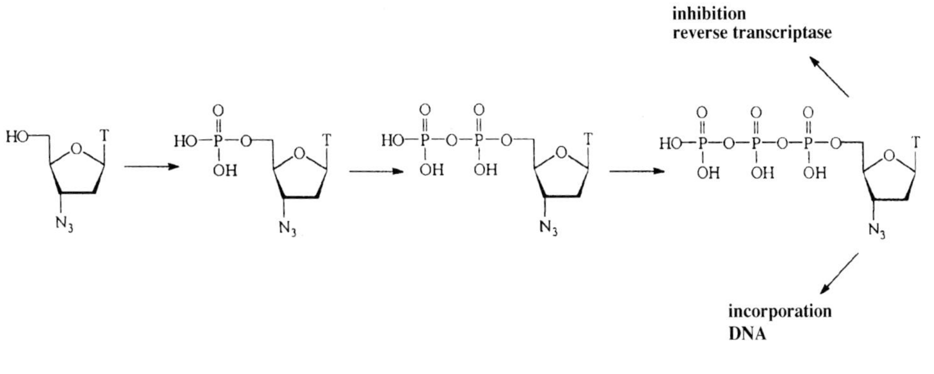

Scheme 16.12

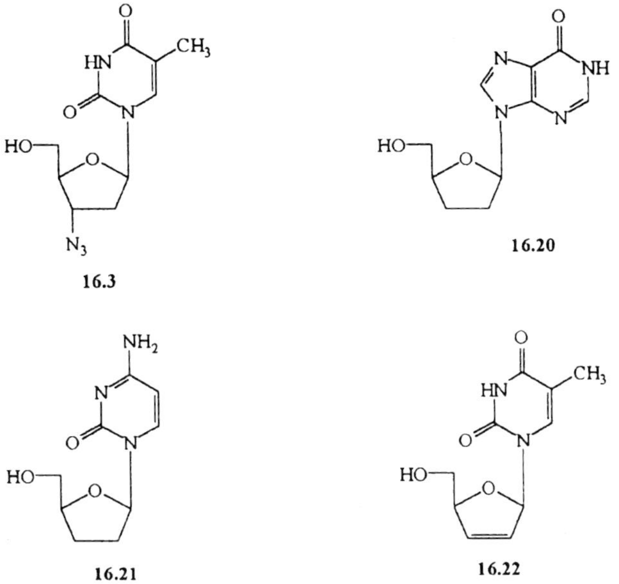

16.3

16.20

16.21

16.22

In its triphosphate form, AZT is a more efficient inhibitor of the reverse transcriptase than of DNA polymerase α, γ and δ. AZT is incorporated into DNA and functions as a chain terminator. $3'$-Azido-$3'$-deoxythymidine (**16.3**) was first synthesized (*vide supra*) starting from thymidine using the pyrimidine base to invert the configuration at the $3'$-position. Later, more efficient ways have been developed for the synthesis of (**16.3**) from thymidine. An interesting example is the two step conversion using 2-chloro-1,1,2-trifluorotriethylamine and lithium azide, respectively (Scheme 16.13).

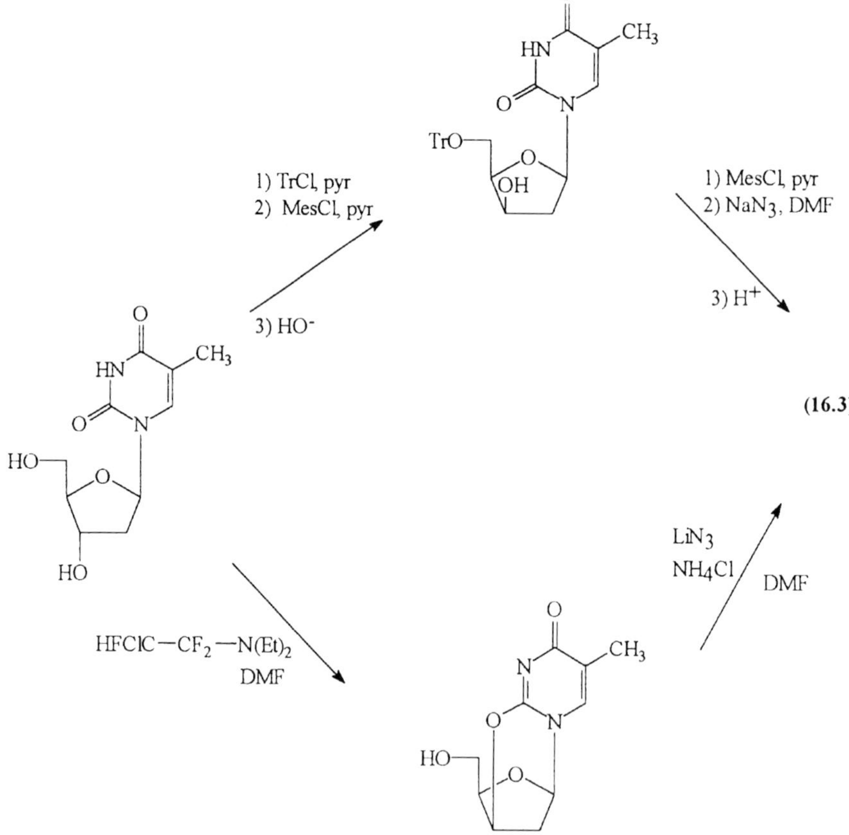

Scheme 16.13

The active metabolite of dideoxyinosine (DDI) (**16.20**) is dideoxyadenosine-5′-triphosphate. Dideoxyinosine is first converted to dideoxyinosine-5′-monophosphate. Through a sequential action of adenylosuccinate synthetase and lyase, dideoxyadenosine-5′-monophosphate is formed which is further converted to the above mentioned triphosphate. Dideoxycytidine (DDC) and didehydrodideoxythymidine (D4T) are alo converted intracellularly to their active triphosphates. All these triphosphates inhibit DNA polymerase α, β and γ to a lesser extent than reverse transcriptase and, once incorporated, all these nucleosides may function as chain terminators. AIDS patients may benefit from a therapy with AZT, DDI, DDC or D4T. An improvement of virological, immunological and clinical parameters and an increase in survival rate has been observed with these compounds. However, dideoxynucleosides are not ideal drugs. These drugs may lead to the emergence of drug-resistant virus strains and toxicity has been observed for all of them: AZT (anemia, neutropenia, thrombocytopenia), DDC (peripheral neuropathy), D4T (peripheral neuropathy), and DDI (acute pancreatitis and peripheral neuropathy).

16.2 DESIGN OF NEW ANTIVIRAL AGENTS

16.2.1 Carbocyclic nucleosides

As mentioned in the preceding section, nucleosides are sensitive to phosphorolytic cleavage of their N-glycosidic linkage by purine or pyrimidine nucleoside phosphorylases. This degradation problem can be overcome by using carbocyclic analogues of nucleosides. In these carbocyclic nucleosides, the furanose oxygen is replaced by a methylene group.

(16.23)   (16.24)

The carbocyclic analogue of cytidine (carbodine) (**16.23**) is active against influenza and various other viruses *in vitro*. The carbocyclic analogues of IdUrd (**16.25**), IdCyd (**16.27**), BVdUrd (**16.26**), BVdCyd (**16.28**), 2′-deoxyguanosine (**16.29**) (Scheme 16.14) and 2,6-diaminopurine ribofuranoside (**16.24**) show marked anti-herpes activity.

(**16.30**) R=H
(**16.31**) R=COCH$_2$OCH$_3$

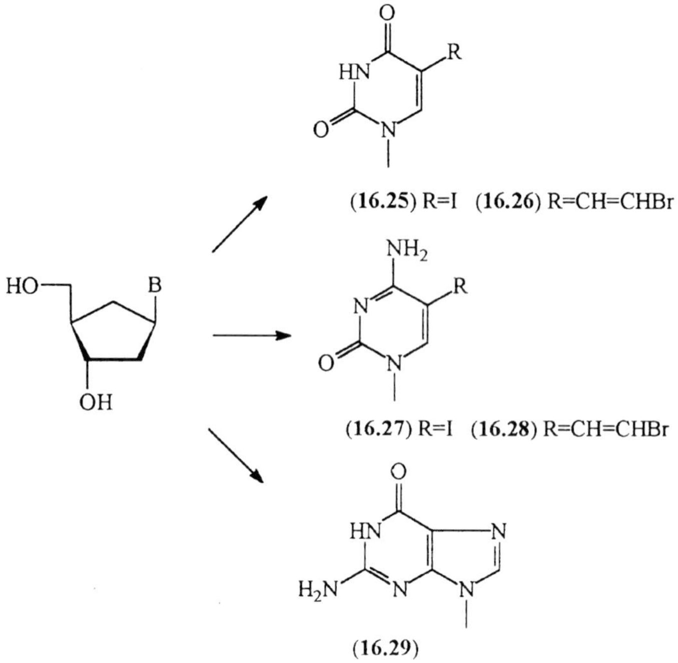

(16.25) R=I (16.26) R=CH=CHBr

(16.27) R=I (16.28) R=CH=CHBr

(16.29)

Scheme 16.14

Another example of a carbocyclic compound is cyclaradine (**16.30**). This compound is resistant to adenosine deaminase and less toxic than ara-A. The 5-methoxyacetyl derivative of cyclaradine (**16.31**) has proved more effective than acyclovir in the topical treatment of genital HSV-2 infection in animal models.

16.2.2 Nucleoside prodrugs

The activity of a compound *in vivo* is highly dependent on the formulation in which the compound is presented. Active research is focused on developing prodrugs with optimal bioavailability. Apart from the classical approach of using esters as prodrugs (see Chapter 13), other approaches are based on the knowledge of the different enzymes involved in nucleoside metabolism. One of the oldest examples in the nucleoside field is the use of the 5'-monophosphate of ara-A (**16.32**) (Scheme 16.15). Ara-A has a very low solubility in water (approximately 0.5 mg/ml). Administration of ara-A by infusion requires large volumes (2 liter for an adult person). The greater solubility of ara-A monophosphate permits the use of smaller infusion volumes.

Another enzyme which has proved valuable in the prodrug design is xanthine oxidase. Guanine nucleosides are very insoluble in water because of the strong intermolecular associations through hydrogen bonds between the base moieties. As a consequence, compounds such as acyclovir (**16.14**) are quite insoluble in body fluids. The 6-deoxy

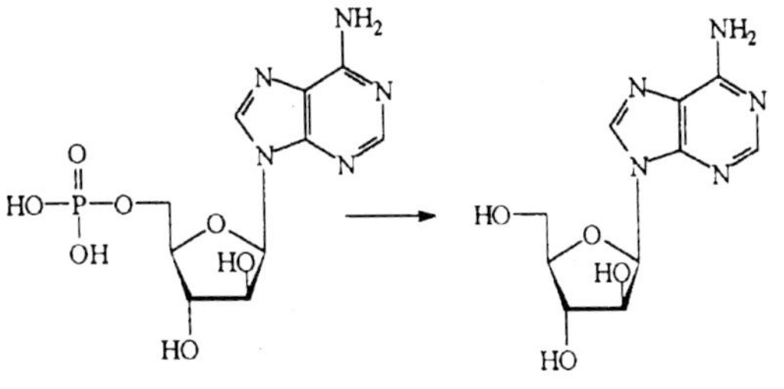

(16.32)

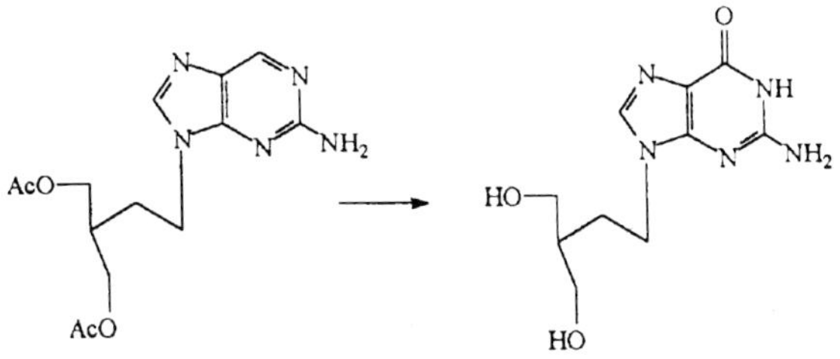

(16.34)

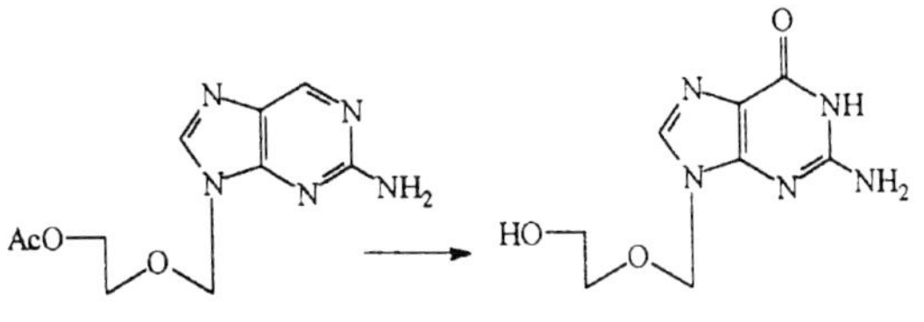

(16.33)

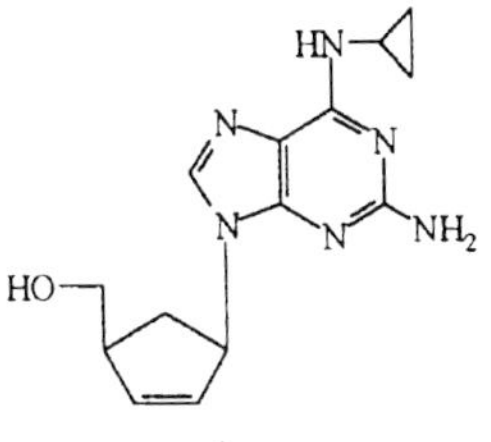

(16.35)

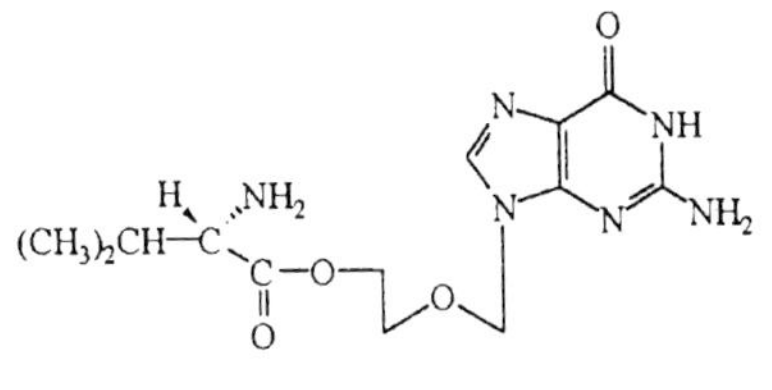

(16.36)

Scheme 16.15

analogue of acyclovir (desiclovir) (**16.33**) is more soluble and is metabolized *in vivo* by xanthine oxidase to acyclovir. When administered orally, 6-deoxyacyclovir gives the same blood levels of acyclovir as those obtained with intravenous acyclovir. An analogous approach has also proved successful for penciclovir (**16.16**). The diacetyl derivative of the 6-deoxy analogue of penciclovir (**16.34**) gives peak plasma concentrations after 1 h which are ten-fold higher than those detected following an equivalent oral dose of penciclovir.

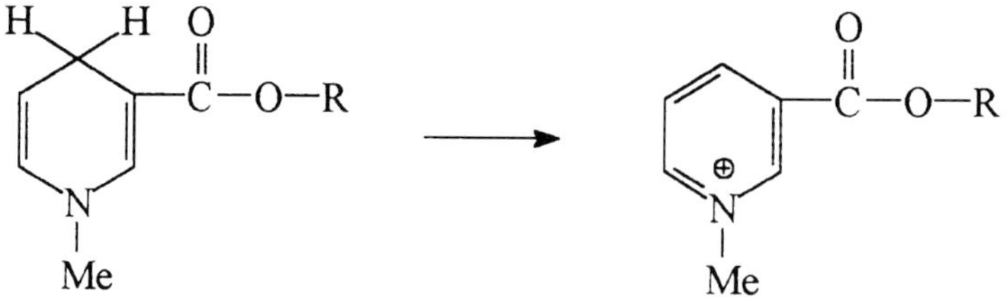

Scheme 16.16

This prodrug has been given the name of famciclovir, which has been launched for the systemic (i.e. oral) treatment of HSV and VZV infections. 1592 U89 (**16.35**) is an example of another prodrug form of a purine nucleoside. This compound is intracellularly activated to (−)-carbovir triphosphate by several metabolic steps.

The potential therapeutical armamentarium of acyclic anti-HSV and anti-VZV nucleosides has recently been extended to the L-valyl ester of acyclovir (valacyclovir) (**16.36**). This drug is a prodrug of acyclovir and has been developed because of the low oral bioavailability of the parent compound. It will be used for the systemic (i.e. oral) treatment of HSV and VZV infections.

One of the most attractive approaches for the delivery of drugs across the blood-brain barrier is based on the dihydropyridine-pyridinium salt redox system. The dihydropyridine drug precursor is taken up into the brain and oxidized to the pyridinium salt (Scheme 16.16). The charged compound is trapped within the brain where the drug is slowly released *via* enzymatic hydrolysis. This system has been used in attempts to target anti-HIV drugs such as azidothymidine (AZT) and 2′,3′-didehydro-2′,3′-dideoxythymidine (D4T) to the brain.

16.2.3 Analogues of 5′-monophosphates

As most, if not all, nucleosides need to be phosphorylated to exert their antiviral activity, an interesting approach would be based upon the use of the phosphorylated derivatives themselves.

The main problem associated with this approach, however, is that the phosphorylated derivatives are as such not taken up by cells (Scheme 16.17). Furthermore, 5′-O-phosphates of nucleosides are easily dephosphorylated by esterases which thereby release the parent nucleosides. The cyclic monophosphate of ganciclovir (**16.15**), however, is taken up intact by the cell and opened intracellularly to the (S)-enantiomer of ganciclovir-monophosphate (Scheme 16.18), which is then further phosphorylated to the triphosphate.

This compound (2′-norcGMP) (**16.37**) shows a broad-spectrum activity against DNA viruses (i.e. HSV-1, HSV-2, CMV, VZV and also against TK⁻ HSV strains) *in vitro*. It is also effective orally and topically in preventing orofacial HSV-1 infection and genital HSV-2 infection in mice.

A logic pursuit of this approach has led to the development of the nucleoside phosphonate derivatives. In designing such compounds, one should take into account that a glycosidic bond is *a priori* sensitive to chemical and enzymatic degradations whereas an alkylated purine or pyrimidine base should not have this problem. Thus, a new series of

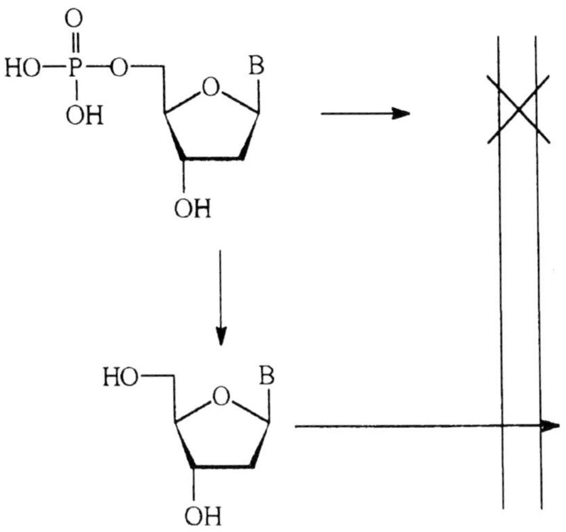

Scheme 16.17

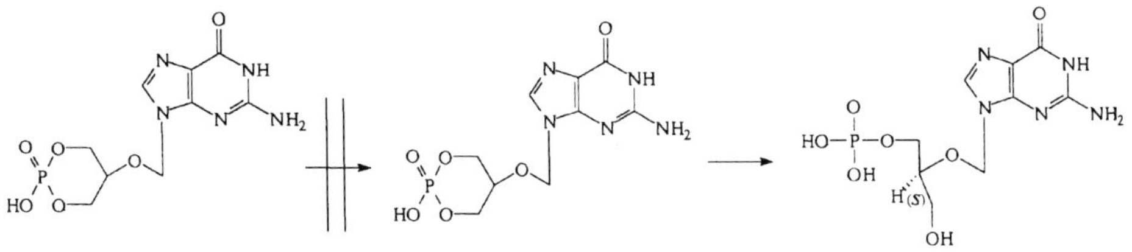

(16.37)

Scheme 16.18

purine and pyrimidine derivatives with an aliphatic side chain and a phosphonate group attached to it was developed. The first compound of this series, (S)-HPMPA or (S)-9-(3-hydroxy-2-phosphonylmethoxypropyl)adenine (**16.39**) was conceived after another acyclic nucleoside, (S)-DHPA or (S)-9-(2,3-dihydroxypropyl)adenine (**16.38**), that had been synthesized earlier and shown to inhibit the multiplication of several DNA viruses (i.e. vaccinia virus) and RNA viruses (i.e. vesicular stomatitis virus) *in vitro*.

(S)-HPMPA has a broad-spectrum activity against DNA viruses (i.e. HSV-1, TK⁻ HSV-1, HSV-2, VZV, TK⁻ VZV, CMV, EBV, vaccinia virus and adenoviruses). The most interesting features of this compound are that, on the one hand, it is stable against metabolic degradation and, on the other hand, it can penetrate cells thus circumventing the need for phosphorylation by dThd kinase (or other nucleoside kinases). Within the cell, (S)-HPMPA is further phosphorylated by cellular enzymes (i.e. AMP kinase and/or PRPP synthetase) to its diphosphoryl derivative. (S)-HPMPA inhibits viral DNA synthesis at a concentration

NH₂ (adenine ring)
|
CH₂
|
(S) CHOH
|
CH₂OH

(S)-DHPA

(16.38)

NH₂ (adenine ring)
|
CH₂
|
(S) CH—O—CH₂—P(=O)—OH
| |
CH₂OH   OH

(S)-HPMPA

(16.39)

NH₂ (adenine ring)
|
(CH₂)₂
|
O
|
CH₂   O
| ‖
O=P—OCH₂OC—Buᵗ
|
O
|
CH₂
|
O
|
C=O
|
Buᵗ

(16.40)

which is by several orders of magnitude lower than the concentration required for inhibition of cellular DNA synthesis. Two compounds derived from (S)-HPMPA, and showing even more interesting activity, are PMEA (**16.5**) and (S)-HPMPC (**16.4**). PMEA shows potent anti-retrovirus activity *in vitro* and *in vivo* (mice, cats, lambs, monkeys and man) and is a promising candidate for the treatment of HIV and HBV infections. Because of the low bioavailability of PMEA, an oral prodrug i.e. bis(POM)PMEA (**16.40**), is now under clinical investigation for the treatment of HIV infections in man. The conversion of an acid into its pivaloyloxymethyl ester to increase its bioavailability has already been demonstrated to be very useful in the antibiotic field (i.e. pivampicillin). (S)-HPMPC (**16.14**) is the most potent and selective inhibitor of the *in vitro* CMV replication that has been described to date. Of particular interest also is the activity of (S)-HPMPC against herpes viruses other than CMV, as well as adeno- and papillomaviruses.

16.2.4 Nucleosides which do not need phosphorylation to exert antiviral activity

As mentioned in the introduction, any nucleoside that is phosphorylated within the cell has the potential of interacting with the cellular DNA polymerases and may eventually be incorporated into the DNA of the cells. To avoid this potential problem, one may envisage molecular targets with which the nucleoside analogues can as such interact without having to be phosphorylated.

S-Adenosylhomocysteine (SAH) hydrolase is a key enzyme in transmethylation reactions depending on S-adenosylmethionine (SAM) as the methyl donor. Such methyltransferases are required for the maturation of viral mRNA, i.e. for 5′-capping. As SAH is not only the product but also an inhibitor of the SAM-dependent transmethylation reaction, inhibitors of SAH hydrolase may be expected to interfere with viral mRNA methylation through the accumulation of SAH (Scheme 16.19).

The prototype inhibitor of SAH hydrolase is (S)-DHPA (**16.38**). It is active against some (−)RNA (rabies, measles, parainfluenza), (±)RNA (reo) and DNA (vaccinia) viruses.

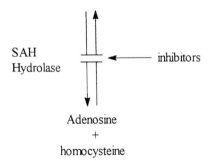

S-adenosylmethionine

maturation of
viral mRNA ← Methyltransferases

S-adenosylhomocysteine

SAH
Hydrolase ← inhibitors

Adenosine
+
homocysteine

Scheme 16.19

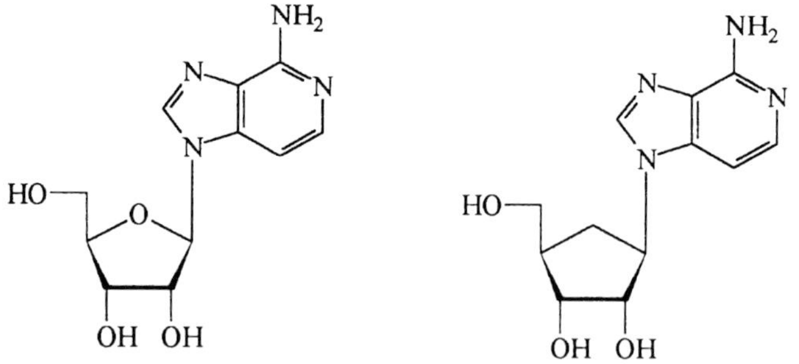

(16.41)   (16.42)

More potent inhibitors of SAH hydrolase are found among the carbocyclic analogues of 3-deazaadenosine.

3-Deazaadenosine (**16.41**) is neither deaminated nor phosphorylated. It is a substrate for SAH hydrolase which means that the resulting 3-deazaadenosylhomocysteine can act as an inhibitor of the methylation reaction. However, 3-deazaadenosine is antivirally active at concentrations which are only 5- to 10-fold lower than its cytotoxic concentration. The carbocyclic analogue of 3-deazaadenosine 3-deazaaristeromycin (C-c^{3}Ado) (**16.42**), is a more potent inhibitor of SAH hydrolase than 3-deazaadenosine (**16.41**). It is active against the same spectrum of viruses as (*S*)-DHPA (**16.38**) at concentrations ranging from 0.2 μg/ml to 1 μg/ml.

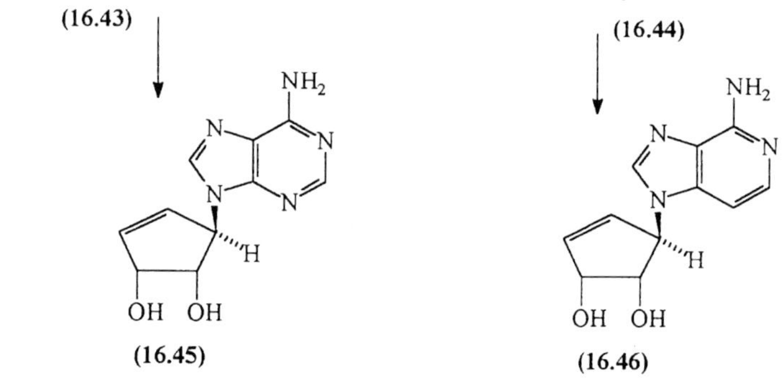

(16.43)   (16.44)

(16.45)   (16.46)

Scheme 16.20

Neplanocin A (**16.43**) (Scheme 16.20), a naturally occurring nucleoside, is even more potent as an inhibitor of SAH hydrolase than C-c^{3}Ado. It also is a more potent antiviral agent, but rather toxic and not very active *in vivo*. The 3-deaza analogue of neplanocin A (**16.44**) has been synthesized. Again, this compound is a powerful inhibitor of SAH hydrolase and a potent antiviral agent.

For these adenosine analogues, to act preferentially at the SAH hydrolase level, they should not be phosphorylated nor deaminated. Phosphorylation would make the compound cytotoxic and deamination would make them biologically inert. Both phosphorylation and deamination require an intact 5′-hydroxyl group. Removal of the 5′-CH$_2$OH group leads to compounds (**16.45**) and (**16.46**) with increased selectivity as SAH hydrolase inhibitors. This is a nice example of rational drug design.

There are plenty of examples of nucleoside analogues which are very active *in vitro* but not efficacious as antiviral agents *in vivo*, primarily because of toxicity. A typical example is pyrazofurin (**16.47**) (Scheme 16.21). This compound belongs to the most potent and selective *in vitro* inhibitors of orthomyxo (i.e. influenza) and paramyxo (i.e. measles, respiratory syncitial) virus infections which have ever been described. Yet, its systemic use *in vivo* is impeded by toxicity. Perhaps, pyrazofurin may be useful in the topical treatment (i.e. as an aerosol) of respiratory tract virus infections.

Toxic compounds could also be used as model compounds in attempts to separate activity from toxicity. For example, tubercidin (**16.48**) (Scheme 16.21), the 7-deaza analogue of adenosine, is highly toxic to mammalian cells and of no use as an antiviral drug. Modification of the *ribo* to the *xylo* configuration results in a product (9-β-D-xylofuranosyl-7-deazaadenine) (**16.49**) which has lost much of its toxicity, yet retained potent activity against HSV-1 and HSV-2.

Recently benzimidazole nucleosides have been described with potent and selective activity against human cytomegalovirus. The prototype of this series is 2-bromo-5,6-dichloro-1-(β-D-ribofuranosyl)benzimidazole (**16.50**) (Scheme 16.21). This compound prevents the appearance of unit lengths DNA and high molecular weight head-to-tail concatamers are formed. Normally, these concatamers are processed to unit length DNA during the DNA packaging process.

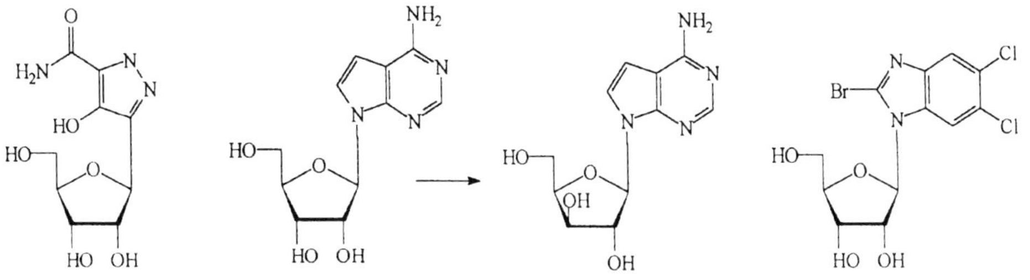

(16.47)   (16.48)   (16.49)   (16.50)

Scheme 16.21

16.2.5 Nucleosides with the non-natural L-configuration

All nucleosides which have been described before have a carbohydrate fragment corresponding to the D-series. Till recently, it was generally accepted that nucleosides belonging to the L-series will not be accepted as substrates for enzymes and, thus, will not be active. Surprising results, however, were obtained with these "mirror-image" nucleosides.

(16.51) X = H   (16.53) X = H
(16.52) X = F   (16.54) X = F

Dideoxycytidine (16.21) is very active against HIV (EC$_{50}$:0.01 μM), but is also quite toxic (CC$_{50}$:10 μM). Its L-isomer (16.51) is somewhat less active against HIV (EC$_{50}$:0.02 μM) but has markedly lower toxicity (CC$_{50}$:100 μM). This difference has also been observed with 3'-thiacytidine. The activity (EC$_{50}$) and toxicity (CC$_{50}$) of the compound with the "natural" structure is 0.25 μM and 1 μM, respectively. The "unnatural" (−)-isomer (16.53) is as active (0.2 μM) but less toxic (>100 μM). Clinical trials with this compound (3TC, lamivudine), have been carried out. A striking characteristic of 16.51 and 16.53 and of their 5-fluorinated congeners (16.52) and (16.54) is that they are not only active against HIV but also HBV, which extends their potential use to the treatment of this latter disease. It has been suggested that the low toxicity of the L-series is due to the fact that these non-natural compounds are not transported in mitochondria. Part of the toxicity of the anti-HIV nucleosides AZT (16.13), DDC (16.21) and DDI (16.20) could be due to the inhibition of mitochondrial DNA synthesis.

16.2.6 Non-nucleoside antivirals

Numerous non-nucleoside compounds have been described that show *in vitro* antiviral activity against a wide variety of viruses. Some of these compounds have been marketed. Methisazone (16.55) has been advocated for prophylactic use against smallpox and therapeutic use against the complication of cowpox vaccination. There is at present no need for such prophylaxis or therapy.

Amantadine (16.57) and rimantadine (16.58) are used in the prophylaxis and early treatment of influenza A virus infections; in this regard rimantadine is as efficacious as amantadine and less prone to toxic side effects (i.e. for the central nervous system). Phosphonoformic acid (PFA) (16.56) is pursued for its potential in the treatment of CMV

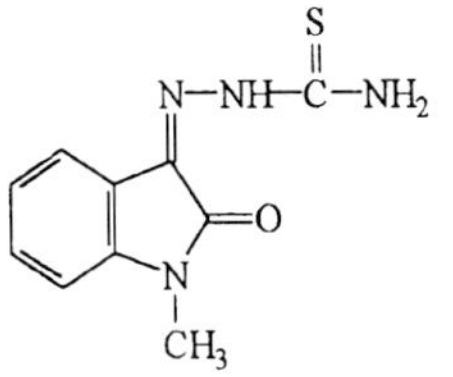

(16.55)

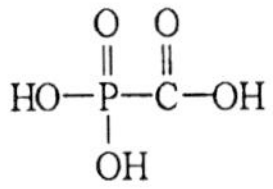

(16.56)

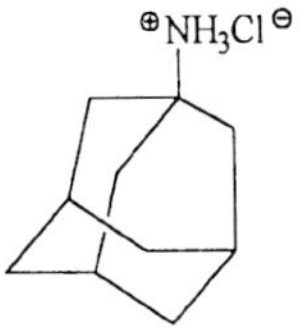

(16.57)

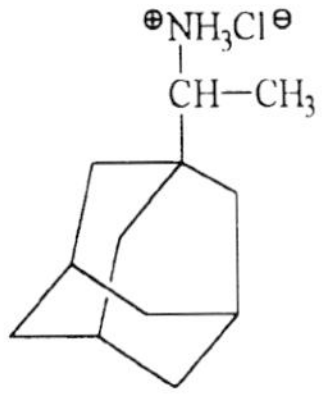

(16.58)

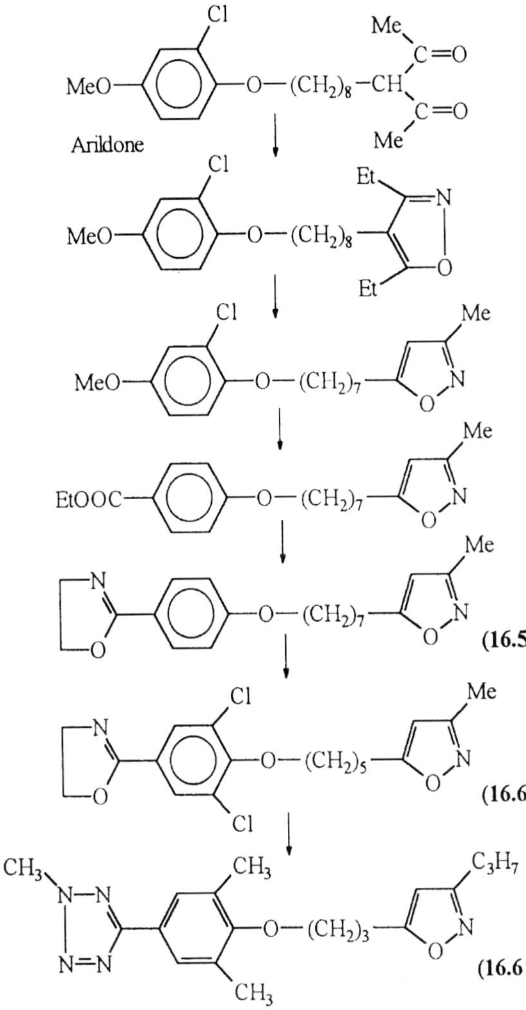

Arildone

(16.59)

(16.60)

(16.61)

Scheme 16.22

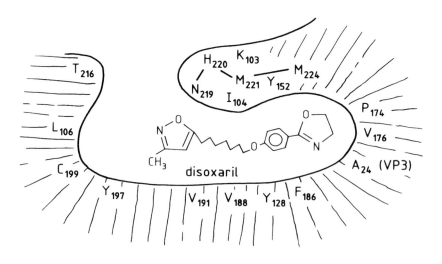

Figure 16.1

infections (particularly retinitis) in immunocompromised patients, as an alternative to ganciclovir (**16.15**) treatment.

Interferons have been proposed for the treatment of several viral infections, i.e. due to rhinovirus, influenza A virus, herpes viruses, papilloma virus, adenovirus, hepatitis B virus, hepatitis C virus and others, but their usefulness has remained controversial. Disoxaril (**16.59**) and its 4-methyloxazoline analogue exhibit broad-spectrum activity both against rhinoviruses and enteroviruses. These compounds are derived from arildone, a compound which is quite active against poliovirus but only marginally active against rhinoviruses. Systematic variation of the substituents on the phenyl ring and introduction of different heterocyclic rings on the "other side" has led to the discovery of disoxaril (**16.59**) as a potent antirhinovirus compound (Scheme 16.22).

These compounds specifically bind to the viral capsid and inhibit uncoating of the viral RNA. The interaction of these compounds with the viral capsid protein VP1 of rhinovirus-14 has been studied by X-ray crystallographic analyses. These compounds fit into a specific hydrophobic pocket, which corresponds to the cell receptor binding site and interacts with domains 1 and 2 of ICAM-1 (Fig. 16.1). Elucidation of the mode of action of the compounds at the molecular level may lead to compounds with greater activity and selectivity. Following this lead, an analogue of disoxaril, WIN 54954 (**16.60**) was shown to be more effective than disoxaril. The acid lability, however, of the oxazoline ring could explain the short half-life of these molecules. New analogues with a tetrazole ring were, therefore, designed. These molecules likewise demonstrate a broad spectrum of activity (15 human rhinovirus serotypes tested) at $\pm 0.02 \ \mu M$ (**16.61**).

A problem in the development of antirhinovirus compounds is the number of different serotypes (>100). Given the relative harmlessness of the common cold infection, any candidate drug has to be absolutely free of toxic side effects to be acceptable for clinical use. Nevertheless, a good antirhinovirus compound will be of great value because of the

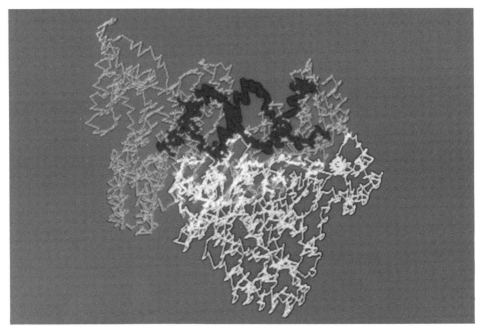

Figure 16.2 The structure of HIV reverse transcriptase. (See Color Plate VII.)

socio-economic impact of this disease. The problem with the above mentioned compounds is that they do not demonstrate significant clinical effects against rhinoviruses if administered after the onset of symptoms. However, they are able to reduce the symptoms of the infection when used prophylactically (i.e. disoxaril (**16.59**) and WIN 54954 (**16.60**) against human Coxsackie A21 virus infection).

16.2.7 Anti-AIDS compounds

Since the discovery of the human immunodeficiency virus type 1 (HIV-1) as the causative agent of the acquired immunodeficiency syndrome (AIDS), there has been an intensive search for HIV inhibitors. The number of promising compounds is already overwhelming and it will be a difficult task to select the best candidate compounds for the clinical trials.

The replicative cycle of HIV-1 offers a wealth of possible targets for antiviral agents.

The most potent anti-HIV-1 agents that so far have been identified interact with either the reverse transcriptase, viral protease or viral adsorption. Polyanionic substances such as sulfated polysaccharides interfere with the virus adsorption process. These compounds inhibit the replication of HIV *in vitro* at concentrations which are 3 to 4 orders of magnitude below their cytotoxicity threshold. Since HIV adsorption to the cells requires a specific interaction of the viral envelope glycoprotein, gp 120, with the CD4 receptor of the cell membrane, the viral absorption process can also be blocked by soluble CD4 constructs.

The uncoating of the virus can be inhibited by bicyclams from which a representative example is given (**16.62**). These compounds inhibit HIV replication at concentrations in the nanomolar range, which are $\geq 10^5$ lower than the cytotoxic concentrations.

Possible targets for anti-HIV therapy

Target	Potential anti-HIV agent
Virus adsorption	CD4 constructs, polysulphates, -sulfonates, -carboxylates and -oxometalates
Virus-cell fusion	plant lectins, negatively charged albumins, betulinic acids
Virus uncoating	bicyclams
Reverse transcriptase (Fig. 16.2)	nucleosides as substrate analogues
	non-nucleoside inhibitors
DNA replication	antigene oligonucleotides
Transcription	antisense oligonucleotides, tat-inhibitors
Translation	antisense oligonucleotides, ribozymes
Maturation	protease, myristoylation and glycosylation inhibitors
Virus budding	interferon-α

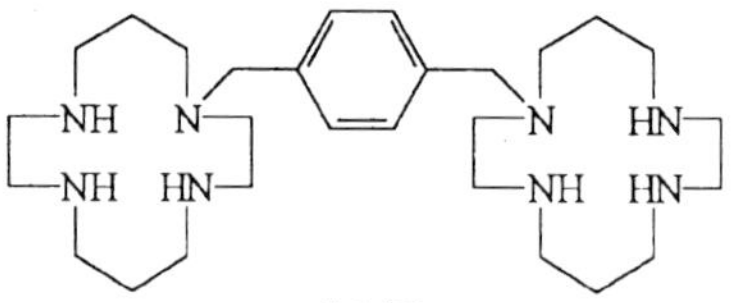

(16.62) 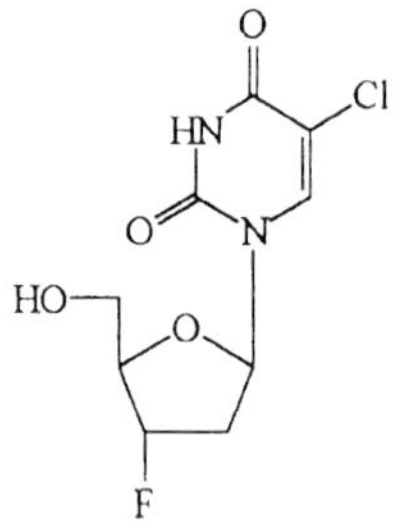   (16.63)

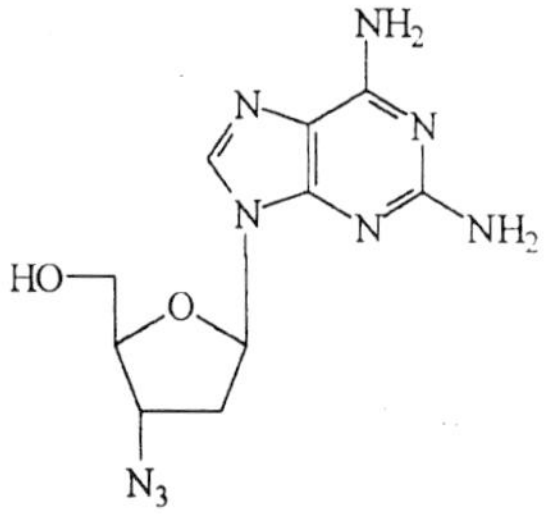

(16.64) 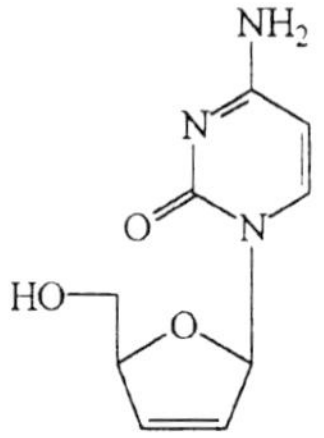   (16.65)

The most important nucleosides that inhibit HIV replication have already been mentioned (AZT, DDI, DDC, D4T, lamivudine, PMEA). Except for PMEA, these compounds can be considered as $2',3'$-dideoxynucleosides, or their $2',3'$-unsaturated counterparts, or $2',3'$-dideoxynucleosides with an azido- or fluoro substituent in the $3'$-erythro configuration, or $3'$-thianucleotides. Some of these compounds have selectivity indexes that approach or exceed that of AZT. Interesting congener which have not yet been tested in the clinic are $3'$-fluoro-5-chloro-dideoxyuridine (**16.63**), $3'$-azido-2-amino-$2',3'$-dideoxyadenosine (**16.64**) and $2',3'$-didehydro-$2',3'$-dideoxycytidine (**16.65**).

An increasing number of molecules of the non-nucleoside type that are targeted at the HIV-reverse transcriptase has been described. These non-substrate inhibitors bind tightly to the enzyme and inhibits its function. The structures of these inhibitors are very diverse. Rapid emergence of drug-resistant virus, however, may limit the effectiveness of mono-therapy with these compounds. Representative examples are TIBO (i.e. R-82913, **16.66**) nevirapine (i.e. BI-R6-587, **16.67**), α-anilinophenylacetamides (i.e. R-89439, **16.68**), pyridinones (i.e. L-697661, **16.69**), bis(heteroaryl)piperazines (i.e. U-90152, **16.70**) and phenylethylthioureathiazoles (i.e. LY-297345, **16.71**).

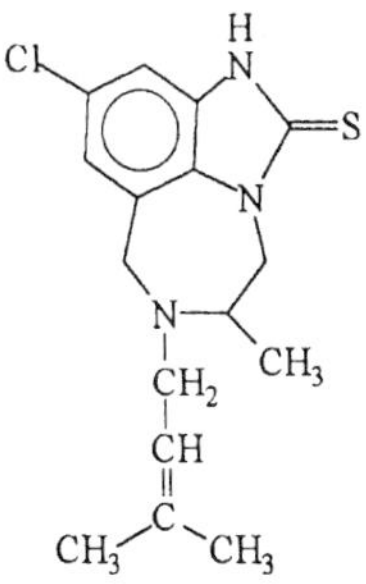

(16.66)

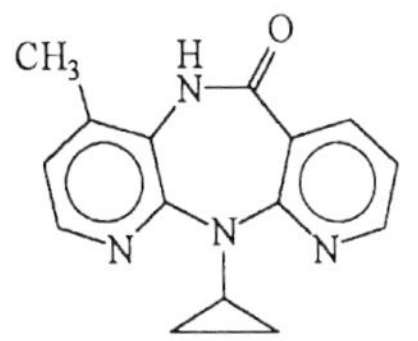

(16.67)

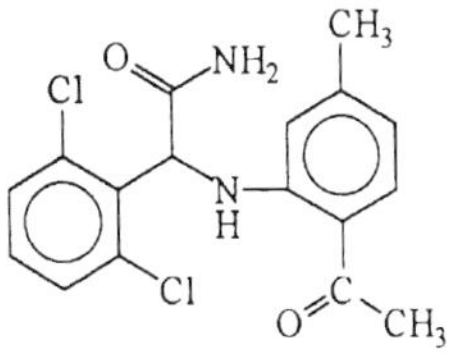

(16.68)

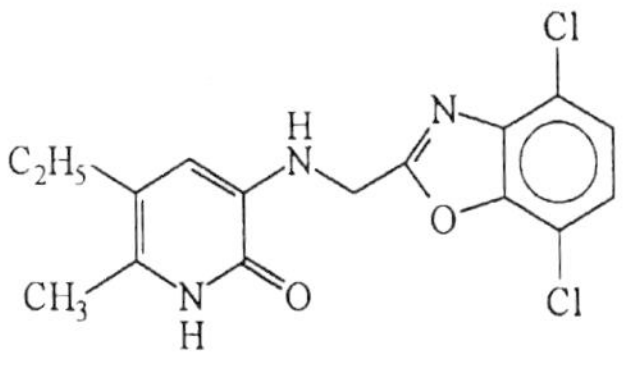

(16.69)

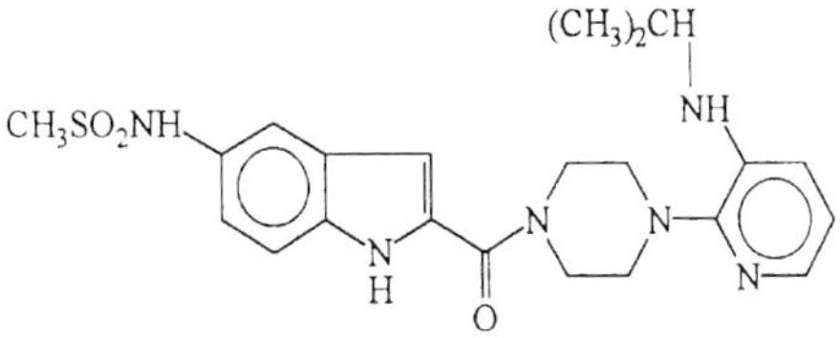

(16.70)

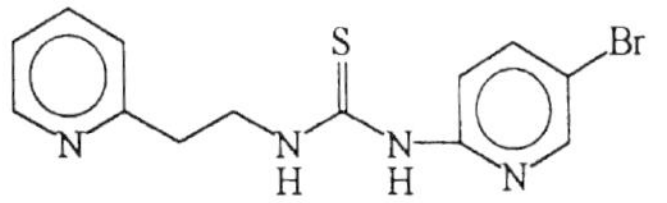

(16.71)

The maturate gag and pol proteins of HIV are formed from cleavage of precursor proteins (Pr55 and Pr160) by the action of aspartyl protease. As the HIV protease is required for viral infectivity, HIV protease inhibitors might be effective antivirals. The protease is composed of 99 amino acids. A structural aspect of the protease is the formation of a C_2-symmetric homodimer which generates the catalytic center and the substrate binding pocket. The X-ray structure of HIV protease has been resolved (Fig. 16.3) and complex formation with several inhibitors has been thoroughly investigated. The number of protease inhibitors, which have been identified by now, is of the same magnitude as the number of non-nucleoside reverse transcriptase inhibitors reported.

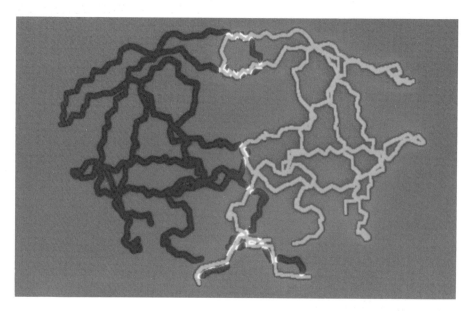

Figure 16.3   The structure of HIV-protease. (See Color Plate VIII.)

(16.72)

(16.73)

(16.74)

Some examples of protease inhibitors are shown. The Tyr(Phe)-Pro peptide linkage is the most frequent cleavage site for retroviral proteases. A number of hydroxyethylamine transition state isosteres as mimics of this natural substrate cleavage site have been described (i.e. Ro 318959, **16.72**). Potent inhibitors have been designed that match the symmetry of the enzyme. They consist of a central linker between two symmetrical moieties having substrate binding elements (i.e. A 77003, **16.73**). An example of a non-peptide protease inhibitor is the cyclic urea PMP 323 (**16.74**). Here the cyclic urea carbonyl oxygen atom mimics the hydrogen-bonding feature of a structural water molecule found in the HIV protease-inhibitor complexes. Clinical trials with several protease inhibitors are underway, the most advanced being those initiated with Ro 318959 (saquinavir).

After ten years of intensive anti-HIV research it is clear that the chemotherapy of HIV infections will require multi-drug combinations so as to maximally suppress virus replication and prevent drug-resistant virus from emerging.

FURTHER READING

Sidwell, R.W., Revankar, G.R. and Robins, R.K. (1985) Ribavirin: review of a broad spectrum antiviral agent. In *International Encyclopedia of Pharmacology and Therapeutics*, D. Shugar (ed.), **2**, 49–107.

Diana, G. and Dutko, F.A. (1990) A model for compounds active against human rhinovirus-14 based on X-ray crystallography data. *J. Med. Chem.*, **33**, 1306–1311.

Sachs, M.K. (1992) Antiretroviral chemotherapy of Human Immunodeficiency Virus infections other than azidothymidine. *Arch. Intern. Med.*, **152**, 485–501.

De Clercq, E. (1993) Antiviral agents: characteristics activity spectrum depending on the molecular target they interact with. In *Advances in Virus Research*, K. Maramorosch, F.A. Murphy and A.J. Shatkin (eds.), vol. 42, Academic Press, Orlando, Florida, pp. 1–55.

Herdewijn, P., Balzarini, J. and De Clercq, E. (1993) 2′,3′-Dideoxynucleoside analogues as anti-HIV agents. In *Advances in Antiviral Drug Design*, vol. 1, E. De Clercq (ed.). JAI Press Inc., Greenwich, Connecticut, pp. 233–318.

Balzarini, J. and De Clercq, E. (1994) Biochemical pharmacology of nucleoside analogues active against HIV. In *Textbook of AIDS Medicine*, S. Broder, T.C. Marigan and D. Bolognesi (eds.). Williams and Wilkins, Baltimore, Maryland, pp. 751–772.

Herdewijn, P. (1994) 5′-Substituted-2′-deoxyuridines as anti-HSV-1 agents: synthesis and structure activity relationship. *Antiv. Chem. Chemother.*, **5**, 131–146.

Balzarini, J. and De Clercq, E. (1995) Antiviral activity of acyclic purine nucleoside phosphonate derivatives. In *Antiviral Chemotherapy*, D.J. Jeffries and E. De Clercq (eds.). John Wiley and Sons Ltd., West Sussex, England, pp. 41–63.

17. ANTICANCER AGENTS

INGRID KJØLLER LARSEN

CONTENTS

17.1 DNA AS TARGET FOR ANTICANCER DRUGS

The DNA molecule is essential for the growth of all living cells, and so far it has been the main target for anticancer drug action. Some of these drugs act directly on the DNA molecule, either by drug induced DNA damage or by some kind of alteration of DNA (Section 17.1.1), whereas other drugs prevent nucleic acid synthesis by inhibiting one or more of the enzymes involved in the DNA synthesis, or by disturbing the DNA function by incorporation of "wrong pieces" into the DNA molecule (Section 17.1.2).

The DNA interacting drugs prevent cell growth, but not only cancer cell growth. Unfortunately, the growth of normal cells is also blocked. The cytotoxic effect is most serious on rapidly dividing cells, i.e. in addition to tumour cells the cells of normal bone marrow, gut, skin epithelium, and mucosa of the mouth.

The lack of selectivity of cancer drugs is one of the main problems in cancer chemotherapy. All the known abnormal biological phenomena of cancer cells (e.g. excessive cell proliferation, loss of tissue-specific characteristics, invasiveness, and metastasis) seem to be based on normal biological functions of the cells, e.g. by use of normal enzyme systems. The abnormality of malignant tumour growth is connected to the regulation of cell growth and caused by mutations in control genes, which are converted to oncogenes. The introduction of gene therapy might be a very important step forward in the treatment of cancer in the future. In most gene therapies full, healthy genes are introduced as substituents for wrong versions, but blocking of bad genes by a drug might also be possible (cf. Section 17.1.1.5).

It should be noticed that most anticancer drugs interfering with DNA or DNA synthesis also exhibit a variety of actions on other targets in the cells. The classification of anticancer drugs in this chapter is based on the mode of action of the specified anticancer agents, which is generally believed to be responsible for the cytotoxic activity.

All drugs with action directly on the DNA molecule affect all fast growing cells without preference for a special phase of the cell cycle (phase non-specific agents). They are, however, usually more effective against proliferating cells than against resting cells, where no DNA replication may occur for long periods of time. Drugs interfering with one or more of the enzymes involved in DNA synthesis are most effective in one phase of the cell cycle, i.e. the S phase of the cell cycle, which is the period of DNA synthesis (S phase specific agents).

One of the most serious problems in cancer chemotherapy is the development of drug resistance. Most drugs are initially very effective, but subsequent therapy may fail because the tumour cells have become non-sensitive to the drug. In many cases the mechanisms of resistance to antitumour drugs are known and are discussed later in this chapter under the individual classes of drugs.

In recent years the existence of multidrug resistance (MDR) has been recognized. MDR is characterized by cross-resistance to a group of structurally and mechanistically distinct antitumour agents including the anthracyclines (daunomycin and adriamycin), the vinca alkaloids (vincristine and vinblastine), colchicine and podophyllotoxins, and actinomycin D. However, this resistance does not extend to all anticancer agents, for example antimetabolites (e.g. methotrexate, cytarabine, and thioguanine) and alkylating agents (e.g. carmustine and cyclophosphamide) are not affected.

There are probably several different mechanisms by which cells can be cross-resistant to multiple drugs. However, MDR is commonly associated with high levels of a membrane associated phosphoglycoprotein (Pgp), which is a transport protein with extensive homology with bacterial transport proteins. Pgp functions as an energy (ATP) dependent drug efflux pump. It has been shown that the drug efflux from cells, in which the gene for Pgp is expressed, increases with resistance. The detailed mechanism by which Pgp pumps drugs out of cells is not fully understood.

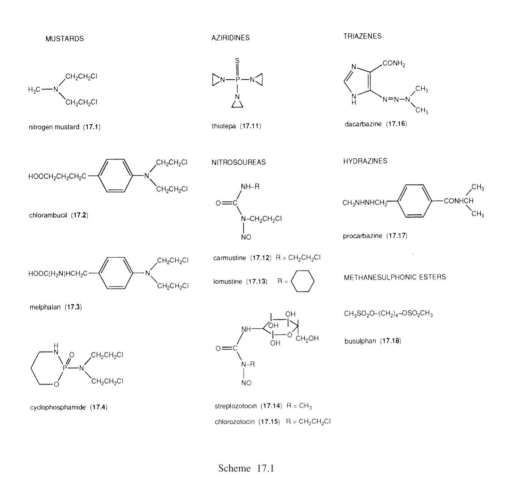

Scheme 17.1

17.1.1 Drugs interacting directly with DNA

The functions of the DNA molecule can be influenced by drugs in different ways. Damage to DNA, where covalent bond formation is involved, is performed by the category of compounds usually called alkylating agents, including some anticancer antibiotics (Section 17.1.1.1), and by *cis*-platinum complexes (Section 17.1.1.2). Breakdown of the DNA molecule (DNA strand scission) is caused by other antibiotic agents (Section 17.1.1.3). The intercalating agents (Section 17.1.1.4) disturb DNA function by intercalating between the base pairs, but normally without bond breakage or formation. Antisense anticancer agents (Section 17.1.1.5) are designed to perform their action on nucleic acids (canceling of specified base sequences) by a combination of intercalating and alkylating abilities, in addition to hydrogen bonding and hydrophobic interactions.

17.1.1.1 Alkylating agents
At least six major classes of alkylating agents are employed in cancer chemotherapy (cf. Scheme 17.1, where representative structures are given). All these compounds undergo a reaction in which an alkyl group becomes covalently linked to some cellular constituent, preferably the DNA molecule.

NITROGEN MUSTARDS

Nitrogen mustard (**17.1**), mustine, mechlorethamine, di(2-chloroethyl)methylamine is a volatile liquid, but it is administered clinically as the chloride. The salt is crystalline, but hygroscopic, and has to be dissolved in water immediately before use (intravenous saline infusion), because it is unstable in aqueous solution. The compound is very irritating (vesicant) to skin and mucous membranes, thus the acute side effects are severe and painful. The most serious delayed side effect is bone marrow depression, as also for all other alkylating agents. Nitrogen mustard has a very rapid alkylating effect and is therefore valuable in life-threatening situations.

Nitrogen mustard was the first drug used in cancer chemotherapy. It was discovered during the Second World War that the war gas *sulphur mustard* $[S(CH_2-CH_2-Cl)_2]$ and the isosterically related compound nitrogen mustard have antitumour activity. The sulphur mustard is too reactive and toxic for clinical use. Nitrogen mustard is also a very reactive drug with a number of toxic side effects, but it has proved to be a very useful drug, and it is still in clinical use, often in combination with other drugs.

The proposed mechanism of action of nitrogen mustard is shown in Scheme 17.2. The molecule forms a reactive cyclic intermediate, an aziridinium ion, by release of a chloride ion. This aziridinium ion is an electrophile, which attacks electron-rich centres (nucleophiles) in biological macromolecules. The reaction is an S_N2 process, as the bimolecular reaction with the nucleophile is the rate controlling step, which obeys second-order kinetics. The formation of the aziridinium ion is a very fast unimolecular reaction, when CH_3 (or another alkyl group) is connected to the N atom of the nitrogen mustard.

The nucleophilic groups, which can be attacked by the electrophile formed from nitrogen mustard, may be amino, hydroxyl, sulphhydryl or imidazole moieties in proteins and nucleic acids. The reaction of major importance in the cytotoxic effect of nitrogen mustards is the formation of a covalent bond with the N-7 of a guanine base of DNA. N-7 is thought to be the preferred position for purine alkylation, because it is more accessible than N-3, and N-1 is involved in hydrogen bonding in a Watson-Crick base pair.

The other chloroethyl side chain of nitrogen mustard can undergo a similar cyclization and react with another nucleophilic group. If this second reaction involves an N-7 of a guanine base from an opposite strand of the double helix, the result is cross-linking between the DNA strands. Intra-strand cross-links can also be formed, and, in addition, reactions between monoalkylated DNA and another nucleic acid or a protein are possible. There is a good correlation between DNA cross-linking and inhibition of cell growth, and DNA cross-links are generally believed to be responsible for the antitumour activity of bifunctional alkylating agents, e.g. nitrogen mustards. However, as many cellular constituents, including membrane proteins, can be alkylated, it might be assumed that the cytotoxicity is a result of many diverse effects.

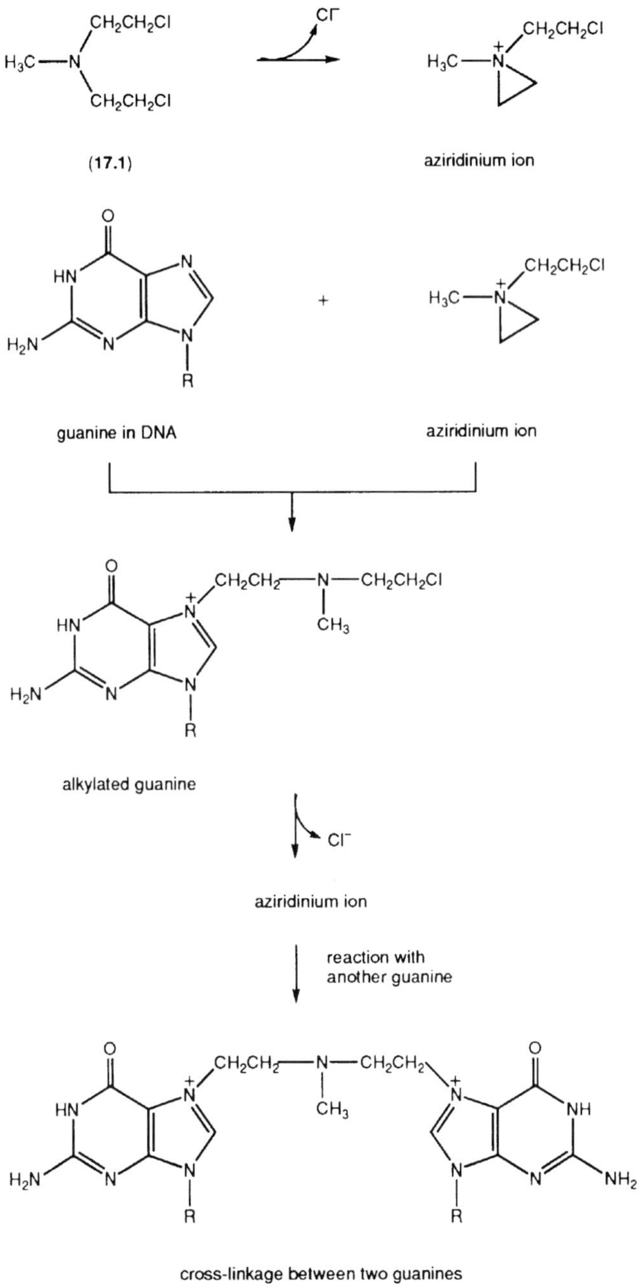
CH2CH2Cl
H3C—N
CH2CH2Cl
Cl⁻
(17.1)
aziridinium ion
guanine in DNA
aziridinium ion
alkylated guanine
aziridinium ion
reaction with
another guanine
cross-linkage between two guanines

Scheme 17.2

Nitrogen mustard is easily hydrolysed. This happens when the initially formed aziri-dinium ion reacts with a water molecule instead of a nucleophilic group of a biomacro-molecule. In this case the inactive hydroxy form of the compound [CH_3–$N(CH_2CH_2OH)_2$] is formed. A considerable amount of the injected drug is actually inactivated before reaching the biological targets.

Evidence for the formation of cross-links between two different DNA strands of the double helix has been obtained from different experiments. Alkylation of DNA bases, and especially intra- and interstrand cross-linking, disturbs the functions of the DNA molecule in different ways. The cross linkages prevent separation of the individual strands, thereby mainly inhibiting DNA replication, but DNA transcription will also be influenced. In addition, the operation of DNA polymerases may be affected.

All living cells can repair DNA damage, whether accidentally arisen or due to alkylating agents, by the DNA repair system, involving several enzymes (e.g. endonucleases, repair polymerase and ligase). Drug resistance of cells treated with nitrogen mustards (or other cross-linking agents) is due to an increased ability of the resistant cells to excise the cross-linked residues in DNA and repair the defect.

Chlorambucil (**17.2**), 4-[bis(2-chloroethyl)amino]benzenebutanoic acid, is a synthetically prepared, crystalline compound. This aromatic nitrogen mustard was introduced at an early stage of cancer therapy. It has a milder effect than nitrogen mustard, no serious acute side effects, and it can be given orally. The long term toxicity is bone marrow depression.

Melphalan (**17.3**), 4-[bis(2-chloroethyl)amino]-L-phenylalanine, is another crystalline nitrogen mustard with an aryl group attached to the N-atom. This drug was also developed as a drug with less reactivity (see below) than nitrogen mustard. In addition, it was originally synthesized in support of the idea that attachment of a mustard group to a naturally occurring carrier (in this case phenylalanine) might increase the effectiveness, because of increased affinity for certain biological sites. Since phenylalanine is a precursor for melanin, it was hoped that melphalan would preferentially accumulate in melanomas and thereby produce a selective effect. This early attempt on site-directed mustard effect was not successful, but still melphalan is a widely used drug, because of its pharmacological properties.

The mechanism of action of chlorambucil and melphalan is similar to that of nitrogen mustard (see Scheme 17.2). One of the advantages of nitrogen mustards, as compared to sulphur mustard, is that the third substituent (CH_3 in nitrogen mustard) can be varied in order to introduce some variation of the reactivity of the drug. Attachment of an aromatic ring to the nitrogen atom, as in chlorambucil and melphalan, decreases the rate of alkylation. The electron withdrawing effect of the ring, and/or delocalization of the lone pair electrons, makes the nitrogen atom less nucleophilic and the rate of cyclization much slower than for alkyl nitrogen mustards. This step (formation of aziridinium ion by first order cyclization) is probably the rate limiting step in the case of aryl nitrogen mustards, and the reaction is believed to be an S_N1 type process.

The decreased reactivity of aromatic nitrogen mustards can be advantageous for several reasons. The drug can be given orally, whereas nitrogen mustard has to be given intravenously. The higher stability allows time for absorption and wide distribution before degradation (hydrolysis) and before extensive alkylation. Finally, the acute side effects are much less severe. The biological effects are the same.

Cyclophosphamide (**17.4**), 1-bis(2-chloroethyl)amino-1-oxo-2-aza-5-oxaphosphoridine, is a nitrogen mustard with an oxazaphosphorine ring attached to the N-atom. It was synthesized originally as a transport form (prodrug) for nornitrogen mustard [normustine, $HN(CH_2CH_2Cl)_2$], which is also an active alkylating agent, but too toxic and with a low therapeutic index. The biochemical rationale behind this early approach to the development of a selective, target-directed prodrug was that the compound should be enzymatically converted into the active compound *in vivo* by phosphoramidase. Later it was demonstrated, however, that simple enzymatic cleavage is not the reason for the bioactivation of cyclophosphamide.

Cyclophosphamide (CPA) is one of the most effective alkylating agents with a wide application in cancer chemotherapy against many different neoplastic diseases. It can be given either orally or intravenously and its side effects are less severe and easier to control than those of nitrogen mustard (**17.1**). Immunosuppression is a side effect, which has led to its use to prevent transplant rejection. In addition, CPA has a number of undesirable side effects, some of which are probably caused by one or more of the metabolites.

CPA has to be metabolically activated in the body before it can alkylate cellular constituents. CPA by itself is not cytotoxic to cells in culture (*in vitro*), but cells are killed, when incubated with both the drug and a liver homogenate, which can convert it into the active form. The mechanism of the metabolic activation of CPA has been extensively studied. The metabolic degradation pathway is considered to be as shown in Scheme 17.3. The oxidation product 4-hydroxy-CPA (**17.5a**) either undergoes further oxidation (detoxification) into 4-keto-CPA (**17.6**) or tautomerizes into the open-chain aldehyde aldophosphamide (**17.5b**). Aldophosphamide may be oxidized into carboxy-CPA (**17.7**), a detoxification reaction, or the enol form of **17.5b** may undergo a spontaneous β-elimination (reverse Michael addition) to give acrolein (**17.8**) and phosphoramide mustard (**17.9**). In addition, nornitrogen mustard (**17.10**) is formed as a decomposition product (hydrolysis, non-enzymatic) of several of the above mentioned compounds.

Phosphoramide mustard (**17.9**) is generally believed to be the biologically active agent. Neither of the two major urinary metabolites (**17.6**) and (**17.7**) is significantly cytotoxic and represents inactivated excretion products. Acrolein (**17.8**) and phosphoramide mustard are produced in equimolar amounts during the metabolism of CPA. Because of the known toxicities of acrolein one might expect it to contribute to the final cytotoxicity of CPA. This is unlikely, however, as phosphoramide mustard is cytotoxic at levels considerably below the level of acrolein required for cytotoxicity. Some roles for acrolein in the pharmacology of CPA cannot be excluded, however. Thus, the bladder toxicity observed in patients treated with CPA is caused by acrolein and can be diminished by administration of the drug together with an alkyl sulphide (e.g. MESNA, sodium 2-mercaptoethanesulphonate) to remove acrolein by a Michael's reaction.

Phosphoramide mustard as well as nornitrogen mustard are powerful cytostatic agents, also *in vitro*, and high levels of both compounds can be detected in plasma 1–10 h after CPA infusion. Phosphoramide mustard is considered to be the ultimate alkylating agent for several reasons, e.g. because it is a more powerful alkylating agent than nornitrogen mustard. In addition, nornitrogen mustard is a sec. amine and may, after formation of an aziridinium ion, deliver H^+ to solvent, thereby forming the uncharged chloroethylaziridine, which is relatively resistant to nucleophilic attack.

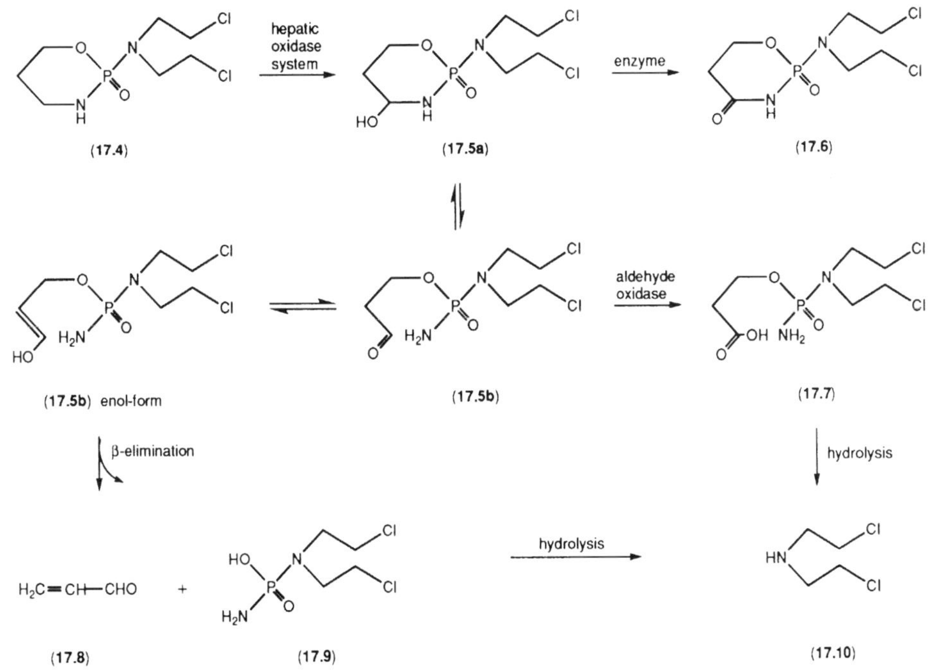

Scheme 17.3

Phosphoramide mustard (**17.9**) is an alkylating agent because of its ability to form an aziridinium ion in contrast to CPA (**17.4**), where the withdrawing electronegative effect of the ring, and delocalization of the lone pair electrons, makes the N atom less nucleophilic and the rate of initial cyclization very slow. In phosphoramide mustard, which is ionized at physiological pH (pKa of the OH group is 4.75), the nucleophilic effect of the N atom is not decreased because of strong contributions of the resonance forms with the negative charge on the two oxygen atoms of the phosphoramide group and therefore negligible delocalization of the lone pair on the N atom with the chloroethyl substituents.

The biological effect of CPA is the same as that of nitrogen mustard, i.e. formation of DNA cross-links by alkylation of guanine N-7. The initial phosphoramide-DNA adduct is unstable and converted to the corresponding nornitrogen mustard adduct G-nor-G. Monoalkylation also occurs. Many different methods have been used in order to obtain detailed understanding of the mechanism of cyclophosphamide cytotoxicity, including multinuclear (^{31}P, ^{13}C, ^{2}H, and ^{1}H) Fourier-transform NMR spectroscopy.

AZIRIDINES

Thiotepa (**17.11**), triethylenethiophosphoramide, tris(1-aziridinyl)phosphine sulphide, is a hexasubstituted triamide of thiophosphoric acid. Thiotepa is unstable in acid and is poorly absorbed from the gastrointestinal tract. It is therefore given intravenously or used topically, e.g. to treat papillary carcinoma of the bladder. The major side effect is bone marrow depression.

Thiotepa is not a nitrogen mustard, but contains aziridine rings. It has been developed as an analogue of the reactive aziridinium ions formed from nitrogen mustard, in order to obtain a deactivated alkylating agent. The aziridine ring is less attractive to nucleophiles because of the lack of a positive charge. However, if the third substituent on the N-atom of the aziridine ring is an electron-withdrawing group, some positive charge (electron deficiency) arises on the C-atoms of the aziridine ring, due to polarization of the bonds.

NITROSOUREAS

Carmustine (**17.12**), BCNU, N,N'-bis(2-chloroethyl)-N-nitrosourea, and the structural analogue *lomustine* (**17.13**), CCNU, N-(2-chloroethyl)-N'-cyclohexyl-N-nitrosourea, are developed as a result of the observation of promising antileukemic properties of N-methyl-N-nitrosourea in routine screening of this compound. The compounds are rather unstable in acidic and alkaline aqueous solutions. BCNU has to be given intravenously, whereas CCNU can be administered orally.

The nitrosoureas are unionized at physiological pH and consequently they have much higher lipid solubility than the nitrogen mustards and other alkylating agents. Their ability to pass the blood-brain barrier renders them especially useful in the treatment of central nervous system neoplasm (e.g. brain tumours and metastases). BCNU and CCNU both produce nausea and vomiting, and the delayed side effects are bone marrow depression, leukopenia, and thrombocytopenia. BCNU is the more toxic of the two compounds.

A number of theories on the mechanism of action of the nitrosoureas has been proposed. It is evident that these drugs are alkylating as well as carbamoylating agents and that cross-linking of DNA is a consequence of alkylation.

The proposed mechanisms for the alkylation and carbamoylation, which are outlined in Scheme 17.4, are based on the mechanism of decomposition of nitrosoureas in aqueous solution at pH 7.4. Base abstraction of the amide hydrogen atom produces an unstable intermediate, which rapidly decomposes to yield the corresponding alkylisocyanate and 2-chloroethanediazohydroxide. The isocyanate formed is capable of carbamoylating proteins, e.g. lysine and cysteine residues. By spontaneous decomposition of the diazohydroxide a chloroethyl carbocation is formed, which attacks a nucleophilic centre of base X. Both N-7 and O-6 of guanine may be alkylated (β-chloroethylated), and an ethylene bridge with the cytosine (base Y) on the complementary strand is then formed more slowly by elimination of a chloride ion. DNA-protein cross-links as well as monoalkylated nucleic acids and proteins can also occur as the result of alkylation with nitrosoureas. The relative contribution of alkylation *versus* carbamoylation to the cytotoxicity of the nitrosoureas is not known.

Streptozotocin (**17.14**), an anticancer antibiotic isolated from *Streptomyces achromogenes*, is a nitrosourea derivative with a glucose moiety at one N-atom and a methyl group at the other. By substitution of this methyl group with a chloroethyl group *chlorozotocin* (**17.15**) was obtained, which shows lower toxicity (myelosuppression) than streptozotocin.

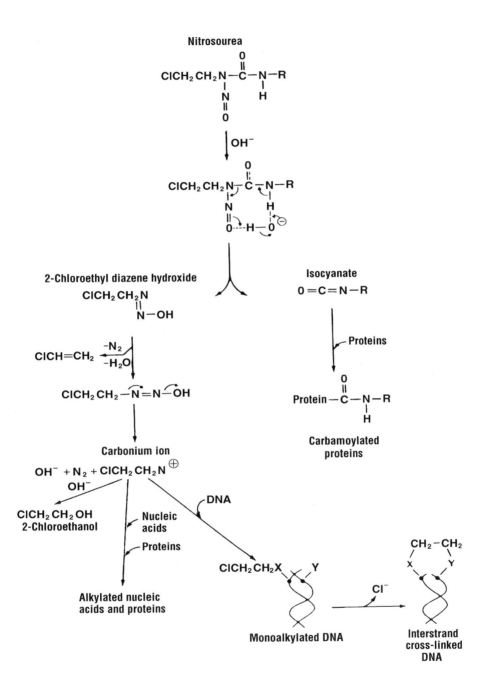

Scheme 17.4 (Scheme 17.4 with the following footnote: This scheme is reproduced from Pratt, W.B. and Ruddon, R.W.: "The Anticancer Drugs". Oxford University Press, Oxford 1979, with permission by Oxford University Press).

The drugs are retained in the β-cells of the islets of Langerhans and can be used experimentally to induce diabetes in laboratory animals. Insulin chock is a dangerous acute toxicity. Because of the β-cell effect the drugs can be used against metastatic islet cell carcinoma. The compounds probably act by alkylation of nucleophilic sites, but the precise mechanism has not been well worked out. The glucosamine moiety of the drug may be important by providing some specificity of uptake into β-cells.

TRIAZENES

Dacarbazine (**17.16**), DTIC, 5-(3,3-dimethyl-1-triazenyl)-1-*H*-imidazole-4-carboxamide, is a compound, which is stable in solution, but has to be protected against light. The drug is given intravenously and produces severe nausea and vomiting and sometimes a flu-like syndrome or fever. Dacarbazine has appeared to be particularly suitable for the treatment of malignant melanoma.

Dacarbazine was originally developed as a structural analogue of 5-aminoimidazole-4-carboxamide, an intermediate in purine biosynthesis. It is, however, now known that the cytotoxicity of the drug is due to its alkylating (methylating) action, rather than to inhibition of purine biosynthesis. The generally accepted mechanism (metabolism and subsequent chemical decomposition) is shown in Scheme 17.5.

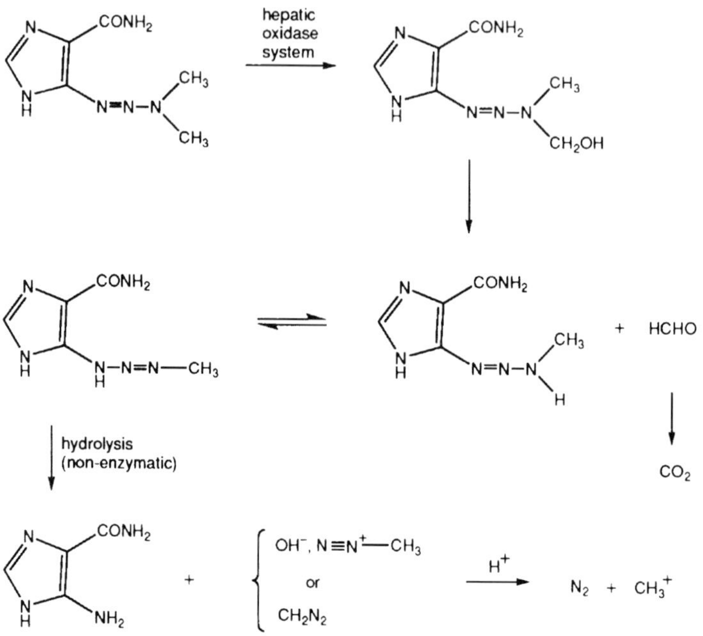

Scheme 17.5

The monomethyl derivative produced *via* the corresponding hydroxymethyl derivative by enzymatic oxidation decomposes spontaneously (non-enzymatically) to form 5-aminoimidazole-4-carboxamide (the major metabolite excreted in the urine) and the methylating agent, which is methyl carbocations, formed from either diazomethane (CH_2N_2), or methyldiazonium hydroxide ($CH_3N_2^+OH^-$). The methyl carbocations can attack nucleophilic groups in DNA and other cellular constituents. An important site of *in vivo* alkylation is the N-7 position of guanine, and the 7-methylguanine product has been identified in the urine of patients given ^{14}C-methyl-dacarbazine.

Many triazenes have been investigated in which the imidazole ring has been replaced by other heterocyclic systems or phenyl derivatives in a search for second-generation antitumour triazenes with enhanced selectivity and activity. The studies have shown that the nature of the aromatic moiety does not affect the activity markedly. Substitution of one of the methyl groups of the triazene moiety has no effect on antitumour activity, provided that the replacement alkyl group can undergo oxidative dealkylation (depends e.g. on chain length and bulkyness of the alkyl group). If both methyl groups of the triazene N atom are substituted by other alkyl groups, total loss of activity is observed. It is not yet fully understood why methyl substituents predispose so decisively towards the activity of the triazenes.

HYDRAZINES

Procarbazine (**17.17**), *N*-(1-methylethyl)-4-[(2-methylhydrazino)methyl]benzamide, is used as the chloride of the hydrazine. This compound was synthesized as a potential monoamine oxidase (MAO) inhibitor, but it was later shown to have antitumour effect. It is clinically used both in combination drug therapy and in various drug protocols to treat e.g. melanoma and Hodgkin's disease. Procarbazine can penetrate into the cerebrospinal fluid and has been used to treat malignant brain tumours. Its side effects are similar to those of typical alkylating agents, but it also causes psychopharmacological effects consistent with its ability to inhibit MAO.

Procarbazine is inactive *in vitro* and requires enzymatic activation before it shows antitumour activity. *In vivo* it is rapidly converted to azo-procarbazine, CH_3–N=N–CH_2–C_6H_4–CONHCH(CH_3)$_2$, probably by hepatic microsomal enzymes. Several pathways have been proposed for the conversion of this intermediate to the major urinary metabolite *N*-isopropylterephthalamic acid, HOOC–C_6H_4–CONHCH(CH_3)$_2$. Methane is observed as a minor metabolite, and it has been suggested that methyl radicals or methyl carbocations are the biologically active methylating agent.

METHANESULPHONATE ESTERS

Busulphan (**17.18**), myleran, 1,4-bis(methanesulphonyloxy)butane is unstable in aqueous solution, but can still be given orally and is well absorbed from the gastrointestinal tract. If is excreted in the urine as methanesulphonic acid and several metabolites, which are derived from the alkylating butylene moiety. It is a very mild alkylating agent with no acute side effects, and it is useful mainly in the treatment of patients with chronic granulocytic leukemia. A number of long term side effects are observed, among those bone marrow depression.

Busulphan is a bifunctional alkylating agent, which has a reactivity considerably lower than that of nitrogen mustard. The mechanism of the alkylation is believed to be similar to that of nitrogen mustards. The alkyl-oxygen bond splits with the methanesulphonate moiety as the leaving group. The carbocation formed reacts with nucleophilic centres of the cell constituents, including N-7 of guanine bases, but also with sulphhydryl groups of cysteines in proteins. Diguanyl derivatives can be formed as a reaction product between busulfan and nucleotides, and cross-linking of DNA is believed to be the main reason for the cytotoxic activity of busulphan.

17.1.1.2 Metal complex binding to DNA

Platinum coordination complexes with the formula cis-PtA_2X_2 where X is a uninegative, readily exchangeable group, and A is ammonia or an amine, have been known for many years to exhibit antitumour properties. The initial trials were very promising, but the toxic side effects, e.g. renal toxicity, appeared to be a serious limitation of the use of the Pt-complexes as anticancer agents. Improved administration procedures have now resulted in large-scale clinical application of cis-Pt-complexes, especially in combination treatment of testicular cancer. The antitumour properties of cis-Pt-complexes are now accepted to be mainly based on interactions of these compounds with DNA. Introduction of Pt-complexes is regarded as one of the most important acquisitions in cancer chemotherapy of the last decade.

cisplatin (**17.19**)   carboplatin (**17.20**)   ormaplatin (**17.21**)

A = NH₃   X = Cl

Cisplatin (**17.19**), *cis*-diammine-dichloroplatinum(II), is routinely administered by intravenous infusion, and supplied as a lyophylized powder, because of the low solubility in water. Cisplatin is particularly used in combination therapy (e.g. with taxol and bleomycin) in the treatment of testicular cancer, but good response in the treatment of several other cancer forms has been observed. The toxic side effects are diminished by improved administration of the drug.

Several methods have been used in order to elucidate the mechanism of action of cisplatin and other Pt-complexes. It is known that cisplatin interacts with DNA by specific binding to the guanine N-7 sites. Binding to cytidine N-3, adenine N-1, and adenine N-7 is also possible, but is less common. A second binding interaction readily takes place on the same strand of DNA, most frequently at another guanine base being a next-neighbour. Interstrand cross-linking is also possible.

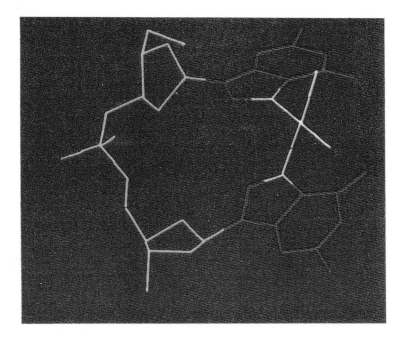

Plate 17.1   Structural model of the Pt(NH$_3$)$_2$ (d(GpG)) adduct, determined from analysis of the NMR spectra. From Reedijk, J. in "NMR Spectroscopy in Drug Research". Eds. J.W. Jaroszewski, K. Schaumburg and H. Kofod. Munksgaard, Copenhagen 1988, with permission by Munksgaard. (See Color Plate IX.)

Detailed information on the nature of the binding of cisplatin to DNA has been obtained from studies of the model complexes consisting of cisplatin bound to short DNA fragments. The accurate structure in solution of the adduct *cis*-Pt(NH$_3$)$_2$- [d(GpG)]$^+$ has been studied using high-resolution NMR techniques, and the solid state structure of the very similar adduct *cis*-Pt(NH$_3$)$_2$- [d(pGpG)] was solved using X-ray diffraction (see Plate 17.1). The geometry of the two adducts (in solution and in the solid state) were shown to be substantially the same. Pt binds to the two guanine bases of the dinucleotide by coordination through N-7, and the conformational changes of the overall structure of the nucleotide are limited to small changes in the position of the sugar ring at the 5′ side of d(GpG) and of the dihedral angle between the guanine bases. The distortion of the DNA structure, after chelation of cisplatin to a GG sequence, should therefore be rather small.

NMR studies of the double helix model compound, prepared from the Pt chelate of the decanucleotide d(TCTCGGTCTC) by addition of the complementary strand d(GAGACC-GAGA), show that normal Watson-Crick type hydrogen bonding remains possible after platination. In addition, the model studies suggest a helix distortion, which can best be described as a kink or a bend in the helical axis of about 40 $^\circ$ (see Plate 17.2). The biological consequences of the rather small DNA distortion is not quite clear, but it appears to be large enough to hamper cell replication. The cytotoxic effects of cisplatin might, however, be considered to be due to the combined effects of various lesions.

It has also been known for some time that *trans*-PtA$_2$X$_2$, e.g. *trans*-diamminedichloro-platinum(II), binds to DNA, but these complexes have much lower cytotoxic effect and

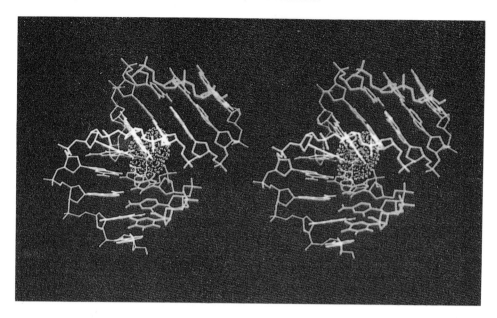

Plate 17.2   Stereo projection of a possible distorted helical DNA structure after chelation of cisplatin to the central GG bases of the same strand. (From Reedijk, J. – see legend to Plate 17.1). (See Color Plate X.)

no anticancer activity. As the binding affinities to the nucleobases are quite comparable with those of the *cis*-complexes, the different activity must originate from differences related to the bifunctional binding. NMR studies have shown that *trans*-Pt compounds can chelate to GNG sequences (N = A, T or C) through the guanine N-7 atoms, but the distortion of DNA after such *trans* binding is larger. This has prompted the hypothesis that repair enzymes recognize and remove the *trans* compound easier than the *cis* compound. It has been shown recently, however, that planar ligands, e.g. pyridines, dramatically enhances the cytotoxicity of *trans*-Pt-complexes. The reason for this is not known.

Several thousands of analogues of cisplatin has been synthesized and tested in order to enhance the therapeutic index. So far most analogues are found to be so-called "me too" versions of cisplatin. The only one, which has provided definite advantage over cisplatin is *carboplatin* (**17.20**), *cis*-diamine-1,1-dicyclobutanedicarboxylatoplatinum(II). Carboplatin has, however, afforded benefit only in reducing some of the toxic side effects. It has the same spectrum of anticancer activity, and it is not active in cisplatin-resistant cancers.

SAR studies has been performed on *cis*-platinum compounds with the following conclusions:

(1) The nature of the leaving group X in PtA_2X_2 determines the rate of the substitution reactions. Introduction of very labile groups, such as H_2O or NO_3^-, gives rise to very toxic compounds with little or no antitumour activity. On the other hand, strongly bound groups, such as thiocyanate, are inactive in biological systems.

(2) The nature of the amine group A coordinated to platinum also influences anti-cancer activity. Active compounds have at least one hydrogen atom at the N atom of the amine ligand, which should not be too large. *Ormaplatin* (**17.21**), 1,2-

diaminecyclohexanetetrachloroplatinum(IV), is an analog with platinum(IV) configuration and with a rather bulky amine substituent. Ormaplatin is in clinical trial and
is of interest because of a broad spectrum of antitumour activity, and because it is also
active against cisplatin-resistant cell lines and less nephrotoxic than cisplatin.

(3) The net-charge of the complexes has to be zero. Presumably charged complexes are
unable to cross the cell membranes.

17.1.1.3 Degradation of DNA

Anticancer agents of a wide range of structural types have been observed to produce
strand breaks in DNA *in vivo* and *in vitro*. These include some of the earlier mentioned
categories of compounds, e.g. nitrosoureas, but this is not the primary cytotoxic action of
these compounds, as it appears to be in the case of *bleomycin*. This drug binds to DNA
and causes strand scission by an oxidative attack involving chelated iron and free radical
species.

Bleomycin (**17.22**). Bleomycins are a group of related glycopeptide antibiotics isolated
from *Streptomyces verticillus*. Bleomycin A$_2$ (Scheme 17.6) is the major component of
the bleomycin employed clinically (as the sulphate). The various bleomycins differ only in
their terminal amine moieties R. In bleomycinic acid, which is inactive, the terminal amine
moiety is replaced by a hydroxyl group.

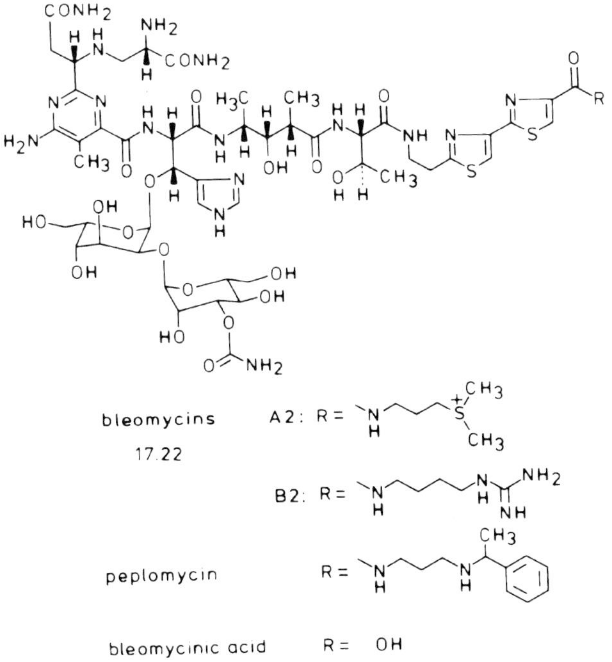

Scheme 17.6

Bleomycin (BLM) can be given by a number of parenteral routes, but it is most commonly injected intravenously. The drug is widely distributed in the tissues, except in brain tissue. Apparently BLM cannot enter the cerebrospinal fluid in any significant concentration. The highest concentrations of active drug are found in skin and lung. This is important because these two sites are very susceptible to BLM toxicity. The most common acute side effects involve the skin and mucous membranes, and the most severe, dose-limiting BLM toxicity is the pulmonary toxicity. BLM is unique among the available antitumour antibiotics by producing very little bone marrow depression. For this reason it is particularly useful in combination therapy with nearly all major anticancer drugs.

The chemistry and biological effects and mechanism of action of BLM have been extensively studied. The glycopeptide contains several unusual amino acids and sugars, a pyrimidine ring, an imidazole ring, and a planar bithiazole ring system. X-ray structure determination of BLM has not been reported, and the structure shown in Scheme 17.6 is based on conventional methods and confirmed by high-resolution, two-dimensional NMR spectroscopy.

The right part of the BLM molecule is the DNA-binding domain, and the left part is the metal chelating domain, where the reaction with DNA is initiated. The bithiazole moiety is believed to bind in the minor grove of DNA with specific DNA sequences leading to sequence specificity in DNA cleavage. Computer analysis and modelling of a DNA-BLM complex has been performed, but the structure of the complex has not yet been confirmed by X-ray analysis. The reaction by which DNA strand scission is effected by BLM has been found to require Fe(II) and O_2 as cofactors. The ultimate agent of DNA damage is an active BLM dioxygen species ("activated BLM").

BLM forms one-to-one complexes with several metals, e.g. copper, zinc, iron, and cobalt. The BLM-Cu(II) complex is the most stable complex and also the natural form produced by fermentation. It is inactive and resistant to BLM hydrolase, a BLM inactivating enzyme. BLM hydrolase is present in cells and hydrolyses metal-free BLM, resulting in inactivation of BLM.

After injection of BLM (metal-free) it binds to Cu(II) ions in blood to form the stable BLM-Cu(II) complex. Inside the cells, the copper of the complex is removed reductively and trapped by other proteins, leaving BLM free to form the active iron complex (or to be inactivated enzymatically). Thus, the Cu(II) complex of BLM has two biological functions, (1) to protect against inactivation, and (2) to provide transport and distribution in the body in an inactive form.

The structure of the BLM-Cu(II) complex is shown in Scheme 17.7, together with the BLM-Fe(II)-O_2 complex. The structures are proposed structures, as no metal-BLM structure has yet been solved by the X-ray method. The structure of the copper complex is, however, based on the X-ray structure of a model compound, i.e. a smaller part of the BLM molecule, lacking the sugar and bithiazole moieties. The BLM-Fe(II) structure is believed to be similar, but in the oxygenated complex there is strong evidence suggesting that dioxygen is the sixth ligand.

In the cells the oxygenated complex, BLM-Fe(II)-O_2, is further converted into a transient ferric species called "activated BLM", which slowly decays to BLM-Fe(III). Activated BLM is believed to be the ultimate agent of DNA damage. The structure of the active complex is not known with certainty, but it has been shown to be a Fe(III) complex. By transfer of one electron from Fe(II) to the molecular oxygen ligand a resonance form with a superoxide

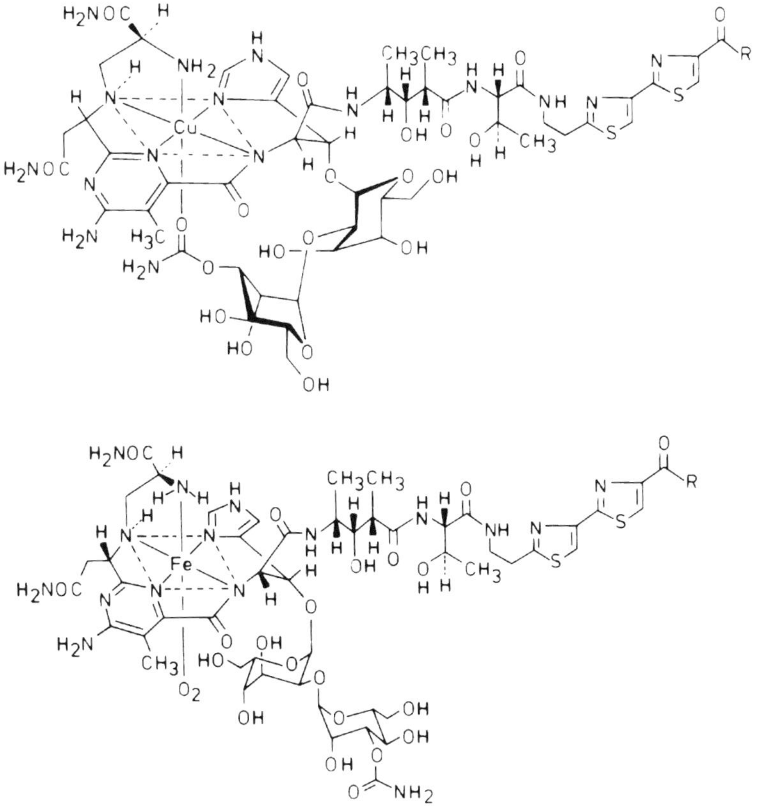

Scheme 17.7

anion ligand is formed [BLM-Fe(III)-O$_2^{\cdot-}$]. One-electron reduction of the complex yields activated BLM, and the active complex is probably BLM-Fe(III)-O$_2^{2-}$, i.e. with a peroxide anion ligand. Activated BLM can also be formed anaerobically from BLM-Fe(III) and H$_2$O$_2$.

The degradation of DNA by BLM, which has been studied by identification of the products (DNA fragments) formed, is initiated by an attack on the ribose sugar ring (abstraction of the 4′ H atom), and, while degrading the deoxyribose, BLM releases the bases undamaged. This is compatible with a site-specific generation of an oxygen radical species close to a susceptible site on the deoxyribose moiety and remote from the bases.

One of the disadvantages of BLM treatment is the development of pulmonary fibrosis. A lot of semi-synthetic BLM analogues have been prepared in order to find an active drug with lower pulmonary toxicity, e.g. *peplomycin*, a BLM with a synthetic terminal amine (see Scheme 17.6). Semi-synthetic BLM analogues can be prepared by reaction of the Cu(II) complex of BLM acid (Scheme 17.6) with the amine in the presence of a coupling reagent for peptide synthesis. BLM acid is prepared enzymatically from native BLM in order to avoid cleavage also of other peptide bonds in the molecule. The Cu(II) coordination protects the primary amino group in the α-position of the terminal β-aminoalanine moiety and prevents inter- and intramolecular coupling.

As earlier mentioned, Cu(II) coordination also protects against BLM hydrolase inactivation, as the terminal β-aminoalanine carboxamide is the recognition site of the enzyme. Several attempts have been performed in order to achieve drugs resistant to enzymatic hydrolysis. N-alkylation of the primary amino group in the α-position leads to diminished anticancer activity, probably due to difficulty in coordination of the amino group with metal. It appeared to be a better idea to transform the carboxamide group into a secondary amide.

17.1.1.4 Intercalating agents

Several compounds bind reversibly to double-stranded DNA by intercalation, i.e. by squeezing in between adjacent base pairs of DNA. Such compounds have to be rather planar and are most often aromatic ring systems, which are held between the flat purine and pyrimidine rings by van der Waals' forces and charge-transfer complex formation. Some of the compounds also bind covalently, in some cases after metabolic transformation, e.g. *benzopyrene*, which is a carcinogen. Intercalating drugs can be primarily antibacterial (e.g. *aminoacridines*), antimalarial (e.g. *mepacrine*), or carcinostatic agents (e.g. *actinomycin D, daunomycin* and *adriamycin*). In this chapter only the anticancer agents will be considered.

Several techniques have been used to characterize the interactions of intercalating agents with DNA. Evidence for binding to DNA can be obtained by determination of the association constant and number of binding sites. Intercalating agents give rise to increase in the length of DNA, as shown diagrammatically in Figure 17.1. This unwinding property of intercalators can be used in several ways to demonstrate that drugs bind to DNA by intercalation. One method is to investigate the effect of the drugs on the supercoiling of closed circular duplex DNA, by monitoring the rate of sedimentation, which decreases by unwinding. The anticancer antibiotic *mithramycin* is an example of a drug, which binds to DNA in a different way, as it does not change DNA supercoiling. Detailed information on the nature of the binding of intercalating agents to DNA can be obtained by studying model drug-DNA complexes by NMR methods or – if crystalline complexes are available – by X-ray structure determinations. In addition, molecular modelling methods have become increasingly significant in recent years.

DNA intercalation has various biological consequences, e.g. inhibition of DNA replication and transcription, probably due to prevention of DNA/RNA polymerase activity. The cytotoxicity of intercalating agents is believed to be primarily a consequence of the DNA interaction, but DNA damage (strand scissions), produced by some of the drugs, probably contributes to the cytotoxicity and may play an important role in their mutagenic and carcinogenic activity.

Actinomycin D (**17.23**), dactinomycin, AMD, is an anticancer antibiotic isolated from *Streptomyces* species. Several other actinomycins have been isolated from natural sources or developed by chemical modifications, but AMD is the only one used clinically. It is given by rapid flowing infusion, because injection is accompanied by severe local reaction. Because of additional serious and painful side effects, both acute and delayed, it has got limited clinical application, but has been extensively used as a research tool.

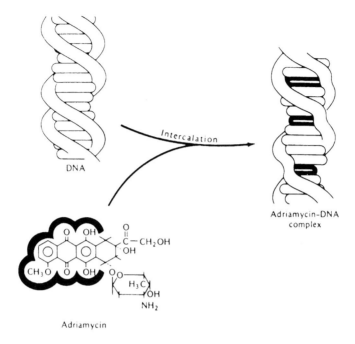

Adriamycin

Figure 17.1 Diagrammatic model of intercalation of the flat part of the adriamycin molecule (in black) into DNA, showing local unwinding of the helical structure. From Lerman, L.S. *J. Cell. Comp. Physiol.*, **64**, Suppl. 1:1 (1964) with permission by LISS (Alan R. Liss, Inc.). New York.

actinomycin D (**17.23**)

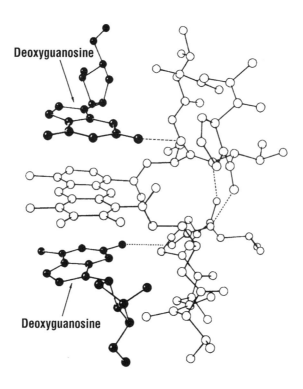

Figure 17.2 The X-ray structure of the actinomycin-deoxyguanosine complex. The two deoxyguanosine molecules stack on alternate sides of the phenoxazone ring. Hydrogen bonds are indicated by dashed lines. (Redrawn from Sobell, H.M., *et al. Nature New Biol.*, **231**, 200 (1971), with permission by Macmillan Journals Ltd).

The AMD molecule consists of an aminophenoxazone ring system, to which two identical cyclic pentapeptides are attached. The first and the last amino acids are linked by the formation of a lactone ring. It seems reasonable to expect that the aromatic ring system is the intercalating part of the molecule. Information on the binding of AMD to DNA was originally obtained from the X-ray structure determination of a drug-nucleoside model complex, namely the co-crystallized complex of AMD and deoxyguanosine (see Fig. 17.2).

The study showed that the planar phenoxazone ring of AMD in the model complex is squeezed in between the planar guanine bases of two deoxyguanosine molecules. Strong hydrogen bonds connect the 2-amino groups of guanine and the carbonyl oxygen of threonine residues in the cyclic peptides and contribute to the strong binding of AMD to DNA together with the "stacking forces" (charge-transfer complex formation). The structure of this and other model complexes suggest that AMD recognizes 5'-GpC-3' sites of DNA. In addition, based on model building the cyclic peptides were suggested to lie in the minor grove of DNA. This has recently been confirmed by structure determination of a model complex consisting of AMD and the self-complementary double

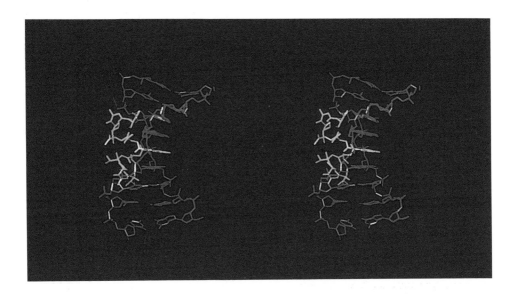

Plate 17.3   Stereoview of the AMD-d(GAAGCTTC) complex. The AMD molecule is shown in magenta, the DNA octamer in green. This side view of the complex shows the intercalation of the chromofore in the G5C5 site and the cyclic peptides of AMD in the minor groove. The structure was generated using the programme SYBYL with coordinates from Brookhaven Protein Data Base. (See Color Plate XI.)

helix DNA octamer d(GAAGCTTC), see Plate 17.3. The numerous van der Waals interactions between the peptide side chains and DNA contribute considerably to the tight binding of AMD.

Structure-activity studies on AMD analogues have shown that replacement of *N*-methylvaline with valine leads to reduced activity due to the strong hydrophobic binding of *N*-methylvaline to DNA. Replacement or removing of the amino group or the quinone function of the phenoxazone ring also leads to loss of activity. The model structure AMD-d(GAAGCTTC) shows that the amino group is important, as it is hydrogen bonded to two ribose oxygen atoms of one of the DNA strands. The quinone imine chromophore of AMD is probably reduced enzymatically in the cells and the free radical species formed is believed to cause chromosomal damage and DNA fragmentation. This effect contributes to the cytotoxicity of AMD.

Daunomycin (**17.24**), daunorubicin and *adriamycin* (**17.25**) doxorubicin, are both anthracycline antibiotics isolated from various *Streptomyces peucetius* species. The compounds are unstable in alkaline and acidic aqueous solution and cannot be given orally. Although daunomycin and adriamycin are nearly identical structurally, adriamycin is more cytotoxic and has a wider spectrum of antitumour activity. The reasons for these differences in activity are not quite clear. Both drugs bind tightly to DNA with comparable association constants (ca. 10^5 M^{-1}). The differences in potency and clinical use may be due to differences in uptake, transport and distribution of the drugs.

daunomycin (**17.24**) R = H

adriamycin (**17.25**) R = OH

Adriamycin has the broadest range of clinical usefulness of all the anticancer drugs in routine clinical use. It has established activity against several solid tumours, which earlier had been relatively unresponsive to chemotherapy. Daunomycin is primarily used to treat acute leukemia. The side effects of the two anthracycline drugs are similar, e.g. nausea and vomiting, alopecia, myelosuppression and cardiotoxicity (cardiomyopathy). The cardiotoxicity is the most serious side effect, which limits the doses and the duration of the treatment. This effect seems to be connected to the quinone moiety of the aromatic ring system, which, after reduction to a semiquinone radical species, induces lipid peroxidation by a free radical mechanism. Thousands of analogues have been synthesized and tested in order to find effective drugs without – or with lower – cardiotoxicity.

The anthracyclines daunomycin and adriamycin have a characteristic four-ring structure (rings A–D), the aglycon chromophore, which is linked, *via* a glycoside bond, to an amino sugar, daunosamine. The rings B–D constitute the anthracycline nucleus. The only difference between the structures of the two drugs is in the C-9 side chain of ring A, where CH_3 in daunomycin is replaced by CH_2OH in adriamycin.

The interaction of daunomycin and adriamycin with DNA by intercalation has been demonstrated by several methods. Detailed information on the daunomycin-DNA interactions has been obtained from X-ray structure determinations of several model complexes, e.g. of daunomycin co-crystallized with the self-complementary DNA hexamer fragment d(CGTACG). The six-base pair fragment of the double helix of DNA binds two molecules of daunomycin (plus several water molecules and two sodium ions). The structure of part of this model compound is shown in Figure 17.3, which focuses on four base pairs of the hexamer with daunomycin intercalated.

In the model complex the planar anthracycline part of the daunomycin molecule is squeezed in between the layers of C-G base pairs of the right-handed DNA double helix (B-DNA), at the CpG sites of both ends of the hexamer duplex (cf. the structure of the adriamycin-DNA hexamer complex shown in Plate 17.4). The long axis of the anthracycline aglycon is almost perpendicular to the direction of the base pair hydrogen bonds. This is in contrast to model complexes of other drugs, e.g. *proflavine* in the complex of this drug with

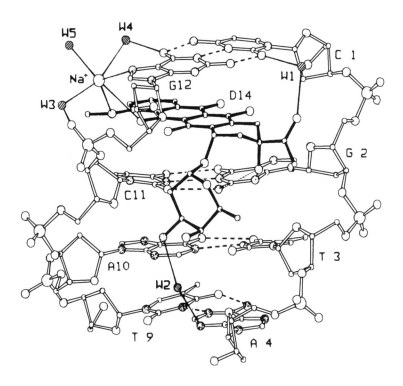

Figure 17.3   Diagram of daunomycin (D14) intercalated into the DNA hexamer. Four base pairs are shown (G12:C1, C11:G2, A10:T3, and T9:A4). Hydrogen bonds in base pairs are represented by dashed lines, other hydrogen bonds by dotted lines (those involving O-9) or thin lines (those involving bridging water molecules, W1 and W2). From Wang, H.-J., *et al. Biochemistry*, **26**, 1152 (1987), with permission by The American Chemical Society.

the dinucleotide d(CpG), where the long axis of the proflavine molecule is parallel to the base pair hydrogen bonds (parallel overlap). As a result of the non-parallel intercalation of the daunomycin aglycon, the amino sugar ring is placed in the minor groove of DNA, while the ring D of the anthracycline moiety protrudes on the major groove side. The distance between the base pairs of the intercalation site is increased from the normal 3.4 to 6.8 Å, and this can be achieved by adjusting the torsion angles of the phosphate ester backbones, resulting in a slightly distorted DNA fragment (unwinding of the DNA double helix).

The model complex shows that the cyclohexane ring A of the daunomycin aglycon is almost planar, with the exception of C-9, which is displaced in the same direction as the amino sugar relative to the plane of the aglycon. This arrangement, in combination with the axially placed hydroxyl group at C-9, gives rise to several specific hydrogen bonding interactions, which stabilize the binding of daunomycin. The hydroxyl oxygen atom O-9

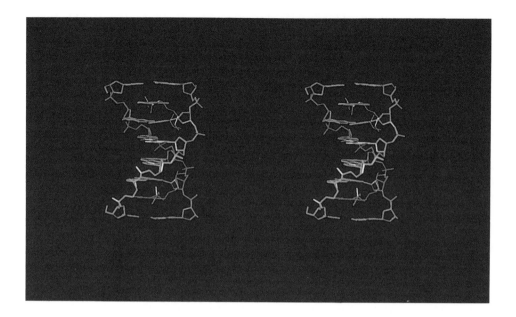

Plate 17.4   A stereoview of the adriamycin-d(CGATCG) complex. The two antibiotic molecules are shown in green, the DNA hexamer in red. The structure was generated using the programme SYBYL with coordinates from Brookhaven Protein Data Base. (See Color Plate XII.)

is involved in two hydrogen bonds, both to nitrogen atoms of the guanine base G2 below the intercalator. Another hydrogen bonding system is seen on the other side of the aglycon ring system involving the C-13 oxygen atom O-13. This carbonyl oxygen is hydrogen bonded *via* a water molecule (W1) to a carbonyl oxygen atom of the cytosine ring C1 in the base pair above the intercalator. In this way the OH group and the side chain at C-9 of ring A together serves as an anchor for the daunomycin molecule and contributes considerably to the stability of the binding complex, in addition to the "stacking forces" due to the intercalation.

The amino sugar portion of daunomycin is held in a proper orientation by the hydrogen bonding system of the C-9 substituents. It fits snugly into the minor groove, but this position excludes any interaction between the positively charged amino group of the sugar ring and the negatively charged phosphate oxygen atoms of the backbone. The X-ray results show that the sugar ring is very mobile, probably due to the lack of strong specific hydrogen bonding as well as ionic interactions. It has been proposed that this "anchored flexibility" may allow the functional groups of the sugar to interact non-productively with DNA polymerase, while at the same time blocking productive interaction of the polymerase with DNA and thereby inhibiting replication.

The X-ray structures of the model complexes consisting of the related DNA hexamer d(CGATCG) and daunomycin and adriamycin, respectively, have been solved recently, and both are almost isostructural with the daunomycin-d(GGTACG) complex. In all of the three structures the anthracycline antibiotic intercalate with d(CpG) as the intercalation step, indicating some sequence specificity of the drugs. Theoretical as well as experimental studies indicate that the third base pair is also of importance and should preferably be an A-T base pair (triplet recognition). In the adriamycin complex the O-14 hydroxyl group is hydrogen bonded to a nearby phosphate group *via* a water molecule.

Structure-activity studies, involving numerous synthetic, semisynthetic as well as natural anthracycline analogues, have been performed with the aim of finding structural analogues with reduced toxicity and/or a wider spectrum of activity. The testing for anticancer activity of compounds with modifications in the amino sugar moiety showed relatively low limitations for structural variations in this part of the drug molecule. The chirality of the 4'-position can be changed, *epirubicin* (4'-epidoxorubicin) has antitumour activity comparable to doxorubicin. The therapeutic index of the compound is more favourable because of reduced cardiotoxicity when compared to doxorubicin and epirubicin is now in clinical use. *Esorubicin* (4'-deoxydoxorubicin), which also has favourable pharmacological properties, is undergoing clinical trials. Both drugs have been crystallized complexed with DNA hexamers. In the epirubicin complex the inverted (O-4') hydroxyl is hydrogen bonded to an adenine base below the intercalation step.

The presence of a cationic charge on the sugar ring seems to be of importance. Acylation of the amino group leads to markedly lower potency as is the case when the amino group is replaced by a hydroxy group. In the anticancer antibiotic *aclacinomycin A* a trisaccharide is coupled to the anthracycline aglycon. This trisaccharide can be fitted easily in the minor groove of the double helix, reflecting the flexibility and low structural requirements of the amino sugar of these drugs.

mitoxanthrone (**17.26**)

$R_1 = R_2 = NHCH_2CH_2NHCH_2CH_2OH$

The more recent anticancer agent, *mitoxanthrone* (**17.26**), is an aminoalkyl-substituted anthraquinone, i.e. a derivative where the amino sugar, as well as ring A, are replaced by side chains with several possibilities for hydrogen bonding and protonation (hydroxy and amino functions). X-ray structure determination of a mitoxantrone-nucleotide model complex has not been published, but computer modelling and energy calculations have shown that this compound, as well as several analogues, can also bind intercalatively with DNA, and that the aminoalkyl substituents are used to anchor the molecules. Mitoxanthrone is an example of a drug designed on the basis of knowledge on drug-DNA interactions obtained from model complexes.

The methoxy group on C-4 of ring D of the anthracycline moiety of daunomycin and adriamycin is not required for anticancer activity, *idarubicin* (4-demethoxydaunorubicin) is a highly active compound. This is in accordance with the model, which shows that ring D protrudes out into the major groove without direct interaction with the DNA helix. *Carminomycin*, in which the methoxy group is replaced with an OH group, also has antitumour activity. The hydroquinone system is more sensitive to structural changes. The overlap of the rings B and C with base pairs is relatively small, but the oxygen atoms on each side of the rings may play a stabilizing role by being stacked with the bases. Methylation of the hydroxy groups results in loss of potency and lower affinity to DNA.

The geometry and substitutions of ring A are most important for the activity of anthracycline antibiotics. This is in full agreement with the model, which shows that this part anchors the molecules by hydrogen bonding to the bases on either side of the intercalator. The chirality at C-9 and C-7 cannot be changed without loss of activity. Substitution of the C-9 hydroxyl group with a methyl group also leads to inactive compounds, and when the hydroxy group is removed, compounds with reduced affinity to DNA and lowered potency and anticancer efficacy are obtained. Ring A cannot be 9,10-dehydrogenated without loss of activity, probably because the proper "sofa"-conformation of the ring is thereby hindered. The C-9 side chain has to be of small size and with one or two oxygen atoms, which can provide for the hydrogen bonding to the base pair above the intercalator molecule.

Several drug design studies are aimed at developing sequence-specific DNA intercalators, e.g. bis-intercalators in which two intercalating ligands are bridged by a central linking chain, in order to obtain specific effects and stronger binding to DNA. Such compounds might become of interest in gene therapy.

17.1.1.5 Antisense agents

Nucleic acids are the targets for the so-called antisense agents, which are under design and development for anticancer or antivirus chemotherapy. Antisense RNA and DNA is a new and emerging technique for selective manipulation of gene activity. In this technique an "antisense" sequence (inverted piece of the gene code) complementary to the coding strand is used to specifically lock unto potentially dangerous genetic messengers, canceling their ability to do harm. The bad gene could be a cancer-causing oncogene, and this is one of the potential roles of antisense agents in cancer therapy.

Antisense agents normally target the gene's messenger RNA (mRNA), as they are designed to bind with and block the specific piece corresponding to the bad gene on DNA (see Fig. 17.4). Translation of the genetic information is thereby blocked, and the ribosomal production of the corresponding protein is prevented. In principle, it should also be possible to use the double helix of DNA itself as target for antisense agents. In this case the compounds (oligonucleotides, "oligos") preferably are called antigene agents, as they block the gene by binding directly to DNA, forming a local triple helix.

The major technical problems in using antisense agents as drugs are to figure out (1) how to penetrate into the cells, (2) how to prevent degradation of the oligos by nucleases, and (3) how to obtain effective binding to the target sense mRNA sequence. Improvement of stability and cellular uptake of oligos have been obtained by chemical changes in the phosphodiester group. Oligos with covalently linked groups (e.g. intercalators and/or alkylators) are developed in order to obtain strong and specific binding to mRNA.

Recently it has been discovered that peptide nucleic acids (PNA's), which are oligonuc-leotides in which the backbone is replaced by a peptide-like backbone of N-(2-ethyl)glycine units, bind much stronger to complementary parts of DNA/RNA than the complementary

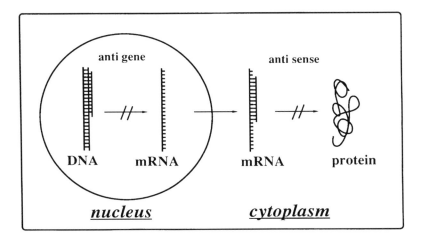

Figure 17.4   Schematic illustration of the antisense/antigene DNA principle. (The drawing was kindly provided by Professor Peter E. Nielsen, Research Center for Medical Biotechnology, University of Copenhagen, Denmark).

oligonucleotides themselves. The PNA's are easy to prepare, water soluble and stable at biological conditions, and the basis for the development of gene-specific drugs of decisive value in gene therapy seems to be excellent.

This new approach in anticancer and antivirus research, based upon mRNA (or duplex DNA) as the primary drug target, is very promising and might lead to the desired goal in chemotherapy: selective cell death.

17.1.2 Drugs interfering with DNA synthesis

A number of different enzymes are involved in the synthesis of DNA and these are potential targets for anticancer (as well as antibacterial and antiviral) drug action. Inhibitors of these enzymes, which are often also called antimetabolites, block more or less crucial steps in DNA synthesis. Most of the drugs so far used in cancer chemotherapy were found by routine screening of the compounds and their mechanism of action was established later. Now several of the structures of the enzymes involved in DNA synthesis are known from X-ray structure determinations, and new drugs are being designed and developed using this knowledge. Anticancer agents with effect as inhibitors of enzymes involved in DNA synthesis are specific for the S-phase of the cell cycle.

17.1.2.1 Inhibition of tetrahydrofolate synthesis
Folic acid analogues have for several years been used in the chemotherapy of infectious and neoplastic diseases. These drugs act by inhibiting the enzyme dihydrofolate reductase (DHFR). This enzyme, which is widely distributed in nature (from bacteria, protozoa and plants to man), converts dihydrofolic acid to tetrahydrofolic acid in the presence of NADPH as a cofactor (see Scheme 17.8).

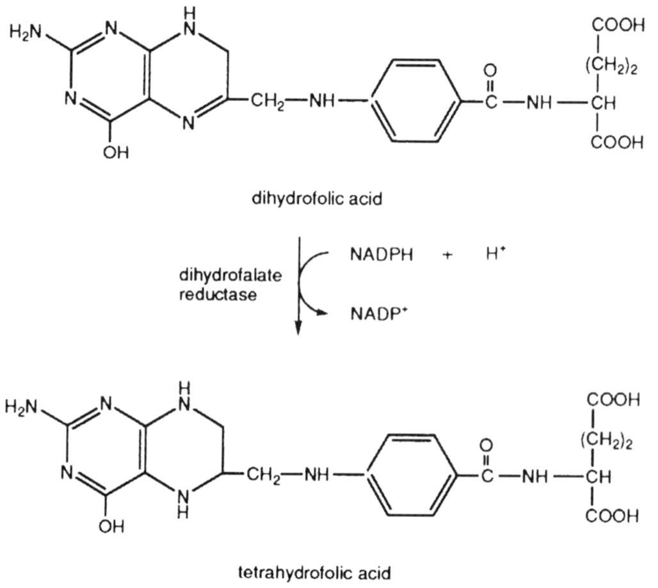

dihydrofolic acid

dihydrofalate
reductase

NADPH + H⁺

NADP⁺

tetrahydrofolic acid

Scheme 17.8

DHFR is one of the enzymes, which has been most thoroughly studied, and the three-dimensional structure of the protein is known from X-ray structure determinations of DHFR from several sources (e.g. *E. coli*, *L. casei*, and chicken liver). Some of the structures are known both without and with inhibitor and/or cofactor (NADPH) bound to the enzyme in a binary or ternary complex, showing the interactions between the drug and its "receptor" (the biomacromolecule). Some of the inhibitors of DHFR have become useful in the treatment of cancer, e.g. *methotrexate*, others as antibacterial drugs, e.g. *trimethoprim*, while *pyrimethamine* is used as an antimalarial drug. Only the anticancer drug methotrexate will be discussed in more detail. The other drugs will be mentioned for comparison in an attempt to understand the differential use of the drugs.

Methotrexate (**17.27**), MTX, is closely related to folic acid (cf. Scheme 17.9), and the compound can be prepared synthetically. MTX has a low aqueous solubility, and the risk of nephrotoxicity can be minimized in patients on high dose therapy by alkalinizing the urine. MTX is widely used in cancer chemotherapy, most often in combination with other drugs. MTX has serious side effects, both acute effects, e.g. ulceration, and delayed toxicities such as bone marrow depression and – particularly with high doses – hepatic toxicity.

MTX and other folic acid analogues are potent competitive inhibitors of DHFR ($K_i < 10^{-9}$ M). There are several consequences of inhibiting the synthesis of tetrahydrofolate, since this compound is further converted *in vivo* to N^5,N^{10}-methylenetetrahydrofolate (methylene-THF, see Scheme 17.9), which functions as a cofactor for various enzymes involved in one-carbon transfer reactions, e.g. for the enzyme thymidylate synthase

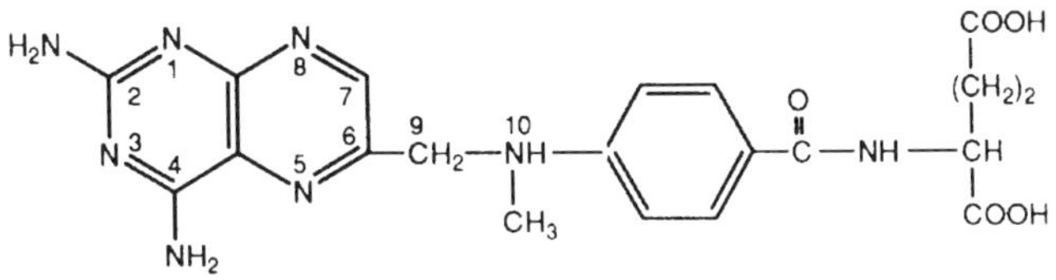

methotrexate (17.27)

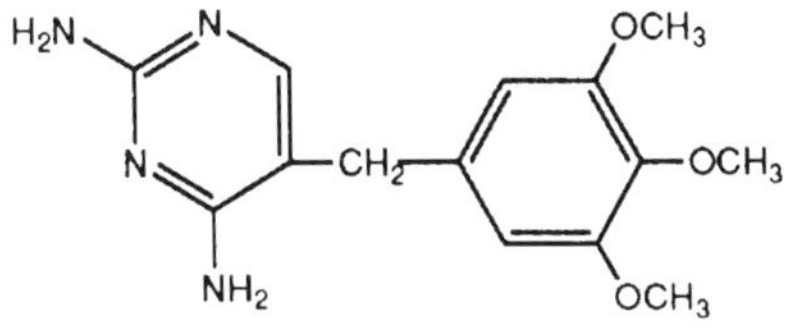

trimethoprim

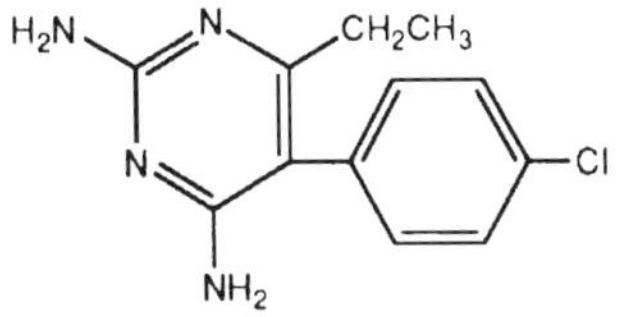

pyrimethamine

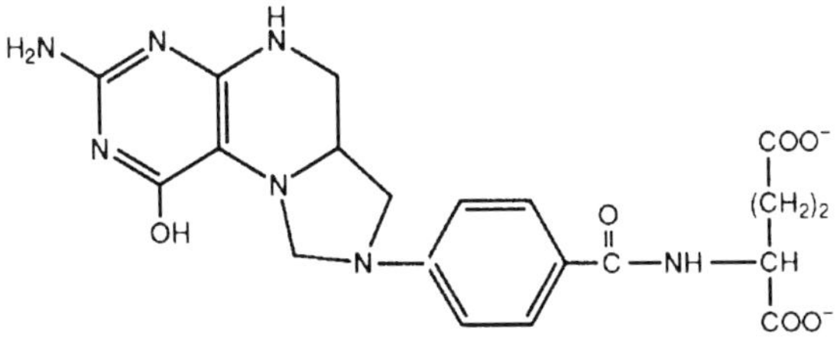

N^5,N^{10}-metyhylenetetrahydrofolate

Scheme 17.9

(cf. Fig. 17.7). The most critical effect leading to cell death after exposure to MTX is probably the indirect inhibition of the action of thymidylate synthase and thereby blocking of the production of deoxythymidylate, which is required for the synthesis of DNA. MTX is actively transported into the cells, and the ability of various tumour cells to transport MTX seems to be related to their ability to respond to the drug. Increased cellular content of DHFR due to increased rate of enzyme synthesis is probably the main reason for resistance to MTX.

The amino acid sequences for a number of DHFRs (i.e. enzymes from several different sources) have been determined, and, as expected, they have common features. The sequence homology between enzymes from different vertebrates is in the region of 75–90%, between the vertebrate enzymes and the bacterial enzymes, on the other hand, only about 20–30%. Nevertheless, crystallographic studies of some of the DHFRs have shown that there is a high degree of resemblance in the folding of the main chains of these enzymes. As an example of this, the tertiary structures of DHFR from chicken liver and from E. coli are shown in Figure 17.5.

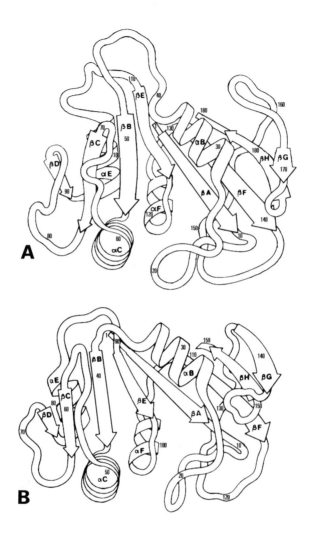

Figure 17.5   Schematic illustration of the folding of the main chain, A of chicken liver, and B of *E. coli* DHFR (From Beddell, C.R. in "X-Ray Crystallography and Drug Action", ed. A.S. Horn and C.J. De Ranter, Oxford University Press, Oxford 1984 with permission by Oxford University Press).

Common to these, and other known DHFR structures, is a central 8-stranded β-sheet area with the strands denoted βA–H. In addition, the molecules contain four helical regions, αB, αC, αE and αF. The molecules have a bi-lobed appearance, as the active site forms a 15 Å deep cleft in the central part of the molecule between the B and C helices. The width of this cleft has been observed to be 1.5–2.0 Å greater in the vertebrate enzymes than that in the bacterial enzymes. In addition to that, the foldings mostly differ in the loop areas at the surface of the enzyme. Nevertheless, it seems evident that the structural differences between enzymes are responsible for the highly selective inhibition of E. coli DHFR exhibited by trimethoprim and the particular selectivity of pyrimethamine for DHFR of the malarial protozoan *Plasmodium berghei*.

X-ray crystallographic studies of the enzyme-inhibitor complex of e.g. DHFR from E. coli and MTX show the binding interactions between drug and protein (see Fig. 17.6A). As it appears from the figure, there are good contacts to side chains of amino acids at the active site of the protein. The pteridine ring interacts with Asp-27 through the electrostatic interactions at N-1, and the 2-amino group (salt bridges or "charge-assisted" hydrogen bonds). The pKa value for N-1 of MTX has been shown to be much higher in the complex than in free MTX (10 and 5.7, respectively), which implies that in the complex the pteridine ring is protonated at physiological pH. In addition to inhibitor binding, Asp-27 appears to play an important functional role in the reduction of the enzyme substrate. The 4-amino group of the pteridine ring is hydrogen bonded to backbone carbonyl groups behind the drug (not shown). The α-carboxylic group of the glutamate moiety of MTX is involved in strong hydrogen bonding (charge-assisted) with the guanidinium group of Arg-57, whereas the γ-carboxylic group is not directly bonded to the protein. The benzene moiety of MTX is sandwiched between Ile-50 and Leu-28 forming hydrophobic (or van der Waals) contacts to these residues.

In Figure 17.6B the X-ray structure of the trimethoprim (TMP) complex with E. coli DHFR is illustrated. As it can be seen, there are qualitative similarities between the binding of the two drugs, MTX and TMP. The 2,4-diaminopyrimidine rings bind in the same manner, the benzene rings are involved in hydrophobic interactions, and charged-assisted hydrogen bonds are formed to Asp-127 in both cases. However, TMP does not have a carboxylic group and cannot interact electrostatically with Arg-57. On the other hand, the trimethoxyphenyl ring fits very favourably into the more narrow active site cleft of E. coli DHFR. The relatively subtle structural differences are apparently largely responsible for the 3000-fold difference in affinity for TMP of E. coli compared to chicken liver enzyme.

The structure of the E. coli DHFR-TMP complex has been used for modelling studies with the aim of designing analogues of TMP with higher affinities for the enzyme. TMP analogues in which one *meta*-methoxy group was replaced by carbalkoxy substituents of varying lengths were designed (cf. Scheme 17.10). Modelling experiments using computer graphics indicated that the compound with five methylene groups in the chain was able to interact particularly well with Arg-57 in the same way as methotrexate.

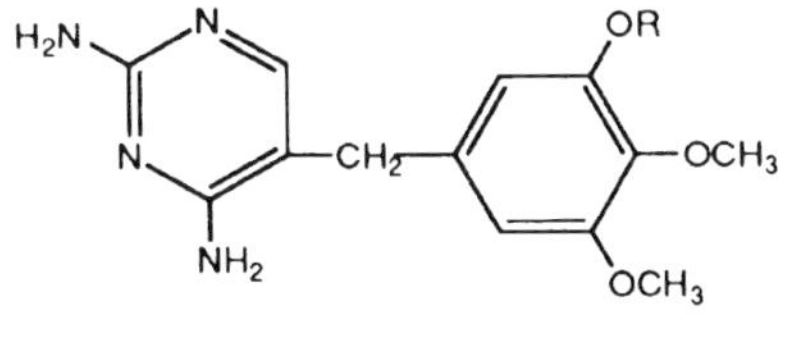

R = (CH$_2$)$_n$–COOH   n = 1 – 6

Scheme 17.10

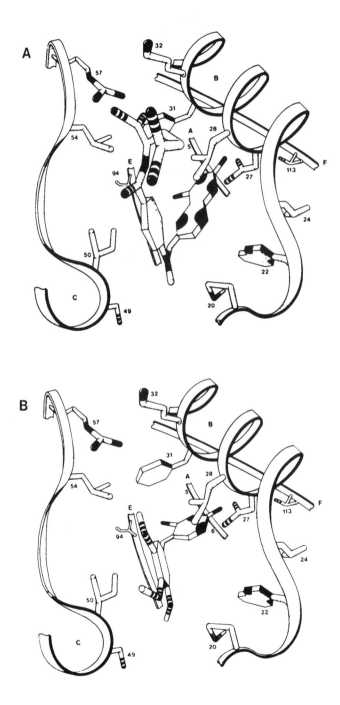

Figure 17.6   Schematic illustration of the active site of *E. coli* DHFR; A with bound methotrexate, and B with bound trimethoprim. Selected atoms of drugs and protein side chains are highlighted: oxygen by stripes, nitrogen in black, and sulphur by hatching. (From Beddell, C.R. — see legend to Fig. 17.5).

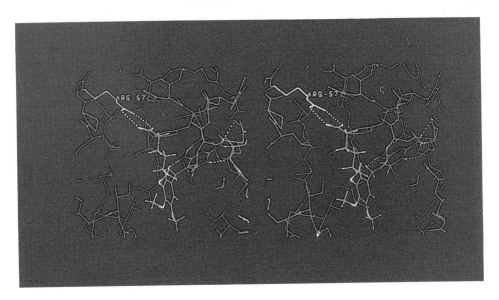

Plate 17.5   The active site of *E. coli* DHFR with a carbalkoxy analogue of trimethoprim bound (C, green; H, white; N, blue; O, red). (From Hitchings, G.H., *et al.* in "Design of Enzyme Inhibitors as Drugs" Eds. M. Sandler and H.J. Smith. Oxford University Press, Oxford 1989, with permission by Oxford University Press. (See Color Plate XIII.)

The compounds were synthesized and tested for enzyme affinity, and the compound with five methylene groups was found to be most active. X-ray structure determination of *E. coli* DHFR complexed with this carbalkoxy analogue was performed in order to determine the actual position of the analogue in the active site. The study shows that the compound is binding as modelled (see Plate 17.5). Because of unfavourable biopharmaceutical properties the analogue did not become a new antibacterial drug, but similar analogues might have been developed.

Other methods, e.g. classical QSAR combined with molecular graphics, have been used for rational design and analysis of inhibitors of DHFR. However, the most obvious approach to the design of novel inhibitors is the utilization of the three-dimensional structures of the enzyme. With detailed knowledge of the structure of the enzymes of different origin (vertebrate, bacterial, etc.) the opportunities for rational design of selective inhibitors are not only present, but as good as possible.

17.1.2.2 Inhibition of purine and pyrimidine synthesis
Analogues of purine and pyrimidine block one or more steps in the purine/pyrimidine synthesis. Both categories of compounds have to be converted in the cells into the corresponding nucleotides before they become active. Several analogues of purine and pyrimidine nucleotides are important as antiviral agents and are discussed in Chapter 16.

6-Mercaptopurine (**17.28**), 6-MP, and *6-thioguanine* (**17.29**), 6-TG, are purine analogues, which can be given orally, and are used in the treatment of leukemias. Bone marrow depression is the principal toxic effect of both drugs. Allopurinol can be given to inhibit xanthine oxidase degradation of 6-MP into thiouric acid, thereby preventing renal damage.

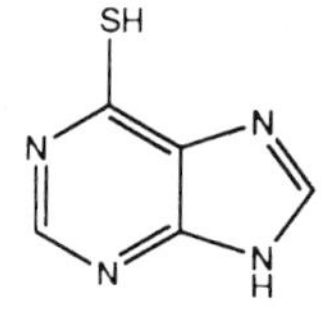

6-mercaptopurine (**17.28**) 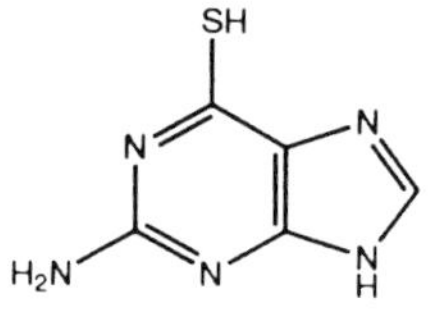   6-thioguanine (**17.29**) 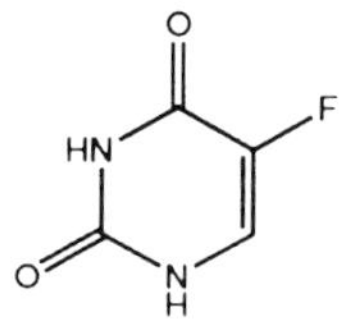   5-fluorouracil (**17.30**)

6-MP acts as a normal substrate for the enzyme hyoxanthine-guanine phosphoribosyl transferase and is thus converted into the nucleotide 6-mercaptopurine ribose phosphate (6-MPRP). This nucleotide interferes with an early step in the purine biosynthesis by inhibiting the enzyme phosphoribosylpyrophosphate (PRPP) amidotransferase. In addition, several other enzymatic pathways are inhibited, and cell death may be the result of a combination of different events. 6-TG is also converted *in vivo* to the nucleotide (6-TGRP), but it has a much weaker inhibitory effect on the enzymes involved in purine synthesis, e.g. the amidotransferase. The cytotoxic action of 6-TG seems to be primarily due to incorporation into DNA of the nucleotide 6-TGRP after further phosphorylation into the triphosphate.

Fluorouracil (**17.30**), 5-FU, is a synthetically prepared pyrimidine analogue with a close structural relationship to the natural base uracil. The drug can be given orally or intravenously. It is effective against several types of solid tumours, in these cases usually administered intravenously, since absorption from the gastrointestinal tract is incomplete and unpredictable. 5-FU has severe side effects, both acute and delayed.

Like the thiopurines, 5-FU has to be converted *in vivo* into a nucleotide, 5-fluoro-2'-deoxyuridine-5'-monophosphate (FdUMP), before it becomes active as a cytotoxic drug. This conversion can be accomplished *via* different pathways involving various enzymes, and resistance to 5-FU has been shown to be due to decreased activity of some of these enzymes.

FdUMP blocks DNA synthesis by inhibition of the enzyme thymidylate synthase (TS). This enzyme catalyzes the conversion of dUMP into dTMP, which subsequently is incorporated into DNA (see Fig. 17.7). FdUMP inhibits the enzyme irreversibly after acting as a normal substrate through part of the catalytic cycle. First, a sulphhydryl group of the enzyme reacts with C-6 of FdUMP (see Scheme 17.11). The cofactor methylene-THF

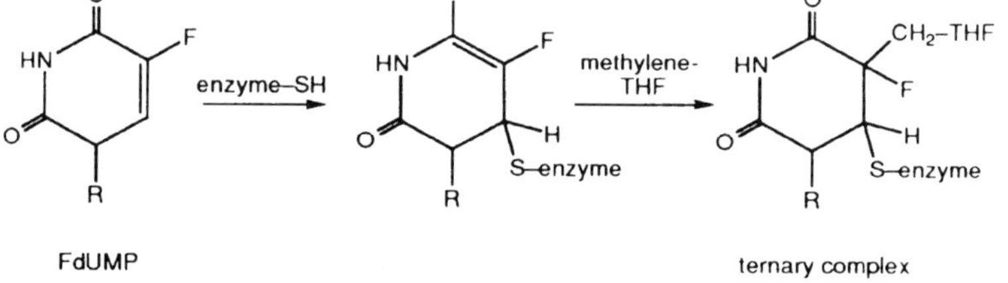

FdUMP   ternary complex

Scheme 17.11

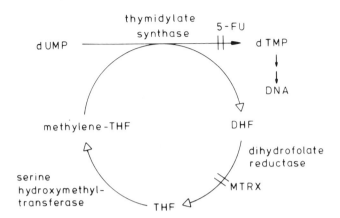

Figure 17.7 Schematic representation of the conversion of dUMP (deoxyuridine monophosphate) into dTMP (deoxythymidine monophosphate). DHF = dihydrofolate, THF = tetrahydrofolate, and methylene-THF = N^5, N^{10}-methylenetetrahydrofolate. Fluorouracil (5-FU) inhibits the methylation of dUMP, and methotrexate (MTRX) blocks the regeneration of THF from DHF.

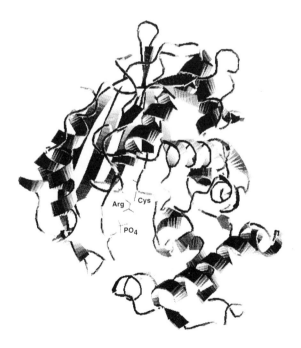

Figure 17.8 Schematic representation of the folding of the main chain of TS. Important residues and a bound phosphate ion in the active site cleft are shown. The structure is generated using the programme "O" with coordinates from Brookhaven Protein Data Base.

then adds to C-5, and, in the case of the substrate dUMP, a proton is removed from C-5 of the bound nucleotide. However, the C-F bond of the bound inhibitor FdUMP cannot be broken, and the catalysis is blocked at the stage where a ternary covalent complex is formed, consisting of enzyme, FdUMP and cofactor.

This mechanism has been confirmed recently by the X-ray structure determinations of TS from several sources, e.g. from *E. coli* and *L. casei*, both with and without inhibitor and/or cofactor or cofactor analogue. In the native enzyme the cysteine residue (Cys-198), which reacts with C-6 of FdUMP, can be seen in the active site cleft (see Fig. 17.8). Cys-198 is activated (more acidic) due to hydrogen bonding to the base Arg-218. In complexes with inhibitor and cofactor (or an analogue) covalent bonds connect the inhibitor with enzyme and cofactor (short distances are observed, see Plates 17.6 and 17.7).

5-FU is often given in combination with other anticancer drugs, e.g. with 4′-epirubicin and cyclophosphamide. In addition, co-administration of leucovorin (5-formyl-THF) is now frequently used. Leucovorin is rapidly converted *in vivo* to 5-methyl-THF and further to methylene-THF. Excess of this cofactor ensures the tight binding of FdUMP to the enzyme, the result being optimal inhibition of TS and increased cytotoxic effect of 5-FU.

TS is an important target for structure-based drug design by advanced computer methods. A molecular docking computer programme (DOCK) has been used recently to screen all the compounds of a data base of commercial available compounds (about 55,000) for molecules that fit to the active site of *L. casei* TS. In addition to retrieving the substrate and several known inhibitors, some previously unknown putative inhibitors were proposed, e.g. phenolphthalein analogues. These compounds, which were found to inhibit TS in the micromolar range, do not resemble the substrate dUMP. X-ray structure determinations of the TS-drug complexes showed that the compounds bind in the active site cleft in another binding region 6–9 Å displaced compared to the substrate. The phenolphthalein analogues are a novel family of tight-binding specific TS inhibitors, found by the use of the known target protein structure, which might lead to the development of new drugs in chemotherapy.

17.1.2.3 Inhibition of DNA/RNA polymerases

DNA polymerases catalyze the step-by-step addition of deoxynucleotide units to the new DNA strand during DNA replication and are potential targets for anticancer and antiviral drug action. Very few inhibitors of DNA polymerases are in clinical use in cancer therapy, whereas several inhibitors (substrate analogues) have become useful in curing virus infections (see Chapter 16). The compounds are purine or pyrimidine analogues, and some of them are also incorporated into DNA.

Cytarabine (**17.31**), cytosine arabinoside, Ara-C, is a pyrimidine nucleoside analog with a structural change in the ribose ring. The drug is poorly absorbed orally, and it is routinely given intravenously or by continuous infusion methods because of rapid hepatic deamination by cytosine deaminase into inactive ara-U (uracil arabinoside). It is used primarily in the treatment of acute leukemias. The principal toxicities are nausea, vomiting, and bone marrow depression. Ara-C is converted *in vivo* into the active nucleotide triphosphate Ara-CTP by enzymes that treat Ara-C as a normal substrate. Ara-CTP is an analogue of the deoxycytidine triphosphate substrate of DNA polymerase and inhibits this enzyme competitively. As a consequence, DNA synthesis and cell growth is inhibited. Resistance to Ara-C is probably associated with high levels of deaminase activity.

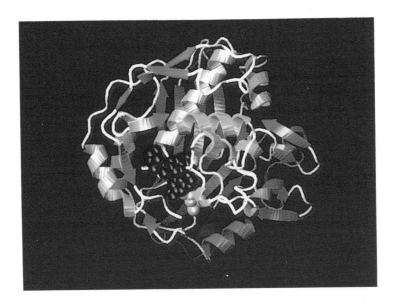

Plate 17.6   The structure of TS of *E. coli* with substrate (in magenta) and cofactor analogue (in blue) bound in active site. The structure was generated using the programme "O" with coordinates from Brookhaven Protein Data Base. (See Color Plate XIV.)

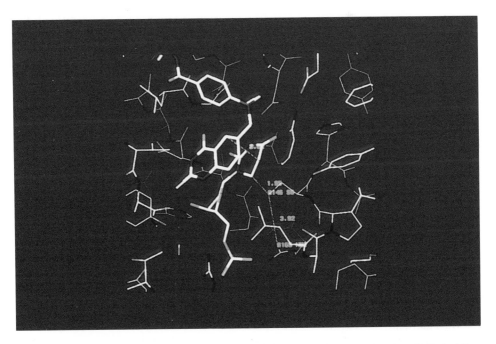

Plate 17.7   The active site of TS with substrate and cofactor analogue bound (N, blue; O, red). Dashed lines indicate short distances. The structure was generated using the programme "O" with coordinates from Brookhaven Protein Data Base. (See Color Plate XV.)

cytarabine (**17.31**)

vidarabine (**17.32**)

Vidarabine (**17.32**), adenine arabinoside, Ara-A, is a purine nucleoside analogue with a similar mechanism of action as Ara-C, but this drug is primarily used as an antiviral agent. Structural modifications of Ara-A and Ara-C, as well as co-administration of a deaminase inhibitor, have been used in order to avoid inactivation of the drugs.

17.1.2.4 Inhibition of ribonucleotide reductase

The enzyme ribonucleotide reductase (RNR) is an essential component of all living cells. The function of the enzyme is to participate in the synthesis of DNA by catalyzing the conversion of all of the four ribonucleotides into the corresponding deoxyribonucleotides, see Scheme 17.12. This is the only pathway for the formation of deoxyribonucleotides, and the reaction is believed to be a rate limiting step in DNA synthesis. Consequently, RNR is an obvious target for anticancer as well as antibacterial and antiviral drug action. The only RNR inhibitor in clinical use is *hydroxyurea*, but other compounds are in clinical trial. Design and development of selective antiviral agents will also be possible, as some viruses (e.g. herpes simplex virus, HSV) code for their own enzyme system. Structural differences between host and virus enzymes exist and is being utilized in drug design.

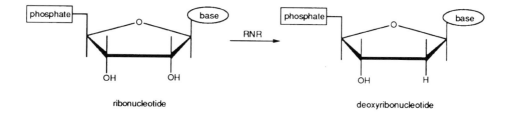

Scheme 17.12

Hydroxyurea (**17.33**), *N*-hydroxyurea, hydrea, is a crystalline compound, which is routinely given orally, as it is water soluble and well absorbed from the gastrointestinal tract. It is excreted very rapidly and has to be given in very high and frequent doses. Hydroxyurea is primarily used to treat chronic myelogenous leukemia, but has also demonstrated activity in malignant melanoma and other solid tumours. The acute side effects are mild and bone marrow depression is the dose limiting toxicity. Resistance to hydroxyurea is mainly due to overproduction and increased activity of RNR.

Hydroxyurea inhibits RNR by interfering with the smaller of the two proteins, of which the enzyme consists (protein R2, see Fig. 17.9). R2 is unusual in containing a free radical group (a tyrosyl radical), which is essential for catalysis. This radical is destroyed (reduced to a normal tyrosine residue) by hydroxyurea, and the enzyme function is thereby prevented. Hydroxyurea is an iron chelator, but the iron centres of protein R2 are not affected by the drug. The function of the iron is to generate and stabilize the free radical group.

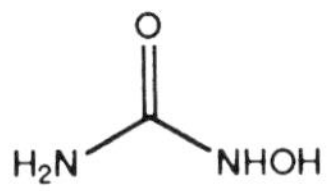

hydroxyurea (**17.33**)

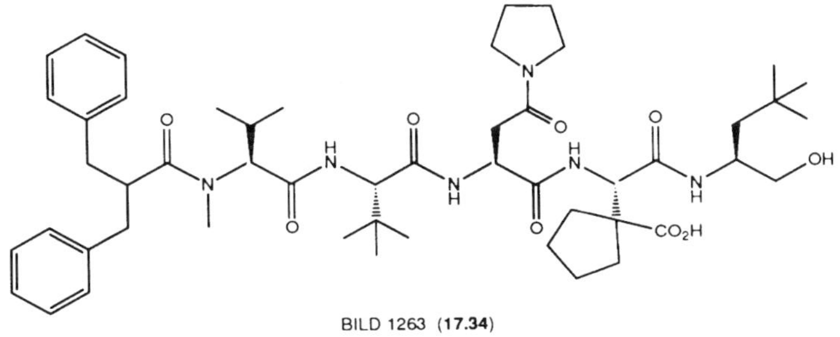

BILD 1263 (**17.34**)

Studies on analogues of hydroxyurea have indicated that inhibitors of this type (radical scavengers) have to be rather small and flat molecules. The reason for this has not yet been fully elucidated. X-ray structure determination of protein R2 of the enzyme of *E. coli* has shown that the tyrosyl radical (and iron center) is buried in a hydrophobic pocket in the protein. In R2 of mammalian RNR the radical/iron center seems to be more accessible. The structure of the R1 subunit of *E. coli* RNR has also been determined recently, and the R1R2 holoenzyme complex has been modelled on the basis of the two separate protein structures (see Plate 17.8).

The carboxy terminal of R2 is known to be involved in the R1R2 association. Consequently, peptidomimetics, i.e. analogues of oligopeptides with amino acid sequences corresponding to the carboxy terminal of the R2 subunit of RNR of HSV, have recently been developed as selective antivirus agents. These compounds inhibit the enzyme by interfering with the interphase between the subunits, thereby preventing association of the subunits. BILD 1263 (**17.34**) is the first HSV R1R2 subunit association inhibitor published with

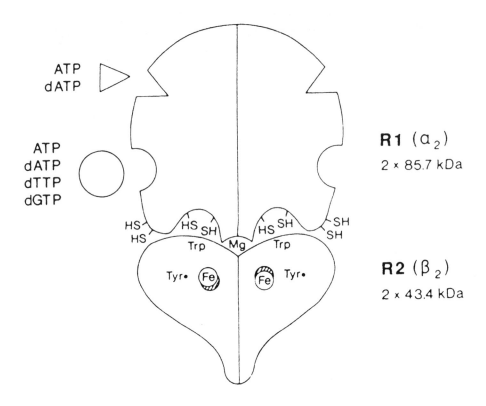

Figure 17.9   Model drawing of ribonucleotide reductase of *E. coli* showing the two homodimeric proteins, R1 and R2, the effector sites and the redox-active sulphhydryl groups on R1, and the iron centres and tyrosyl radicals on R2. (The drawing was kindly provided by Professor Britt-Marie Sjöberg, Department of Molecular Biology, University of Stockholm, Sweden).

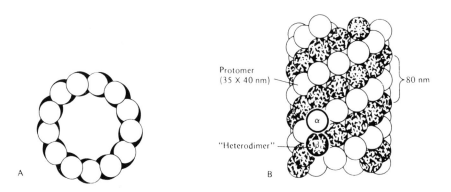

Figure 17.10   Schematic model of a microtubule, showing the pattern of tubulin subunits. A is a cross-sectional view showing the arrangement of the thirteen protofilaments. B is a longitudinal view showing the surface lattice of α and β subunits. (From Bryan, J. *Fed. Proc.*, **33**, 152 (1974) with permission by the Federation of American Societies for Experimental Biology).

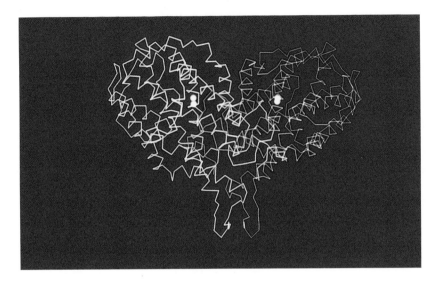

Plate (A)

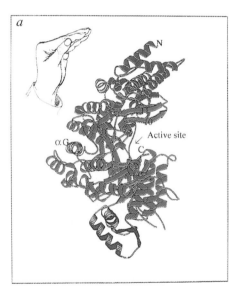

Plate (B)

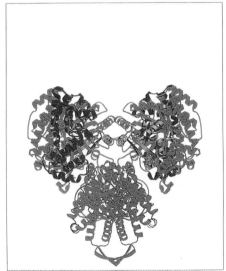

Plate (C)

Plate 17.8 The structures of (A) protein R2 of *E. coli* RNR as the dimer (in green and magenta) with the iron atoms in red; (B) protein R1 of *E. coli* RNR as the monomer. The colours illustrate different domains of the protein; (C) the R1R2 holoenzyme modelled on the basis of the seperate X-ray structures of R1 and R2. The R2 dimer is coloured in red. The figures were kindly provided by Professor Hans Eklund, Department of Molecular Biology, Biomedical Center, Uppsala, Sweden. (See Color Plate XVI.)

antiviral activity *in vivo*. The compound does not affect mammalian RNR, in which the R2 carboxy terminal is different. Disruption of protein-protein interactions is a relatively new strategy of inhibitor design for the development of chemotherapeutic agents.

17.2 MITOTIC APPARATUS AS TARGET FOR DRUGS

The mitotic inhibitors act by interfering with the mitosis of cells and thereby inducing mitotic arrest. Mitosis takes place during the M phase of the cell cycle, and drugs that prevent cell division by interfering with mitosis are M phase specific. Mitotic arrest is induced because of damage to the spindle apparatus. Consequently, the chromatides, which are separated in the metaphase, are prevented from being pulled toward opposite poles in the following anaphase.

The separate threads of the spindle apparatus are built as a microtubule system. Microtubules are hollow, cylindrical structures built up of the protein tubulin, which consists of two similar subunits, α- and β-tubulin. The cylinder consists of thirteen rows of tubulin heterodimers, the protofilaments. The microtubule cylinder can also be regarded as consisting of a helical array of alternating α- and β-tubulin subunits (see Fig. 17.10). Most of the mitotic inhibitors disrupt microtubule assembly by binding with high affinity to tubulin. Some of the drugs have a common binding site (the *vinca alkaloids*) and others a different, but probably common, binding site (*podophyllotoxin* and *colchicine*). *Taxol*, on the other hand, promotes the assembly of tubulin to microtubules, and prevents depolymerization by binding to tubulin.

Microtubules are found as a ubiquitous substituent in cells and have several other functions than being elements in mitosis. Microtubules are part of the cytoskeleton, and take part in intracellular transport and communication. Some of the toxic side effects of the mitotic inhibitors may be due to disturbance of these phenomena.

17.2.1 Drugs interfering with the vinca alkaloid binding site of tubulin

Vinblastine (**17.35**) and *vincristine* (**17.36**) are constituents of the Madagascar periwinkle *Vinca rosea* Linn. Vinblastine (VBL) is found in much larger quantity than vincristine (VCR), but it is easily converted synthetically into the clinically more useful drug VCR (conversion of a methyl group into a formyl group). VBL and VCR are used as the sulphates and are given intravenously because of bad and unpredictable absorption from the gastrointestinal tract. The compounds are highly irritating to tissue and great care has to be taken to avoid extravasation and contact with eyes. The dose-limiting toxicity of VBL is bone marrow depression, whereas VCR is considered to be bone marrow sparing compared to most anticancer drugs. Neurotoxicity is dose-limiting for VCR, on the other hand, while this is a less frequent and serious problem with VBL. The reasons for these differences in toxicity of the structurally very similar compounds are not fully understood.

The clinical use of the drugs is also different. VCR is given in combination therapy to induce remission in acute lymphocytic leukemia of childhood, and it has actually revolutionized the therapy of this disease, as 90–100% of the patients are achieving complete remission. Very high percentages of remission are also achieved in the treatment of Hodgkin's disease with combinations of drugs including VCR or VBL. Both drugs are used in the treatment of several other cancer diseases.

vinblastine (**17.35**) R = CH₃

vincristine (**17.36**) R = CHO

The vinca alkaloids are known to bind to tubulin at a common binding site. As a result of this binding, the tubulin units cannot polymerize to form microtubules, a reversible reaction, which normally occurs in the presence of Mg^{2+} and GTP in addition to the microtubules-associated proteins (MAPs). Only when GTP is bound to tubulin the filament can grow, and only from one end. Thus, the normal microtubules are in dynamic instability. When VBL (or VCR) is bound to tubulin new GTP-tubulin units cannot be added to the filaments, and the growth is thereby prevented. Dissociation of tubulin units can still occur, and the result is rapid disappearance of the spindle apparatus.

Very little is known on the nature of the binding of the vinca alkaloids to tubulin. The amino acid sequences of α- and β-tubulin are known, but the X-ray structures have not been reported. Several semisynthetic compounds have been derived from VBL in order to obtain drugs with lower neurotoxicity.

17.2.2 Drugs interfering with the colchicine binding site of tubulin

The two drugs mentioned below are not commonly used in cancer therapy, but are considered for comparison with the vinca alkaloids and taxol.

Podophyllotoxin (**17.37**) can be isolated from extracts of the roots of *Podophyllum peltatum* L. (American mandrake), and is primarily used in the treatment of condyloma. *Colchicine* (**17.38**) is the major alkaloid of the meadow saffron *Colchicum autumnale* L. It is an active antimitotic drug, but the toxicity of the compound has limited its use to the treatment of gout and related inflammatory disease states.

podophyllotoxin (**17.37**)   colchicine (**17.38**)

As the vinca alkaloids, podophyllotoxin (PODO) and colchicine (COL) both inhibit mitosis by binding to tubulin and thereby preventing microtubule assembly. The two drugs share a common binding site, which is distinct from the VBL binding site. It has been proposed that, while VBL/VCR prevent longitudinal interactions between tubulin subunits, COL and PODO seem to prevent microtubule assembly by inhibiting lateral interactions between subunits in adjacent protofilaments. The binding of both COL and PODO to tubulin is tight, but, although practically irreversible, probably non-covalent in nature. Details on the nature of the bindings are not yet known.

taxol (**17.39**)

17.2.3 Drugs interfering with the assembled microtubules, taxol

Taxol (**17.39**) is a plant product isolated from the cortex of the western yew *Taxus brevifolia*. The compound has a very low solubility in water, and this has caused serious problems related to its formulation. Now it is used as an emulsion with Cremophor EL (a polyethoxylated castor oil) as the surfactant, but this formulation is far from ideal. The allergic reactions observed in some patients are probably caused by the solvent. However, improved administration procedures, including premedication with glucocorticoides and antihistamines, have reduced this problem.

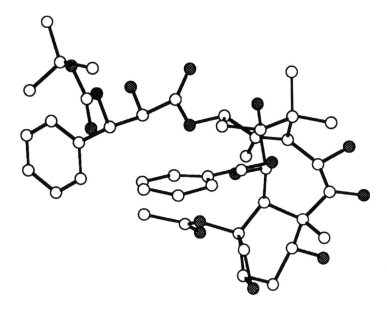

Figure 17.11   The X-ray structure of taxotere (generated using the programme SYBYL with coordinates from Cambridge Structural Data Base).

Another problem is the very low yield of taxol from the cortex of *T. brevifolia*. Now most of the compound is produced semisynthetically from a precursor that can be obtained in higher yield. Taxol is now in phase III trials, and in clinical use against ovarian cancer and breast cancer. Taxol also has effect against a variety of other cancer diseases. The major side effect of taxol, in addition to hypersensitivity, is neurotoxicity.

Taxol (**17.39**) is a taxane diterpenoid characterized by its ester side chain at C-13 (the *N*-benzoyl-β-phenylisoserine ester of the compound *baccatin III*) and by its oxetane ring D. No X-ray structure of taxol has been reported, but the X-ray structure of *taxotere*, an analogue with the *N*-benzoyl group replaced by a *t*-butoxycarbonyl group, clearly shows a cup-like shape of the taxane skeleton (see Fig. 17.11). Taxotere is also a promising anticancer drug and is progressing through clinical trials.

Unlike other plant-derived antimitotic agents (colchicine, podophyllotoxin and the vinca alkaloids), which inhibit microtubule assembly, taxol actually promotes the assembly of tubulin and stabilizes the microtubules formed against depolymerization. The drug binds to tubulin dimers, and recent photo affinity labeling experiments provide clear evidence for binding to the N-terminal amino acids of the β-subunit of tubulin. The cytotoxicity of taxol is related to the microtubule-mediated interruption of mitosis, resulting in distortion of the mitotic spindle.

An understanding of the binding of taxol to microtubules would be useful in the development of improved taxol analogues by facilitating the design of molecules that fit to the binding site. Such information might be obtained by X-ray structure determination of tubulin co-crystallized with taxol, but, as mentioned earlier, no crystal structure of tubulin, or of tubulin-drug complexes, has been reported. However, some information has been obtained indirectly by SAR studies.

Beccatin III, without the ester side chain at C-13, is significantly less active than taxol, indicating the importance of this side chain for the activity. An N-acyl group is required in the side chain (benzoyl in taxol, and t-butoxycarbonyl in taxotere). Various taxol analogues that lacks the 3′-phenyl group of the side chain are significantly less active than taxol. A free 2′-hydroxy group (or a hydrolysable ester) is required, and a change of the chirality at 2′ and 3′ leads to less active compounds.

Structural variations along the upper part (C-6–C-12) of the taxol molecule (e.g. acylation or removal of an OH group) do not greatly affect the bioactivity of taxol, suggesting that this region is not intimately involved in binding to tubulin. The lower part, on the other hand, including C-14, C-1–C-5 and the unusual oxetane ring at C-4–C-5, appears to be a region, which is crucial to the activity of taxol, as structural changes have major effects on activity. Opening of the oxetane ring with electrophilic reagents yields products, which are less active than taxol, and also the benzoyloxy group at C-2 is required. The oxetane ring is relatively inert chemically, and it has been suggested that its role simply may be to act as a lock to maintain the conformation of the diterpenoid ring system of taxol.

FURTHER READING

Wilman, D.E.V. and Connors, T.A. (1983) Molecular structure and antitumour activity of alkylating agents. In *Molecular Aspects of Anti-cancer Drug Action*, edited by S. Neidle and M.J. Waring, pp. 233–282. London: The Macmillan Press.

Lown, J.W. (1983) The chemistry of DNA damage by antitumour drugs. In *Molecular Aspects of Anti-cancer Drug Action*, edited by S. Neidle and M.J. Waring, pp. 283–314. London: The Macmillan Press.

Pratt, W.B. and Ruddon, R.W., Eds. (1979) *The Anticancer Drugs*. Oxford: Oxford University Press.

Friedman, O.M., Myles, A. and Colvin, M. (1979) Cyclophosphamide and related phosphoramide mustards. Current status and future prospects. In *Advances in Cancer Chemotherapy*, Vol. 4, edited by A. Rosowsky, pp. 143–204. New York: Marcel Dekker.

Mirkes, P.E., Brown, N.A., Kajbaf, M., Lamb, J.H., Farmer, P.B. and Naylor, S. (1992) Identification of cyclophosphamide-DNA adducts in rat embryos exposed *in vitro* to 4-hydroperoxocyclophosphamide. *Chem. Res. Toxicol.*, **5**, 382–385.

McCormick, J.E. and McElhinney, R.S. (1990) Nitrosoureas from chemist to physician: Classification and recent approaches to drug design. *Eur. J. Cancer*, **26**, 207–221.

Reedijk, J. (1988) Structure determination of platinum antitumour compounds and their adducts with DNA. In *NMR Spectroscopy in Drug Research*, edited by J.W. Jaroszewski, K. Schaumburg and H. Kofod, pp. 341–357. Copenhagen: Munksgaard.

Weiss, R.B. and Christian, M.C. (1993) New cisplatin analogues in development. A review. *Drugs*, **46**, 360–377.

Sugiura, Y., Takita, T. and Umezawa, H. (1985) Bleomycin antibiotics: Metal complexes and their biological action. In *Metal Ions in Biological Systems*, Vol. 19, edited by H. Sigel, pp. 81–108. New York: Marcel Dekker.

Dedon, P.C. and Goldberg, I.H. (1992) Free-radical mechanisms involved in the formation of sequence-dependent bistranded DNA lesions by the antitumor antibiotics bleomycin, neocarzinostatin, and calicheamicin. *Chem. Res. Toxicol.*, **5**, 311–332.

Arcamone, F. (1984) Structure-activity relationships in antitumour anthracyclines. In *X-Ray Crystallography and Drug Action*, edited by A.S. Horn and C.J. De Ranter, pp. 367–388. Oxford: Clarendon Press.

Wang, A.H.-J. (1992) Intercalative drug binding to DNA. *Curr. Opin. Struct. Biol.*, **2**, 361–368.

Joshua-Tor, L. and Sussman, J.L. (1993) The coming age of DNA crystallography. *Curr. Opin. Struct. Biol.*, **3**, 323–335.

Cohen, J., Ed. (1989) *Oligodeoxynucleotides Antisense Inhibitors of Gene Expressions*. London: The Macmillan Press.

Nielsen, P.E., Egholm, M. and Buchardt, O. (1994) A DNA mimic with a peptide backbone. *Bioconjugate Chemistry*, **5**, 3–7.

Champness, J.N., Kuyper, L.F. and Beddell, C.R. (1986) Interaction between dihydrofolate reductase and certain inhibitors. In *Topics in Molecular Pharmacology*, Vol. 3, edited by A.S.V. Burgen, G.C.K. Roberts and M.S. Tute. Amsterdam: Elsevier.

Kuyper, L.F. (1989) Inhibitors of dihydrofolate reductase. In *Computer-Aided Drug Design. Methods and Applications*, edited by T.J. Perun and C.L. Propst, pp. 327–364. New York: Marcel Dekker.

Hardy, L.W., Finer-Moore, J.S., Montfort, W.R., Jones, M.O., Santi, D.V. and Stroud, R.M. (1987) Atomic structure of thymidylate synthase. Target for rational drug design. *Science*, **235**, 448–455.

Shoichet, B.K., Stroud, R.M., Santi, D.V., Kuntz, I.D. and Perry, K.M. (1993) Structure-based discovery of inhibitors of thymidylate synthase. *Science*, **259**, 1445–1450.

Larsen, I.K. (1990) Inhibition of the enzyme ribonucleotide reductase. In *Frontiers in Drug Research. Crystallographic and Computational Methods*, edited by B. Jensen, F.S. Jørgensen and H. Kofod, pp. 47–57. Copenhagen: Munksgaard.

Nordlund, P. and Eklund, H. (1993) Structure and function of *Escheria coli* ribonucleotide reductase protein R2. *J. Mol. Biol.*, **232**, 123–164.

Liuzzi, M., Déziel, R., Moss, N., Beaulleu, P., Bonneau, A.-M., Bousquet, C., Chafouleas, J.G., Garneau, M., Jarmillo, J. Krogsrud, R.L., Lagacé, L., McCollum, R.S., Nawooy, S. and Guindon, Y. (1994) A potent peptidomimetic inhibitor of HSV ribonucleotide reductase with antiviral activity *in vivo. Nature*, **372**, 695–698.

Iwasaki, S. (1993) Antimitotic agents: Chemistry and recognition of tubulin molecule. *Med. Res. Rev.*, **13**, 183–198.

Kingston, D.G.I. (1994) Taxol: The chemistry and structure-activity relationships of a novel anticancer agent. *TIBTECH*, **12**, 222–227.

18. DRUG DEVELOPMENT: FROM DISCOVERY TO MARKETING

JOSEPH P. YEVICH

CONTENTS

18.1 INTRODUCTION

Successful drug development entails the highly coordinated interaction of numerous groups of individuals working in disciplines ranging from the basic sciences to the legal and medical professions. The average overall cost of bringing a drug to market is now well in excess of 300 million dollars and the developmental time frame can be a decade or longer. There is roughly a 1 in 10,000 chance of a compound's achieving the arduous trek from the laboratory to the marketplace. The basic research aspects (synthetic-medicinal chemistry, pharmacology, molecular biology, etc.) of drug discovery may occur within the context of academic institutions, government-sponsored agencies or the pharmaceutical industry. However, for all practical purposes, the costly and lengthy enterprise of developing an active lead compound to a marketed drug can be most efficiently achieved by pharmaceutical companies which command the necessary financial and interdisciplinary manpower resources to get the job done.

This chapter will deal with the various components of drug discovery and development in the U.S. pharmaceutical industry. Drug development outside the United States is similar for the most part, the major differences being in the requirements of various countries' registrational authorities with respect to drug approval. Although the ensuing discussion of such complex topics as pharmacokinetics and toxicity is admittedly superficial, the main emphasis is upon how they fit into the comprehensive picture of drug development.

18.2 OVERVIEW OF THE DRUG DEVELOPMENT PROCESS

The overall scheme of drug development from initial discovery to marketing is depicted in Figure 18.1 along with approximate time frames. The identification of novel chemical leads in a given target area is typically followed by structure analog synthesis in order to elucidate structure-activity relationships (SAR) within the series. This synthetic work is directed toward optimizing the therapeutic index, i.e., the ratio of drug dosage causing undesirable side effects or toxicity to that which achieves the desired biological effect. Computer assisted drug design (CADD), if not utilized in the initial lead discovery, may be implemented at this stage to minimize the number of analogs to be synthesized. In-depth biological evaluation of the refined leads is conducted for the purpose of characterizing their complete pharmacological profile, gaining mechanism-of-action insight, and ultimately choosing a preferred clinical candidate. The reader is referred to Chapter 1 for a more detailed discussion of drug discovery.

During the time frame of lead optimization, the patent-filing process will be expedited to provide the company with the necessary proprietary rights to the compound(s) and its use. A variety of other activities also ensue with the selection of a clinical drug candidate: the company's chemical process development group undertakes the synthesis of bulk quantities of the raw drug substance; the drug substance is formulated by the pharmaceutical development group, providing suitable dosage forms for clinical purposes; toxicity studies in several animal species are initiated; the metabolic disposition and pharmacokinetic parameters of the drug are investigated in animals. These interdisciplinary studies span several years and culminate in a preclinical data package which provides the basis for carrying the drug into clinical trials. Of course any untoward findings, especially unacceptable levels of toxicity, would obviate further development.

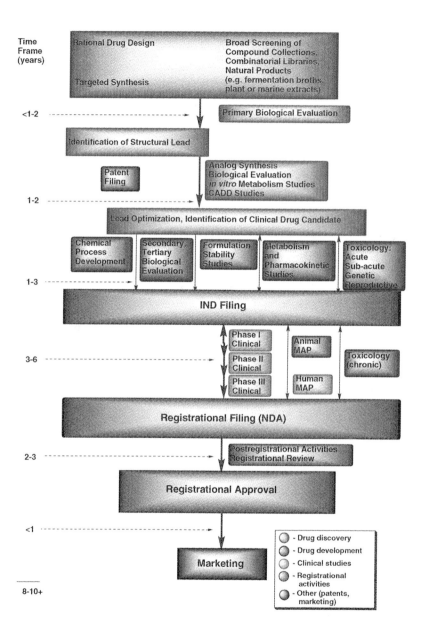

Figure 18.1 Discovery to marketing of a drug. The various steps in the path from the discovery of a potential new drug to its approval and marketing are indicated along with approximate time frames. Color-coding indicates related activities. Various activities necessary for IND filing continue beyond the IND and may even continue after registrational (NDA) filing. As indicated by doubleheaded arrows, MAP and toxicity findings may lead to reformulation of clinical dosage form or to the synthesis of improved analogs. (See Color Plate XVII.)

If the drug candidate survives such studies, the next customary step in the U.S. is the sponsoring firm's filing of an Investigational New Drug (IND) application with the Food and Drug Administration (FDA). This is, in essence, a formal request to begin clinical investigation of the drug in man. The company submits a plan of its intended human studies including details of the clinical protocols. In order to ensure that the plan complies with ethical medical practices and that the safety and welfare of clinical subjects will not be compromised, the proposed studies are carefully reviewed by an Independent Review Board (IRB) which typically consists of a doctor, an attorney and perhaps a minister and several other members of the lay community.

Phase I clinical trials are initiated in healthy volunteers in order to establish the drug's safety and appropriate dosage levels. Assuming that no compromising side effects are observed in Phase I, the drug advances to Phase II patient studies which are designed to evaluate its therapeutic effectiveness. Subsequent and more extensive Phase III studies are conducted to verify efficacy and monitor possible adverse reactions from chronic administration. Depending upon the drug and the nature of the disease it treats, the overall clinical trial period may last from three to six years, sometimes longer. If the results of clinical investigation are supportive of the drug having a useful therapeutic effect with minimal side effects, the voluminous compilation of preclinical and clinical data is submitted to the FDA as a New Drug Application (NDA). The scrupulous review of the registrational submission takes on average about three years and, in favorable cases, results in approval of the drug to be marketed. It should be emphasized that registrational approval is usually contingent upon the drug exhibiting some distinct advantages over existing therapeutic agents. So-called "me-too" agents which fail to exceed already-marketed drugs in terms of efficacy and/or safety are not likely to be sanctioned.

The foregoing discussion addressed the steps of drug development in the United States. However, major multi-national pharmaceutical companies, whether U.S. based or not, seek to market their new drugs on a world-wide basis. In addition to the U.S., EEC countries of western Europe and Japan are major targets for approval. This often entails the need to conduct clinical trials within these key market countries and to accommodate the particular requirements of the countries' registrational authorities. The components of the drug development process will now be considered in some greater detail.

18.3 LEAD DISCOVERY

The identification of patentably-novel chemical entities having potentially useful pharmacological properties can arise from the testing of synthesized compounds which have been rationally-designed to interact with some specific biological target, such as a receptor or enzyme, or from the broad-based, high-throughput screening of natural products (e.g. fermentation broths, plant extracts), compound collections or combinatorial libraries. Chapter 1 presents a comprehensive discussion of lead discovery and optimization.

18.4 PATENTS

The "lifeblood" of a pharmaceutical company is the patent rights which it holds both on its approved and experimental drugs. These rights provide the basis for exclusivity

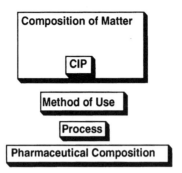

Figure 18.2   Types of patents.

for the manufacture, use and sale of such agents and thus allow return on the significant investment of time and money required for drug development. Following the expiration of patent coverage of one of its marketed drugs, a company loses its patent-related exclusivity and the drug becomes part of the public domain. Generic versions of the drug can then be manufactured and sold by competitors following appropriate approval (in the U.S., an Abbreviated New Drug Application (ANDA) is submitted to the FDA for approval).

18.4.1 Types of patents

Figure 18.2 shows the general types of patents which are most commonly obtained on pharmaceutical agents: (1) composition of matter; (2) method of use; (3) process; (4) pharmaceutical composition.

Of these, the "composition of matter" or "product" patent is generally of greatest value. Such patents include a specific description and claim to some chemical entity or structurally-related series of entities. The patent will also disclose their physical properties, method of preparation, and some designated utility. In addition to adequate disclosure, the basic requirements for any patent are novelty, utility, and unobviousness of the invention. As it pertains to "composition of matter" patents, the novelty criterion requires that the compounds which comprise the subject matter of the patent not have been rendered part of the public domain by prior publication or other disclosure. While utility of the compounds may be demonstrated with clinical data, frequently such demonstration involves a display of biological activity in some preclinical test relevant to the claimed utility. A "composition of matter" patent application can be rejected as being obvious because of close prior art. If chemical compounds differ but slightly, as with a substituent group, from previously-reported agents having a related utility, the patent office may judge the compounds to be obvious extensions of prior art and deny the patent.

In the U.S., inventors can expand the claimed subject matter by filing a continuation in part (CIP) application relating to the original application. The CIP application must be filed before the parent patent application is abandoned or a patent is issued on it. However, if foreign patents are to be filed, then the CIP should be filed within one year after filing the original application so that the foreign filings can be based on the more extensive CIP application. With the expected implementation of patent law modifications due to GATT/TRIPS international agreements, CIP patents and other areas of current U.S. practice may undergo a change.

"Method of use" patents can be filed on known compounds which are part of the public domain including those covered by existing patents. The basis of a "use" patent is a convincing demonstration of previously unreported and unobvious pharmacological activity for known compounds. Companies may obtain "use" patents on their own drugs which may effect a broadening of the scope and extension of the time frame of their exclusivity; they may also claim new uses for competitors' drugs.

"Process" patents describe a novel and/or improved method of synthesis often of a previously described compound. Most often, the patent discloses a preparative method which is amenable to pilot plant or manufacturing scale. Companies usually seek to obtain "process" patents on marketed drugs or those under active development.

"Pharmaceutical composition", also known as "formulation" patents, disclose specific formulations of a drug or drugs; formulations may be of proprietary importance insofar as they solve a problem of drug delivery, bioavailability, etc.

18.4.2 U.S. vs. foreign (non-U.S.) patents

The recent U.S. ratification of the General Agreement on Tariffs and Trade (GATT) treaty has necessitated some significant changes in U.S. patent law. Whereas U.S. patents filed prior to mid-1995 had terms of seventeen years from the date of their issuance, those patents filed after June 8, 1995 will (like most non U.S. patents) have terms of twenty years from the filing dates. In cases where more than one party claims the same invention, the U.S. will continue to award the patent to the first-to-invent regardless of who was first to file a patent application; most other nations grant patents on a "first-to-file" basis. However legislative changes now permit prefiling inventive activity in any WTO country to establish priority of invention for U.S. patents rather than limiting such activity to that done in the U.S. The amended U.S. Patent Act also allows the filing of a new type of patent application, i.e. the "provisional application". The latter has fewer formal requirements and lower fees than do standard applications. An applicant has twelve months from filing a provisional application to file a standard utility patent application on the subject matter and has the advantage of the priority date of the provisional filing even though the intervening year will not count against the term of the issued patent.

18.4.3 Biotechnology patents

Unique patent-related issues have emerged as the result of rapid progress in biotechnology over the past decade. Until as recently as 1980, U.S. patent law did not consider living organisms as patentable entities. However, recombinant DNA technology employs or generates living organisms to produce commercially important products. Thus, since 1980, several court decisions have led to modifications in patent law which now allow the patenting of living species from microorganisms to plants and animals arising from transgenic experiments. As the result of the liberalized patent laws, biotechnology products such as human insulin and growth hormone are already being sold, and numerous other proteins are in various stages of commercial development. The basic laboratory methods of biotechnology research can also be patented although due to the dynamic changes in the field, today's novelty often becomes tomorrow's obviousness.

18.5 CHEMICAL PROCESS DEVELOPMENT

Whenever a synthetic compound is selected for clinical trial, a major issue becomes the preparation of the compound in bulk quantity. The responsibility for preparing the compound in the kilogram amounts needed for toxicological evaluations and subsequent clinical use is usually shifted to a chemical process development group. The task of the developmental chemist is to adapt and modify, as necessary, the research chemist's synthetic process in order to obtain bulk drug in an efficient, cost-effective manner. Whereas initial chemical development work is usually conducted in over-sized glassware, the ultimate process must be compatible with the logistical limitations of batch operations in pilot plant reactors. Because of such considerations, development chemists may need to forgo expedients enjoyed by their research counterparts such as the use of costly starting materials and reagents, employment of very high or low temperature conditions, and chromatographic means of isolation and purification. While the research chemist may have had the luxury of accepting a few low-yield steps, in order to obtain sufficient material for testing, the development chemist must endeavor to maximize yield for the sake of cost. Various experimental manipulations which are fairly trivial when carried out at the laboratory bench of the research chemist can be cumbersome in the pilot plant setting. For example, while such isolation procedures as solvent-solvent extraction and filtration are feasible on large scale, they are best minimized. Collection of a solid reaction product by centrifugation followed by decantation of solvent is often a viable alternative to bulk filtration.

Purity of the bulk drug supplies is critical. With few exceptions, the drug substance prepared for toxicological evaluation and especially for human studies must be of very high (>99%) purity. The toxicity of reagents, from the standpoint of both human exposure and waste disposal, is also of much greater concern when working on the developmental scale. As a consequence of these practical considerations, the bulk drug synthesis, which may become the method of manufacture, can differ considerably from that used to initially prepare the compound.

In many countries, the syntheses of drug substances for human administration must be conducted in compliance with governmental regulations. In the U.S., the FDA mandates that such preparations be performed under Good Manufacturing Practices (GMP) protocols. While these are too extensive to detail here, they include guidelines for the sanitation of the workplace and equipment, the storage and testing of raw materials, and the packaging and labeling of the final drug substance. Facilities and operations are subject to governmental inspection.

18.6 METABOLISM AND PHARMACOKINETICS (MAP)

18.6.1 Drug absorption and bioavailability

Among the critical factors which must be determined for an experimental drug are its absorption, distribution, metabolism, and elimination (ADME). The absolute bioavailability of a given dose is the amount of drug which reaches the systemic circulation after administration by a particular route relative to that which reaches the systemic circulation after i.v. administration. The i.v. route circumvents absorption factors and first-pass liver metabolism and results in immediate and optimal plasma concentrations.

The most traditional, convenient, and cost-effective means of drug administration is by the oral route as tablet, capsule, solution, or suspension formulations. Orally-given drugs enter the circulatory system by absorption primarily from the small intestine and, to a lesser extent, from the stomach. The absorption of a chemical substance from the gastrointestinal (GI) tract is primarily a function of its lipophilicity and the extent of its ionization but is also affected by its complexation with ingested food and the rate of dissolution of tablet or capsule formulations. Chemical entities which enter the bloodstream from the GI tract are passed through the portal vein into the liver where they can undergo considerable metabolic conversion.

The area under the curve (AUC) of a plot of time vs. plasma concentration is a measure of a drug's systemic exposure for a specific route of administration. Absolute bioavailability after oral administration is given by

$$\frac{AUC\ p.o.}{AUC\ i.v.} \times \frac{Di.v.}{Dp.o.} \times 100$$

where (AUC) i.v. defines the drug's area under the plasma concentration-time curve after i.v. administration and Di.v. and Dp.o. are the intravenous and oral doses respectively.

Bioavailability studies should be conducted as early as possible in the developmental process since lack of the desired clinical response may be attributable to an agent's inability to reach therapeutic concentration in the circulation. Such findings could warrant the synthesis of suitably modified or latentiated derivatives or the development of alternative dosage formulations to maximize bioavailability (see Chapter 13).

18.6.2 Distribution and elimination

Drugs in the circulatory system are distributed throughout various fluid compartments of the body and are eventually eliminated from the body either as unchanged drug or metabolites. Depending upon its structural characteristics, a drug can reversibly bind to plasma or tissue proteins which act as storage depots in which bound drug is in equilibrium with free drug in the tissue and plasma. Tissue distribution studies in animals employing radiolabeled (^{3}H or ^{14}C) drug serve to determine if the agent reaches the target organ and whether it accumulates at various sites. Radiolabeled drug may also be employed in material-balance studies in animals and in man (but only using ^{14}C-labeled drug in man) to establish the routes and time course of elimination. Drugs are eliminated in the urine and bile either as parent drug or after conversion to metabolites. The half-life of elimination of a drug, which can serve as a measure of its duration of action, can be derived from the plasma concentration vs. time curves.

18.6.3 Metabolism

Metabolism most often leads to inactivation of a drug and the formation of more polar, hydrophilic compounds which can be more readily excreted. Not infrequently, however, active metabolites are formed and in some cases the activity of the parent drug may be largely or solely attributable to an active metabolite. Metabolic enzymes can transform the parent drug by oxidative, reductive or hydrolytic reactions, and the polar metabolites thus formed can couple with carbohydrates or other endogenous substrates to form biologically-inactive and readily-excretable conjugates. The metabolic enzymes are fairly ubiquitous throughout the body but are particularly abundant in the liver. Thus preparations of liver homogenates or microsomes or hepatocyte cell cultures are used to conduct *in vitro* studies of a drug's metabolism. Human tissues are now commonly employed in such studies in order to predict how man will metabolize a compound. The use of radiolabeled and stable isotopically-labeled (^{2}H, ^{13}C, ^{15}N) drugs in both animals and man is an important means of identifying metabolites when coupled with methodologies such as GLC-MS and HPLC-MS. Metabolite identification is important for registrational purposes and can also provide the insight to synthesize analogs having improved pharmacokinetic properties.

18.7 TOXICOLOGY

Ideally, one would like to introduce into clinical trial drugs having no toxicity or side effect liability. From a realistic perspective, however, all drugs manifest toxic effects at some dose levels and thus the more practical objective is to identify dose ranges that can achieve therapeutic benefit with minimal toxicity. Even though the safety and tolerance to side effects of a drug must, like its efficacy, be ultimately determined by clinical evaluation, it is mandatory to conduct extensive preclinical toxicological studies prior to and during the drug's testing in man. It should be noted however that many drugs for the treatment of life-threatening diseases, such as cancer, are recognized as having intrinsically high toxicity and it is unnecessary to evaluate such agents in the same manner as drugs for the therapy of more benign disorders. Specific types of toxicity studies are discussed in the following sections and are summarized in Table 18.1.

18.7.1 Genetic toxicology

The primary objective of genetic toxicity studies is to satisfy safety and regulatory requirements for assessing the mutagenic (DNA damaging) potential of drug candidates. These studies consist of a battery of *in vitro* assays conducted in either bacterial strains or isolated mammalian cells. The most commonly used assay is the Ames test in which drugs are tested for the induction of mutations in several strains of *Salmonella*. Various concentrations of drug are tested both with and without metabolic activation, for even if the drug molecule itself is non-mutagenic one of its metabolites may be. A positive result (i.e., induction of mutagenesis) in the Ames test or other such assay is often sufficient to curtail the development of a clinical drug candidate. Since *in vitro* toxicology tests are relatively quick and inexpensive and because the information they impart is so critical, it is prudent to conduct such testing in the early stages of a drug's development.

18.7.2 Acute to chronic *in vivo* toxicity testing

In vivo toxicity studies in animals establish whether a drug is sufficiently safe for administration to humans and provide a recommendation of the maximum allowable clinical dose. Acute toxicity testing is generally performed in a rodent and non-rodent species and involves administration of single doses of the experimental agent. The test animals are observed for several weeks after dosing. Range-finding studies of up to a month are conducted for the purpose of establishing the appropriate dosage levels to be used in subsequent subchronic and chronic toxicity evaluations.

Subchronic and chronic toxicity testing is performed in several species, both rodent and non-rodent, in order to determine whether adverse effects occur upon repeated daily dosing of the experimental agent. The duration of such studies depends upon the plans for initial clinical evaluation of the drug. In the U.S., FDA guidelines require that Phase I clinical trials, in which individuals are administered single doses over a few days, be supported by a minimum of two to four weeks of subchronic animal testing, whereas, three months of toxicity testing are needed for Phase II trials of one to three months. Chronic toxicity studies of six to twelve months are necessary to support longer term clinical trials as well as to fulfill registrational requirements.

During the course of any toxicity study, the animals are closely observed for changes in such parameters as body weight, food consumption, behavior, hematology, and liver/kidney function. Following completion of an extended toxicity study, the animals are sacrificed, necropsied and major organs are subjected to both gross and microscopic examination to detect the occurrence, if any, of drug-induced abnormalities.

18.7.3 Reproductive toxicity testing

In order to avert the catastrophe of horrible birth defects such as those attributable to the use of thalidomide several decades ago, most countries require evaluation of a drug's possible reproductive toxicity. This is especially important for drugs taken by women of childbearing potential. In the U.S., a battery of segment studies (summarized in Table 18.1) are conducted to assess reproductive toxicity.

18.8 PHARMACEUTICS

The primary responsibility of pharmaceutics in the drug development process is the formulation of the raw drug substance into an optimally-effective delivery system for clinical usage. Essential preformulation work includes characterization of the physical chemical properties of the new chemical entity, investigating rates and mechanisms of its degradation and establishing dosage-form specifications and storage conditions to assure developmental reproducibility. For example, the raw drug substance in the solid state or in solution as well as clinical formulations are subjected to extended storage under varying combinations of temperature and exposure to light and air. Samples are then analyzed to determine whether any appreciable deterioration has occurred.

Drugs for oral administration are in most cases formulated as capsules containing the various dosage levels needed for clinical study. A practical consideration especially for agents administered in solution or suspension is the palatability of the drug substance. Patient compliance in taking the medication can be negatively impacted by bitter or otherwise unpleasant taste and flavoring agents are often required to mask such properties.

Table 18.1   Toxicity tests.

Toxicity Test	Time Frame	Number and Type of Required Species	Purpose
Genetic	Variable.	*In vitro* tests in bacteria and mammalian cells (e.g. Ames test).	Detection of gene mutations and primary DNA damage.
Acute	Single dose; animals observed for 14 days after dosing.	Rodent- rat or mouse: 3–10/sex/dose level. Nonrodent- dog, rabbit or primate: 1–3/sex/dose level.	Determination of adverse effects within short time frame of single dose administration.
Range-finding	2–4 weeks of repeated daily dosing.	Rodent: 5/sex/dose level. Nonrodent- usually dog or primate: 1/sex/dose level.	Establish dosage levels for subsequent toxicity studies.
Subchronic	1–3 months.	Rodent: 10–15/sex/dose level. Nonrodent- usually dog or primate: 2–3/sex/dose level.	Determination of adverse effects resulting from repeated daily dosing.
Segment I	Dosing of males for 60–80 days prior to mating. 14 days for females prior to mating and during gestation and lactation.	Rat: 25 males and 25 females/dose level.	Assess effects on fertility and general reproductive performance.
Segment II	About 1 month. Dosing conducted during sensitive period of organogenesis.	Rats: 25 females/dose level. Mice: 25 females/dose level. Rabbits: 15 females/dose level.	Determine potential drug-induced embryotoxicity and teratogenicity.
Segment III	Dosing from last gestation day (day 16–17) to end of weaning. If reproductive capacity of offspring is evaluated, study duration is 5–6 months.	Rat or mouse: 20 pregnant females/dose level.	Determine drug effects on late fetal development, labor, delivery, lactation and newborn viability.
Chronic	>3 months; usually 6–12 months.	Rodent: 25/sex/dose level. Nonrodent- usually dog or primate: 4–5/sex/dose level.	Determine chronic toxipathological effects of a drug.
Carcinogenicity	18 or 24 months.	Rat and mouse or hamster: 50/sex/dose level and 100/sex/control group.	Determine potential tumorigenic effects of drug when given over significant portion of animal's lifetime.

Intravenously administered drugs, such as certain antibiotics and cancer therapy agents, must be solubilized in a physiologically-acceptable medium under highly sterile conditions. Less common delivery modes may be developed for certain drugs such as inhalation formulations for anti-asthmatics and trans-dermal patches for cardiovascular agents. Sustained release dosage forms can significantly prolong the duration of action of drugs having short half-lives.

18.9 CLINICAL EVALUATION

Regardless of how promising a drug candidate may appear based upon its pharmacological and toxicological evaluation in species up to and including primates, the approvability of the drug is contingent on demonstration of its efficacy and safety in man.

The scope and duration of clinical drug trials can vary widely, depending upon the nature of the drug and its therapeutic application. This section will cover only some general aspects of clinical testing and the reader is referred to texts such as those edited and authored by Kato and Spilker, respectively, for a comprehensive discussion of the topic.

18.9.1 Phase I

Phase I clinical trials are generally conducted in about 20–100 healthy volunteers, mainly young males. Exceptions are trials involving drugs for cancer and AIDS in which the Phase I studies are most often carried out in patients. Phase I trials, which normally last 3–6 months, have the objective of gauging the safety and appropriate dosage of the experimental agents. The drug is initially administered in single acute doses and subsequently in repeated doses up to three or four times a day. Phase I clinical protocols usually plan for a gradual increase in the size of both single and total daily doses to levels supported by subchronic toxicological studies or until unacceptable side effects are observed.

The volunteers are closely monitored during the course of their participation in the study and vital signs such as blood pressure, pulse, and temperature are measured regularly. Blood and urine samples are collected frequently in order to check for any untoward drug-induced changes in composition and to allow researchers the opportunity to assess the drug's pharmacokinetic parameters including plasma levels of unchanged drug and metabolites and rate of drug excretion.

Approximately 70% of experimental agents succeed in passing Phase I trials and those that fail usually do so because they elicit one or more unacceptable side effects. A drug can also fail in Phase I due to an unsatisfactory pharmacokinetic profile; i.e. it may not attain blood plasma levels sufficient to achieve a pharmacological effect.

18.9.2 Phase II

The dual purpose of Phase II trials is to ascertain the appropriate dosing regimen for the experimental drug and whether it is effective in treating the target disease. Phase II clinical studies are thus conducted in patients and typically several hundred patients may be enrolled, often at multiple sites. The duration of Phase II development ranges from six months to two years.

Drug range-finding and proportionality studies are most conveniently conducted in an open, non-blinded format in which all patients are knowingly administered test drug. These studies are conducted in order to determine a dosing regimen that will achieve maximum therapeutic benefit with minimal side effects.

Most Phase II efficacy studies are "multiple-arm" in design. In a typical two-arm study, groups of patients are administered either drug or placebo which serves as a negative control. If approved drugs are available for the condition in question, then the clinical protocol can be designed to include an additional arm, i.e., a patient group on the approved drug as a positive control. Multiple-armed studies are most often done under a blinded format. In single-blind studies, patients are unaware as to whether they are receiving drug or placebo, whereas in double-blind studies, neither patients nor the clinical investigators are cognizant of which patients are being administered experimental drug, placebo, or positive control. The administered dosage forms are carefully coded by persons other than those conducting the investigation and upon conclusion of the study, the identity of the drug or non-drug given to each individual patient is revealed. The purpose of blinded studies is to eliminate, as much as possible, patient or investigator bias in evaluation of the test agent. The measured clinical end point in efficacy studies is of course contingent upon the disease being treated.

Efficacy trials must be conducted in a sufficient number of patients so that individual variability (due to age, gender, metabolism, etc.) "averages out" over all treatment groups. Following the completion of trials, a critical event becomes the biostatistical analysis of the decoded clinical data. Such analyses determine whether the experimental drug has shown a statistically-significant difference from placebo and/or positive control with respect to both efficacy and side effects.

Approximately 33% of drugs that enter human clinical studies pass Phase II trials. Those that fail in Phase II usually do so because of a lack of significant efficacy.

18.9.3 Phase III

Phase III clinical trials can involve anywhere from several hundred to several thousand patients and can last from 1–5 years. The objectives of Phase III studies are to verify the drug's effectiveness, to monitor the development of tolerance or adverse reactions arising from long-term use, and to ascertain that the medication does not cause complications in patients having other illnesses. Very often, special studies in various patient sub-groups such as children, the elderly and the renally or hepatically-impaired may be performed in Phase III. Drug interaction studies may also be done in patients taking concomitant medications.

Roughly 25% of experimental drugs survive Phases I–III. Upon the completion of Phase III and the compilation and analyses of all clinical data, the sponsoring firm submits the NDA and/or the corresponding registrational filing in countries other than the U.S. If the drug is approved for marketing, Phase IV studies are subsequently undertaken. The purpose of Phase IV is to accumulate an ever-larger database on the drug and, in particular, to monitor the occurrences of adverse effects. Adverse effects having a low incidence may not have occurred during Phases I–III but could emerge within the much larger patient population receiving the marketed drug.

18.10 PLANNING

Once a compound is identified in the laboratory setting as having pharmacological properties that warrant clinical evaluation, then a developmental plan must be formatted. Quite commonly, an interdisciplinary team comprised of both preclinical and clinical personnel, will be assembled and assigned the responsibility of devising the developmental plan and monitoring its progress. The plan must emphasize two critical factors: time and cost.

Owing to the long time frame of drug development, it is essential that the plan identifies rate-determining components and provides for mutually-independent steps (e.g. toxicology studies and pharmaceutical formulation studies) to be conducted simultaneously. Planning must be conducted within the practical constraints of available manpower and budgetary resources.

Once the wheels of the project have begun turning, the most essential function of the team is to insure that the plan remains on schedule and on target. Potential bottlenecks must be anticipated, if possible, and alleviated if and when they occur.

A major pharmaceutical company is bound to have a number of different investigational drugs in its pipeline at any point in time. Since a finite quantity of resources must be distributed among all projects, the progress of any given drug in the pipeline is a function of its judged importance relative to the other drugs under development. It is the job of upper research management, often in conjunction with a formal planning group, to weigh various economic, logistical and ethical factors in order to prioritize the company's project drugs and allocate resources accordingly.

18.11 REGISTRATION

The "final exam" which a drug must pass in the U.S. is registrational approval by the FDA. Prior to submission of an NDA, meetings are held between the sponsoring firm and the FDA to discuss the registrational format. The sponsor's clear understanding of the FDA expectations with regard to a suitable NDA, can minimize delays in the subsequent review.

Documentation which averages 40,000–60,000 pages is then submitted to substantiate the application. This includes comprehensive reports of both preclinical and clinical studies as well as case report forms on each individual human subject or patient involved in drug trials. The lengthy review process then begins. During the course of the review, the FDA is likely to ask numerous questions about any facet of the drug, perhaps request additional data, and may even require that additional studies be conducted. Proof of safety and efficacy are minimal criteria for approval; the FDA may also wish to see tangible evidence for advantages of the drug over existing therapy. If these requirements are satisfied, the drug is approved for marketing. The registrational process is similar in other countries, differing in the stringency of specific requirements.

18.12 MARKETING

The commercial success of an approved drug becomes the responsibility of a company's marketing and sales forces. Marketing strategy for a new drug must be mapped out well in advance of its post-approval launch and is based upon careful consideration of many important factors. Chief among these are the following:

(1) the clinically-determined profile of the drug;
(2) the size of the existing and potential market;
(3) competitors' drugs and/or alternative means of therapy.

Marketing strategy must aim to achieve a reasonable market share for the new drug by emphasizing its perceived advantages; these can include enhanced efficacy, faster onset of action, longer duration of action (hence, less frequent dosing), or fewer side-effects relative to competitive drugs.

Marketing personnel will encourage the publication of relevant scientific manuscripts and may arrange scientific symposia focusing upon both preclinical and clinical findings in order to establish awareness of the particular drug within the scientific/medical community. Following its approval, the drug will be advertised, mainly in technical journals and trade magazines read by health care professionals. The company's sales representatives, thoroughly schooled in the medically-pertinent information on the drug, will visit physicians, pharmacists, and others involved in the sale or purchase and dispensing of prescription drugs. Both before and after launch, it is vitally important that marketing provides reasonably accurate estimates of sales volume so that adequate (but not highly excessive) supplies of the drug are manufactured and distributed.

The involvement of marketing should not be limited to approved drugs. Collaboration and communication between research and developmental groups and marketing should be maintained during all phases of the drug discovery/development process. By defining unmet therapeutic needs and providing projections of changes in disease prevalence, marketing can inform basic research groups of the areas in which their drug discovery efforts will best be spent. As mentioned earlier, marketing should be kept abreast of the developmental progress of an exploratory drug in order to avoid any unpleasant surprises as the agent nears registration.

18.13 ORPHAN DRUGS

Pharmaceutical companies most often endeavor to develop drugs to treat diseases having a high prevalence. This is logical from the standpoint of both public health welfare and economics. For the purpose of encouraging the development of agents for the treatment of rare diseases (over 5,000 disorders are considered rare), the U.S. Congress passed the Orphan Drug Act in 1983. This legislation defines orphan drugs as agents intended for use in disorders affecting fewer than 200,000 persons in the U.S. and/or for which reasonable recovery of the sponsoring firm's research and development expenditures is not expected within the first seven years of sales. The act provides various incentives to pharmaceutical manufacturers to develop and market orphan drugs including tax credits equal to 50% of the costs of human clinical trials and seven years of exclusive marketing rights even if the drug is non-patentable.

During the decade prior to the passage of the Orphan Drug Act, only 10 medicinal agents were approved in the U.S. for what are now recognized as orphan diseases whereas over 60 drugs were approved by the FDA for orphan indications in the 10 years following the legislation. Examples of approved orphan drugs are: pentamidine (Pentam 300®), which has been shown to be safe and effective therapy for pneumonic infections in AIDS patients; chenodiol (Chenix®) for dissolution of gallstones; clofazimine (Lamprene®) for therapy of resistant leprosy; pimozide (Orap®) for Tourette syndrome; the genetically-engineered somatrem (Protropin ®) for growth hormone deficiency.

18.14 CONCLUDING REMARKS

The powerful tools afforded by modern molecular and cell biology, computer-assisted drug design and combinatorial chemistry will combine to facilitate the discovery of exciting new drugs well into the 21st century. However, once a novel chemical entity is found to have biological properties which warrant the evaluation of its therapeutic effects in man, it must then run the complex gauntlet of developmental studies that have been described in this chapter. As time-consuming and costly as these studies may be, they are essential to bringing effective and safe drugs to the market.

FURTHER READING

Knoop, S.J. and Worden, D.E. (1988) The pharmaceutical drug development process: an overview. *Drug Information Journal*, **22**, 259–268.

Spilker, B. (1989) *Multinational Drug Companies: Issues in Drug Discovery and Development*. John Wiley & Sons, New York.

Williams, M. and Malick, J.L. (1987) *Drug Discovery and Development*. Humana Press, New York.

Maynard, J.T. and Peters, H.M. (1991) *Understanding Chemical Patents: A Guide for the Inventor*, 2nd edition, American Chemical Society, Washington, D.C.

Wegner, H.C. (1992) *Patent Law in Biotechnology, Chemicals and Pharmaceuticals*. Stockton Press, New York.

Bisis, A. and Kabel, R.L. (1985) *Scaleup of Chemical Processes: Conversion from Laboratory Scale Tests to Successful Commercial Size Design*. John Wiley & Sons, New York.

Roth, H.J. and Kleeman, A. (1988) *Pharmaceutical Chemistry, Volume I: Drug Synthesis*. John Wiley & Sons, New York.

Racz, I. (1989) *Drug Formulation*. John Wiley & Sons, New York.

Gibaldi, M. (1984) *Pharmaceutics and Clinical Pharmacokinetics*. Lea and Fibiger, Philadelphia.

Hawkins, D.R., ed., (1988–1992) *Biotransformations, Volumes I–IV*. Royal Society of Chemistry, London.

Hayes, A.W., ed. (1994) *Principles and Methods of Toxicology*, 3rd edition, Raven Press, New York.

Spilker, B. (1984) *Guide to Clinical Studies and Developing Protocols*. Raven Press, New York.

Cato, A.E., ed., (1988) *Clinical Drug Trials and Tribulations*. Marcel Dekker, New York and Basel.

Prine, R.F. and Robinson, D.S. (1994) *Clinical Evaluation of Psychotropic Drugs*. Raven Press, New York.

Asbury, C.H. (1991) The orphan drug act, the first seven years. *Journal of the American Medical Association*, **265**, 893–897.

Index

1592 U89, 446
4C3HPG, 243
A 77003, 459
Abbreviated New Drug Application (ANDA), 512
ABPA, 247
Absorption, distribution, metabolism and elimination/excretion (ADME), 30, 514
ABT 418, 27
ACE, 305, 402
    inhibitor monotherapy, 308
    inhibitors, 306, 402
    zinc metalloprotein enzyme, 306
3-Acetoxyquinuclidine, 85
Acetylcholine (ACh), 276
Acetylcholinesterase (AChE), 275
Acetylcholinesterase inhibitors, 283
    clinical studies, 283
    dyflos, 283
    eserine, 283
    insecticides, 283
    nerve gas, 283
    organophosphorus inhibitors, 283
    physostigmine, 283
    tacrine, 283
    treatment of Alzheimer patients, 283
Acetyl-CoA:choline-O-acetyltransferase (ChAT), 275
N_3-Acetyl-5-fluorouracil, 363
N-Acetyl-γ-glutamylsulphamethoxazole, 378
Acetylsalicylic acid, 39, 319
ACh, 276
AChE, 275
ACPD, 243
Acrolein, 466
Acromelic acid, 242
Actinomycin D, 478-9
Actinomycin-deoxyguanosine complex, 480
Active conformation, 70
Active principle, 16
Acyclovir, 435
AD/SDAT patients, 277
    neuroprotective drugs, 277

    neuroprotective treatments, 277
    symptomatic treatment, 277
    therapies, 277
Adenosine A_{2a} receptor, 24
Adenosine kinase, 15, 440
Adenosine receptor, 23
S-Adenosylhomocysteine (SAH) hydrolase, 448
S-Adenosylmethionine (SAM), 448
Adeno-viruses, 447-8
ADME, 30, 514
Adrenocorticotropic hormone (ACTH), 387
Adriamycin, 479
    -d(CGATCG) complex, 484
    -DNA complex, 479
    intercalation of, 479
AF-DX, 116, 279
African green monkey kidney (COS) cells, 143
4-AHCP, 250
AIDS, 154, 440
    vaccine, 145
Alaproclate labelling, 184
Aldophosphamide, 466
Aldosterone, 305
[(Alkoxycarbonyl)-oxy]alkyl esters, 357
Allupurinol, 370
    prodrugs, 384
Alzheimer's disease (AD), 275, 331
AMAA, 239, 244
    pharmacology, 247
Amantadine, 452
AMD, 478
AMD-d(GAAGCTTC), 481
Amide isosteres, 396
Amine oxidases, 344
Amino acids, 388
    conformationally restricted analogues, 395
p-Aminobenzoic acid (PABA), 313
2-Amino-4-hydroxy-6-methylpterin, 313
5-Aminoimidazole-4-carboxamide, 470
4-Aminopentanoic acid, 258

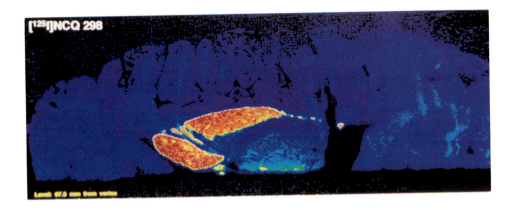

Color Plate I (See Chapter 7, p.198. Halldin and Högberg.)

Figure 7.4 [^{125}I]NCQ 298 ([^{125}I]**7.18**) binding to dopamine D$_2$ receptors in a post-mortem human brain using whole hemisphere autoradiography. The figure was kindly provided by Dr Håkan Hall, Karolinska Institutet, Sweden.

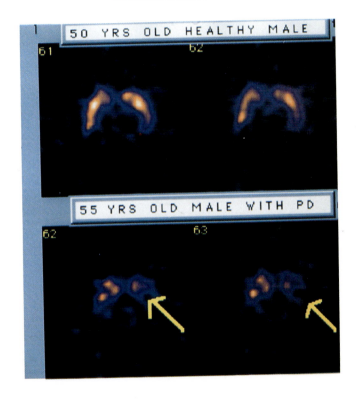

Color Plate II (See Chapter 7, p.199. Halldin and Högberg.)

Figure 7.5 SPECT images taken 21 hours after injection of [^{123}I]β-CIT ([^{123}I]**7.19**) in a healthy male (top) and a patient with Parkinson's disease (bottom). The images demonstrate highly reduced uptake in the patient with Parkinson's disease (arrow). The figure was kindly provided by Dr Jyrki Kuikka, Kuopio University Hospital, Finland.

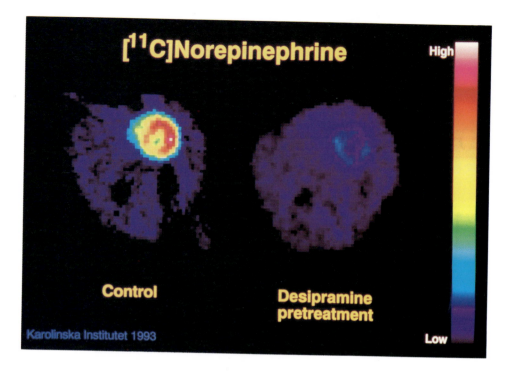

Color Plate III (See Chapter 7, p.202. Halldin and Högberg.)

Figure 7.7   PET images showing distribution of radioactivity in the chest of a monkey after injection of $[^{11}C]$norepinephrine ($[^{11}C]$**7.39**) in a control experiment (left) and a pretreatment experiment with desipramine (right). The figure was kindly provided by Dr Lars Farde, Karolinska Institutet, Sweden.

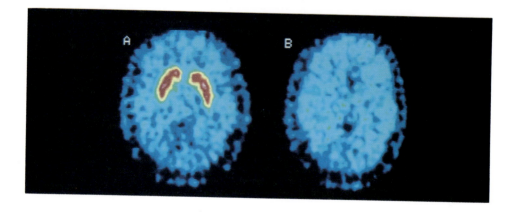

Color Plate IV (See Chapter 7, p.203. Halldin and Högberg.)

Figure 7.9   PET images showing distribution of radioactivity in the brain after injection of $[^{11}C]$raclopride ($[^{11}C]$**7.41**) (A) and the inactive enantiomer ($[^{11}C]$**7.43**) (B). The figure was kindly provided by Dr Lars Farde, Karolinska Institutet, Sweden.

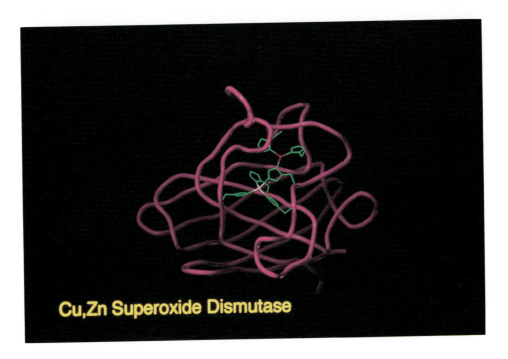

Color Plate V (See Chapter 12, p.344. Jøn and Johansen.)

Figure 12.4   Structural model of superoxide dismutase displaying the zinc and copper centers.

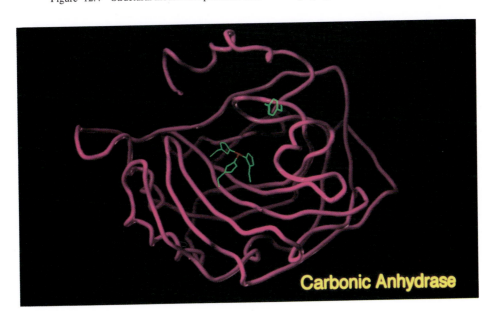

Color Plate VI (See Chapter 12, p.345. Jøn and Johansen.)

Figure 12.5   Structural model of the zinc enzyme, carbonic anhydrase.

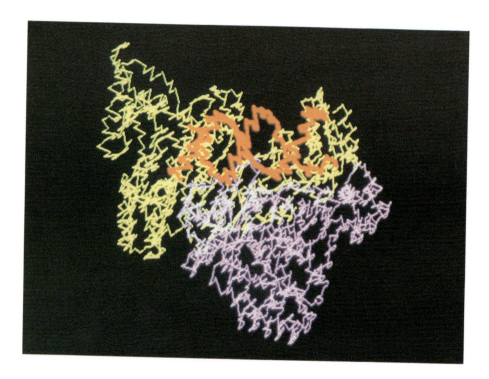

Color Plate VII (See Chapter 16, p.455. Herdewijn and Clercq.)

Figure 16.2   The structure of HIV reverse transcriptase.

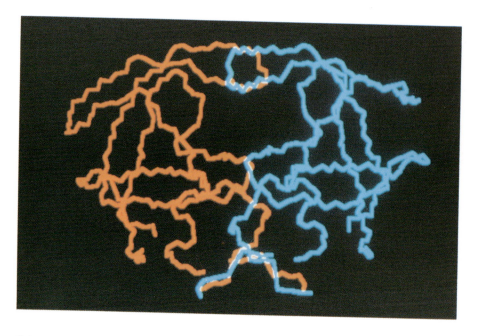

Color Plate VIII (See Chapter 16, p.458. Herdewijn and Clercq.)

Figure 16.3   The structure of HIV-protease.

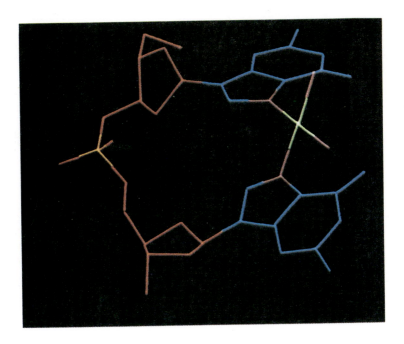

Color Plate IX (See Chapter 17, p.473. Larsen.)

Plate 17.1 Structural model of the Pt(NH$_3$)$_2$ (d(GpG)) adduct, determined from analysis of the NMR spectra. From Reedijk, J. in "NMR Spectroscopy in Drug Research". Eds. J.W. Jaroszewski, K. Schaumburg and H. Kofod. Munksgaard, Copenhagen 1988, with permission by Munksgaard.

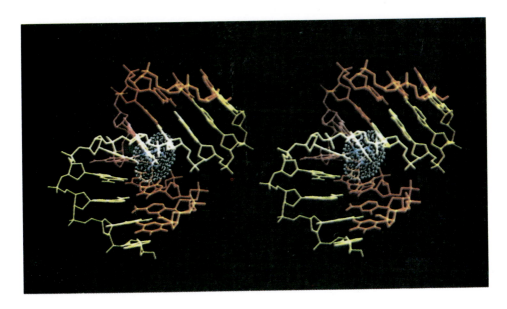

Color Plate X (See Chapter 17, p.474. Larsen.)

Plate 17.2 Stereo projection of a possible distorted helical DNA structure after chelation of cisplatin to the central GG bases of the same strand. (From Reedijk, J. — see legend to Plate 17.1).

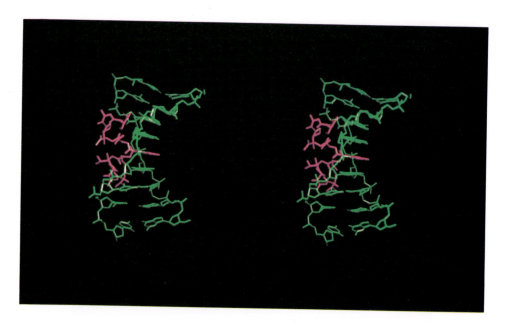

Color Plate XI (See Chapter 17, p.481. Larsen.)

Plate 17.3   Stereoview of the AMD-d(GAAGCTTC) complex. The AMD molecule is shown in magenta, the DNA octamer in green. This side view of the complex shows the intercalation of the chromofore in the G5C5 site and the cyclic peptides of AMD in the minor groove. The structure was generated using the programme SYBYL with coordinates from Brookhaven Protein Data Base.

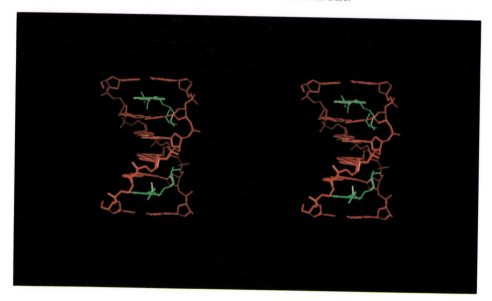

Color Plate XII (See Chapter 17, p.484. Larsen.)

Plate 17.4   A stereoview of the adriamycin-d(CGATCG) complex. The two antibiotic molecules are shown in green, the DNA hexamer in red. The structure was generated using the programme SYBYL with coordinates from Brookhaven Protein Data Base.

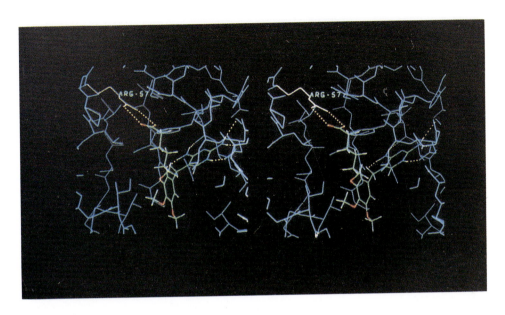

Color Plate XIII (See Chapter 17, p.493. Larsen.)

Plate 17.5   The active site of *E. coli* DHFR with a carbalkoxy analogue of trimethoprim bound (C, green; H, white; N, blue; O, red). (From Hitchings, G.H., *et al*. in "Design of Enzyme Inhibitors as Drugs" Eds. M. Sandler and H.J. Smith. Oxford University Press, Oxford 1989, with permission by Oxford University Press.

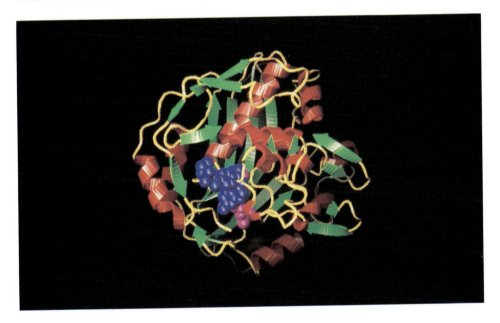

Color Plate XIV (See Chapter 17, p.497. Larsen.)

Plate 17.6   The structure of TS of *E. coli* with substrate (in magenta) and cofactor analogue (in blue) bound in active site. The structure was generated using the programme "O" with coordinates from Brookhaven Protein Data Base.

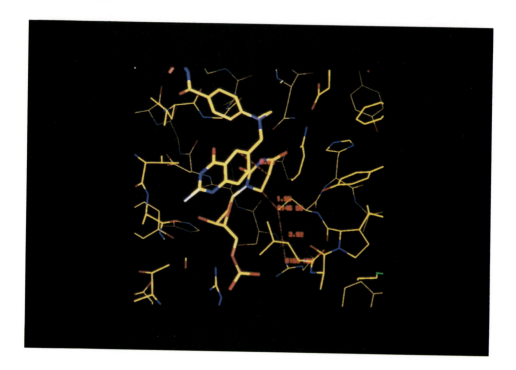

Color Plate XV (See Chapter 17, p.497. Larsen.)

Plate 17.7   The active site of TS with substrate and cofactor analogue bound (N, blue; O, red). Dashed lines indicate short distances. The structure was generated using the programme "O" with coordinates from Brookhaven Protein Data Base.

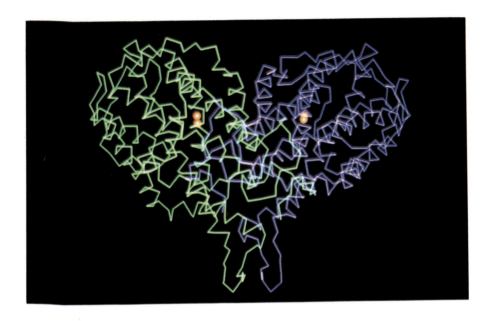

Plate (A)

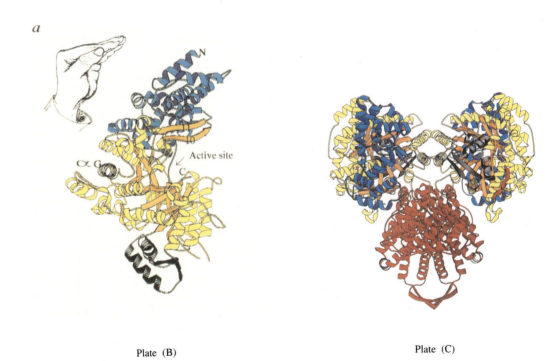

Plate (B)

Plate (C)

Color Plate XVI (See Chapter 17, pp. 501, Larsen.)

Plate 17.8   The structures of (A) protein R2 of *E. coli* RNR as the dimer (in green and magenta) with the iron atoms in red; (B) protein R1 of *E. coli* RNR as the monomer. The colours illustrate different domains of the protein; (C) the R1 R2 holoenzyme modelled on the basis of the seperate X-ray structures of R1 and R2. The R2 dimer is coloured in red. The figures were kindly provided by Professor Hans Eklund, Department of Molecular Biology, Biomedical Center, Uppsala, Sweden.

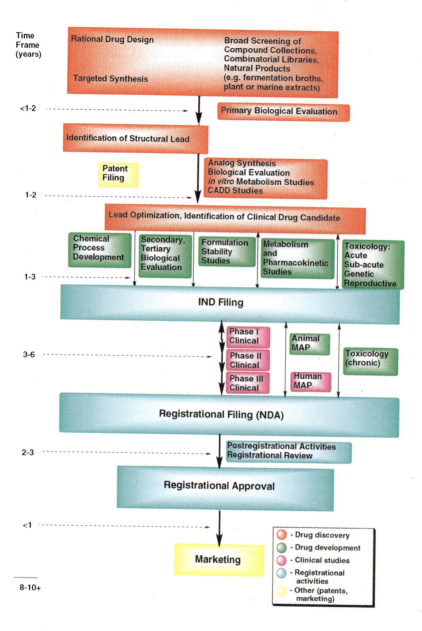

Color Plate XVII (See Chapter 18, p.510. Yevich.)

Figure 18.1 Discovery to marketing of a drug. The various steps in the path from the discovery of a potential new drug to its approval and marketing are indicated along with approximate time frames. Color-coding indicates related activities. Various activities necessary for IND filing continue beyond the IND and may even continue after registrational (NDA) filing. As indicated by doubleheaded arrows, MAP and toxicity findings may lead to reformulation of clinical dosage form or to the synthesis of improved analogs.